ROUTLEDGE HANDBOOK
OF
ERGONOMICS IN
SPORT AND EXERCISE

Ergonomics is concerned with the 'fit' between people and their work. With an increasing number of people becoming conscious about their health and participating in sport or physical activity, ergonomics has become an increasingly prominent concern within the sport and exercise sciences. From the design of footwear and artificial playing surfaces, to studies of proprioception by obese children, the way in which people interact with their environment – designed and natural – has important implications for performance sport and for the design of safe and beneficial forms of physical activity.

The Routledge Handbook of Ergonomics in Sport and Exercise is the first book to offer a comprehensive and in-depth survey of cutting-edge scientific research into ergonomics in sport and exercise. Written by world-leading international scientists and researchers, the book explores key topics such as:

- Musculoskeletal adaptation to sports and exercise
- Environmental factors of injury and fatigue
- Load weight and performance
- Ergonomics in adapted sports and exercise
- Measurement in sports and exercise
- Modelling and simulation in ergonomics design
- Influence of playing surface, footwear and equipment design

Bridging the gap between fundamental scientific research in sport and exercise and applications in sport and exercise contexts, this is an important reference for all advanced students, researchers and professionals working in sport and exercise science, kinesiology, sports technology, sports engineering, ergonomics and product design.

Youlian Hong is a Professor in the Department of Sports Medicine, Chengdu Sports University, China. He received his PhD from the German Sports University of Cologne. He is also Editor-in-Chief of *Research in Sports Medicine: An International Journal*, and Fellow, Live Member and former President and Geoffrey Dyson Lecturer of the International Society of Biomechanics in Sports.

ROUTLEDGE HANDBOOK OF ERGONOMICS IN SPORT AND EXERCISE

Edited by Youlian Hong

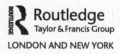

LONDON AND NEW YORK

First published 2014
by Routledge
2 Park Square, Milton Park, Abingdon, Oxon OX14 4RN

and by Routledge
711 Third Avenue, New York, NY 10017

This paperback edition published in 2016
by Routledge

Routledge is an imprint of the Taylor & Francis Group, an informa business

© 2016 Youlian Hong

British Library Cataloguing in Publication Data
A catalogue record for this book is available from the British Library

Library of Congress Cataloging in Publication Data
Hong, Youlian, 1946–
Routledge handbook of ergonomics in sport and exercise/edited by Youlian Hong.
pages cm
1. Sports – Physiological aspects. 2. Human engineering. 3. Human mechanics. I. Title.
RC1235.H66 2014
613.7′1 – dc23
2013012964

ISBN: 978–0–415–51863–5 (hbk)
ISBN: 978–1–138–65710–6 (pbk)
ISBN: 978–0–203–12335–5 (ebk)

Typeset in Bembo
by Florence Production Ltd, Stoodleigh, Devon

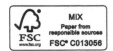

Printed and bound in Great Britain by
TJ International Ltd, Padstow, Cornwall

I dedicate this book and all my work to
the loving memory of my mother and father,
CHEN Hui Shen and HONG Qi Ming,
who have been my inspiration in my academic endeavours.
Without their unwavering guidance, influence and support,
I would not be where I am today.

CONTENTS

SECTION 9

Modelling and simulation in sports and exercise   **469**

SECTION 10

Measurement in adapted sports and exercise   **535**

INTRODUCTION

Ergonomics is concerned with the 'fit' between people and their work. As more people become conscious about their health and participate in sports or physical activities, ergonomics has become a prominent concern in sports and exercise sciences. From the design of footwear and artificial playing surfaces to studies of proprioception by obese children, people's interaction with their environment – designed and natural – significantly influences their performance in sports and design of safe and beneficial forms of physical activity. This book intends to provide a comprehensive and in-depth survey of cutting-edge scientific research on ergonomics in sports and exercise. Written by leading scientists and researchers worldwide, the book comprises 10 sections that explore key topics focused on ergonomics in sports and exercise.

Section 1, 'Muscular adaptation to sports and exercise', includes four chapters. In the first chapter, David Bentley *et al.* examine the relationship among different types of training, endurance and strength combined with resistance training and endurance performance. Gordon J. Bell subsequently reviews the literature on the role of breathing entrainment and respiratory muscle training on various physiological adaptations specific to rowing exercise. William A. Braun examines the neuromuscular adaptations proposed to confer economical advantages relevant to endurance running performance. David J. Pearsall *et al.* finally explore biomechanical adaptations from walking and running, to skating locomotion, focusing on differences in lower limb kinematics coordination, muscle recruitment and propulsion dynamics.

Section 2, 'Environmental factors of injury and fatigue', is divided into four chapters. In Chapter 5, Matt Greig *et al.* investigate the acute risks of playing soccer within a 90-minute match and the possibility of sustaining an injury. In Chapter 6, Beat Knechtle explores the influence of various factors such as environmental circumstances (heat, cold), overuse injuries of the lower limbs, and gastrointestinal problems on performance in ultra-endurance racing. Chapter 7 presents a review by Jochen D. Schipke *et al.* of environmental factors related to fatigue and injury in both breath-hold diving and scuba. Finally, Kazuhiko Watanabe examines the biomechanical and physiological approaches to adapting to cold environment and presents the Rating of Perceived Cold Stress to evaluate cold stress in peripheral parts of the body.

Section 3, 'Environmental condition and sports performance', also consists of four chapters. Chapter 9 by Martin Burtscher addresses the effects of environmental conditions such as winter clothing, nutrition and acclimatization on performance and maintaining well-being in winter sports. Michael D. Kennedy and William N. Lampe examine the concepts and ongoing challenges of minimizing drag while maximizing power output during cycling. In Chapter 11, Joshua Guggenheimer *et al.* examine the influence of equipment, hydrodynamic influences, techniques and water quality on corresponding injury and performance during competitive swimming. Finally, Billy Sperlich and Dennis-Peter Born address the most important psychophysiological responses when playing soccer in hot and cold environments, as well as at altitude.

Section 4, 'Effects of load weight on body posture and performance', also comprises four original studies. In the first study, Youlian Hong *et al.* explore spine posture alteration in children carrying school bags while walking on stairs. A symmetrical backpack with a load not exceeding 20 per cent or an asymmetrical school bag with a load not exceeding 10 per cent of the body weight are recommended. The second study, contributed by Liam Corrigan and Jing Xian Li, investigates the electromyography of the trunk and lower limbs during unilateral load carriage. Tarkeshwar Singh and Michael Koh also examine changes in spatio-temporal and kinematic parameters, as well as changes in trunk and pelvic coordination in load carriage. Finally, Yun Wang and Kazuhiko Watanabe report findings on differences in plantar forces associated with changes in backpack load and gait speed during treadmill walking.

Section 5, 'Measurement in sports and exercise', comprises five chapters. In Chapter 17, Marie C. McCormick and Julien S. Baker address resistive force selection and upper body contraction dynamics in relation to anaerobic cycle ergometry performance. Rae S. Gordon *et al.* review the measurement systems used in determining the required parameters to calculate work and power, as well as the different techniques and procedures in calculating work and power, particularly for the Wingate Anaerobic Test. In Chapter 19, Craig E. Broeder highlights the essential components to ensure that a sports performance metabolic testing centre provides reliable and accurate results for every athlete tested. In Chapter 20, the same author discusses how cycling power meter technologies provide a more accurate and real-time quantification of a rider's training or race load demands versus traditional heart rate measurements. Finally, Gongbing Shan *et al.* introduce the selection of dominant factors by using ground-reaction-force measurement and 3D motion capture to develop biofeedback training for golf swing.

Section 6, 'Influence of playing surface on sports and exercise', consists of five chapters. First, in an original study, Lin Wang *et al.* compare plantar loads during running on natural grass, concrete and synthetic rubber surfaces. Caroline Martin and Jacques Prioux provide an overview of the recent results from scientific research on physiological, biomechanical and epidemiological effects of playing surfaces in tennis to help players and coaches enhance performance. Chapter 24 by Kevin R. Ford thoroughly reviews studies on the effects of playing surface on injury risk, athletic performance and movement biomechanics in football at youth and professional levels. Federico Formenti illustrates how technical and material development, with empirical understanding of muscle biomechanics and energetics, led to one of the fastest forms of human-powered locomotion on ice surface. Finally, Lars Karlöf *et al.* review the factors influencing alpine skiing performance, in which snow conditions and the interaction between skis and snow are emphasized.

Section 7, 'Influence of footwear on sports and exercise', comprises six chapters. Chapter 27 by Youlian Hong *et al.* investigates possible differences in the perceived comfort, plantar pressure and rearfoot motion between laced running shoes and elastic-covered running shoes. Lin Wang *et al.* investigate the durability of prototype running shoes with ethylene vinyl acetate and polyurethane midsoles in 500 km running. The cushioning and energy return characteristics of each shoe were measured using a standard impact tester before and after each 50 km run. Chapter 29 by Uwe G. Kersting explores how calcaneal movement in running is not directly affected by changes in midsole hardness within the normal range of running shoes available on the market. Following this chapter is that in which Ewald M. Hennig and Katharina Althoff suggest a functional traction test to analyse the grip of soccer shoes. They indicate that shoe constructions influence maximum ball velocity, especially accuracy of kicking. In Chapter 31, Ki-Kwang Lee investigates the effect of heel modifications of footwear on shock attenuation and joint loading during extreme lunge movements among elite badminton players. Finally, the chapter by Edward C. Frederick reviews scientific literature on weight effects, as well as other studies on various biomechanical properties of footwear, which affect the energetic economy of movement.

Section 8, 'Influence of implements and protective devices in sports and exercise', contains five chapters. First, Andrew Post *et al.* examine the mechanism and quantification of head injuries by using linear and rotational acceleration, as well as brain deformation metrics, through finite element modelling and how current helmet technologies work to prevent injury. Sergej M. Ostojic *et al.* address the applicability of functional knee braces in reinjury prevention and athletic performance, as well as the design of functional braces. Duane Knudson *et al.* review how racket properties and engineering affect tennis play. In Chapter 36, Richard M. Smith *et al.* present an original study on compressive force in the lumbar spine while rowing on ergometers with both fixed and sliding ergometer subassemblies. The last chapter in this section, contributed by Kevin Laudner and Robert C. Lynall, details the extensive advancement in sport-related headgear design and construction since the introduction of the first helmet in the late 1800s.

Section 9, 'Modelling and simulation in sports and exercise', also contains five chapters. In Chapter 38, Pui Wah Kong examines previous modelling and simulation research applied in springboard diving. This chapter is followed by the chapter in which Luisa Consiglieri summarizes the non-linear mathematical model adopted to yield dynamic descriptions for rowing exercise. Parisa Saboori and Ali M. Sadegh present the issues of mechanotransduction of head influence to the brain, highlighting the role of material modelling of the subarachnoid space. Chapter 41 by Mikhail P. Shestakov introduces transition management of a biomechanical system from an initial state to the predetermined final state by the self-learning feature of a neural network in a simulation. Finally, Kim Nolte addresses the application of three-dimensional musculoskeletal modelling in assessing resistance training equipment in terms of injury risk, exercise efficacy and ability to accommodate the anthropometric dimensions of the end-user or exerciser.

Section 10, 'Measurement in adapted sports and exercise', is composed of four chapters. First, Siobhán Strike explores the joint coordination pattern adopted by unilateral transtibial amputees on the intact and residual sides while performing a maximum vertical jump. Weerawat Limroongreungrat and Yong Tai Wang present an original research on three-dimensional pushrim forces during three different speeds of racing wheelchair propulsion. In Chapter 45, Kayoko Ando and Shinji Sakurai introduce the development, application and results of the wheelchair tennis fitness test involving Japanese players who have recently dominated the wheelchair tennis world. The book ends with the chapter in which Justin Keogh and Brendan Burkett review kinematics studies on shot-put, discus and javelin throwing in Paralympic athletes.

This project aimed to bridge the gap between fundamental scientific research in sports and exercise and their applications. The contributors hope the book becomes an important reference for students, researchers and professionals working in sports and exercise science, kinesiology, sports technology, sports engineering, ergonomics and product design. The editor sincerely acknowledges deep appreciation for the contributors who devoted precious time to this endeavor. Finally, gratitude is extended to Professor Lin Wong for the time and effort invested in editing original submissions of all chapters.

Youlian Hong
Chengdu Sports University, Sichuan, China

SECTION 1

Muscular adaptation to sports and exercise

1

RESISTANCE TRAINING AND ENDURANCE PERFORMANCE

Physiological adaptations and recommendations for performance enhancement

David Bentley,[1] Glen Deakin[2] and Lars R. McNaughton[3]

[1]UNIVERSITY OF ADELAIDE, ADELAIDE
[2]JAMES COOK UNIVERSITY, CAIRNS
[3]EDGE HILL UNIVERSITY, ORMSKIRK

Introduction

Athletes, coaches and sports scientists typically define training into two distinct areas: weight or resistance training, and aerobic or cardiovascular training. Traditionally, the former is taken to be the realm of the athlete and the latter the realm of the health-conscious individual, though clearly each are used by both groups of individuals. The ability of all humans, however, to perform activities of daily life is clearly related to maintenance of the main elements of health-related physical fitness; for example, aerobic capacity, strength and power production, and mobility (Faulkner and Eston, 2007; Fleg *et al.*, 2005; Stathokostas *et al.*, 2004). These fitness parameters can be positively modified with specific training objectives that may differ between resistance or endurance training modes.

It is generally accepted that in order to maximize physiological adaptations and to avoid overtraining, appropriate management and progression of training programme variables, including the intensity, frequency and volume of exercise, for both strength and endurance training, is required. Hence, in order to accomplish performance improvements, training that incorporates several modes has become popular in order to prevent overtraining. This mix of both weight and endurance training has been termed 'concurrent training' (Hickson, 1980).

The aim of this chapter is to provide a contemporary summary of the acute physiological responses related to performance of resistance-type training after endurance exercise and vice versa. Additionally, the chronic performance-related outcomes in terms of endurance performance, as well as the factors associated with these adaptations, will be examined. In both cases, recommendations will be made outlining different strategies for prescribing resistance exercises to improve endurance performance. While significant adaptations to musculoskeletal and cardiovascular systems occurs with either resistance or endurance training variations, this chapter will focus specifically on the endurance performance-related changes that take place due to concurrent training.

The physiological effects of resistance training on endurance performance

Humans are the only group of animals for whom exercise is unique; we do it because we can, not because we have to. In the main, cardiovascular or endurance exercise is beneficial (except possibly for ultra-endurance events; see Green et al., 2008).

Resistance training can vary based on the load (per cent maximum strength), frequency (sessions per week) and the velocity of contractions employed within a training intervention, each with different potential muscle contractile performance outcomes (Deschenes and Kraemer, 2002; Fry, 2004). The studies examining the physiological adaptations of resistance training on endurance performance have varied considerably in terms of training variables, as well as the length of the resistance training intervention (ranging from 4 to 14 weeks) and the type of resistance training employed (Mikkola et al., 2011; Rønnestad et al., 2010a, 2010b, 2012a, 2012b, 2012c; Taipale et al., 2010). The training stimulus has generally been described as either 'heavy' maximal strength-orientated or 'explosive' with the frequency of training (range 1–4 times per week). Typically, resistance training incorporating heavy loads of > 8 RM (or ~ 80 per cent of 1 RM) have generally resulted in the largest improvements in endurance performance, although explosive-type resistance training has also been shown to improve running, cycling and cross-country ski performance (Losnegard et al., 2011; Mikkola et al., 2007a, 2007b, 2011; Millet et al., 2002; Taipale et al., 2010). For example, Rønnestad et al. (2010a, 2010b) found that a 12-week intervention involving heavy resistance training twice per week, starting at 10 RM and progressing to 6 RM, resulted in increases in the cross-sectional area (CSA) of the knee flex/extensor muscle groups in national-level cyclists. Increases in maximal isometric squat strength and improvement in peak power output during an incremental exercise test, as well as 40-minute cycle time trial performance were also observed. Mikkola et al. (2011) found that 8 weeks of either explosive-type resistance training incorporating loads of 40 per cent of 1 RM or heavy resistance training performed at an intensity of 4–6 RM improved endurance running performance, although the explosive training intervention resulted in the greatest improvement in endurance running performance. Another study also performed using endurance runners with similar loading variations found similar improvements in running economy and time to fatigue at the velocity associated with VO_2 max (vVO_2 max) (Støren et al., 2008). Paton and Hopkins (2005) found the addition of explosive resistance-type training (three sessions per week for 4 weeks of single-leg squat jumps) and high-intensity interval training resulted in improvement in endurance performance as measured by peak power output and submaximal metabolic (lactate) response during an incremental cycle test to exhaustion. The findings of this study using more explosive-type training have been replicated in cross-country skiers and runners (Paavolainen et al., 1991; Støren et al., 2008). This supports the notion that explosive 'body weight-loaded' training or using conventional resistance-based equipment with low to moderate loading performed at high velocity may facilitate improvements in endurance performance. In resistance training research, studies have shown that load optimization, specifically low-intensity resistance (30 per cent of 1 RM) results in greater improvements in muscle explosive power (Wilson et al., 1993). Therefore, it seems that this loading amount may also be appropriate in improving power performance, as well as endurance performance in athletes of different modes, although the observed changes in explosive/power performance may not be as great as pure power-based athletes and may even plateau after only a short training period in endurance athletes (Paavolainen et al., 1999; Rønnestad et al., 2012b).

The traditional resistance training frequency used to promote gains in muscle strength is usually 2–4 times per week for a given muscle or muscle group (Deschenes and Kraemer,

2002; Tan, 1999). However, in order to promote optimal gains in endurance performance and eliminate potential negative training responses due to an excess in the resistance training stress (combined with the endurance training), an approach often taken is to reduce the frequency of resistance training; this is especially true in periods of competition. Indeed, a number of studies have shown that improvements in muscular strength and endurance performance can be achieved by using a frequency of as little as two times per week (Aagaard *et al.*, 2011; Rønnestad *et al.*, 2010b). However, it has been shown that strength improvements may reach a plateau or are not as great as that compared to a resistance training-only group (Rønnestad *et al.*, 2010b, 2012a). This may be due to the lower volume of resistance training that is achievable with a combined resistance/endurance training regime. However, the effects of variation of resistance training and/or endurance training volume on strength and endurance outcomes are not well known. Conversely, the important consideration is that resistance training volume (and accompanying training variables) for an endurance athlete may not be the same as a strength training athlete and should be carefully planned and prioritized at different training stages. It should also be considered that large increases in muscular strength performance may not be observed, despite positive changes in endurance performance.

The primary outcome of any training regime is to evoke optimal race performance during a competition period. Therefore, the focus of training in this period is to optimize the endurance training stress and improve competition skills. Hence, providing resistance training to improve muscular strength may not be a priority in this stage of training. In one study of well-trained cyclists, it was shown that considerable gains in muscular strength and endurance performance could be reached after a 12-week period of resistance training and that these gains could be maintained on as little as one training session per week (Rønnestad *et al.*, 2010a). Hence, the practical implications of this finding is that appropriate progression of resistance training should occur, then prioritizing of training should be made, and this could include a reduction in the volume and frequency of resistance training performed within the overall training plan of an endurance athlete.

Adaptations to resistance training will vary depending upon the initial status of the person, with very large increases in muscular strength occurring in the early phase of resistance training in untrained subjects (Deschenes and Kraemer, 2002). Studies examining the effects of resistance training on endurance performance have used either endurance-trained subjects with mixed ability and subjects that have not been exposed to any prior resistance training stress, which could lead to inferior or limited gains in either strength or endurance performance (Bastiaans *et al.*, 2001; Bishop *et al.*, 1999; Ferrauti *et al.*, 2010; Jackson *et al.*, 2007; Kelly *et al.*, 2008; Levin *et al.*, 2009; Taipale *et al.*, 2010). Therefore, one issue with inclusion of resistance training within the overall plan of an endurance athlete is the potential dramatic increase in training load and stress, which may potentially negate the positive adaptations to the training. This, in part, could be due to prolonged and chronic residual fatigue (see page 11). In this situation, the optimal structure and progression of training is important. Indeed, there have been contradictory reports to the positive benefits of resistance training on endurance performance associated with suboptimal training stress. Levin *et al.* (2009) found that a relatively short (6-week) period of resistance training (6–12 RM) did not result in any improvement in 30 km cycle time trial performance despite improvement in 1 RM maximal strength. These authors concluded that the increase in total training stress with the addition of the resistance training intervention and the inability of the athletes to tolerate this training was linked to the lack of positive findings. It is also possible, of course, that the time trial performance measure is not sensitive to such changes in training. Indeed, the appropriate management and progression of resistance training within an overall plan of an endurance athlete is an important practical consideration when attempting to optimize endurance performance outcomes through resistance training. In another study, Jackson *et al.* (2007) found no significant effects of either a 10-week heavy resistance or low-intensity/high-repetition training programme on incremental cycling performance. However, this study was conducted in cyclists of mixed ability. The authors also concluded that it appeared the resistance training volume was of significant magnitude to promote ongoing acute residual fatigue, which could have impacted on the results of the study. The study crucially highlights the important practical consideration of appropriate acute planning of resistance training and minimizing/controlling residual fatigue from both forms in order to maximize performance outcomes.

There are very few studies that have examined the influence of resistance training on endurance performance in young or female athletes. Bishop *et al.* (1999) investigated the effects of lower limb heavy resistance training (12 weeks; 2–8 RM) on 1-hour cycling performance in moderately trained female athletes. The authors found that the resistance training intervention was associated with improvements in lower limb maximal strength but endurance performance remained unchanged. The authors concluded that increased leg strength was not associated with improvement in endurance cycle performance in female athletes. In another study, Kelly *et al.* (2008) investigated the effects of heavy resistance-type training on 3 km running performance. The authors reported minimal worthwhile effects of this training on 3 km running performance in these recreational-level participants. It would appear that female athletes with limited training history in endurance or resistance training may respond negatively to the combined regime of strength and endurance training, especially if the training is not well periodized. However, more studies are required examining the effects of resistance training in female endurance athletes. In another study, Aagaard *et al.* (2011) found that in U23 national-level cyclists, both 5-minute all-out and 45-minute cycle time trial performance was improved after a period (16 weeks) of resistance training (two times per week), which progressed from a load of 10 RM to 5 RM over the course of the training intervention. While this study did not highlight how much endurance training was performed in the subjects who completed the resistance training, it did indicate that with appropriate progression, endurance performance gains can be facilitated in younger athletes with heavy-type resistance training. In a study examining running performance, Mikkola *et al.* (2007a, 2007b) found contrary findings and showed that a group of runners aged 16–18 years who supplemented ~ 20 per cent of their training with high-velocity, low-load, explosive-type training found no significant change in endurance running performance. While this study could be interpreted as being a negative finding, these authors showed that anaerobic running performance was improved with the resistance training intervention.

The potential improvement in endurance performance due to resistance training may be a function of the intensity and duration of the endurance event (Aagaard and Andersen, 2010). Furthermore, the mode (and accompanying biomechanical characteristics) of the endurance exercise that the performance improvement is desired may also be an important consideration when interpreting whether there are positive effects of resistance training for endurance athletes. The majority of studies have assessed the changes in endurance performance in cycling and running of different distances following a period of resistance training, each with different general outcomes. In general, endurance cycling performance of short duration appears to be improved the greatest in resistance training involving heavy loads over periods ranging from 6 to 16 weeks (Yamamoto *et al.*, 2010). The adaptations associated with a resistance training intervention on running endurance performance have been equivocal (Ferrauiti *et al.*, 2010; Mikkola *et al.*, 2011; Millet *et al.*, 2002). For example, in one study, no positive effect was shown on submaximal physiological parameters (anaerobic threshold, VO_2 at fixed running speeds) after a period of heavy-type strength training, despite improvements in leg strength (Ferrauti *et al.*, 2010). However, in this study, the subject cohort was not well controlled and comprised older runners of varying ability and gender. In another study, well-trained runners demonstrated a similar improvement in running economy after a 4-week period of either explosive strength training or traditional heavyweight strength training (Guglielmo *et al.*, 2009). Millet *et al.* (2002) investigated the effects of a 14-week heavy resistance training programme (twice per week; 90 per cent of 1 RM) on subsequent 3 km running performance. The authors found that lower limb muscle strength improved and this was associated with improvements in endurance running performance. One Finnish group has conducted a number of studies examining the effects of different resistance training variations (heavy or explosive-type training) on endurance running performance (Mikkola *et al.*, 2007a, 2007b, 2011; Taipale *et al.*, 2010, 2012). In two separate studies by the same research group (Mikkola *et al.*, 2007a, 2007b, 2011), no improvement in endurance running performance was found in senior and junior runners as measured by the maximal and submaximal physiological responses during an incremental running test to exhaustion, despite improvements in anaerobic running performance and maximal muscle strength. While it could be concluded that endurance performance was unchanged by the resistance training intervention, most studies have focused on changes in running economy or responses during incremental exercises testing, with no actual time trial used as a measure of endurance running performance. These studies generally show that endurance running performance remains unchanged after a period of resistance training. However, this could be a function of the type of resistance training employed, either heavy or explosive-type training, or that the time trials used as a performance measure are not suitably sensitive to show a significant performance difference. Paavolainen *et al.* (1999) have demonstrated that 9 weeks of explosive-type resistance training resulted in improved 5 km running performance. Saunders *et al.* (2006) subsequently found beneficial changes in running economy at 18 km.h^{-1} following a short-term period of plyometric training. Distance runners who replaced a portion of their usual competitive phase training consisting of explosive single-leg and resisted treadmill sprints showed improvements in the running speed corresponding to lactate threshold and 5 km time trial speed (Hamilton *et al.*, 2006). In another study, Taipale *et al.* (2012) investigated the effects of either maximum strength, explosive strength training or a combination of training on a number of strength, power and endurance components. While it was shown that physiological variables obtained during a maximal exercise testing improved with training over an 8-week period, resistance training intervention produced no better gains in strength-, power- and endurance-performance. Therefore, the majority of the available evidence indicates that explosive-type training using low loads compared to heavier-type resistance training is more beneficial for improving endurance performance. Hence, a consideration in planning resistance training for endurance athletes is to consider the biomechanical considerations of the endurance mode, which could be influenced by the type of resistance training employed. Other studies have shown contrary results to this opinion in terms of training aimed at improving muscular power. For example, Støren *et al.* (2008) also found that running economy and time to fatigue at maximal aerobic running speed improved following an 8-week heavy resistance training (5 RM) intervention in well-trained runners.

A number of investigations have shown that endurance performance can be improved with heavy resistance-type activity, and this is associated with an increase in muscular strength without large changes in hypertrophy (Hickson *et al.*, 1988; Rønnestad *et al.*, 2010a, 2010b, 2012a). Generally, the studies examining the effects of resistance training on endurance performance have also presented little information on the potential mechanisms of the endurance performance improvement. A number of researchers have concluded one significant mechanism behind the improvement in endurance performance is a delay in the fast-twitch muscle fibre recruitment during the time endurance performance task (Hickson *et al.*, 1988; Paton and Hopkins, 2005; Rønnestad *et al.*, 2010a, 2010b). Hickson *et al.* (1988), in one of the first controlled studies to explore the effects of resistance training on endurance performance, showed that a 10-week progressive intervention comprising a 'heavy' training intervention comprising five sets of five repetitions at 80 per cent of 1 RM of lower-body isotonic exercises resulted in leg-strength improvements of 30 per cent without any change in muscle size, and this was associated with an improvement in endurance time to exhaustion while cycling at 80 per cent of VO$_2$ max. The authors concluded that endurance performance was associated with modification of muscle recruitment patterns during the exercise task. While this suggests that a component of any positive (endurance) adaptation to a resistance training stimulus is of neurological origin, other studies have proposed the negative 'interference effect' resulting from combined strength and endurance training (Docherty and Sporer, 2000; Häkkinen *et al.*, 2003; Wilson *et al.*, 2011). This model suggests that there is a reduced capacity of the neuromuscular system to adapt to the conflicting resistance endurance training stimulus of the concurrent training regime, which is typically not observed when resistance training is employed in isolation. However, this interference effect is typically observed during a muscle function/strength test performed before and after training. In contrast to this observation, and in keeping with the hypothesis that muscle fibre recruitment patterns are positively modified during endurance cycling following resistance exercise, there are studies that have shown, using electromyographic (EMG) signals in muscle during exercises, that muscle recruitment patterns change after a period of resistance training, which is associated with fatigue resistance (Hausswirth *et al.*, 2010). While these investigators used heavy resistance-type training, it remains to be confirmed with other resistance training forms, such as high-velocity resistance training, whether muscle recruitment patterns are associated with improved performance after resistance training.

A considerable factor influencing endurance performance is skeletal muscle oxidative capacity and slower fibre-type phenotype changes (Bentley *et al.*, 2009; Coyle *et al.*, 1991). Resistance training, especially heavier-type training, results in no change in muscle oxidative capacity or slow-twitch muscle fibre type with increases in muscle fibre area (Deschenes and Kraemer, 2002). Very little research has examined the effects of resistance training and endurance performance and related skeletal muscle phenotype (Aagaard *et al.*, 2011; Bishop *et al.*, 1999). In one study, 16 weeks of heavy strength training in young elite cyclists resulted in significant increases in type IIa muscle fibre type and reciprocal decreases in type IIx fibres. Furthermore, no significant changes were observed in muscle fibre area of capillarization. In another study, a 12-week resistance training programme aimed at improving maximal muscle strength resulted in no changes in fibre type diameter, fibre type percentage or muscle oxidative capacity in a group of mixed-ability-level female cyclists (Bishop *et al.*, 1999). These studies indicate resistance training has a limited effect on muscle oxidative phenotype when combined with endurance training in athletes, and supports the concept that changes in endurance performance with resistance training are due largely to modifications in muscle fibre recruitment patterns. However, additional research is required to further explore some of the conflicting molecular adaptations of skeletal muscle to combined resistance and endurance training (Hawley, 2009; Nader, 2006).

Acute physiological responses with concurrent training

Regardless of whether the intention of training is for strength or endurance adaptation, the accumulation of the acute responses to a training stimulus is what will ultimately determine the resultant level of adaptation. Unfortunately, the majority of research into concurrent training to date has focused on 'training studies' that have looked at strength and endurance adaptations over varying periods of time (e.g. 6–22 weeks). Consequently, there is limited information in respect of the acute effect that one concurrent training session has on another performed either on the same day or subsequent days.

Effect of a bout of endurance or strength exercise on the acute strength response

In respect of the acute effect of endurance activity on the acute strength response, the recovery of muscle force generation capacity (MFGC) is not immediate following exercise, but may take hours (Bentley *et al.*, 1998) to days (Sherman *et al.*, 1984) to recover. What appears to determine the extent and speed of recovery of MFGC following endurance exercise is the intensity and duration of the endurance exercise, with shorter-duration, high-intensity exercise (e.g. < 1 hour, Bentley *et al.*, 1998) having faster recovery times of MFGC (less than 24 hours) than longer-duration but moderate-intensity exercise (e.g. > 1 hour, Sahlin and Seger, 1995; Sherman *et al.*, 1984). Similarly, the effect of a single bout of resistance exercise on the acute strength response, measured as MFGC, has also been found to produce significant reductions in muscle function, and while greatest immediately post-exercise, can persist for periods up to 96 hours (4 days) post-exercise (Gibala *et al.*, 1995). Again, the extent and speed of recovery of MFGC is dependent on the intensity and volume/duration of the exercise (Behm and St-Pierre, 1997). Consequently, the acute hypothesis of strength deprivation put forward by Craig *et al.* (1991), suggesting that the residual fatigue generated from a prior bout of endurance exercise can have detrimental influences on a subsequent bout of strength exercise, due to a reduction in the ability to generate tension during the strength element of a concurrent training programme, may be true and apply not only to the acute effect of endurance training on the strength response, but the effect of strength training on endurance exercise.

The above-mentioned scenario has been found to be the case in the few studies that have examined the acute effects of concurrent training sessions. Deakin (2004), Palmer and Sleivert (2001) and Twist and Eston (2005) have all shown an attenuated performance and/or increased physiological cost of submaximal cycling, submaximal running or maximal running performance 3, 8 and 24 hours post a bout of moderate- to high-intensity strength training, respectively. However, it should also be mentioned that there have been studies that have shown no detrimental influences on endurance running performance (Doma and Deakin, 2012a; Marcora and Bosio, 2007) in the hours following strength training. The difference in outcomes between the studies that found detrimental influences and those that did not seem to be related to differences in training variables. That is, the intensity and volume of the strength training exercises performed (including training of same or different muscle groups), the intensity of the endurance exercise undertaken (submaximal versus maximal) and the time period between the bout of strength training and the subsequent endurance exercise. High-intensity, high-volume strength training, coupled with moderate- to high-intensity endurance training within 24 hours, appears to produce the greatest influence not only on the level of muscular fatigue post-exercise and its duration, but the physiological cost of the endurance exercise performed.

Order of concurrent training sessions

Based on the above evidence, it seems that irrespective of the order of concurrent training sessions, there is the potential for some form of residual fatigue to be carried forward from one session to the next, and that this level of fatigue is determined by the intensity and volume/ duration of the initial and subsequent training session, as well as the time period between the training sessions. Given that some concurrent training adaptation studies (Bell *et al.*, 1988; Gravelle and Blessing, 2000) have found one order of concurrent training sessions to be more conducive to minimizing the detrimental effects of combining the two forms of training, then the order of concurrent training sessions may be an important factor in determining the acute training response.

In one of the first studies to compare the acute effects of the order of concurrent training on exercise and post-exercise recovery, Deakin (2004) found that there was an order effect when high-intensity strength training and moderate-intensity endurance cycle training sessions were separated by 3 hours of recovery. Even though all sessions completed second in the training sequence experienced an increased physiological cost (e.g. higher heart rate, blood lactate concentrations), performing the order of strength then endurance training produced a greater level of fatigue (indicated by a slower recovery of MFGC) and high physiological cost of exercise 3 hours post than performing the reverse order. While the above is only one study, the findings do suggest that there may be an interaction between the order in which the concurrent training sessions are completed and the degree of fatigue/physiological cost of training sessions and speed of recovery. Hence, the combination of the two training sessions in a particular order may produce a compound effect, resulting in a greater level of fatigue being carried forward from one training day to the next; a point that has been shown to be the case in a recent study by Doma and Deakin (2012b), who examined the acute effects of completing strength training on alternate days combined with endurance running on four consecutive days. Ten moderately trained runners completed four consecutive days of running sessions consisting of a combination of 20 minutes of submaximal and maximal running (time to exhaustion), 10 and 24 hours following a strength training session on the first and third days. The outcome was a significant reduction in running time to exhaustion at the maximal level in both running sessions, completed the days following the combined strength and endurance training sessions, when compared to the baseline session. This corresponded with impaired MFGC of the quadriceps muscle prior to each running session compared to a pre-strength training baseline. Even though the submaximal cost of running was unaffected, the results showed the runners were in a chronic state of muscular fatigue for each training session.

The significance of the above research is that the order of concurrent training sessions and the optimal recovery time between training sessions may need to vary depending on the type (strength or endurance) and intensity (high, medium or low) of training, with exercise such as high-intensity strength or endurance training requiring a greater recovery time period than low-intensity strength or aerobic endurance training. Furthermore, days where strength and endurance training sessions are both undertaken may require a greater period of recovery than days were only one type of training session is completed. The practical implications of this are that the performance of another training session in the hours following an initial training session using the same muscle groups may be adversely affected if sufficient recovery has not taken place. If an athlete is still in the process of recovering, then there will be a carry forward of fatigue, as well as an increase in energy expenditure both during and in the recovery from the second bout of exercise. In addition, the continual presence of fatigue over days of training could lead to athletes overreaching and possibly overtraining.

The other practical implication of insufficient recovery between training sessions is that if heart rate or a similar physiological parameter (e.g. oxygen uptake, blood lactate) is the criteria used to set exercise intensity, then an elevated heart rate following the first training session could mean that the intensity of the subsequent training session is conducted below the designated level. In light of the above, consideration must be given to the timing of a second bout of exercise where multiple training sessions are completed within the same day or on adjacent days. The intensity and duration of these respective training sessions and the method employed to prescribe exercise intensity also need to be carefully considered.

Influence of athlete training status on acute concurrent training responses

A variable that may influence the speed of recovery between concurrent training sessions, irrespective of whether they are on the same day or different days, is the training experience and level of adaptation of the athlete. Athletes that have a higher strength training experience have a smaller disturbance of homeostasis, owing to greater training adaptations and to more efficient exercise techniques, than lesser trained athletes (Thornton and Potteiger, 2002). Similarly, the recovery rates of endurance-trained athletes have been found to be faster than lesser-trained/untrained individuals from the same relative and absolute work rates (Short and Sedlock, 1997). It is thought that trained athletes have a faster regulation of post-exercise metabolism, as well as experience lesser stress resulting from the exercise stimulus than that incurred by lesser-trained athletes. Subsequently, the design of concurrent training regimes (i.e. recovery period between sessions and combination of the intensity and duration of training sessions) may need to be varied according to the level of athlete being trained.

Sources of residual fatigue

Even though a number of acute sources of residual fatigue have been proposed to explain the influence that one concurrent training session has on another, not all are thought to be major contributors.

Accumulation of metabolites

The reduction in level of tension generated by muscles immediately post-training has been attributed to muscular fatigue resulting from an accumulation of metabolites including lactate (Allen *et al.*, 1992). This level of accumulation has been linked with increases in exercise intensity (Baker *et al.*, 1993). Even though there is evidence to suggest that muscular fatigue may not be directly associated with the accumulation of metabolites such as lactate (Webster *et al.*, 1993), the accumulation of metabolites are unlikely to be a factor in concurrent training regimes where there are hours of rest between training sessions because such metabolites are generally dispersed within a short time after the cessation of exercise (Baker *et al.*, 1993). However, the accumulation of metabolites may play a part in concurrent training regimes where one mode of training session immediately precedes another, particularly if the preceding training session involves periods of high-intensity exercise.

Muscle damage

While it is possible that endurance exercise involving relatively large amounts of eccentric muscle activity may impair performance in a subsequent strength training session, this source of fatigue has been considered unlikely to affect long-term impairment of strength development (Leveritt *et al.*, 1999) for two reasons. First, because muscle damage after repeated bouts of either strength or endurance exercise, termed the 'repeated bout effect' (Hortobágyi and Denahan, 1989), is reported to be minimal compared with the initial exercise bout (McHugh,

1999). Second, the level of damage after strength training would be greater than that induced after endurance training, and as such strength-trained groups would experience impaired strength development similar to the concurrent-trained groups, yet this is not a common occurrence (Leveritt *et al.*, 1999). Even though this source of muscle fatigue has been questioned, it cannot be ruled out completely.

Glycogen depletion

The depletion of muscle glycogen has been proposed as a contributing factor to muscle fatigue because of the well-documented evidence that indicates that an acute bout of endurance (Costill *et al.*, 1971; Sherman *et al.*, 1984) or strength (Pascoe *et al.*, 1993; Robergs *et al.*, 1991) exercise can considerably reduce muscle glycogen levels. Consequently, the performance of exercise using the same muscle groups in the period of time before muscle glycogen levels have been replenished after a prior bout of exercise would be restricted, either in the level of force generation (exercise intensity) or time duration of the exercise (Grisdale *et al.*, 1990). Therefore, it is plausible that strength training performance following endurance exercise or vice versa would be impaired. However, this line of reasoning has been questioned because of the findings of a number of concurrent training studies whereby the level of training undertaken by subjects in one study (e.g. Dudley and Djamil, 1985) was considerably less than that undertaken by the subjects in another study (Hickson, 1980), yet both experienced impeded strength development. While this suggests that muscle glycogen depletion was not a factor in the impeded strength development, the findings may simply reflect an insufficient volume or intensity of training to significantly reduce muscle glycogen stores to a level that would impede endurance development, but enough to influence strength development. The rate of muscle glycogen resynthesis after depletion is dependent on the type of diet (Ivy, 1991) and the timing of food ingestion post-exercise (Ivy *et al.*, 1988). A carbohydrate-rich diet immediately following exercise restores muscle glycogen levels faster than a low-carbohydrate diet with delayed ingestion. In light of the above, the timing of food ingestion both during and after exercise may have implications for concurrent training sessions, particularly if performed on the same day, by determining the extent of muscle glycogen depletion during exercise and the speed and extent of recovery between training sessions.

Neuromuscular fatigue

Of the four proposed sources of acute fatigue influencing concurrent training, neuromuscular fatigue seems to be the most likely candidate. Neuromuscular fatigue can stem from a failure at any link in the command chain for voluntary muscular activity that starts in the brain and finishes with the formation of a muscle contraction (Maclaren *et al.*, 1989). Through the use of MFGC in conjunction with EMG, a variety of forms of endurance exercise including cycling (Bentley *et al.*, 1998; Lepers *et al.*, 2000) and running (Paavolainen *et al.*, 1999) of varying durations have shown significant reductions in MFGC and maximal EMG of the exercising muscles immediately post-exercise. Similar findings have also been found following heavy resistance exercise (Häkkinen, 1992, 1993; Linnamo *et al.*, 1998). Both types of training have shown that while these parameters have improved over the hours to days following exercise, it is common for them to still be below pre-training levels for days post-training. The reductions in MFGC and maximal EMG are attributed to both the central nervous system and peripheral mechanisms.

Even though it is unlikely that any one source is solely responsible for the acute fatigue that may be carried forward from one concurrent training session to the next, anything that can be done to minimize the impact that one training session has on another or speed recovery should be implemented, including:

- maximizing of recovery times between concurrent training sessions;
- offsetting the scheduling of intensity and duration of concurrent training sessions on the same day or utilizing alternating days for high-intensity, high-volume/long-duration training;
- ensuring an adequate dietary routine is in place while performing and recovering from concurrent training sessions;
- employing active and passive recovery techniques to enhance the recovery process; and
- monitoring athletes for signs/symptoms of insufficient recovery from concurrent training sessions, particularly for those athletes that are less trained.

Conclusion

It would appear that concurrent training, a distinct mix of both weight or resistance training and endurance training, is in use in a variety of sports, but as yet research would provide contradictory results with respect to the adaptations and performance improvements. The studies examining physiological adaptations of resistance training on endurance performance have varied considerably in terms of training variables, as well as the length of the resistance training intervention and the type of resistance training employed. However, based upon the current research, there is support for the notion that explosive 'body weight loaded' training or using conventional resistance-based equipment with low to moderate loading, performed at high velocity, may facilitate improvements in endurance performance. The potential improvement in endurance performance due to resistance training may also be a function of the intensity and duration of the endurance event. Athletes and coaches therefore need to be mindful of the inclusion of resistance training within the overall plan of an endurance athlete, as this may lead to dramatic increases in training load and stress, which may potentially negate the positive adaptations to the training.

High-intensity, high-volume strength training, coupled with moderate- to high-intensity endurance training within 24 hours, appears to produce the greatest influence not only on the level of muscular fatigue post-exercise and its duration, but the physiological cost of the endurance exercise performed. Based on research evidence, it seems that irrespective of the order of concurrent training sessions, there is the potential for some form of residual fatigue to be carried forward from one session to the next, and that this level of fatigue is determined by the intensity and volume/duration of the initial and subsequent training session, as well as the time period between the training sessions. Hence, the order of concurrent training sessions and the optimal recovery time between training sessions may need to vary depending on the type (strength or endurance) and intensity of training, with exercise such as high-intensity strength or endurance training requiring a greater recovery time period than low-intensity strength or aerobic endurance training. Furthermore, days where strength and endurance training sessions are both undertaken may require a greater period of recovery than days were only one type of training session is completed. Subsequently, the design of concurrent training regimes (i.e. recovery period between sessions and combination of the intensity and duration of training sessions) may need to be varied according to the level of athlete being trained.

Areas that require further work include the effects of resistance training in female endurance athletes and the acute effect that one concurrent training session has on another performed either on the same day or subsequent days.

References

Aagaard, P. and Andersen, J. L. (2010) 'Effects of strength training on endurance capacity in top-level endurance athletes', *Scandinavian Journal of Medicine and Science in Sports*, 20(2): 39–47.

Aagaard, P., Andersen, J. L., Bennekou, M., Larsson, B., Olesen, J. L., Crameri, R., Magnusson, S. P. and Kjaer, M. (2011) 'Effects of resistance training on endurance capacity and muscle fiber composition in young top-level cyclists', *Scandinavian Journal of Medicine and Science in Sports*, 21(6): e298–307.

Allen, D. G., Westerblad, H., Lee, J. A. and Lännergren, J. (1992) 'Role of excitation-contraction coupling in muscle fatigue', *Sports Medicine*, 13(2): 116–26.

Baker, A. J., Kostov, K. G., Miller, R. G. and Weiner, M. W. (1993) 'Slow force recovery after long-duration exercise: metabolic and activation factors in muscle fatigue', *Journal of Applied Physiology*, 74(5): 2294–300.

Bastiaans, J. J., van Diemen, A. B., Veneberg, T. and Jeukendrup, A. E. (2001) 'The effects of replacing a portion of endurance training by explosive strength training on performance in trained cyclists', *European Journal of Applied Physiology and Occupational Physiology*, 86(1): 79–84.

Behm, D. G. and St-Pierre, D. M. M. (1997) 'Effects of fatigue duration and muscle type on voluntary and evoked contractile properties', *Journal of Applied Physiology*, 82(5): 1654–61.

Bell, G. J., Petersen, S. R., Quinney, H. A. and Wenger, H. A. (1988) 'Sequencing of endurance and high-velocity strength training', *Canadian Journal of Sport Science*, 13(4): 214–19.

Bentley, D. J., Roels, B., Thomas, C., Ives, R., Mercier, J., Millet, G. and Cameron Smith, D. (2009) 'The relationship between monocarboxylate transporters 1 and 4 expression in skeletal muscle and endurance performance in athletes', *European Journal of Applied Physiology*, 106(3): 465–71.

Bishop, D., Jenkins, D. G., Mackinnon, L. T., McEniery, M. and Carey, M. F. (1999) 'The effects of strength training on endurance performance and muscle characteristics', *Medicine and Science in Sports and Exercise*, 31(6): 886–91.

Costill, D. L., Bowers, R., Branam, G. and Sparks, K. (1971) 'Muscle glycogen utilization during prolonged exercise on successive days', *Journal of Applied Physiology*, 31(6): 834–8.

Coyle, E. F., Feltner, M. E., Kautz, S. A., Hamilton, M. T., Montain, S. J., Baylor, A. M., Abraham, L. D. and Petrek, G. W. (1991) 'Physiological and biomechanical factors associated with elite endurance cycling performance', *Medicine and Science in Sports and Exercise*, 23(1): 93–107.

Craig, B. W., Lucas, J., Pohlman, R. and Stelling, H. (1991) 'The effects of running, weightlifting and a combination of both on growth hormone release', *Journal of Applied Sport Science Research*, 5(4): 198–203.

Deakin, G. B. (2004) 'Concurrent training in endurance athletes: the acute effects on muscle recovery, physiological, hormonal and gene expression responses post-exercise', unpublished doctoral thesis, Southern Cross University.

Deschenes, M. R. and Kraemer, W. J. (2002) 'Performance and physiologic adaptations to resistance training', *American Journal of Physical Medicine and Rehabilitation*, 81(l): S3–16.

Docherty, D. and Sporer, B. (2000) 'A proposed model for examining the interference phenomenon between concurrent aerobic and strength training', *Sports Medicine*, 30(6): 385–94.

Doma, K. and Deakin, G. B. (2012a) 'Investigation of running economy 6 hours post full body and lower body strength training', *Journal of Australian Strength and Conditioning*, 20(1): 94–6.

Doma, K. and Deakin, G. B. (2012b) 'The cumulative effects of strength and endurance training on running performance', *Proceedings of the National Strength and Conditioning Association Conference*, Rhode Island: National Strength and Conditioning Association.

Dudley, G. A. and Djamil, R. (1985) 'Incompatibility of endurance- and strength-training modes of exercise', *Journal of Applied Physiology*, 59(5): 1446–51.

Faulkner, J. and Eston, R. (2007) 'Overall and peripheral ratings of perceived exertion during a graded exercise test to volitional exhaustion in individuals of high and low fitness', *European Journal of Applied Physiology*, 101(5): 613–20.

Ferrauti, A., Bergermann, M. and Fernandez-Fernandez, J. (2010) 'Effects of a concurrent strength and endurance training on running performance and running economy in recreational marathon runners', *Journal of Strength and Conditioning Research*, 24(10): 2770–8.

Fleg, J. L., Morrell, C. H., Bos, A. G., Brant, L. J., Talbot, L. A., Wright, J. G. and Lakatta, E. G. (2005) 'Accelerated longitudinal decline of aerobic capacity in health older adults', *Circulation*, 112(5): 674–82.

Fry, A. C. (2004) 'The role of resistance exercise intensity on muscle fibre adaptations', *Sports Medicine*, 34(10): 663–79.

Gibala, M. J., MacDougall, J. D., Tarnopolsky, M. A., Stauber, W. T. and Elorriaga, A. (1995) 'Changes in human skeletal muscle ultrastructure and force production after acute resistance exercise', *Journal of Applied Physiology*, 78(2): 702–8.

Gravelle, B. L. and Blessing, D. L. (2000) 'Physiological adaptation in women concurrently training for strength and endurance', *Journal of Strength and Conditioning Research*, 14(1): 5–13.

Green, D. J., Naylor, L. H., George, K., Dempsey, J. A., Stickland, M. K. and Katayama, K. (2008) 'Cardiovascular and pulmonary adaptations to endurance training', in N. A. S. Taylor and H. Groeller (eds), *Physiological Basis of Human Performance During Work and Exercise*, Edinburgh: Churchill Livingstone, pp. 49–70.

Grisdale, R. K., Jacobs, I. and Cafarelli, E. (1990) 'Relative effects of glycogen depletion and previous exercise on muscle force and endurance capacity', *Journal of Applied Physiology*, 69(4): 1276–82.

Guglielmo, L. G., Greco, C. C. and Denadai, B. S. (2009) 'Effects of strength training on running economy', *International Journal of Sports Medicine*, 30(1): 27–32.

Häkkinen, K. (1992) 'Neuromuscular responses in male and female athletes to two successive strength training sessions in one day', *The Journal of Sports Medicine and Physical Fitness*, 32(3): 234–42.

Häkkinen, K. (1993) 'Neuromuscular fatigue and recovery in male and female athletes during heavy resistance exercise', *International Journal of Sports Medicine*, 14(2): 53–9.

Häkkinen, K., Alen, M., Kraemer, W. J., Gorostiaga, E., Izquierdo, M., Rusko, H., Mikkola, J., Häkkinen, A., Valkeinen, H., Kaarakainen, E., Romu, S., Erola, V., Ahtiainen, J. and Paavolainen, L. (2003) 'Neuromuscular adaptations during concurrent strength and endurance training versus strength training', *European Journal of Applied Physiology*, 89(1): 42–52.

Hamilton, R. J., Paton, C. D. and Hopkins, W. G. (2006) 'Effect of high-intensity resistance training on performance of competitive distance runners', *International Journal of Sports Physiology and Performance*, 1(1): 40–9.

Hausswirth, C., Argentin, S., Bieuzen, F., Le Meur, Y., Couturier, A. and Brisswalter, J. (2010) 'Endurance and strength training effects on physiological and muscular parameters during prolonged cycling', *Journal of Electromyography and Kinesiology*, 20(2): 330–9.

Hawley, J. A. (2009) 'Molecular responses to strength and endurance training: are they incompatible?', *Applied Physiology, Nutrition, and Metabolism*, 34(3): 355–61.

Hickson, R. C. (1980) 'Interference of strength development by simultaneously training for strength and endurance', *European Journal of Applied Physiology*, 45(2–3): 255–63.

Hickson, R. C., Dvorak, B. A., Gorostiaga, E. M., Kurowski, T. T. and Foster, C. (1988) 'Potential for strength and endurance training to amplify endurance performance', *Journal of Applied Physiology*, 65(5): 2285–90.

Hortobágyi, T. and Denahan, T. (1989) 'Variability in creatine kinase: methodological, exercise, and clinically related factors', *International Journal of Sports Medicine*, 10(2): 69–80.

Ivy, J. L. (1991) 'Muscle glycogen synthesis before and after exercise', *Sports Medicine*, 11(1): 6–19.

Ivy, J. L., Katz, A. L., Cutler, C. L., Sherman, W. M. and Coyle, E. F. (1988) 'Muscle glycogen synthesis after exercise: effect of time of carbohydrate ingestion', *Journal of Applied Physiology*, 64(4): 1480–5.

Jackson, N. P., Hickey, M. S. and Reiser, R. F. (2007) 'High resistance/low repetition vs. low resistance/high repetition training: effects on performance of trained cyclists', *Journal of Strength and Conditioning Research*, 21(1): 289–95.

Kelly, C. M., Burnett, A. F. and Newton, M. J. (2008) 'The effect of strength training on three-kilometer performance in recreational women endurance runners', *Journal of Strength and Conditioning Research*, 22(2): 396–403.

Lepers, R., Hausswirth, C., Maffiuletti, N., Brisswalter, J. and van Hoecke, J. (2000) 'Evidence of neuromuscular fatgiue after prolonged cycling exercise', *Medicine and Science in Sports and Exercise*, 32(11): 1880–6.

Leveritt, M., Abernethy, P. J., Barry, B. K. and Logan, P. A. (1999) 'Concurrent strength and endurance training: a review', *Sports Medicine*, 28(6): 413–27.

Levin, G. T., Mcguigan, M. R. and Laursen, P. B. (2009) 'Effect of concurrent resistance and endurance training on physiologic and performance parameters of well-trained endurance cyclists', *Journal of Strength and Conditioning Research*, 23(8): 2280–6.

Linnamo, V., Häkkinen, K. and Komi, P. V. (1998) 'Neuromuscular fatigue and recovery in maximal compared to explosive strength loading', *European Journal of Applied Physiology*, 77(1–2): 176–81.

Losnegard, T., Mikkelsen, K., Rønnestad, B. R., Hallen, J., Rud, B. and Raastad, T. (2011) 'The effect of heavy strength training on muscle mass and physical performance in elite cross country skiers', *Scandinavian Journal of Medicine and Science in Sports*, 21(3): 389–401.

McHugh, M. (1999) 'Can exercise induced muscle damage be avoided?', *British Journal of Sports Medicine*, 33(6): 377.

Maclaren, D. P. M., Gibson, H., Parry-Billings, M. and Edwards, R. H. T. (1989) 'A review of metabolic and physiological factors in fatigue', *Exercise and Sport Sciences Reviews*, 17: 29–66.

Marcora, S. M. and Bosio, A. (2007) 'Effect of exercise-induced muscle damage on endurance running performance in humans', *Scandinavian Journal of Medicine and Science in Sports*, 17(6): 662–71.

Mikkola, J., Rusko, H., Nummela, A., Pollari, T. and Häkkinen, K. (2007a) 'Concurrent endurance and explosive type strength training improves neuromuscular and anaerobic characteristics in young distance runners', *International Journal of Sports Medicine*, 28(7): 602–11.

Mikkola, J., Rusko, H. K., Nummela, A. T., Paavolainen, L. M. and Häkkinen, K. (2007b) 'Concurrent endurance and explosive type strength training increases activation and fast force production of leg extensor muscles in endurance athletes', *Journal of Strength and Conditioning Research*, 21(2): 613–20.

Mikkola, J., Vesterinen, V., Taipale, R., Capostagno, B., Häkkinen, K. and Nummela, A. (2011) 'Effect of resistance training regimens on treadmill running and neuromuscular performance in recreational endurance runners', *Journal of Sports Sciences*, 29(13): 1359–71.

Millet, G. P., Jaouen, B., Borrani, F. and Candau, R. (2002) 'Effects of concurrent endurance and strength training on running economy and VO_2 kinetics', *Medicine and Science in Sports and Exercise*, 34(8): 1351–9.

Nader, G. A. (2006) 'Concurrent strength and endurance training: from molecules to man', *Medicine and Science in Sports and Exercise*, 38(11): 1965–70.

Paavolainen, L., Häkkinen, K. and Rusko, H. (1991) 'Effects of explosive type strength training on physical performance characteristics in cross-country skiers', *European Journal of Applied Physiology*, 62(4): 251–5.

Paavolainen, L., Häkkinen, K., Hämäläinen, I., Nummela, A. and Rusko, H. (1999) 'Explosive-strength training improves 5-km running time by improving running economy and muscle power', *Journal of Applied Physiology*, 86(5): 1527–33.

Palmer, C. D. and Sleivert, G. G. (2001) 'Running economy is impaired following a single bout of resistance exercise', *Journal of Science and Medicine in Sport*, 4(4): 447–59.

Pascoe, D. D., Costill, D. L., Fink, W. J., Robergs, R. A. and Zachwieja, J. J. (1993) 'Glycogen resynthesis in skeletal muscle following resistive exercise', *Medicine and Science in Sports and Exercise*, 25(3): 349–54.

Paton, C. D. and Hopkins, W. G. (2005) 'Combining explosive and high-resistance training improves performance in competitive cyclists', *Journal of Strength and Conditioning Research*, 19(4): 826–30.

Robergs, R. A., Pearson, D. R., Costill, D. L., Fink, W. J., Pascoe, D. D., Benedict, M. A., Lambert, C. P. and Zachwieja, J. J. (1991) 'Muscle glycogenolysis during difffering intensities of weight-resistance exercise', *Journal of Applied Physiology*, 70(4): 1700–6.

Rønnestad, B. R., Hansen, E. A. and Raastad, T. (2010a) 'Effect of heavy strength training on thigh muscle cross-sectional area, performance determinants, and performance in well-trained cyclists', *European Journal of Applied Physiology*, 108(5): 965–75.

Rønnestad, B. R., Hansen, E. A. and Raastad, T. (2010b) 'In-season strength maintenance training increases well-trained cyclists' performance', *European Journal of Applied Physiology*, 110(6): 1269–82.

Rønnestad, B. R., Hansen, E. A. and Raastad, T. (2012a) 'High volume of endurance training impairs adaptations to 12 weeks of strength training in well-trained endurance athletes', *European Journal of Applied Physiology*, 112(4): 1457–66.

Rønnestad, B. R., Hansen, E. A. and Raastad, T. (2012b) 'Strength training affects tendon cross-sectional area and freely chosen cadence differently in noncyclists and well-trained cyclists', *Journal of Strength and Conditioning Research*, 26(1): 158–66.

Rønnestad, B. R., Kojedal, O., Losnegard, T., Kvamme, B. and Raastad, T. (2012c) 'Effect of heavy strength training on muscle thickness, strength, jump performance, and endurance performance in well-trained Nordic Combined athletes', *European Journal of Applied Physiology*, 112(6): 2341–52.

Sahlin, K. and Seger, J. Y. (1995) 'Effects of prolonged exercise on the contractile properties of human quadriceps muscle', *European Journal of Applied Physiology*, 71(2–3): 180–6.

Saunders, P. U., Telford, R. D., Pyne, D. B., Peltola, E. M., Cunningham, R. B., Gore, C. J. and Hawley, J. A. (2006) 'Short-term plyometric training improves running economy in highly trained middle and long distance runners', *Journal of Strength and Conditioning Research*, 20(4): 947–54.

Sherman, W. M., Armstrong, L. E., Murray, T. M., Hagerman, F. C., Costill, D. L., Staron, R. C. and Ivy, J. L. (1984) 'Effect of a 42.2-km footrace and subsequent rest or exercise on muscular strength and work capacity', *Journal of Applied Physiology*, 57(6): 1668–73.

Short, K. R. and Sedlock, D. A. (1997) 'Excess postexercise oxygen consumption and recovery rate in trained and untrained subjects', *Journal of Applied Physiology*, 83(1): 153–9.

Stathokostas, L., Jacob-Johnson, S., Petrella, R. J. and Paterson, D. H. (2004) 'Longitudinal changes in aerobic power in older men and women', *Journal of Applied Physiology*, 97(2): 781–9.

Støren, O., Helgerud, J., Støa, E. M. and Hoff, J. (2008) 'Maximal strength training improves running economy in distance runners', *Medicine and Science in Sports and Exercise*, 40(6): 1087–92.

Taipale, R. S., Mikkola, J., Nummela, A., Vesterinen, V., Capostagno, B., Walker, S., Gitonga, D., Kraemer, W. J. and Häkkinen, K. (2010) 'Strength training in endurance runners', *International Journal of Sports Medicine*, 31(7): 468–76.

Taipale, R. S., Mikkola, J., Vesterinen, V., Nummela, A. and Häkkinen, K. (2012) 'Neuromuscular adaptations during combined strength and endurance training in endurance runners: maximal versus explosive strength training or a mix of both', *European Journal of Applied Physiology*, doi: 10.1007/s00421-012-2440-7.

Tan, B. (1999) 'Manipulating resistance training program variables to optimize maximum strength in men: a review', *Journal of Strength and Conditioning Research*, 13(3): 289–304.

Thornton, M. K. and Potteiger, J. A. (2002) 'Effects of resistance exercise bouts of different intensities but equal work on EPOC', *Medicine and Science in Sports and Exercise*, 34(4): 715–22.

Twist, C. and Eston, R. (2005) 'The effects of exercise-induced muscle damage on maximal intensity intermittent exercise performance', *European Journal of Applied Physiology*, 94(5–6): 652–8.

Webster, M. J., Webster, M. N., Crawford, R. E. and Gladden, L. B. (1993) 'Effect of sodium bicarbonate ingestion on exhaustive resistance exercise performance', *Medicine and Science in Sports and Exercise*, 25(8): 960–5.

Wilson, G. J., Newton, R. U., Murphy, A. J. and Humphries, B. J. (1993) 'The optimal training load for the development of dynamic athletic performance', *Medicine and Science in Sports and Exercise*, 125(11): 1279–86.

Wilson, J. M., Marin, P. J., Rhea, M. R., Wilson, S. M., Loenneke, J. P. and Anderson, J. C. (2011) 'Concurrent training: a meta analysis examining interference of aerobic and resistance exercise', *Journal of Strength and Conditioning Research*, 26(8): 2293–307.

Yamamoto, L. M., Klau, J. F., Casa, D. C., Kraemer, W. J., Armstrong, L. E. and Maresh, C. M. (2010) 'The effects of resistance training on road cycling performance among highly trained cyclists: a systematic review', *Journal of Strength and Conditioning Research*, 24(2): 560–6.

2

BREATHING ENTRAINMENT AND RESPIRATORY MUSCLE TRAINING FOR ROWING

Gordon J. Bell

UNIVERSITY OF ALBERTA, EDMONTON

Introduction

Traditional rowing is a sport performed on water in racing shells built to accommodate one (single) to eight athletes. The Olympic and Paralymic rowing race distances are 2,000 and 1,000 m, respectively, but race distances can vary at other competitions such as head races or 'sprints'. On-water rowing is accomplished by either sculling with two oars or 'sweep', in which each rower only uses one oar (Nolte, 2005). There is also an indoor rowing competition using stationary rowing machines (e.g. Concept 2®) and there is a 2,000 m international championship hosted annually using these same devices (C.R.A.S.H.-B Sprints, 2012). Thus, rowing exercise is performed in two general ways, on water or using stationary exercise on a rowing ergometer or machine. As well, rowing exercise is not only performed by rowers, but has also become popular for recreation, fitness training and rehabilitation (Gillies and Bell, 2000; Smart et al., 2012; Urhausen et al., 2009; Wheeler et al., 2002). Finally, past research has examined various physiological and biomechanical aspects of both on-water and stationary rowing exercise and training (Bompa, 1980; Di Prampero et al., 1971; Hagerman, 1984; Martindale and Robertson, 1984; Secher, 1993; Steinacker, 1993; Webster et al., 2006).

The rowing stroke begins in the catch position, where the rower is seated, holding the handle (or oar) with the arms extended. The trunk is flexed forward and the knees are bent so that the shins are vertical and the feet are dorsiflexed at the ankle joint and strapped to foot stops. The rowing stroke is initiated at the catch by increasing the force on the handle primarily with leg and hip extension initially, followed by trunk extension and arm flexion forcing the handle to the chest (Bell et al., 2013; Mazzone, 1988; Nolte, 2005; Webster et al., 2006). This sequence is basically reversed when returning to the catch position (see Figure 2.1). Thus the movement pattern of the rowing stroke includes the catch, drive, finish and recovery phases (Mazzone, 1988; Nolte, 2005). As a result of this sequence of body movement, rowing exercise places a unique demand on the mechanics of breathing (Cunningham et al., 1975; Siegmund et al., 1999). This is partly because the respiratory auxiliary muscles are also needed to support the torso and assist with maintaining a proper body posture during the rowing stroke. In addition to this, when the rower is in the catch position, there is an increase in intra-abdomenal pressure that can compromise the movement of the diaphragm (Cunningham et al., 1975). This has been shown to reduce forced vital capacity in the catch position (Siegmund et al., 1999). To compensate for any restriction to breathing during rowing exercise, rowers generally adopt two different breathing patterns: exhalation during the drive phase of the stroke and inhalation during the recovery, or vice versa (MacLennan *et al.*, 1994; Webster *et al.*, 2010). Regardless of the pattern of breathing, there is usually a brief Valsalva manoeuvre performed at the start of the drive phase just prior to the generation of force to initiate the stroke (Rosiello *et al.*, 1987), followed by a variety of breathing patterns depending on the individual and intensity of the rowing exercise. Individuals that row have been shown to entrain their breathing, which includes one breathing cycle per stroke (1:1), 2:1 or even 3:1 at near maximal intensities (MacLennan *et al.*, 1994; Mahler *et al.*, 1991; Siegmund *et al.*, 1999; Webster *et al.*, 2010; Wily *et al.*, 2001).

Although it has been suggested that the lung is 'overbuilt' for exercise (Dempsey, 1986), it is possible that clinical conditions such as exercise-induced bronchospasm (EIB) or asthma (EIA) can limit exercise performance (Dempsey *et al.*, 2003). As well, McKenzie (2012) outlined

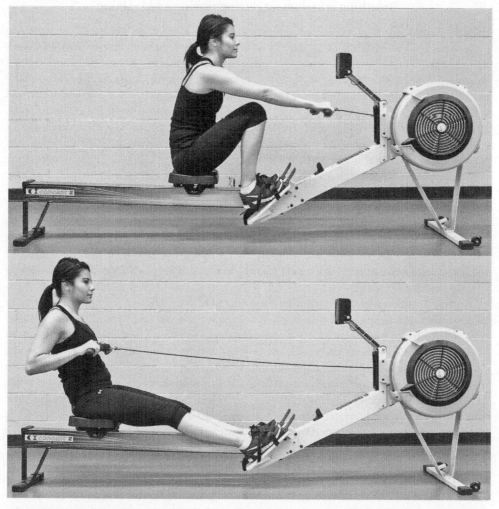

Figure 2.1 The position of the rowing stroke at the catch (top panel) and at the finish (bottom panel) (photo courtesy of Zoltan Kenwell).

four possible factors that may link limits in the respiratory system of a healthy individual to decreases in exercise performance, including arterial hypoxaemia experienced during high intensity exercise, expiratory flow limitations, vocal cord dysfunction and respiratory muscle fatigue (McKenzie, 2012). In addition, Harms *et al.* (2000) have suggested that a metabo-reflex may operate during exercise that would reduce blood flow to working muscles during times of respiratory muscle fatigue. The result of any one or combination of these factors would be a greater onset of fatigue and reduced exercise performance. Because of the potential of rowing exercise to be partially limited by the mechanics of breathing that may negatively affect ventilation leading to gas exchange, there have been two primary areas of focus that have been examined in an attempt to improve breathing mechanics, reduce respiratory muscle fatigue and thereby promote gas exchange and hopefully performance in rowers. These are the use of breathing entrainment during rowing exercise and the implementation of respiratory muscle training.

Breathing entrainment during rowing and training

Breathing entrainment or locomotor-respiratory coupling is the coordination of the breathing cycle with limb movements in an attempt to decrease the metabolic cost of muscular work during exercise and therefore improve economy (MacLennan *et al.*, 1994; Mahler *et al.*, 1991; Siegmund *et al.*, 1999; Webster *et al.*, 2010). It has been seen to occur during acute rowing exercise and breathing entrainment patterns, including one breath per stroke (1:1), 2:1 and 3:1, and has been observed during both on-water and stationary rowing (MacLennan *et al.*, 1994; Mahler *et al.*, 1991; Siegmund *et al.*, 1999; Webster *et al.*, 2010). As well, during maximal rowing exercise at the limits of fatigue such as that experienced during a 2,000 m rowing race, breathing can become sporadic and uncoordinated (Webster *et al.*, 2010). This coupling of the rowing stroke to the breathing cycle is thought to limit interference of the required posture and muscular exertion during rowing exercise on ventilation and potentially improve the efficiency and thereby reduce the overall metabolic cost of rowing exercise (Bonsignore *et al.*, 1998; Webster *et al.*, 2010). Despite these observations of breathing entrainment patterns during acute rowing exercise, there have been few studies that have pursued whether specific breathing entrainment patterns performed during chronic rowing training may provide additional respiratory muscle adaptations that would contribute to improved physiological responses during rowing exercise.

Because of this paucity, we compared the effects of two different breathing entrainment patterns used during training on various physiological responses to rowing exercise (Webster *et al.*, 2010). It was hypothesized that if rowers trained for 8 weeks with breathing frequencies of either 1:1 or 2:1 breaths per stroke, the respiratory muscle support would adapt in such a way that there would be greater improvements in submaximal exercise responses compared to training with no breathing entrainments. We found that rowing economy was improved when the 1:1 and 2:1 breathing patterns were used during submaximal rowing and ventilation was lower when using a 2:1 breathing pattern after training. There were similar improvements in breathing frequency, rowing performance and maximal oxygen uptake regardless of which breathing pattern was used. However, there was a greater increase in tidal volume observed during the first 1,000 m of a simulated 2,000 m rowing race after training in the group that trained with the 1:1 breathing pattern. It was concluded that exercise economy was greatest during submaximal rowing exercise when using a breathing entrainment pattern of either one or two breaths per stroke and that training with breathing controlled at a rate of 1:1 can increase tidal volume during high-intensity exercise. Certainly, breathing entrainment can provide some physiological benefits to rowing exercise that may be partially related to improved respiratory muscle adaptations. However, further research is recommended to investigate this latter contention and examine whether breathing entrainment used during rowing exercise training at a variety of exercise intensities can provide any greater benefits.

Respiratory muscle training in rowing

Respiratory muscle (RM) training refers to some form of repetitive overload stimulus in an attempt to improve the strength and/or endurance of the muscles involved in the support of breathing such as the diaphragm, intercostals and other accessory muscles. There are two types of RM training that differ in their focus; that is, the development of repetitive, low- to moderate-intensity performance (i.e. endurance) or the maximum force capabilities (i.e. strength) of the respiratory support muscles (Illi *et al.*, 2012; Sheel, 2002). RM endurance training is usually performed by performing high sustained rates of voluntary ventilation at a low force that are repeated several times a week for several weeks in an attempt to improve the endurance capabilities of the breathing support muscles and reduce their fatigue. RM strength training is conducted by breathing against a high resistance, usually with the aid of a resistive breathing device, for a certain number of repetitions and sets much like a strength training prescription used for other skeletal muscle groups. This latter type of training is also performed several days a week for several weeks to improve the ability to forcefully breathe. Some resistive breathing devices are designed to provide variable resistance to inspiration only, while others provide resistance to both inspiration and expiration. Thus, there should be a distinction made between whether the goal of the RM training is to improve the endurance or strength capabilities of the respiratory support musculature and whether the RM is targeting inspiratory versus expiratory breathing or both. Two recent reviews of the effects of RM training on a variety of physiological and exercise performance responses in healthy individuals have been published (Illi *et al.*, 2012; Sheel, 2002).

The majority of research investigating RM training in rowers has used respiratory muscle training devices and has focused on strength and endurance performance while performing inspiratory only (IMT), expiratory only (EMT) and combined inspiratory and expiratory muscle training (COMT). With few exceptions, many studies have found that all three types of RM training prescriptions improve maximal inspiratory PI_{max} (Bell *et al.*, 2013; Forbes *et al.*, 2011; Griffiths and McConnell, 2007; Klusiewicz *et al.*, 2008; Riganas *et al.*, 2008; Volianitis *et al.*, 2001) and expiratory PE_{max} (Bell *et al.*, 2013; Forbes *et al.*, 2011; Griffiths and McConnell, 2007) pressure measured at the mouth. Data from our laboratory shows that increases in both PI_{max} and PE_{max} at rest occur after training with either IMT, EMT or COMT (see Figure 2.2). Respiratory muscle fatigue as measured by the recovery of PI_{max} or PE_{max} after rowing exercise has been shown to be reduced after IMT (Bell *et al.*, 2013; Volianitis *et al.*, 2001), EMT (Bell *et al.*, 2013) and COMT (Forbes *et al.*, 2011). However, this latter effect is not universal (Griffiths and McConnell, 2007). Ratings of perceived breathing exertion and the perception of dyspnea during and after acute rowing exercise have been shown to improve with RM training in some research (Griffiths and McConnell, 2007; Volianitis *et al.*, 2001), but not all (Forbes *et al.*, 2011; Riganas *et al.*, 2008). It is relatively clear that RM training in trained rowers has no appreciable effect on inspiratory or expiratory spirometry measurements, submaximal or maximal ventilatory parameters during rowing exercise or on aerobic fitness (Bell *et al.*, 2013; Forbes *et al.*, 2011; Griffiths and McConnell, 2007; Klusiewicz *et al.*, 2008; Riganas *et al.*, 2008; Volianitis *et al.*, 2001). An exception is that Riganas *et al.* (2008) observed a significant increase in maximum voluntary ventilation (MVV) with 6 weeks of IMT; however, we did not observe a change in MVV after 10 weeks of IMT, EMT or COMT in rowers

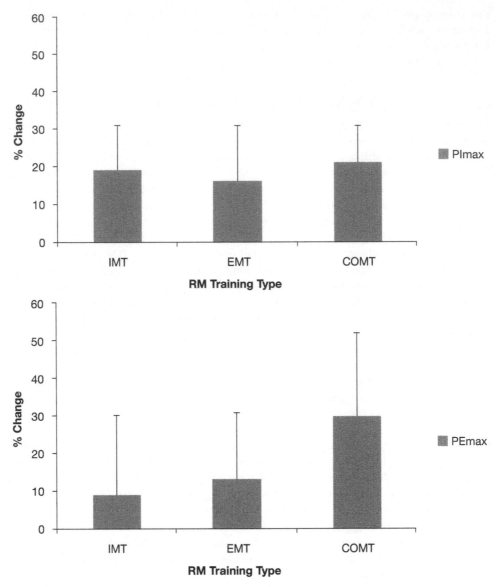

Figure 2.2 Per cent change in resting maximum inspiratory pressure (PI_{max}; top graph) and maximum expiratory pressure (PE_{max}; bottom graph) after inspiratory only training (IMT), expiratory only training (EMT) or using combined inspiratory and expiratory training (COMT) in rowers. Data modified from our laboratory (Bell *et al.*, 2013; Forbes *et al.*, 2011).

(Bell *et al.*, 2013; Forbes *et al.*, 2011). It is important to note in the above literature that all studies used RMT as an adjunct to other physical training being performed by the rowers.

With respect to rowing performance, prescribing RM training as an adjunct to other physical training that rowers perform during their annual training programmes in an attempt to influence performance is controversial. Previous research has shown that IMT in addition to rowing training resulted in a greater distance rowed during a 6-minute rowing test and a greater decrease in time to complete 5,000 m of rowing in comparison to a placebo group (Volianitis *et al.*, 2001). As well, Griffiths and McConnell (2007) reported a significant improvement in mean rowing power and distance rowed with an initial 4-week IMT programme. However, other studies have failed to show a significant improvement in rowing performance using a simulated 2,000 m rowing race after IMT, EMT or COMT (Bell *et al.*, 2013; Forbes *et al.*, 2011; Riganas *et al.*, 2008). One reason for this discrepancy may be due to the RM training prescription. Volianitis *et al.* (2001) and Griffiths and McConnell (2007) both used IMT that involved 30 inspiratory efforts, which would be considered a muscular endurance training prescription. In comparison, our research (Bell *et al.*, 2013; Forbes *et al.*, 2011) investigated IMT only, EMT only and COMT using an 8–10 repetition maximum breathing strength training prescription designed to improve maximal strength of the respiratory support muscles. Other reasons for the variable effects of RM training on rowing performance may be the differences in the type of rowing performance test used in the previous research and the differences in the type of adjunct physical training the rowers were performing in conjunction with the RMT. As athletes, rowers commonly perform a combination of training modalities at different times of their annual training calendar that most often includes some form of rowing endurance and strength training. Thus, the majority of the RM training research conducted on rowers to date has involved the addition of the RM protocol to other physical training programmes followed by the rowers. This may influence the adaptive potential of the respiratory support musculature. Thus, caution must be advised in interpretation of the current literature.

Summary

Rowing exercise is unique in that it requires a combination of various muscle groups developing force across a variety of joints while maintaining a particular posture on the rowing machine. As a result, rowing exercise may challenge breathing efficiency and this can possibly have negative consequences and limit rowing performance. Breathing entrainment during rowing exercise and during training may improve economy and some ventilatory responses during submaximal rowing exercise. Respiratory muscle training has also been used as an adjunct to other types of physical training normally performed by rowers and has shown to be effective at improving forceful breathing performance and reducing respiratory muscle fatigue after exercise. However, it is unlikely that RMT as an adjunct training modality in rowers improves pulmonary function or aerobic fitness and it is controversial as to whether RMT can positively influence rowing performance. Future research may improve on past in regards to these controversial findings.

References

Bell, G., Game, A., Jones, R., Webster, T., Forbes, S. and Syrotuik, D. (2013) 'Inspiratory and expiratory respiratory muscle training as an adjunct to concurrent strength and endurance training provides no additional 2000 m performance benefits to rowers', *Research in Sports Medicine*, 21: 264–79.

Bompa, T. O. (1980) 'Technique and muscle force', *Canadian Journal of Sport Sciences*, 5(4): 245–9.

Bonsignore, D. M., Morici, G., Abate, P., Romano, S. and Bonsignore, G. (1998) 'Ventilation and entrainment of breathing during cycling and running in triathletes', *Medicine and Science in Sport and Exercise*, 30(2): 239–45.

C.R.A.S.H.-B Sprints (2012) *World Indoor Rowing Championships, Cambridge, MA*, available at: www.crash-b.org (accessed 5 April 2012).

Cunningham, D. A., Goode, P. B. and Critz, J. B. (1975) 'Cardiorespiratory response to exercise on a rowing and bicycle ergometer', *Medicine and Science in Sports*, 7(1): 37–43.

Dempsey, J. A. (1986) 'J. B. Wolfe memorial lecture. Is the lung built for exercise?', *Medicine and Science in Sports and Exercise*, 18(2): 143–55.

Dempsey, J. A., Sheel, A. W., Haverkamp, H. C., Babcock, M. A. and Harms, C. A. (2003) 'Pulmonary system limitations to exercise in health', *Canadian Journal of Applied Physiology*, 28: S2–24.

Di Prampero, P. E., Cortili, G., Celentano, F. and Cerretelli, P. (1971) 'Physiological aspects of rowing', *Journal of Applied Physiology*, 31(6): 853–7.

Forbes, S., Game, A., Syrotuik, D., Jones, R. and Bell, G. (2011) 'The effect of inspiratory and expiratory respiratory muscle training in rowers', *Research in Sports Medicine*, 19(4): 217–30.

Gillies, E. and Bell, G. (2000) 'The relationship of physical and physiological parameters to 2000 m simulated rowing performances', *Sports Medicine, Training and Rehabilitation*, 9(4): 277–88.

Griffiths, L. A. and McConnell, A. K. (2007) 'The influence of inspiratory and expiratory muscle training upon rowing performance', *European Journal of Applied Physiology*, 99(5): 457–66.

Hagerman, F. C. (1984) 'Physiology and nutrition for rowing', in D. R. Lamb, H. G. Knuttgen and R. Murray (eds), *Perspectives in Exercise Science and Sports Medicine*, Indianapolis, IN: Cooper Publishing Group, Vol. 7, pp. 221–302.

Harms, C. A., Wetter, T. J., St Croix, C. M., Pegelow, D. F. and Dempsey, J. A. (2000) 'Effects of respiratory muscle work on exercise performance', *Journal of Applied Physiology*, 89(1): 131–8.

Illi, S. K., Held, U., Frank, I. and Spengler, C. M. (2012) 'Effects of respiratory muscle training on exercise performance in healthy individuals. A systematic review and meta-analysis', *Sports Medicine*, 42(8): 707–24.

Klusiewicz, A., Borkowski, L., Zdanowicz, R., Boros, P. and Wesolowski, S. (2008) 'The inspiratory muscle training in elite rowers' *Journal of Sports Medicine and Physical Fitness*, 48(3): 279–84.

McKenzie, D. C. (2012) 'Respiratory physiology: adaptations to high-level exercise', *British Journal of Sports Medicine*, 46(6): 381–4.

MacLennan, S. E., Silvestri, G. A., Ward, J. and Mahler, D. A. (1994) 'Does entrained breathing improve the economy of rowing?', *Medicine and Science in Sport and Exercise*, 26(5): 610–14.

Mahler, D. A., Hunter, B., Lentine, T. and Ward, J. (1991) 'Ventilatory responses and entrainment of breathing during rowing', *Medicine and Science in Sport and Exercise*, 23(2): 186–93.

Martindale, W. O. and Robertson, D. G. (1984) 'Mechanical energy in sculling and in rowing an ergometer', *Canadian Journal of Sport Sciences*, 9(3): 153–63.

Mazzone T. (1988) 'Kinesiology of the rowing stroke', *Strength and Conditioning Journal*, 10(2): 1–4.

Nolte, V. (2005) *Rowing Faster*, Windsor: Human Kinetics.

Riganas, C. S., Vrabas, J. S., Christoulas, K. and Manroukas, K. (2008) 'Specific inspiratory muscle training does not improve performance or VO$_2$max in well trained rowers', *Journal of Sports Medicine and Physical Fitness*, 48(3): 285–92.

Rosiello, R. A. Mahler, D. A. and Ward, J. L. (1987) 'Cardiovascular responses to rowing', *Medicine and Science in Sports and Exercise*, 10(3): 239–45.

Secher, N. H. (1993) 'Physiological and biomechanical aspects of rowing: implications for training', *Sports Medicine*, 15(1): 24–42.

Sheel, A. W. (2002) 'Respiratory muscle training in healthy individuals: physiological rationale and implications for exercise performance', *Sports Medicine*, 32(9): 567–81.

Siegmund, G. P., Edwards, M. R., Moore, K. S., Tiessen, D. A., Sanderson, D. J. and McKenzie, D. C. (1999) 'Ventilation and locomotor coupling in varsity male rowers', *Journal of Applied Physiology*, 87(1): 233–42.

Smart, N., Giallauria, F. and Dieberg, G. (2012) 'Efficacy of inspiratory muscle training in chronic heart failure patients: a systematic review and meta-analysis', *International Journal of Cardiology*, doi:10.1016/j.ijcard.2012.04.029.

Steinacker, J. M. (1993) 'Physiological aspects of training in rowing', *International Journal of Sports Medicine*, 14(1): S3–10.

Urhausen, A., Spieldenner, J., Gabriel, H., Schwarz, L., Schwarz, M. and Kindermann, W. (2009) 'Cardiocirculatory and metabolic strain during rowing ergometry in coronary patients', *Clinical Cardiology*, 17(12): 652–6.

Volianitis, S., McConnell, A. K., Koutedakis, Y., McNaughton, L., Backx, K. and Jones, D. A. (2001) 'Inspiratory muscle training improves rowing performance', *Medicine and Science in Sports and Exercise*, 33(5): 803–9.

Webster, A., Penkman, M., Syrotuik, D., Gervais, P., del la Cruz, L. and Bell, G. (2010) 'Effect of off-season training combined with different breathing entrainment patterns on physiological adaptations and performance in rowers', *Advances in Exercise and Sports Physiology*, 16(1): 15–23.

Webster, T., Gervais, P., Syrotuik, D. and Bell, G. (2006) 'The combined effects of 8-weeks aerobic and resistance training on simulated 2,000-metre rowing performance and the related biomechanical and physiological determinants in men and women', *Advances in Sport and Exercise Physiology*, 12(4): 135–43.

Wheeler, G., Andrews, B., Lederer, R., Davoodi, R., Natho, K., Weiss, C., Jong, J., Bhambhani, Y. and Steadward, R. (2002) 'Functional electrical stimulation-assisted rowing: increasing cardiovascular fitness through functional electrical stimulation rowing training in persons with spinal cord injury', *Archives of Physical Medicine and Rehabilitation*, 83(8): 1093–9.

Wily, L. D., Robinson, J., Reid, D., Shkurhan, G., David, G. J., Coutts, K. D. and McKenzie, D. C. (2001) 'Effects of two entrainment patterns on the physiology and performance of female novice rowers', *Sports Medicine, Training and Rehabilitation*, 10(1): 29–37.

3

NEUROMUSCULAR ADAPTATIONS IN RUNNING

William A. Braun

SHIPPENSBURG UNIVERSITY, SHIPPENSBURG

Introduction

Run training, as with all forms of physical exercise training, stimulates the development of adaptations that should benefit the performance of the task. In the case of distance running, these adaptations often result in improved economy of transport (i.e. lower energy cost to maintain a fixed running speed). Mechanisms behind training-related improvements in running economy fall primarily into two broad categories: metabolic adaptation and neuromuscular adaptation. The focus of this chapter will be on factors that may contribute to neuromuscular adaptations and improvements in running economy primarily in distance runners. In conjunction with this, common training practices will be explored, including: (1) incorporation of resistance training as a means of supporting the performance of running; (2) adaptations that result from chiefly 'run-only' training; and (3) possible influences of barefoot running versus shod running on neuromuscular adaptations that develop from running. The chapter begins with a general exploration of the relationship between endurance run training and neuromuscular factors.

Neuromuscular influences of endurance run training

The specificity of training principle would suggest that slow, continuous aerobic exercise, which is commonly performed by distance runners, will compromise high-velocity force production and power. Endurance-only training also impedes gains in strength and can cause reductions in power due to shifting of fibre-type characteristics towards Type I fibre-type and disuse atrophy effects on Type IIa and IIx muscle fibre (Thayer *et al.*, 2000). In addition, functional adaptations that result from endurance training may be limited to metabolic outcomes (Cohen *et al.*, 2010). As a result, distance runners often incorporate interval-type training and/or strength training as methods for supporting the power-based needs that are often important for success in their sport. Plyometric training has also shown positive benefits for use in distance runners by supporting improvements in running economy (Markovic and Mikulic, 2010; Saunders *et al.*, 2006; Turner *et al.*, 2003). Neuromuscular adaptations that result from these types of training interventions may positively influence motor unit activation and recruitment patterns and alter more commonly assessed factors such as stride length and frequency. Bonacci *et al.* (2009) compiled a comprehensive review of neuromuscular adaptations related to various types of training to which the reader is referred. However, the focus of this chapter will remain on running adaptations.

The quality of running economy may be related to existing (or changes to) elastic properties of the leg muscles in addition to metabolic adaptation. For example, it has been shown that the oxygen cost of running is inversely related to lower limb flexibility in elite marathon runners (Jones, 2002). Those with greater leg stiffness (poorer flexibility) were found to be more economical. Craib *et al.* (1996) made similar observations in a group of sub-elite runners, hypothesizing that greater leg stiffness might confer an economy advantage by improving storage and return of elastic energy generated during the eccentric phase of the stretch-shortening cycle. These findings are also corroborated by Dalleau *et al.* (1998), who found better RE in those runners who possessed greater leg stiffness. The investigators hypothesized that increased leg stiffness develops as a neuromuscular adaptive response to endurance run training. However, stiffness can be acutely affected as well. Stiffness may be increased transiently, leading to a lower energy cost, by avoiding over-flexing the knees during running or by running on a less compliant surface (Dalleau *et al.*, 1998). An adaptive response to running that results in increased leg stiffness may seem counterintuitive, however, as a more rigid muscle might be expected to be more prone to injury resulting from repetitive impact.

Heise *et al.* (2008) found that muscle coactivation of biarticular muscles (rectus femoris and gastrocnemius) during the stance phase leads to increased joint stiffness, which may allow for more efficient use of stored elastic energy. They theorized that coactivation of these muscles may be an adaptive response found in more economical runners. In a group of 16 female runners, muscle coactivation duration was able to explain 45 per cent of the inter-individual variability in running economy; an inverse relationship between running economy and duration of muscle coactivation was noted (Heise *et al.*, 2008). It was also theorized that EMG-based biofeedback might be useful for educating runners about the coactivation process and, thereby, driving higher economy that may result in performance gains.

Few studies have been conducted to explore neuromuscular adaptations that result specifically from endurance training. However, Cohen *et al.* (2010) sought to assess whether such adaptations might be observed in endurance trained adult males and boys. Different aged populations were assessed to gauge whether age-related effects on neuromuscular adaptations could be identified. Trained and untrained subjects from the two age cohorts were assessed for isometric strength of elbow and knee extensors and flexors and EMG activity of the associated agonist and antagonist muscle groups. While age-related and training-related effects were noted for some measures (i.e. higher rate of muscle activation and rate of torque development in adults), there was no clear evidence of neuromuscular adaptation when comparing trained to untrained cohorts. As a result, the authors concluded that endurance training elicits chiefly metabolic adaptations (Cohen *et al.*, 2010).

Indices of neuromuscular adaptation in runners have been reported by other investigators. For example, Paavolainen *et al.* (1999c) showed that 5 km race time was related to neuromuscular characteristics in a homogenous group of elite male orienteers. Specifically, the ability of runners to generate force rapidly during maximal and submaximal running was related to race performance. Similarly, ground contact time was shorter in those with the better race performance. Spending less time during ground contact, especially during the braking phase of contact would, presumably, conserve energy. In support of this, shorter ground contact time was also related to better RE (Paavolainen *et al.*, 1999c). This tends to support the theory proposed by Kram and Taylor (1990) that suggests the energy cost of running is a function of mass and ground contact time. They noted an inverse relationship between the rate at which energy is used during running and the amount of time the foot generates force against the ground. Thus, those runners with better economy tend to also have shorter ground contact time.

Acute neuromuscular effects

Neuromuscular control appears to be modified during the course of sustained running. Paavolainen *et al.* (1999b) found that braking and propulsion components of ground contact times were longer immediately following completion of a 10 km time trial. In addition to these changes, peak and vertical ground reaction forces were significantly reduced and there was a reduction in muscle activation during a 20 m maximal sprint performed after the time trial. The investigators hypothesized that repetitive stretch-shortening cycles reduced the ability of the neuromuscular system to maintain force production and to tolerate impact forces. It was suggested that a decline in muscle stiffness, coupled with a longer transition time between braking and propulsion, led to less conservation of elastic energy. These effects were corroborated by a reduction in IEMG activity during the maximal 20 m runs (Paavolainen *et al.*, 1999b). Thus, acute and high-repetition SSCs have been shown to transiently influence neuromuscular control properties and force production, both of which are important factors in RE. Those runners who were able to better maintain running performance under fatiguing conditions were also found to have higher relative pre-activation and lower relative agonist IEMG-activity during the propulsion phase than the lower caliber runners. This supplies further evidence for the importance of neuromuscular control and conservation of elastic energy via maintenance of muscle stiffness during distance running.

Neuromuscular characteristics were also attributed to success in 5 km race performance (Paavolainen *et al.*, 1999c). Specifically, the ability to produce force quickly was an important factor in maximal and submaximal running. The faster runners tended to demonstrate shorter ground contact time, braking phase time and propulsion phase time than their slower, matched counterparts.

Running economy

Running economy (RE) is a term used to reflect steady-state oxygen uptake under specified conditions (i.e. fixed submaximal treadmill speed at zero grade, controlled environment) (McCann and Higginson, 2008). It has also been defined as the energy demand for a given submaximal velocity (Saunders *et al.*, 2004a). More economical runners will maintain steady-state running at a lower oxygen uptake. Further, when RE is improved through training, the effect is evidenced by a reduction in the oxygen uptake needed to sustain a fixed submaximal running speed. Thus, an increase in RE is reflected by a reduction in total energy cost. Numerous factors have been reported to influence RE. Saunders *et al.* (2004b) provided a schematic that identifies 17 different variables that may impact RE. These variables can be broken into five subsets that include: training, environment, physiology, biomechanics and anthropometry. Much attention has been given to many of these subsets, but teasing apart specific effects and the magnitude of such effects is a complex process. While scientists may be keenly interested in specific slices of the overall outcome and strive to characterize mechanisms for adaptation, trainers and the athletes themselves are more likely to view the big picture outcomes that training provides (i.e. improved performance, better pace maintenance, quality of training). Since RE has been reported to be a better predictor of race performance than aerobic power among elite runners (Costill *et al.*, 1973), it has garnered a great deal of attention from the scientific community. In the following sections, consideration will be given to a variety of training interventions that have been investigated as a means of improving RE and, in some instances, endurance run performance.

Run training-imposed changes in economy

Beyond neuromuscular and metabolic adaptations that result from run training, tissue-specific changes have been reported as well. For example, Fletcher *et al.* (2010) sought to investigate whether run training coupled with isometric training leads to increased triceps-surae tendon stiffness, which is associated with improved running economy. These investigators imposed isometric plantarflexion exercise (working at 80 per cent of MVC) 3 days per week for 8 weeks. Stiffness of the triceps-surae and MVC were assessed every 2 weeks, with RE measured at baseline and upon completion of the 8-week intervention. The group of highly trained middle- and long-distance runners maintained their run training throughout the study. A non-intervention control group of runners was used for comparison. While the training intervention failed to significantly affect tendon stiffness and RE, a significant inverse relationship was found between RE and stiffness of the triceps-surae tendon. This relationship occurred irrespective of group assignment. The investigators observed that acute changes in tendon stiffness and RE can occur and that these changes may happen in tandem. They suggest that less compliant muscle would lower the energy transfer to the tendon, resulting in a lower cost of the muscle activity. Conversely, a more compliant tendon would lead to more muscle fibre shortening and/or an increased velocity of shortening for a given joint movement, which would raise the cost of muscle activity. Whether an increase in tendon stiffness is a function of chronic adaptation or acute high-intensity training is not evident. It is possible that isometric training would be more likely to elicit positive effects on tendon stiffness in moderately trained runners who are not as well adapted as the runners used in this study.

Brisswalter and Legros (1995) applied training overload (300 per cent volume increase over 2 weeks) on well-trained middle-distance runners to gauge impact on running economy and running pattern. Two trends were found to develop: improved economy (~ 9 per cent) was observed only at the running speed that corresponded with the volume overload (which occurred at 80 per cent intensity); the change in economy was associated with individual stride-rate adaptation although stride length was not altered. The improvement in economy was attributed to an adaptation in foot pattern, as well as an improvement in foot stability at the training pace.

Other differences have been reported in mechanical factors that are important to run performance and economy based on sex and training emphasis (i.e. middle distance versus long distance) (Chapman *et al.*, 2012). Chapman *et al.* (2012) found that elite female runners showed significantly shorter ground contact times when running at the same speeds as males. They also had greater stride frequency and shorter stride length compared to male counterparts. However, these differences appeared to be a function of height as when the data were normalized for height, the differences disappeared. The only exception to this was with stride frequency, which remained higher in women across all running speeds. When comparing middle-distance to long-distance trained males, the rate of change in ground contact time differed significantly as the running speed was increased. The long-distance runners showed a significantly larger decline in contact time as running speed increased compared to the middle-distance runners. This effect translated into a 31.1 per cent increase in metabolic cost for the LD runners versus a 25.4 per cent increase for the MD runners when moving from 5 to 7 m.s^{-1}. Based on these findings, the authors suggest that gait differences between distance specialists may be a function of preferred and/or competition speeds and that the preferred speed among LD runners could be driven by economy factors. For information related to neural adaptations and sprint training, the reader is referred to a review by Ross *et al.* (2001). For a more applied review of power training and sport, readers are referred to Young (2006).

Resistance training: effects on run economy

Despite seemingly divergent outcomes based on the principle of specificity, resistance exercise training is a commonly accepted practice among distance runners. Numerous benefits of resistance training for runners have been identified, including better maintenance of form and economy, improved leg power and speed (Paavolainen et al., 1999a), improved sprint ability (Mikkola et al., 2011), attenuation of cardiovascular drift (Hayes et al., 2004), enhanced neuromuscular characteristics (Mikkola et al., 2011) and reduced injury risk. Muscular strength endurance has been linked to better fatigue resistance during distance running as well (Hayes et al., 2011). It has also been suggested that development of power could be impeded as a result of continuous focus on aerobic training in some athletes, which may adversely affect neuromuscular adaptation as well as heighten the risk of overtraining (Elliott et al., 2007).

Tanaka and Swensen (1998) hypothesized that resistance trained distance runners may be better able to sustain performance at fixed submaximal running speeds by either enabling force contribution from each myofibre to be reduced or by requiring fewer myofibres to sustain the work. It was further suggested that resistance training leads to a lesser need for contributions from lower efficiency Type II fibres (Tanaka and Swensen, 1998). These benefits would be achieved by improved quality of the Type I fibre content that may accompany resistance training.

Taipale et al. (2010) examined the effects of differing strength training interventions on measures related to distance running performance, including running economy and VO_2max velocity (vVO_2max). Strength training was performed concurrently with normal run training over a 28-week period in a population of recreational runners. They found that explosive strength training and maximal strength training were more effective than circuit weight training for improving RE and vVO_2max. These benefits were associated with greater strength gains and neuromuscular adaptations (measured via EMG activity of the vastus lateralis and medialis) in the two groups.

Ferrauti et al. (2010) failed to identify improvements in RE or muscle coordination in response to 8 weeks of concurrent run and resistance training in recreational marathon runners despite significant gains in leg strength. Strength training was performed twice weekly and focused on the trunk (for muscular endurance) and lower extremity (high intensity). The high-intensity strength training of the leg muscles was designed to promote motor unit recruitment pattern improvements while minimizing hypertrophic gain in an effort to improve RE. Ground contact time revealed a significant interaction when compared to a run endurance group such that contact time tended to increase in the concurrently trained group while tending to decrease in the run-only group. Despite this interaction, RE remained the same. Stride length and stride frequency, indices of muscle coordination, were unaffected by concurrent training. However, stride length was significantly decreased in the run-only group. Thus, some of the alterations may have been a function of changes to run volume or intensity that occurred in the subjects as they were building towards a marathon competition. The investigators hypothesized that a larger subject pool or longer study duration may have revealed more profound effects (Ferrauti et al., 2010).

Paavolainen et al. (1999b) introduced a 9-week explosive strength training regimen on top of normal endurance training in elite distance runners to study the effects on 5 km race performance. Explosive training included plyometric-type jumping exercises, leg press and leg extension/flexion exercises with low loads and maximal velocity repetitions, and sprint sets. Lifting loads fell below 40 per cent of 1 RM. Significant improvements in 5 km race time (3.1 per cent faster) and in RE were associated with reduced ground contact time during constant velocity running in the strength-trained group. This occurred despite no significant effects on stride rate, stride length or ground reaction force during constant velocity running. Strength training was associated with significant gains in maximal isometric force production of the leg extensors and maximal anaerobic run test velocity (V_{MART}). The improvement in RE (8.1 per cent lower oxygen cost) correlated with the improvement in V_{MART}. VO_2max was not affected by the training intervention. Thus, the gains in performance were attributed to improved neuromuscular function that led to gains in muscle power and a lower cost of steady state transport (Paavolainen *et al.*, 1999b).

Plyometric training and running economy

Plyometric training has been widely used to support and enhance performance in a variety of sport activities (Markovic and Mikulic, 2010). Commonly, this type of training has been advocated for sport tasks that incorporate jumping, agility and explosive power generation. The training technique revolves around the stretch-shortening cycle (SSC) of muscle activation. By challenging the neural and musculotendinous systems that are involved via repeated SSCs, it is believed that more force can be generated over less time, allowing for an increase in power production by the muscle. Thus, plyometric training would theoretically stimulate neuromuscular adaptations that could have application for many types of movement tasks, including distance running. One of the draws for endurance athletes is that plyometric-type training has been reported to induce positive neural adaptations and mechanical advantages with an attenuated hypertrophic response that is commonly associated with heavy resistance training (Häkkinen *et al.*, 1985; Saunders *et al.*, 2006). Plyometric training has also been found to stimulate neuromuscular adaptations (better maintained muscle recruitment pattern) that support the bike-to-run transition in triathletes (Bonacci *et al.*, 2011). However, the neuromuscular adaptations that developed did not translate into improved economy upon completion of the bicycling phase (Bonacci *et al.*, 2011).

SSC training involving plyometrics has focused primarily on the lower body musculature. Saunders *et al.* (2006) examined the effects of 9 weeks of plyometric training on running economy in a population of highly trained distance runners. Plyometric exercises employed fast concentric/eccentric movement patterns and included activities such as straight-leg jumps, squat jumps for height, fast feet drills (where minimum ground contact time and high force production were emphasized), bounding, and high-skipping among others. Running economy (fixed speeds of 14, 16 and 18 km.h^{-1}) was assessed prior to and after 5 and 9 weeks of plyometric training. RE was unchanged at the lower running speeds for any time-point. However, a significant improvement in economy was noted after 9 weeks of plyometric training at the highest running speed (18 km.h^{-1}). The oxygen requirement for this speed was reduced by 4.1 per cent in the plyometric group, while no change was found in the control group. No other cardiorespiratory variables were affected by the training intervention during RE testing. Likewise, no changes in max were found. However, there was a trend for the VO_2 versus running speed slope to be lower in the plyometric group after 9 weeks of training. The plyometric group also tended to show improvement (14.7 per cent) in average power production for a five-jump plyometric test ($p = 0.11$) at 9 weeks. Improved RE was attributed, in part, to improved locomotor muscle metabolism (i.e. improved efficiency of ATP use) and improved recovery of elastic energy (Saunders *et al.*, 2006). It was also speculated that an improvement in whole-body mechanics occurred only with the fastest speed under evaluation, which was deemed more representative of normal training and competition running speed. Finally, since cardiorespiratory substrate use measures were largely unaffected, the improved

RE at the fastest speed was primarily attributed to gains in muscular power and conservation of elastic energy and/or from better gait coordination and technique that accompanied plyometric training (Saunders *et al.*, 2006). While mechanics and changes in gait patterns can be evaluated and quantified, methods for quantifying changes in elastic energy remain elusive (Saunders *et al.*, 2004b). Notably, it has been theorized that those most likely to benefit from interventions designed to boost economy will be the lesser-trained runners (McCann and Higginson, 2008). Thus, plyometric training may be found to elicit more profound and possibly multifaceted effects in less well-trained runners.

For a comprehensive review on plyometric training and performance adaptations, see Markovic and Mikulic (2010).

Barefoot running and neuromuscular adaptation

Barefoot running has gained considerable attention in the past several years. A recent PubMed search using 'barefoot running' revealed that 28 publications have been produced since January 2011 in this general area. Despite the recent heightened attention, a number of sports medicine investigations were conducted in the early to mid 1980s involving barefoot running (Burkett *et al.*, 1985; Robbins and Hanna, 1987; Rodgers and Leveau, 1982). Early investigators explored factors including the potential for barefoot running to help prevent running-related injury (Robbins and Hanna, 1987), and effects of barefoot running on limb kinematics (Burkett *et al.*, 1985). Robbins and Hanna (1987) proposed that running shoes impede sensory input and induce more foot rigidity. These effects of shod running could be associated with a greater injury frequency.

More contemporary investigators have also investigated kinematic adaptations related to barefoot or minimalist running (Divert *et al.*, 2005b; Lieberman, 2012; Perl *et al.*, 2012). Perl *et al.* (2012) studied the effects of footwear on running economy and kinematics. It is commonly found that shod runners are more prone to rearfoot strike while barefoot runners are more likely to show forefoot strike patterns. These differences may influence kinematic and economy factors during steady state running. Perl *et al.* (2012) compared minimalist footwear (Vibram FiveFingers™) to standard running shoes (Asics Gel-Cumulus 10™). Two trials were completed using each style of footwear: forefoot strike (FFS) and rearfoot strike (RFS). Trial order was randomized and expired gases were collected while at steady state (trials were a minimum of 5 minutes). Stride frequency and foot mass were matched between footwear types. Footstrike style (FFS versus RFS) was not found to affect economy within each type of footwear. However, economy was influenced by footwear type within a strike style such that during FFS running, the minimally shod condition was 2.4 per cent more economical. RFS was found to be 3.2 per cent more economical when performed with minimalist footwear. There was wide variability within subjects when minimally shod for economy, ranging from 9.7 per cent more economical to 7.3 per cent less economical; though most subjects were more economical with minimalist footwear. While the mechanisms are yet to be soundly confirmed, economical advantages associated with minimalist footwear were attributed to: (1) greater storage of elastic energy and recoil in the longitudinal arch; (2) less knee flexion during gait (a possible energy conservation adaptation); and (3) increased elastic energy storage in the Achilles tendon (Perl *et al.*, 2012). Further work is needed to investigate each of these proposed mechanisms for enhanced economy in minimalist footwear. Likewise, given the broad variability within subjects under the different conditions, further examination of individual variation is warranted.

Divert *et al.* (2005a) explored stiffness adaptations under shod and barefoot conditions during treadmill running in male runners. They found that vertical stiffness and leg stiffness decreased during 4 minutes of running (3.61 m.s^{-1}) in the shod condition, while in the barefoot condition stiffness was stable. A significant difference between conditions was noted for stride frequency (5 per cent higher in barefoot), while vertical displacement, leg compression and maximal vertical force were significantly lower (15, 5 and 3.5 per cent, respectively) in barefoot running. The lower mean and vertical leg stiffness measures in the shod condition were attributed to the notion that musculotendinous stiffness was not increased adequately to compensate for shoe compliance during the shod running condition (Divert *et al.*, 2005a) Alteration of shoe properties (both acute and chronic) should be considered when examining kinematic and economical measures of runners.

de Koning (1992) suggested that neurologic adaptation may result from barefoot running. He noted significant differences between shod and barefoot running in EMG activity of the tibialis anterior muscle, with higher activity observed during barefoot running. He suggested that this difference may be due to an attempt of the neuromuscular system to attenuate the ground impact force by controlling plantar flexion and/or foot pronation during landing. Barefoot running was also found to elicit a lower landing velocity than shod running. Whether these adaptations are more about protection, comfort or fatigue remains to be answered (de Koning, 1992). Based on early and more contemporary research, it is evident that barefoot

Table 3.1 Summary of key training-specific neuromuscular adaptations and associated economy and performance-related benefits

Training method	Neuromuscular adaptation	Benefit	Reference
Run-only training	Increased leg stiffness	Improved storage of elastic energy and lower metabolic cost	Craib *et al.* (1996) Dalleau *et al.* (1998)
	Improved biarticular muscle coactivation in stance phase	Increased leg stiffness and higher economy	Heise *et al.*(2008)
	Increased rate of force generation and reduced ground contact time	Improved 5 km race performance	Paavolainen *et al.* (1999c)
Concurrent resistance and run training	Increased leg power, leg speed and sprint ability	Improved economy maintenance	Paavolainen *et al.* (1999a)
	Increased EMG activity of *vastus lateralis* and *medius*	Improved economy and vVO$_2$max	Taipale *et al.* (2010)
	Improved Type I fibre quality(?)	More efficient fibre performance	Tanaka and Swensen (1998)
	Reduced ground contact time with constant run velocity	Improved 5 km race time and economy	Paavolainen *et al.* (1999b)
Concurrent plyometric and run training	Improved neuromuscular control	Better transition from cycle to run in triathletes	Bonacci *et al.* (2011)
	Improved leg power, locomotor muscle metabolism, recovery of elastic energy	Improved economy at higher run speeds, but not at slower run speeds	Saunders *et al.* (2006)

running will influence gait pattern, lower extremity muscle activation patterns and leg stiffness, economy and potentially injury incidence. However, neuromuscular adaptations that develop from introduction of barefoot running are yet to be clearly established. Further, whether adaptive responses to barefoot running develop as a result of protection from injury (i.e. shock attenuation) or more from an inherent drive for higher economy of transport is unknown. For further information on the evolutionary influences of barefoot running and its medical implications, Lieberman (2012) provides a review of these topics.

Summary

Numerous factors have the potential to alter running patterns. As with any form of physical training, adaptation will occur. The adaptive response to run training appears to generate several positive outcomes: (1) reduced cost of transport; (2) attenuated impact forces as a means of minimizing injury occurrence; and (3) delayed fatigue development. Neuromuscular adaptations that contribute to these advantages appear to be related to developing increased leg stiffness and reducing knee flexion during gait, which both help to conserve elastic energy. Other neuromuscular factors that may contribute to adaptation include increased stiffness of the Achilles tendon and the tendon surae. Further beneficial adaptations may result from incorporation of resistance, plyometric training or barefoot running. As above, neuromuscular adaptations that result from these types of training are also commonly linked to stiffness changes.

Other factors that should be investigated more thoroughly include the effects of eccentric loading of muscle on neuromuscular adaptations, running surface rigidity and gait alterations, and the effects of footwear rigidity on economy, adaptive response and forces applied to the lower extremity. In addition, clothing that has been designed to support run performance (i.e. elastic compression stockings) should also be studied more thoroughly to clearly elucidate their effects on mechanical and energetic factors of locomotion.

References

Bonacci, J., Chapman, A., Blanch, P. and Vicenzino, B. (2009) 'Neuromuscular adaptations to training, injury and passive interventions: implications for running economy', *Sports Medicine*, 39(11): 903–21.

Bonacci, J., Green, D., Saunders, P. U., Franettovich, M., Blanch, P. and Vicenzino, B. (2011) 'Plyometric training as an intervention to correct altered neuromotor control during running after cycling in triathletes: a preliminary randomized controlled trial', *Physical Therapy in Sport*, 12(1): 15–21.

Brisswalter, J. and Legros, P. (1995) 'Use of energy cost and variability in stride length to assess an optimal running adaptation', *Perceptual and Motor Skills*, 80(1): 99–104.

Burkett, L. N., Kohrt, W. M. and Buchbinder, R. (1985) 'Effects of shoes and foot orthotics on VO_2 and selected frontal plane knee kinematics', *Medicine and Science in Sports and Exercise*, 17(1): 158–63.

Chapman, R. F., Laymon, A. S., Wilhite, D. P., McKenzie, J. M., Tanner, D. A. and Stager, J. M. (2012) 'Ground contact time as an indicator of metabolic cost in elite distance runners', *Medicine and Science in Sports and Exercise*, 44(5): 917–25.

Cohen, R., Mitchell, C., Dotan, R., Gabriel, D., Klentrou, P. and Falk, B. (2010) 'Do neuromuscular adaptations occur in endurance-trained boys and men?', *Applied Physiology, Nutrition, and Metabolism*, 35(4): 471–9.

Costill, D. L., Thomason, H. and Roberts, E. (1973). 'Fractional utilization of the aerobic capacity during distance running', *Medicine and Science in Sports*, 5(4): 248–52.

Craib, M. W., Mitchell, V. A., Fields, K. B., Cooper, T. R., Hopewell, R. and Morgan, D. W. (1996) 'The association between flexibility and running economy in sub-elite male distance runners', *Medicine and Science in Sports and Exercise*, 28(6): 737–43.

Dalleau, G., Belli A., Bourdin, M. and Lacour, J. R. (1998) 'The spring-mass model and the energy cost of treadmill running', *European Journal of Applied Physiology and Occupational Physiology*, 77(3): 257–63.

de Koning, J. J. (1992) 'Adaptations in running kinematics and kinetics due to shoes and playing surfaces', *Proceedings of the Third International Symposium on Sport Surfaces; a Symposium of the University of Calgary*, Calgary: University of Calgary.

Divert, C., Baur, H., Mornieux, G., Mayer, F. and Belli, A. (2005a) 'Stiffness adaptations in shod running', *Journal of Applied Biomechanics*, 21(4): 311–21.

Divert, C., Mornieux, G., Baur, H., Mayer, F. and Belli, A. (2005b) 'Mechanical comparison of barefoot and shod running', *International Journal of Sports Medicine*, 26(7): 593–8.

Elliott, M. C., Wagner, P. P. and Chiu, L. (2007) 'Power athletes and distance training: physiological and biomechanical rationale for change', *Sports Medicine*, 37(1): 47–57.

Ferrauti, A., Bergermann, M. and Fernandez-Fernandez, J. (2010) 'Effects of a concurrent strength and endurance training on running performance and running economy in recreational marathon runners', *Journal of Strength and Conditioning Research*, 24(10): 2770–8.

Fletcher, J. R., Esau, S. P. and Macintosh, B. R. (2010) 'Changes in tendon stiffness and running economy in highly trained distance runners', *European Journal of Applied Physiology*, 110(5): 1037–46.

Häkkinen, K., Komi, P. V. and Alen, M. (1985) 'Effect of explosive type strength training on isometric force- and relaxation-time, electromyographic and muscle fibre characteristics of leg extensor muscles', *Acta Physiologica Scandinavica*, 125(4): 587–600.

Hayes, P. R., Bowen, S. J. and Davies, E. J. (2004) 'The relationships between local muscular endurance and kinematic changes during a run to exhaustion at vVO$_2$max', *Journal of Strength and Conditioning Research*, 18(4): 898–903.

Hayes, P. R., French, D. N. and Thomas, K. (2011) 'The effect of muscular endurance on running economy', *Journal of Strength and Conditioning Research*, 25(9): 2464–9.

Heise, G., Shinohara, M. and Binks, L. (2008) 'Biarticular leg muscles and links to running economy', *International Journal of Sports Medicine*, 29(8): 688–91.

Jones, A. M. (2002) 'Running economy is negatively related to sit-and-reach test performance in international-standard distance runners', *International Journal of Sports Medicine*, 23(1): 40–3.

Kram, R. and Taylor, C. R. (1990) 'Energetics of running: a new perspective', *Nature*, 346(6281): 265–7.

Lieberman, D. E. (2012) 'What we can learn about running from barefoot running: an evolutionary medical perspective', *Exercise and Sport Sciences Reviews*, 40(2): 63–72.

McCann, D. J. and Higginson, B. K. (2008) 'Training to maximize economy of motion in running gait', *Current Sports Medicine Reports*, 7(3): 158–62.

Markovic, G. and Mikulic, P. (2010) 'Neuro-musculoskeletal and performance adaptations to lower-extremity plyometric training', *Sports Medicine*, 40(10): 859–95.

Mikkola, J., Vesterinen, V., Taipale, R., Capostagno, B., Häkkinen, K. and Nummela, A. (2011) 'Effect of resistance training regimens on treadmill running and neuromuscular performance in recreational endurance runners', *Journal of Sports Sciences*, 29(13): 1359–71.

Paavolainen, L., Häkkinen, K., Hamalainen, I., Nummela, A. and Rusko, H. (1999a) 'Explosive-strength training improves 5-km running time by improving running economy and muscle power', *Journal of Applied Physiology*, 86(5): 1527–33.

Paavolainen, L., Nummela, A., Rusko, H. and Häkkinen, K. (1999b) 'Neuromuscular characteristics and fatigue during 10 km running', *International Journal of Sports Medicine*, 20(8): 516–21.

Paavolainen, L. M., Nummela, A. T. and Rusko, H. K. (1999c) 'Neuromuscular characteristics and muscle power as determinants of 5-km running performance', *Medicine and Science in Sports and Exercise*, 31(1): 124–30.

Perl, D. P., Daoud, A. I. and Lieberman, D. E. (2012) 'Effects of footwear and strike type on running economy', *Medicine and Science in Sports and Exercise*, 44(7): 1335–43.

Robbins, S. E. and Hanna, A. M. (1987) 'Running-related injury prevention through barefoot adaptations', *Medicine and Science in Sports and Exercise*, 19(2): 148–56.

Rodgers, M. M. and Leveau, B. F. (1982) 'Effectiveness of foot orthotic devices used to modify pronation in runners', *The Journal of Orthopaedic and Sports Physical Therapy*, 4(2): 86–90.

Ross, A., Leveritt, M. and Riek, S. (2001) 'Neural influences on sprint running: training adaptations and acute responses', *Sports Medicine*, 31(6): 409–25.

Saunders, P. U., Pyne, D. B., Telford, R. D. and Hawley, J. A. (2004a) 'Reliability and variability of running economy in elite distance runners', *Medicine and Science in Sports and Exercise*, 36(11): 1972–6.

Saunders, P. U., Pyne, D. B., Telford, R. D. and Hawley, J. A. (2004b) 'Factors affecting running economy in trained distance runners', *Sports Medicine*, 34(7): 465–85.

Saunders, P. U., Telford, R. D., Pyne, D. B., Peltola, E. M., Cunningham, R. B., Gore, C. J. and Hawley, J. A. (2006) 'Short-term plyometric training improves running economy in highly trained middle and long distance runners', *Journal of Strength and Conditioning Research*, 20(4): 947–54.

Taipale, R. S., Mikkola, J., Nummela, A., Vesterinen, V., Capostagno, B., Walker, S., Gitonga, D., Kraemer, W. J. and Häkkinen, K. (2010) 'Strength training in endurance runners', *International Journal of Sports Medicine*, 31(7): 468–76.

Tanaka, H. and Swensen, T. (1998) 'Impact of resistance training on endurance performance. A new form of cross-training?', *Sports Medicine*, 25(3): 191–200.

Thayer, R., Collins, J., Noble, E. G. and Taylor, A. W. (2000) 'A decade of aerobic endurance training: histological evidence for fibre type transformation', *The Journal of Sports Medicine and Physical Fitness*, 40(4): 284–9.

Turner, A. M., Owings, M. and Schwane, J. A. (2003) 'Improvement in running economy after 6 weeks of plyometric training', *Journal of Strength and Conditioning Research*, 17(1): 60–7.

Young, W. B. (2006) 'Transfer of strength and power training to sports performance', *International Journal of Sports Physiology and Performance*, 1(2): 74–83.

4

BIOMECHANICAL ADAPTATION IN ICE HOCKEY SKATING

David J. Pearsall, René A. Turcotte, Marc C. Levangie
and Samuel Forget

MCGILL UNIVERSITY, MONTREAL

Introduction

The defining trait of the sport of ice hockey is its environment of play and its manner of locomotion: ice and skating. Flat ice surfaces afford both unique physical obstacles and assets to locomotion. Its inherent lower contact friction than normal terrain excludes conventional human walking and running patterns since sufficient ground reaction force (GRF) cannot be generated at the interface of foot and ground to propel the body forward. However, ice surfaces between temperatures of 0 and − 10°C are remarkable (Bowden, 1955; de Koning *et al.*, 1992). They can be etched with sufficient sharp tools, providing the potential for a foothold for push-off. Furthermore, when a sharp blade is moved rapidly across the surface, sufficient frictional energy may be generated to heat then momentarily melt the ice, creating a transient boundary lubrication between blade and ice: that is, the potential to glide. If a tool can be manipulated to alter between these high and low surface friction states, then adapted locomotion patterns are possible. This is the essence of skating: when the blade is oriented more or less perpendicular to the intended direction of motion, adequate GRF is possible for propulsion; when the blade is oriented parallel to the intended direction of motion, remarkably low friction impedance occurs during glide. Of course, ample time and training are required to readapt learned walking and running motor patterns to this more challenging surface; yet the rewards are amazing, exhilarating speeds of movement.

This chapter will examine how exactly the body adapts normal locomotion patterns to that of skating movement. Comparisons between walking and running ground-based locomotion will be made with skating ice-based movement patterns. Differences in the manner of limb kinematics, muscle recruitment and propulsion dynamics will be explored.

Ice hockey: the game

Skating is fundamental to other winter recreational and sport activities: speed and figure skating, as well as cross-country 'skate' skiing. All exhibit the same primary gross movement pattern that we define as skating. It is each environment and strategic contexts that differentiate the skating patterns that have evolved. For example, throw in a puck, net and stick, and several people, and you have one of the fastest chase-and-pursuit games in the world. Forward skating is the common denominator of all skating skills, and thus the most important ability a hockey player must possess to be successful at a competitive level in this sport (Bracko, 2004). Regardless of the activity in which a player is engaged, he or she will need to both move and balance effectively on skates in order to successfully execute other skills such as puck shots and passes, skating transitions including start, stops, turns and pivots and varied directions (forward, backward, crossover), as well as giving and receiving body checks (Pearsall *et al.*, 2000). Skating must be powerful at times and also efficient since during a full length hockey game, an average player will need to cover between 3 and 5 km (Montgomery *et al.*, 2004).

Kinematics of the forward skating stride

The forward skating stride is biphasic, composed of a support phase and a swing phase (Figure 4.1a). The support phase is further subdivided into single and double (limb) support phases of 80 per cent and 20 per cent, respectively, of the total support time (Marino and Weese, 1979). This approximation of total support time may vary significantly when the player accelerates, decelerates or coasts during the game (Pearsall *et al.*, 2000). The forward skating stride begins when a foot contacts the ice with the blade and progresses through the glide, the push-off and the swing (or recovery) phases (de Boer *et al.*, 1986). The glide phase follows initial contact of the blade on the ice, parallel to the intended movement path, and may travel 2–3 m. Towards the end of glide, the blade turns and presses outward, perpendicular to the glide direction but parallel to the opposite skate blade's orientation (Figure 4.1d, 3–4).

For this bipedal motion to occur, the hip, knee and ankle joints will be moved in a characteristic and repeating manner (Novacheck, 1998; Upjohn *et al.*, 2008) (Figure 4.2). Similar range of motion (ROM) values for hip flexion and extension occur during walk, run and skate movement; however, during fast skating the hip remains deeply flexed (50°) during most of the glide and extends only during push-off later in the stride (70 per cent in skating versus 40 per cent in walking and running). With respect to frontal plane motion, land locomotion progresses from 5° adduction (drop to unsupported side), then to neutral or slightly adducted in swing phase. In contrast, during skating the hip rapidly moves into adduction and holds this position until mid-swing. In the transverse plane, walk and run gait typically remain internally rotated throughout the stride, whereas skate gait begins in external rotation (10°) but progressively rotates internally until 50 per cent of the cycle then rapidly counter-rotates externally. In general, the functional consequences of the observed hip movements during skating fulfill the need for greater lateral motion of 50 cm from left to right striding limbs (compared to walking and running that is less than 10 cm) for the skates to reorient themselves for glide to push-off (or from parallel to perpendicular). The gradual outward drift of the skate during glide to push-off is attributed to the lateral flexion (lean) of the trunk over the gliding limb (in hip internal rotation and abduction). The rapid counter-rotation (external rotation) switches the trunk orientation and lean to the opposite limb beginning its glide phase. These two latter actions are critical kinematic adaptations necessary for the sinusoidal tracking characteristic of skating gait. Without these hip movements, sufficient manipulation of skate orientation from glide to push-off would not be possible.

Returning to the sagittal movements of the remaining lower limb joints, the knee ROM estimates range from 5° to 85° for walk, run and skate gait. Walking and running display an early knee flexion (20–40°, respectively) during early stance but quickly extend through push off. Conversely, the skater's knee remains flexed from initial to late stance (50°), then extends at push-off. All gaits display substantial knee flexion during swing (to facilitate rapid replacement

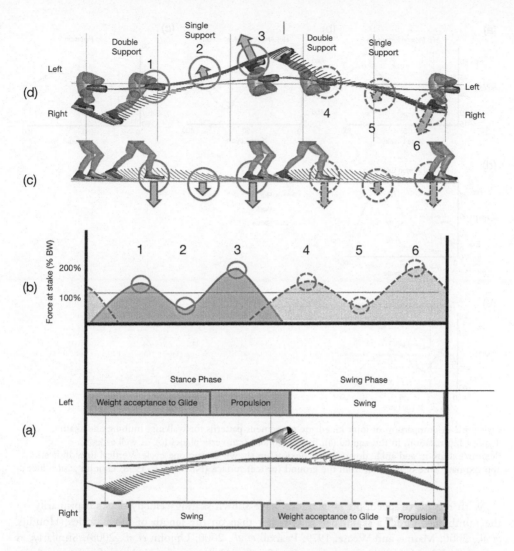

Figure 4.1 Temporal and dynamic phases of the forward skating stride. The lower panel (a) presents the phases that form the basis of skating: stance and swing, as well as the typical motion paths of both left and right skates (Pearsall *et al.*, 2000). The stride begins at stance during initial weight acceptance from the opposite limb side into a glide. The latter part of stance leads to active propulsion. After push-off is the swing phase. During the stance phase, GRF forces are generated perpendicular to the blade's long axis towards the foot (b) (de Boer *et al.*, 1987; Stidwill *et al.*, 2009). The force vectors applied by the skates' blades are both down (c) and in the transverse surface plane (d) of the ice.

of the foot for the next stride, and for easier foot clearance overground). In terms of the ankle, both walking and skating show similar patterns (i.e. dorsi flexed through most of stance then plantar flex at push-off). Running ankle's hopping motion (plantar to dorsi to plantar flexed) is compressed to a short stance window (0–20 per cent). All gaits show dorsi flexion during swing. In summary, the sagittal motions of the hip, knee and ankle remain in a crouched position during most of stance, permitting rapid extension contribution of the gluteal, quadriceps and posterior leg muscle groups (Bracko, 2004; Marino and Weese, 1979; Pearsall *et al.*, 2000).

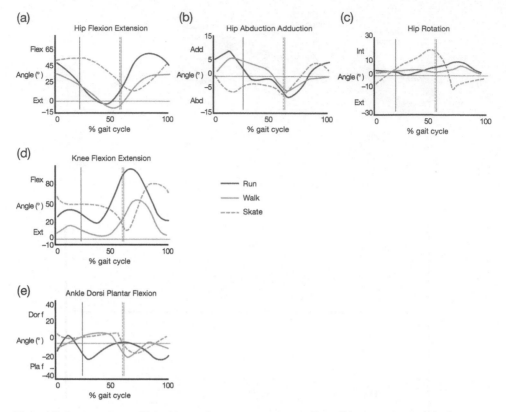

Figure 4.2 A comparison of joint kinematic movement patterns for walking, running and skating. Typical hip rotations in the sagittal (a), frontal (b) and transverse planes (c), as well as knee flexion/extension and ankle dorsi/plantar flexion are shown during one cycle. Vertical lines indicate approximate time of push-off from the ground (or ice) surface (Novacheck, 1998; Upjohn *et al.*, 2008).

With regards to speed, previous studies have shown skating velocity depends primarily on the number of strides a skater performs rather than on the length of those strides (Houdijk *et al.*, 2000; Marino and Weese, 1979; Pearsall *et al.*, 2000; Upjohn *et al.*, 2008). Similarly, as velocity of the skaters increases, the time of contact between the blade of the skate and the ice surface decreases (Turcotte *et al.*, 2001). This is comparable to walking and running, where for a given height (leg length), step length determines the maximum stride length constant. For less experienced players, though, specific training aimed at optimizing lower limb joints' ROM is warranted to obtain the greatest stride length (de Koning *et al.*, 1995).

Muscle recruitment in the forward skating stride

To better understand how the kinematic differences in gait patterns occur between walking, running and skating, estimates of muscle recruitment in terms of effort, timing and duration can be studied. Surface electromyography (sEMG) is often used as a noninvasive means to quantify both the magnitude of muscle activity and the temporal patterns of activation, and infer their kinematic functions.

During the gliding phase, the knee and hip remain deeply flexed prior to push off (de Boer *et al.*, 1987). sEMG of the *peroneus longus* and *tibialis anterior* show increased activity during stance to stabilize the ankle joint and prevent any unwanted inversion or eversion of the limb (Chang *et al.*, 2009). The sEMG of the *vastus medialis*, *bicep femoris* and *gluteus maximus* muscles indicate they are isometrically active to support the body weight and stabilize the knee and hip joints.

During push off the muscle activity is greatest to generate the needed propulsive forces (de Boer *et al.*, 1987; Stidwill *et al.*, 2010). Power at the hip is mainly delivered by the *gluteus maximus*, as seen by sEMG activity peaking just before the end of the stroke (de Boer *et al.*, 1987; de Koning *et al.*, 1991; Chang *et al.*, 2009). This peak corresponds to roughly 90 per cent of the muscles' maximal dynamic contraction (MDC) (de Koning *et al.*, 1991). This both extends and externally rotates the hip by 5–8° (Upjohn *et al.*, 2008). sEMG activity of the quadriceps muscles also peaks (80 per cent of MDC) at the end of the stroke, just prior to toe off (de Boer *et al.*, 1987; Dewan *et al.*, 2004), causing rapid extension of the knee. There is also simultaneous decrease in the activity of *semitendinosus* and *biceps femoris* (Bracko, 2004), presumably to aid in hip extension. The sEMG activity of both the *gastrocnemius* and the *peroneus longus* (Dewan *et al.*, 2004) peak at around 75–90 per cent of MDC just prior to the blade leaving the ice surface. These muscles concentrically contract to plantar flex the ankle.

During the swing or recovery phase, muscles contract to reposition the leg in proper position for the next stride. The sEMG activity of the *adductor magnus* muscle peaks at roughly 70 per cent of MDC during this phase, as it is the principal muscle responsible for the adduction of the lower limb (Chang *et al.*, 2009). sEMG activity of the *tibialis anterior* muscle peaks during the swing phase, as it is responsible for dorsi flexing the ankle, for skate clearance and pre-contact stability (Dewan *et al.*, 2004).

Compared to running, skating is physiologically more efficient (Formenti and Minetti, 2007), but it also requires a very different muscular contribution and different muscle activation patterns. This difference in muscular activity is evident when comparing average sEMG profiles during running (Gazendam and Hof, 2007) and forward skating (van Ingen Schenau *et al.*, 1996) (Figure 4.3). The most notable difference is the large contribution of the *gluteus maximus* prior to push-off during a skating stride, whereas during running the muscle is relatively silent. Additionally, during forward skating the quadriceps muscles peak at the end of the push-off, and just prior to when the skate leaves the ice (Bracko, 2004; de Boer *et al.*, 1987); however, during running the quadriceps muscles peak just after heel strike (Gazendam and Hof, 2007) and are quiet prior to toe off. Skating can be distinguished even further from regular gait by observing the changes in sEMG activity during a simultaneous increase in velocity. It has been shown that the temporal patterns of muscle activation varies with changes in gait velocity, but this has not been noted with increases in skating velocity.

Forces in the forward skating stride

The combined measurements of kinetic parameters with joint and segment kinematics provides for the most complete understanding of the biomechanics of ice skating (de Koning *et al.*, 2000; Lamontagne *et al.*, 1983; Stidwill *et al.*, 2009), as well as how these may differ from more familiar land walking and running. To this end, a few studies have used force transducers between the boot and the blade to estimate ice contact forces in speed skating (de Boer *et al.*, 1987; de Koning *et al.*, 1992; Jobse *et al.*, 1990) and in ice hockey skating (Stidwill *et al.*, 2009). During forward skating, the typical ground reaction forces (GRF, vertical to skate) were bimodal, with the first peak near initial contact in the weight acceptance phase of stance (Figure 4.1b, 1) and the second peak at push-off (Figure 4.1b, 3), with magnitudes between 150 and 200 per cent body weight (BW). These forces were generated primarily through the

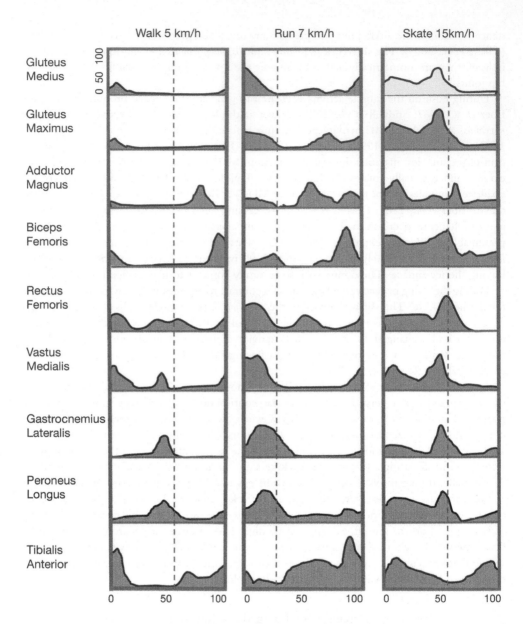

Figure 4.3 Comparison of muscle recruitment patterns during walking, running and skating for selected lower limb muscles (Bracko, 2004; Cappellini *et al.*, 2006; de Boer *et al.*, 1987; Gazendam and Hof, 2007; Novacheck, 1998). Vertical axes indicate per cent maximum sEMG; horizontal axes indicate per cent stride; vertical lines indicate approximate time of push-off.

simultaneous extension of the hip and knee joints. Left and right skate force patterns overlapped by 10 per cent at initial stance and 10 per cent at push off, confirming the double support visually observed during skating. Between peaks (Figure 4.1b, 1, 3), a small dip in force (50–70 per cent BW; Figure 4.1b, 2) is observed due to the momentary downward acceleration of the body's mass. This bimodal force pattern is similar to walking (Keller *et al.*, 1996), but not as seen in running's unimodal impact pattern (Cappellini *et al.*, 2006; Novacheck, 1998).

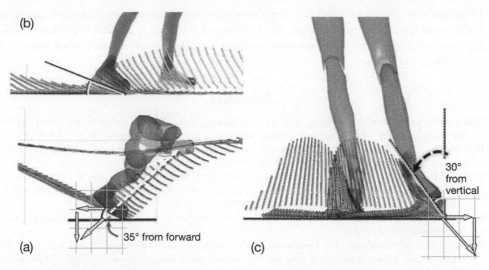

Figure 4.4 Different views of push-off forces top (a), side (b) and rear (c) views.

However, during the first few strides in a skating start, running-like short, single force peaks are observed wherein the athlete needs to push off against a fixed point on the ice so as to accelerate (de Koning *et al.*, 1995; Stidwill *et al.*, 2009).

Based on the previous kinematic and kinetic (Allinger and van den Bogert, 1997; de Boer *et al.*, 1987; Stidwill *et al.*, 2009; Upjohn *et al.*, 2008) measures, the global force vector orientations and magnitudes may be estimated (Figure 4.4). For example, during maximal skating velocity and near the instant of push-off the angle of roll and yaw are ~ 30° from the vertical and 35° from the forward axes. A portion of the total push-off force contributes to supporting the body (Figure 4.4c) and the body's horizontal acceleration towards the next support foot position (Figure 4.4a; Figure 4.1d, 3). These findings corroborate some theoretical estimates of optimal push-off force vectors (Denny, 2011).

Conclusion

Compared to walking and running, skating is physiologically more efficient (Cappellini *et al.*, 2006; Formenti and Minetti, 2007): the bonus of gliding is much more significant than the added cost due to the exaggerated side-to-side movement excursions. The unique ice surface tribology requires substantially adapted footwear, body movement strategies and muscular activation patterns. So what is skating? What is its movement pattern? It appears to be a hybrid of both walking and running. It produces sagittal plane kinematic patterns similar to crouched gait and kinetic vertical GRF patterns such as walking, yet utilizes greater MDC of quadriceps and gastrocnemius muscles similar in magnitude to running and achieves much greater maximal speeds. Skating achieves locomotion through a sinusoidal forward progression achieved by incremental oblique force pulses.

In this chapter, we have demonstrated that by exploring biomechanical aspects of skating, using kinematic, muscular and kinetic markers, we can better understand the fundamental adaptations necessary to achieve movement across ice surfaces. It may also lead to innovations in products. A great case study is the development of the Klapskate in speed skating (de Koning *et al.*, 2000). Inspired by physiological and biomechanical studies (van Ingen Schenau *et al.*,

1996), this new articulated skate led to significant improvements in time performances, breaking many speed skating records following the 1996 season (Houdijk *et al.*, 2000; Versluis, 2005). This is a motivating example of how understanding normal and adapted locomotion behaviour can enhance performance.

References

Allinger, T. L. and van den Bogert, A. J. (1997) 'Skating technique for the straights, based on the optimization of a simulation model', *Medicine and Science in Sports and Exercise*, 29(2): 279–86.

Bowden, F. (1955) 'Some recent experiments in friction: friction on snow and ice and the development of some fast-running skis', *Nature*, 176(4490): 946–7.

Bracko, M. R. (2004) 'Biomechanics powers ice hockey performance', *Biomechanics*, 9: 47–53.

Cappellini, G., Ivanenko, Y. P., Poppele, R. E. and Lacquaniti, F. (2006) 'Motor patterns in human walking and running', *Journal of Neurophysiology*, 95(6): 3426–37.

Chang, R., Turcotte, R. and Pearsall, D. (2009) 'Hip adductor muscle function in forward skating', *Sports Biomechanics*, 8(3): 212–22.

de Boer, R., Schermerhorn, P., Gademan, J., de Groot, G. and van Ingen Schenau, G. (1986) 'Characteristic stroke mechanics of elite and trained male speed skaters', *Journal of Applied Biomechanics*, 2(3): 175–86.

de Boer, R., Cabri, J., Vaes, W., Clarijs, J., Hollander, A., de Groot, G. and van Ingen Schenau, G. (1987) 'Moments of force, power and muscle coordination in speed-skating', *International Journal of Sports Medicine*, 8(6): 371–8.

de Koning, J. J., de Groot, G. and Ingen Schenau, G. J. (1991) 'Coordination of leg muscles during speed skating', *Journal of Biomechanics*, 24(2): 137–46.

de Koning, J. J., de Groot, G. and van Ingen Schenau, G. J. (1992) 'Ice friction during speed skating', *Journal of Biomechanics*, 25(6): 565–71.

de Koning, J. J., Thomas, R., Berger, M., de Groot, G. and van Ingen Schenau, G. J. (1995) 'The start in speed skating: from running to gliding', *Medicine and Science in Sports and Exercise*, 27(12): 1703–8.

de Koning, J. J., Houdijk, H., de Groot, G. and Bobbert, M. F. (2000) 'From biomechanical theory to application in top sports: the klapskate story', *Journal of Biomechanics*, 33(10): 1225–30.

Denny, M. (2011) *Gliding for Gold: The Physics of Winter Sports*, Baltimore: The Johns Hopkins Press.

Dewan, C., Pearsall, D. and Turcotte, R. (2004) *Dynamic Pressure Measurement about the Foot and Ankle*, Montreal: Quebec: McGill University.

Formenti, F. and Minetti, A. E. (2007) 'Human locomotion on ice: the evolution of ice-skating energetics through history', *The Journal of Experimental Biology*, 210(10): 1825–33.

Gazendam, M. G. J. and Hof, A. L. (2007) 'Averaged EMG profiles in jogging and running at different speeds', *Gait and Posture*, 25(4): 604–14.

Houdijk, H., de Koning, J. J., de Groot, G., Bobbert, M. F. and van Ingen Schenau, G. J. (2000) 'Push-off mechanics in speed skating with conventional skates and klapskates', *Medicine and Science in Sports and Exercise*, 32(3): 635–41.

Jobse, H., Schuurhof, R., Cserep, F., Schreurs, A. and de Koning, J. (1990) 'Measurement of push-off force and ice friction during speed skating', *Journal of Applied Biomechanics*, 6(1): 92–100.

Keller, T., Weisberger, A., Ray, J., Hasan, S., Shiavi, R. and Spengler, D. (1996) 'Relationship between vertical ground reaction force and speed during walking, slow jogging, and running', *Clinical Biomechanics*, 11(5): 253–9.

Lamontagne, M., Gagnon, M. and Doré, R. (1983) 'Development, evaluation and application of a dynamometric system of skates', *Canadian Journal of Applied Sport Sciences*, 8(3): 169–83.

Marino, G. and Weese, R. (1979) 'A kinematic analysis of the ice skating stride', in J. Terauds and H. J. Gros (eds), *Science in Skiing, Skating, and Hockey*, Del Mar, CA: Science in Sports Academic Publisher, pp. 65–74.

Montgomery, D., Nobes, K., Pearsall, D. and Turcotte, R. (2004) 'Task analysis (hitting, shooting, passing and skating) of professional hockey players', in D. J. Pearsall and A. B. Ashare (eds), *Safety in Ice Hockey*, West Conshohocken, PA: ASTM International, Vol. 4, pp. 288–96.

Novacheck, T. F. (1998) 'The biomechanics of running', *Gait and Posture*, 7: 77–95.

Pearsall, D. J., Turcotte, R. A. and Murphy, S. (2000) 'Biomechanics of ice hockey', in W. E. Garrett and D. T. Kirkendall (eds), *Exercise and Sport Science*, Philadelphia, PA: Lippincott Williams & Wilkins, pp. 675–92.

Stidwill, T. J., Turcotte, R. A., Dixon, P. and Pearsall, D. J. (2009) 'Force transducer system for measurement of ice hockey skating force', *Sports Engineering*, 12(2) 63–8.

Stidwill, T. J., Pearsall, D. and Turcotte, R. (2010) 'Comparison of skating kinetics and kinematics on ice and on a synthetic surface', *Sports Biomechanics*, 9(1): 57–64.

Turcotte, R. A., Pearsall, D. J. and Montgomery, D. L. (2001) 'An apparatus to measure stiffness properties of ice hockey skate boots', *Sports Engineering*, 4(1): 43–8.

Upjohn, T., Turcotte, R., Pearsall, D. J. and Loh, J. (2008) 'Three-dimensional kinematics of the lower limbs during forward ice hockey skating', *Sports Biomechanics*, 7(2): 206–21.

van Ingen Schenau, G. J., de Groot, G., Wim Scheurs, A., Meester, H. and de Koning, J. J. (1996) 'A new skate allowing powerful plantar flexions improves performance', *Medicine and Science in Sports and Exercise*, 28(4): 531–5.

Versluis, C. (2005) 'Innovations on thin ice', *Technovation*, 25(10): 1183–92.

SECTION 2

Environmental factors of injury and fatigue

5

FATIGUE AND INJURY IN SOCCER

Matt Greig,[1] Colin Johnson[2] and Lars R. McNaughton[1]

[1]EDGE HILL UNIVERSITY, ORMSKIRK
[2]UNIVERSITY OF HULL, HULL

Introduction

Soccer is considered to be not only a high-risk sport, but also a high-risk occupation. Evaluated against criteria used in occupational health, the risk associated with injury in professional soccer has been described as unacceptable (Drawer and Fuller, 2002). An injury audit in soccer, as in most occupations, is considered to be the first stage in a four-step process of injury prevention (Figure 5.1). Having identified that there is a high risk of injury in professional soccer, Hawkins *et al.* (2001) stated that the second phase must be to identify the factors and mechanisms that play a part in the occurrence of the injuries.

Injury risk and the mechanism of injury are influenced by many factors (Hoskins and Pollard, 2005; van Mechelen *et al.*, 1992), with both intrinsic and extrinsic influences/factors having been studied extensively within the athletic population (e.g. Fuller, 2007; Murphy *et al.*, 2003) and in direct relation to soccer (Arnason *et al.*, 2004; Ekstrand, 2008; Engebretsen *et al.*, 2010a, 2010b, 2011; Fousekis *et al.*, 2011, 2012; Ostenberg and Roos, 2000; Rahnama *et al.*, 2002).

The focus of this chapter is the influence of fatigue as an aetiological factor for injury. Fatigue, which has been defined as 'the inability to sustain the required work rate' (Reilly *et al.*, 2008), has been the subject of investigation by all of the cognate disciplines within the

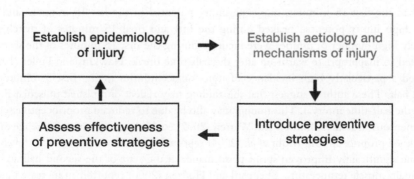

Figure 5.1 A four-step sequence of injury prevention (modified from van Mechelen *et al.*, 1992).

sport and exercise sciences. This chapter considers the varied challenges presented to the modern day footballer, and how fatigue contributes to injury epidemiology. This is considered within a game, over the duration of a game, during periods of the season with high competition volume, over the course of the season, and over the course of a player's career

Instantaneous fatigue in soccer match play

Soccer match play is characterized by an intermittent and irregular activity profile, encompassing all levels from no activity through to maximal, short-term, high-intensity activity. The physical demands of soccer have been well described by notational analyses of evolving complexity (Bangsbo *et al.*, 1991; Di Salvo *et al.*, 2010; Reilly and Thomas, 1976). A total distance covered in the region of 10 km, accounting for positional differences, equates to an average speed of 6.7 km.h^{-1}, equivalent to a fast walk. However, the intermittent activity profile complicates the physical response to exercise, which is characterized by periods of high intensity running interspersed with low activity exercise. A 7:1 ratio of low:high intensity exercise suggests a limited physiological stress; however, the nature of the high intermittent bouts of exercise is such that instantaneous fatigue must be considered.

The average work rate profile suggests a sprint every 2 minutes on average during a game, but more recent and contemporary analyses have suggested a repeated sprint requirement, with clusters of sprints performed (Spencer *et al.*, 2006). Spencer *et al.* (2004) reported that a typical 'cluster' of sprints might comprise 3–7 sprints with a recovery of ~ 15 seconds, and then a longer recovery period between each of the clusters. Such bouts of high intensity exercise will result in elevated acute physiological markers of stress, exacerbated by the mechanical load associated with intermittent exercise. The multi-directional nature of soccer is such that agility is likely to be a greater contributor than linear speed, and as such the physical demands of soccer might be classified as repeat agility ability (RSA; Spencer *et al.*, 2005).

The influence of fatigue has been identified through decreased work rate (Mohr *et al.*, 2003) and increased durations of recovery during the second half of a game (Bangsbo and Mohr, 2005). Periods of high intensity work, both on and off the ball, are also followed by decreases in work rate and prolonged recovery, suggesting the presence of both temporary and cumulative fatigue during match play (Bradley *et al.*, 2009; Mohr *et al.*, 2003, 2005).

The instantaneous nature of fatigue within soccer has also been considered in relation to injury epidemiology. A higher rate of injuries during the last 15 minutes of games will be considered in subsequent sections; however, there are other periods of a game associated with a high risk of injury. Rahnama *et al.* (2002) reported that actions with a mild injury potential peaked in the first 15-minutes, moderate injury potential in the last 15 minutes, and actions with a high injury potential peaked during the first and final 15 minutes of match play. A relatively high number of injuries were incurred during the first 15 minutes of the second half, attributed to inappropriate warm-up after the half-time break. Hawkins and Fuller (1996) also observed a particularly high incidence of non-contact injuries in the first 5 minutes of the second half. These authors suggest that this finding may reflect diminished muscular flexibility during the half-time interval. This finding may also be due to reduced proprioceptive sensitivity in ligamentous structures, Bartlett and Warren (2002) establishing a positive influence of warm-up on knee proprioception. Mohr *et al.* (2004) reported that maintaining activity levels during half-time significantly improved sprint performance at the start of the second half and helped to maintain muscle temperature. Sheppard and Hodson (2006) reported an increased incidence of injuries sustained in the first 15 minutes after half-time in the 2003–4 season relative to the

1997–8 season. The authors advocated performing football-specific activities during half-time to help prevent injury, but failed to account for the relative increase between seasons.

Fatigue over 90 minutes

The incidences of instantaneous fatigue during a game are likely to accumulate, and the temporal pattern of injury occurrence during competition has often highlighted the final 15 minutes of each half as the period of greatest injury potential (Hawkins and Fuller, 1999; Hawkins *et al.*, 2001; Sheppard and Hodson, 2006). Significantly more injuries were observed during the final 15 minutes of the first half and the final 30 minutes of the second half. Figure 5.2 shows the distribution of injuries during match play, as documented by the Football Association injury audit (Hawkins *et al.*, 2001). Woods *et al.* (2004) reported that half of all hamstring strains incurred during games were sustained in the final 15 minutes of each half. The same finding was reported by Woods *et al.* (2003) for ankle sprain injuries.

The activity profile of soccer match play has been well described, and has led to the development of simulation models used to replicate the physical demands of soccer and used subsequently to investigate the influence of fatigue. Such exercise protocols can be classified as free-running (e.g. the LIST protocol of Nicholas *et al.*, 2000) or treadmill-based, using motorized (e.g. Greig *et al.*, 2006) or non-motorized (e.g. Drust *et al.*, 2000) applications. The applications of such laboratory simulations has been diverse, investigating the influence of fatigue on numerous markers of performance and injury. Performance considerations have included the beneficial effects of pre-cooling prior to exercise (Drust *et al.*, 2000) and the influence of carbohydrate ingestion on soccer skill (Ali and Williams, 2009). Applications directed toward investigating the influence of fatigue on injury have considered the primary types of injury sustained in soccer, such as muscle strains and joint sprains (Hawkins *et al.*, 2001). Treadmill protocols designed to replicate the demands of soccer have been used to measure the influence of fatigue on the muscular response to running (Greig *et al.*, 2006; Rahnama *et al.*, 2005), isokinetic strength (Greig, 2008; Rahnama *et al.*, 2003), angles of peak strength (Small *et al.*, 2009), dynamic balance (Greig and Walker-Johnson, 2007), and the biomechanics of soccer techniques (Greig, 2009; Kellis *et al.*, 2006; Russell *et al.*, 2011).

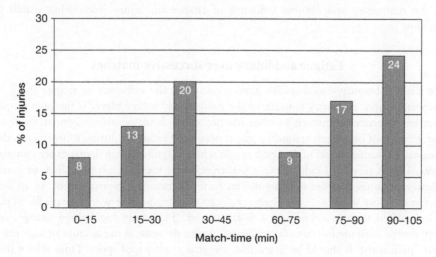

Figure 5.2 Time of injury (from Hawkins *et al.*, 2001).

The relationship between fatigue and markers of injury is a necessary design issue, with actual match play representing a poor research model with no consistency in the physical response. The observations of changes in markers of injury, such as strength, and their direct relation to injury incidence are naturally problematic. There are also a wide range of methodological approaches in the exercise protocol, the participants, and the functional task performed. Often, the exercise protocol is intuitively linked to the task demands. A higher physiological response would suit a study concerned with nutritional interventions, while a protocol with a higher mechanical load is likely to induce a fatigue effect in eccentric hamstring strength. Muscle strength deficits associated with fatigue will increase the susceptibility of injury, and decreases in knee flexor peak torque after intervals of intermittent exercise have been reported (Greig and Siegler, 2009), which mirror the temporal incidence of hamstring strains (Woods *et al.*, 2004). This same finding has been observed in more recent studies using free-running and therefore multidirectional fatigue protocols (Small *et al.*, 2010). Other muscular characteristics such as angle of peak torque and agonist/antagonist ratios were also negatively influenced (Rahnama *et al.*, 2003; Small *et al.*, 2010), further heightening the injury risk of not only muscle but also ligament/associated joint structures (Reilly *et al.*, 2008). The temporal patterns reported very much support the epidemiological studies within the sport and highlight the influence of fatigue.

A fatigued state has also been shown to alter lower limb mechanics and balance strategies regardless of gender (Chappell *et al.*, 2005; Lucci *et al.*, 2011; Sanna and O'Connor, 2008). Greig and Walker-Johnson (2007) investigated the influence of a 90-minute soccer specific fatigue treadmill protocol on a single legged balance task and although no significant changes to lower limb stability were seen across 15-minute increments, there were changes in balance strategy towards the end of each 45-minute period. Small *et al.* (2009) investigated sprint kinematics using a 90-minute, multidirectional soccer fatigue protocol and reported reductions in hip and knee joint angles towards the end of each 45-minute period. Such alterations have also been found utilizing shorter fatigue protocols (Borotikar *et al.*, 2008) and during analysis of more sport specific movements such as kicking (Lees and Davies, 1988) and side stepping (Cortes *et al.*, 2012; Lucci *et al.*, 2011). Borotikar *et al.* (2008) also suggested that the effect of fatigue was more pronounced during unanticipated movements, which are all part of the nature of football. Although differences between methodologies make specific conclusions difficult, the effect of fatigue on different physiological and biomechanical measures simply highlights both the temporary and chronic influence of fatigue on injury risk during match play/ simulation.

Fatigue and injury over successive matches

While many laboratory-based studies have investigated the influence of fatigue using a 90-minute simulation, a primary concern to the modern day soccer player is the high frequency of matches. Recovery between matches has become a fundamental concern in professional soccer. Periods of high game frequency might occur, for example, during tournaments, during pre-season, or during phases of domestic season where league and cup demands are cumulative. Of note, UEFA recently modified the structure of youth tournaments to include an extra rest day between games in order to allow players to recuperate to a greater extent. In an analysis of professional league soccer, Odetoyinbo *et al.* (2008) examined the work rate profile of players who completed three matches over a 5-day period. This study highlighted changes in the activity profile attributed to cumulative fatigue, with a decrease in the amount of high intensity exercise performed. It should be noted that soccer is a self-paced sport. Thus, where there is a high frequency of matches, cumulative fatigue might influence injury epidemiology.

While both international tournaments and domestic league and cup competitions pose a threat of high game volume, there is likely to be a difference in terms of the actual loading incurred by the player. The risk of cumulative fatigue on injury might be modified through a variety of strategies, including recovery modalities, squad rotation, and the training/match ratio, to name but a few. Hawkins and Fuller (1996) reported a 3–4 fold increase in injury risk during match play compared to training.

In a comparison of different types of competition, Hawkins and Fuller (1998) observed an average of 2.76 injuries per game (IpG) during the 1996 European Championship finals, 2.39 IpG during English Premier League games over the 1996–7 season, and 2.87 IpG during matches played in the English First Division over three seasons from 1994 to 1997. Applying the same calculation to the analysis of Hawkins and Fuller (1996) produces an incidence of 2.0 IpG during the 1994 World Cup finals.

Andersen *et al.* (2003) reported a lower incidence at 1.6 incidents per match for the Norwegian U21 team over 35 competitive 'home' matches. There are other factors that might also influence injury epidemiology. Hawkins and Fuller (1996), for example, observed a significantly greater number of injuries in the second half of match play during the 1994 World Cup in the USA, with heat stress proposed to have been a contributing fatiguing factor. Hagglund *et al.* (2009) reported a greater number of contact injuries during the second half of European Championship games from 2006 to 2008, the influence of fatigue being linked to the competitive focus towards the end of the game.

Junge *et al.* (2004a) reported a rate of 81.0 injuries per 1,000 match hours during the 2002 World Cup in South Korea and Japan, this value attributed in part to the nature and format of the competition. Hawkins and Fuller (1996) analysed 44 of the 52 matches played during the 1994 World Cup finals staged in the USA, reporting a total injury incidence of 27.7 per cent per player (number of injuries divided by number of players). Using the same method of calculation, similar values have been reported by Jorgensen (1984) in Scandinavian football (36 per cent) and by Hoy *et al.* (1992) in European football (18 per cent).

The timing of such major tournaments, often shortly after a domestic season, may also contribute to the fatigue of players, again affecting the injury risk but also performance (Hagglund *et al.*, 2009). The finding of injury incidence increasing in the second half has also been consistently observed by research into English (Hawkins and Fuller, 1999; Hawkins *et al.*, 2001; Sheppard and Hodson, 2006) and European football (Arnason *et al.*, 1994; Sandelin *et al.*, 1985).

More recent studies have also investigated the impact of successive matches on performance and injury risk at the professional level (Carling and Dupont, 2011; Dupont *et al.*, 2010; Rey *et al.*, 2010), with no significant difference in performance reported. These perhaps surprising results point towards the footballers' ability to regulate work rate during a game (Rey *et al.*, 2010) as well as possessing the physical capabilities to compete with short durations between matches (Carling *et al.*, 2012). The latter study also reported similar injury rates during a congested eight-match period compared to outside this period. The use of substitutions, tactical changes and, particularly at the higher level of the sport, the influence of squad rotations have also been identified as contributing factors when investigating performance and injury risk across a number of fixtures (Carling *et al.*, 2012; Ekstrand, 2008; Reilly *et al.*, 2008).

There is general consensus in the literature (Hawkins *et al.*, 2001) that competition poses a greater risk of injury, Murphy *et al.* (2003) attributing this to players being more prone to aggressive, risk-taking behaviours that may lead to injury. The risk posed by match play may be deemed non-modifiable, beyond changes to the rule structure and implementation. There is, however, evidence to suggest that training practices may have a great impact on injury incidence, although Reilly *et al.* (2008) highlight the lack of intervention studies looking at training load and the onset of fatigue. Furthermore, it should be noted that research into injury rate must account for exposure, since professional players will spend a greater amount of time in training than in match play.

Hagglund *et al.* (2003) reported that the training/match ratio doubled from 1982 to 2001 in Swedish top division football. Total exposure to football increased by 27 per cent over this period as a result of the increased training, reflecting the move to professionalism. Despite this increased exposure, there was no difference in overall injury risk, Hagglund *et al.* (2003) concluding that increased exposure does not necessarily increase injury incidence, provided it is the amount of training that increases. This supports the recommendation of Ekstrand *et al.* (1983) that a high training/match ratio is beneficial. Hagglund *et al.* (2003) proposed careful consideration of the training week during the competitive season to prevent both physical and mental overload.

Hagglund *et al.* (2005) observed that elite Swedish players had 10.9 hours of training per match hour, compared with 6.6 for the top professional league in Denmark. Thus, Swedish players had greater exposure to training, while exposure to matches did not differ between the countries. The authors observed a higher risk of injury during training in Denmark than Sweden, whereas there was no difference for match play. The distribution of injuries according to type and location was similar between countries, but the risk of incurring a major injury (absence for more than 1 month) was 2.5 fold greater in Denmark. Hagglund *et al.* (2005) attributed the reported differences, at least in part, to the greater training exposure and longer pre-season period in Sweden. This allows greater scope for slow progression to ensure that the musculoskeletal system adapts gradually to an increased physical load.

Fatigue and injury over a season

In those players involved in international competition, typically played over the summer months, the season has become longer and longer. This naturally influences the players' opportunity to recover following a long season, and in some cases disrupts their engagement with pre-season. This might have implications for their physical readiness for the subsequent season. The financial rewards associated with lucrative pre-season tours, particularly when including international travel, can also affect the timing of the season and the physical preparation of players.

Injury rate has typically varied from between 17 (Luthje *et al.*, 1996) and 35 (Arnason *et al.*, 1996; Morgan and Oberlander, 2001) injuries per 1,000 game hours in professional football. This in context with the 81.0 injuries per 1,000 match hours during the 2002 World Cup in South Korea and Japan (Junge *et al.*, 2004b), highlighting the distinction between domestic leagues and structured tournaments. Some associations have enforced a mid-season break, often to align with poor weather. In domestic league soccer, the most comprehensive injury audit (to date) was conducted by the Football Association of England and Wales, which produced an audit of injuries in professional soccer, with medical staff from 91 of the 92 professional football league clubs recording injury data over two seasons. A total of 6,030 injuries were reported over the two seasons (Hawkins *et al.*, 2001). Each player received, on average, 1.3 injuries per season, and each club incurred 39.1 injuries per season. Each injury resulted in an average of 24 days and four competitive matches missed. The implications are numerous and diverse.

It has been reported that between 65 and 91 per cent of players incur an injury during a season (Arnason *et al.*, 1996; Hagglund *et al.*, 2003; Hawkins *et al.*, 2001; Lewin, 1989). Hawkins and Fuller (1999) conducted a longitudinal study over the period November 1994 to May 1997 to establish the causes of occupational injury to players in four English professional football clubs. During each season, between 86 and 100 per cent of players from each club sustained at least one recorded injury, 67 per cent of injuries occurring during competition. Each injury resulted in an average of 14.6 days absence. Previously, Lewin (1989) reported that 91 per cent of players in an English First Division team over one season sustained an injury, 66 per cent of injuries were recorded in competition, and an average of 19.9 days were lost per injury. Similarly, McGregor and Rae (1995) recorded 71–79 per cent of players sustaining at least one injury, 78 per cent of all injuries were sustained during competition, and 27.1 days were lost per injury in a Scottish Premier League team over three seasons. Similar values have been reported for European football. Hagglund *et al.* (2005) reported 81 per cent of players in the top Danish professional league to incur an injury, compared to 67 per cent in the equivalent Swedish league. The mean numbers of days missed per injury were 11.8 and 13.1, respectively.

The study by Hawkins and Fuller (1999), documenting injuries in four league clubs, served as a precursor to an audit commissioned by the Football Association (Hawkins *et al.*, 2001), which represents the largest audit of professional football injuries to date. The audit comprised a prospective epidemiological study of injuries sustained in English professional football over two competitive seasons (from July 1997 to May 1999). A total of 6,030 injuries sustained in training (34 per cent) or competition (63 per cent) were recorded. The average injury rate over the two seasons was 1.3 injuries per player per season. ~75 per cent of players sustained at least one injury and missed an average of 24.2 days and 4.0 matches per injury. Of all injuries recorded, 78 per cent resulted in a minimum of one match missed. Sheppard and Hodson (2006) compared the 1997–8 season with the 2003–4 season in English professional football and reported that while the total number of injuries was not different, the mean number of days missed due to injury increased from 24.6 to 30.7 days. This finding was attributed in part to a greater incidence of major injuries, but also speculated to be due to an increased awareness of injury management techniques allowing a longer period of rehabilitation to ensure full recovery.

Epidemiological research into soccer injuries has also considered temporal issues. Injury incidence has been reported to vary over the playing season, with peak injury rates reported after pre-season training and during match-intensive periods (Ekstrand and Gillquist, 1982; Lewin, 1989; Sandelin *et al.*, 1985). Hawkins *et al.* (2001) also reported a gradual decrease in the incidence of training injuries throughout the season, being significantly higher during the period of pre-season and attributed to a loss in fitness during the close season (Hawkins and Fuller, 1999). Hawkins *et al.* (2001) attributed the high incidence of injury during the first month of the competitive playing season to players failing to reach appropriate levels of fitness. Hagglund *et al.* (2005) reported twice as many muscular strains in Denmark than in Sweden, attributing this difference to the longer pre-season in Sweden. Similarly, Arnason *et al.* (1996) found that injury incidence in elite Icelandic players was reduced in teams with the longest pre-season training period. However, duration must be considered in conjunction with content, Hawkins *et al.* (2001) reporting a higher incidence of training injuries at the start of pre-season, possibly due to the lack of fitness maintenance over the preceding off-season rest period.

Pre-season injuries in English professional football were analysed by Woods *et al.* (2002). An initial epidemiological study (Hawkins *et al.*, 2001) reported an increased frequency of training injuries during pre-season and an increase in match injuries during the early stages of the playing season. Pre-season injuries accounted for 17 per cent of all injuries incurred over two seasons, Woods *et al.* (2002) listing a harder playing surface, rapid progression to a high training intensity, and lack of pre-season preparation as contributory factors. The authors reported that 40 per cent of players sustained at least one injury during pre-season, with an average rate of 0.2 injuries per player. Injuries during pre-season tended to be less severe in comparison to the competitive season. However, this should not be discounted given the propensity for major injury of the same type and location to follow minor injury (Hawkins *et al.*, 2001).

Relative to the competitive season, more muscular strain and tendinous injuries were recorded during preseason, Woods *et al.* (2002) attributing this to the increased duration and intensity of training. In particular, this may be due to increased exposure to running, previously identified as a primary non-contact mechanism of injury. Woods *et al.* (2002) observed that running accounted for 25 per cent of pre-season injuries, compared with 19 per cent of injuries sustained during the competitive season (Hawkins *et al.*, 2001). Woods *et al.* (2002) attributed muscular strains to 37 per cent of pre-season injuries, but in contrast to the predominance of hamstring strains during the competitive season (Hawkins *et al.*, 2001) the *rectus femoris* was the most common site of pre-season muscle strain injuries. The authors attributed this difference to increased exposure to shooting and running activities during the pre-season. The shift in muscular strain predisposition to the *rectus femoris* may suggest that running volume is the critical factor during pre-season, with distance/endurance given priority over speed during the pre-season. The predisposition to hamstring strains during the competitive season would suggest an inappropriate preparation for the increased intensity and exposure to sprinting activities during match play compared with training.

Fatigue and injury over a career

Previous research has reported that football players suffer relatively high rates of injury compared with participants in other sports, and in other occupations (Hawkins and Fuller, 1999). The epidemiology in soccer has been well described, but this has typically been cross-sectional in nature. Just as a succession of matches has been shown to increase injury risk, successive seasons might affect injury aetiology. Drawer and Fuller (2002) reported that the risks associated with injury and lower limb joint osteoarthritis in professional football are unacceptable when evaluated against criteria employed in occupational health. Of 185 retired players, 47 per cent retired because of injury, and 58 per cent of these were chronic injuries. Most of the chronic injuries that led to early retirement were of the knee, lower back and hip. Of all respondents, 32 per cent had been medically diagnosed with osteoarthritis in at least one of the lower limb joints, with more respondents having been diagnosed with osteoarthritis in the knee joints than either the ankle or the hip joints. Roos *et al.* (1994) reported a prevalence of gonarthrosis of 16 per cent in elite football players, 4.2 per cent in non-elite players and 1.6 per cent in controls. Knee injury is identified as a major risk factor for the development of gonarthrosis. Drawer and Fuller (2002) advocated that professional soccer players should be provided with health surveillance during their playing career.

The playing career can start from a very early age. A positive finding was reported by Price *et al.* (2004) regarding the incidence of reinjury in English professional academies. In a sample of players from 9 to 19 years of age, reinjury rate was shown to be very low (3 per cent) in comparison to professional players. The authors attributed this finding, in part, to less pressure in returning young players to competition at the academy level, and while speculative, this is an encouraging observation.

Several studies have reported that injury incidence in soccer increases with age (Chomiak *et al.*, 2000; Ostenberg and Roos, 2000). Intuitively, increased age may be associated with an increased level and intensity of competition, inherent risk factors in injury. However, players at a younger age may be at a greater risk of injury due to the relative immaturity of the musculoskeletal system. Age might therefore be a predisposing factor to particular types of injury. In a study of Australian football players, Orchard (2001) attributed increased age to an increased risk of hamstring strains and calf strains, while age was not a predictive factor in the incidence of quadriceps strains. Similarly, Verrall *et al.* (2001) observed a 1.3 fold increase in hamstring strain risk per year of increased age and Woods *et al.* (2004) showed that English professional soccer players in the youngest age category (17–22 years) had a lower risk of sustaining a hamstring injury.

In an analysis of pre-season injuries in English professional football, Woods *et al.* (2002) reported that younger players (17–25 years) sustained significantly more injuries than older players (26–35+ years). This finding was attributed to an inferior training history in young players and less experience at dealing with both the physical and mental demands of the pre-season phase. This may be of particular importance in the first year of professional football, where players become full-time, since this may represent a substantial increase in training volume. In a case study of English professional soccer academies, Price *et al.* (2004) documented an average injury rate of 0.6 injuries per player per season, resulting in 22.1 days and 2.3 matches absence per injury. The implications of injury in young elite players might not have the same financial impact, but do impinge on technical development. Players from the ages of 9 to 19 were included in the study, with a trend towards more injuries in the older age group. Age is non-modifiable, but such studies do suggest that the exposure to both training and competition might be adapted with consideration for age.

It has been identified that soccer has a characteristic activity profile, and a certain set of skills and techniques. The functional adaptation to this running style and the techniques generic to football may themselves create muscular imbalances, etc. Continued exposure to soccer might therefore exacerbate the risk of certain types of injury. Ekstrand *et al.* (1983) speculated whether it is soccer training itself that can increase injury risk through muscle stiffness. While causality has yet to be proven, it seems reasonable to assume that a lack of flexibility may predispose the muscle or connective tissue to injury (Keller *et al.*, 1987). Ekstrand and Gillquist (1982) found that Swedish amateur football players had lower flexibility than age-matched non-players. Muscle tightness was identified in hip abduction and extension, knee flexion and ankle dorsi-flexion. Two-thirds of the players sampled had one or more tight muscle groups in the lower extremity. These results show clear relation to the epidemiological data regarding the location of soccer injuries. Moller *et al.* (1985) reported that regular soccer training (of duration 1.5 hours) resulted in a decreased range of motion, which persisted for more than 24 hours.

The relationship between skill level and injury has also been considered. Peterson *et al.* (2000) and Chomiak *et al.* (2000) have reported that in an age-matched sample of young players, those with low skill level were at a twofold increased risk of incurring an injury. These findings may reflect greater intensity and aggression at higher skill levels, and may not be of direct consequence to injury incidence in professional football. However, the increasing development of football academies and the implications of incurring injury at a young age make skill level an important consideration to those structuring training and match play activities. Soderman *et al.* (2002) observed an increased risk of anterior cruciate ligament injury when young female players participated at a senior level. These findings, though attributed to age, may also be considered to be due to playing experience, and thus less exposure to technical development. In professional football, Woods *et al.* (2004) observed that significantly more hamstring strains were incurred in the top league and became less common in the lower leagues. Since running has been identified as the predominant mechanism for this type of injury, this frequency pattern was attributed by the authors to the increased physical demands and faster pace of the higher leagues.

The issue of recovery between matches has been considered previously, but there is also the requirement to recover fully post-injury. Previous injury has been shown to be a primary factor in reinjury, with the severity of the reinjury often greater. In the audit of injuries in English professional soccer, Hawkins *et al.* (2001) highlighted the implications of reinjuries. The locations of many subsequent injuries were significantly biased towards the locality of the preceding injury episode, reinjuries attributed to 7 per cent of all injuries. This figure was an average for all injuries, while in follow-up studies hamstring strain reinjuries were recorded at 12 per cent (Woods *et al.*, 2004) and 9 per cent for ankle sprains (Woods *et al.*, 2003). Hawkins *et al.* (2001) reported that of all documented reinjuries, 48 per cent were strains and 18 per cent sprains. Furthermore, reinjuries were more severe than the previous injury, the number of missed training days averaging 25.1 compared with 19.1 days for the initial injury. Woods *et al.* (2003) observed that more ankle sprain reinjuries were attributed to non-contact mechanisms than the initial ankle sprain. Nielsen and Yde (1989) reported a similar pattern, with the initial injury being the result of a major trauma, while only minor trauma causing the reinjury. Increased risk of injury during non-contact mechanisms such as running, turning and landing would suggest incomplete rehabilitation from the initial injury (Arnason *et al.*, 1996).

The impact of reinjuries on the epidemiology of injury incidence is supported by other research. Hawkins and Fuller (1999) reported 22 per cent of all injuries as reinjuries, with 49 per cent being strains and 27 per cent sprains. Similarly, Hagglund *et al.* (2005) attributed 30 per cent of injuries in Denmark and 24 per cent in Sweden to reinjuries. Of these reinjuries, 70 per cent (Denmark) and 82 per cent (Sweden) were classified as overuse injury or muscular strain. Of all major injuries, 37 per cent (Denmark) and 24 per cent (Sweden) were preceded by the same type and location of injury within 2 months. Ekstrand and Gillquist (1982) observed that in 26 per cent of the players who suffered a minor injury, a major injury was incurred within 2 months, 40 per cent of wich were of the same type and location. Chomiak *et al.* (2000) observed that 24 per cent of players to sustain an injury had previously injured the same body part, a third of whom had done so within the past 3 months. Arnason *et al.* (2004) consistently identified previous injury as the most important factor for injury, with a four- to seven-fold increased risk for the four most frequent injury types of knee sprains, ankle sprains, groin strains, and hamstring strains.

The time lost to injury, and reinjury, can have implications for the physical conditioning of the player. Renstrom and Kannus (2000) listed several implications of inactivity and immobilization on the musculoskeletal system: decalcified bones, loss of tensile strength in tendons and ligaments, muscle tissue atrophy, and loss of elasticity in cartilage. A decrease in aerobic capacity, whether over the close season or following an extended period of inactivity due to injury, has been shown to increase the risk of injury (Chomiak *et al.*, 2000) and particularly overuse injuries (Eriksson *et al.*, 1986). Hawkins *et al.* (2001) attributed the increased risk of injury during pre-season to deficits in physiological conditioning. The long-term physical development of the soccer player, and temporal variations in physical fitness, are therefore likely to influence injury risk. Woods *et al.* (2002) observed that younger players were at a greater risk of pre-season injury than older players. The older players, who had a greater history of training, may not suffer as great a detraining effect as those players that are less well trained. This suggestion seems to correlate age to training status, which may not be applicable in all cases.

Summary

Fatigue is seen as a risk factor for injury in many professions including sporting (Pettrone and Ricciardelli, 1987) as well as non-sporting environments (Liberty Mutual Research Institute for Safety, 1995). If fatigue in football is identified as a risk factor for injury, then intervention strategies are required to minimize this risk. The nature of fatigue is diverse, and influenced by the inherent activity profile of soccer, the structure of the competitive season, and the long-term development of the player. An observation that injury incidence increases during the last 15 minutes of match play (Hawkins *et al.*, 2001) attributed injury to insufficient physical fitness. However, soccer is self-paced, and as the players become better conditioned, they run faster and more often, and thus cover greater distances and at a higher physiological intensity. Thus, strategies must be introduced that develop fitness specific to the physical demands of the game, both physiological and biomechanical. Markers of injury reflecting aetiological factors such as strength and balance must be developed so as to become fatigue-resistant to account for the demands of match play. The warm-up and re-warm-up of players should include consideration to injury prevention. Player rotation and the training/match ratio can be optimized to affect the longitudinal distribution of epidemiology over the playing season. The continual evolution of soccer academies provides an additional challenge, when fatigue becomes overreaching, or overtraining. And at the other extreme, the experiences of former footballers and their continued quality of life after playing may harness some interesting questions for the optimal management of players throughout their careers.

References

Ali, A. and Williams, C. (2009) 'Carbohydrate ingestion and soccer skill performance during prolonged intermittent exercise', *Journal of Sports Sciences*, 27(14): 1499–508.

Andersen, T. E., Larsen, O., Tenga, A., Engebretsen, L. and Bahr, R. (2003) 'Football incident analysis: a new video based method to describe injury mechanisms in professional football', *British Journal of Sports Medicine*, 37(3): 226–32.

Arnason, A., Johansson, E., Gudmundsson, A. and Dahl, H. A. (1994) 'Strains, sprains and contusions in Icelandic elite soccer', *Medicine and Science in Sports and Exercise*, 26: S14.

Arnason, A., Gudmundsson, A. and Dahl, H. A. (1996) 'Soccer injuries in Iceland', *Scandinavian Journal of Medicine and Science in Sports*, 6(1): 40–5.

Arnason, A., Sigurdsson, S. B., Gudmundsson, A., Holme, I., Engebretsen, L. and Bahr, R. (2004) 'Risk factors for injuries in football', *American Journal of Sports Medicine*, 32(1): S5–16.

Bangsbo, J. and Mohr, M. (2005) 'Variations in running speed and recovery time after a sprint during top-class soccer matches', *Medicine and Science in Sports and Exercise*, 37: 87.

Bangsbo, J., Norregaard, L. and Thorsoe, F. (1991) 'Activity profile of competition soccer', *Canadian Journal of Sports Science*, 16(2): 110–16.

Bartlett, M. J. and Warren, P. J. (2002) 'Effect of warming up on knee proprioception before sporting activity', *British Journal of Sports Medicine*, 36(2): 132–4.

Borotikar, B. S., Newcomer, R., Koppes, R. and McLean, S. G. (2008) 'Combined effects of fatigue and decision making on female lower limb landing postures: central and peripheral contributions to ACL injury risk', *Clinical Biomechanics*, 23(1): 81–92.

Bradley, P. S., Sheldon, W., Wooster, B., Olsen, P., Boanas, P. and Krustrup, P. (2009) 'High-intensity running in English FA Premier League soccer matches', *Journal of Sports Sciences*, 27(2): 159–68.

Carling, C. and Dupont, G. (2011) 'Are declines in physical performance associated with a reduction in skill-related performance during professional soccer match-play?', *Journal of Sports Sciences*, 29(1): 63–71.

Carling, C., Le Gall, F. and Dupont, G. (2012) 'Are physical performance and injury risk in a professional soccer team in match-play affected over a prolonged period of fixture congestion?', *International Journal of Sports Medicine*, 33(1): 36–42.

Chappell, J. D., Herman, D. C., Knight, B. S., Kirkendall, D. T., Garrett, W. E. and Yu, B. (2005) 'Effect of fatigue on knee kinetics and kinematics in stop-jump tasks', *American Journal of Sports Medicine*, 33(7): 1022–9.

Chomiak, J., Junge, A., Peterson, L. and Dvorak, J. (2000) 'Severe injuries in football players. Influencing factors', *American Journal of Sports Medicine*, 28 (5): S58–68.

Cortes, N., Quammen, D., Lucci, S., Greska, E. and Onate, J. (2012) 'A functional agility short-term protocol changes lower extremity mechanics', *Journal of Sports Sciences*, 30(8): 797–805.

Di Salvo, V., Baron, R., Gonzalez-Haro, C., Gormasz, C., Pigozzi, F. and Bachl, N. (2010) 'Sprinting analysis of elite soccer players during European Champions League and UEFA Cup matches', *Journal of Sports Sciences*, 28(14): 1489–94.

Drawer, S. and Fuller, C. W. (2002) 'Evaluating the level of injury in English professional football using a risk based assessment process', *British Journal of Sports Medicine*, 36(6): 446–51.

Drust, B., Reilly, T. and Cable, N. T. (2000) 'Physiological responses to laboratory-based soccer specific intermittent and continuous exercise', *Journal of Sports Sciences*, 18(11): 885–92.

Dupont, G., Nedelec, M., McCall, A., McCormack, D., Berthoin, S. and Wisloff, U. (2010) 'Effect of 2 soccer matches in a week on physical performance and injury rate', *American Journal of Sports Medicine*, 38(9): 1752–8.

Ekstrand, J. (2008) 'Epidemiology of football injuries', *Science & Sports*, 23(2): 73–7.

Ekstrand, J. and Gillquist, J. (1982) 'The frequency of muscle tightness and injuries in soccer players', *American Journal of Sports Medicine*, 10(2): 75–8.

Ekstrand, J., Gillquist, J., Moller, M., Oberg, B. and Liljedahl, S. O. (1983) 'Incidence of soccer injuries and their relation to training and team success', *American Journal of Sports Medicine*, 11(2): 63–7.

Engebretsen, A. H., Myklebust, G., Holme, I., Engebretsen, L. and Bahr, R. (2010a) 'Intrinsic risk factors for acute ankle injuries among male soccer players: a prospective cohort study', *Scandinavian Journal of Medicine and Science in Sports*, 20(3): 403–10.

Engebretsen, A. H., Myklebust, G., Holme, I., Engebretsen, L. and Bahr, R. (2010b) 'Intrinsic risk factors for groin injuries among male soccer players: a prospective cohort study', *American Journal of Sports Medicine*, 38(10): 2051–7.

Engebretsen, A. H., Myklebust, G., Holme, I., Engebretsen, L. and Bahr, R. (2011) 'Intrinsic risk factors for acute knee injuries among male football players: a prospective cohort study', *Scandinavian Journal of Medicine and Science in Sports*, 21(5): 645–52.

Eriksson, L. I., Jorfeldt, L. and Ekstrand, J. (1986) 'Overuse and distortion soccer injuries related to the player's estimated maximal aerobic work capacity', *International Journal of Sports Medicine*, 7(4): 214–16.

Fousekis, K., Tsepis, E., Poulmedis, P., Athanasopoulos, S. and Vagenas, G. (2011) 'Intrinsic risk factors of non-contact quadriceps and hamstring strains in soccer: a prospective study of 100 professional players', *British Journal of Sports Medicine*, 45(9): 709–14.

Fousekis, K., Tsepis, E. and Vagenas, G. (2012) 'Intrinsic risk factors of noncontact ankle sprains in soccer: a prospective study of 100 professional players', *American Journal of Sports Medicine*, 40(8): 1842–50.

Fuller, C. (2007) 'Managing the risk of injury in sport', *Clinical Journal of Sport Medicine*, 17(3): 182–7.

Greig, M. (2008) 'The influence of soccer-specific fatigue on peak isokinetic torque production of the knee flexors and extensors', *American Journal of Sports Medicine*, 36(7): 1403–9.

Greig, M. (2009) 'The influence of soccer-specific activity on the kinematics of an agility sprint', *European Journal of Sport Science*, 9(1), 23–33.

Greig, M. and Walker-Johnson, C. (2007) 'The influence of soccer-specific fatigue on functional stability', *Physical Therapy in Sport*, 8(4): 185–90.

Greig, M. and Siegler, J. C. (2009) 'Soccer-specific fatigue and eccentric hamstrings muscle strength', *Journal of Athletic Training*, 44(2): 180–4.

Greig, M. P., McNaughton, L. R. and Lovell, R. J. (2006) 'Physiological and mechanical response to soccer-specific intermittent activity and steady-state activity', *Research in Sports Medicine*, 14(1): 29–52.

Hagglund, M., Walden, M. and Ekstrand, J. (2003) 'Exposure and injury risk in Swedish elite football: a comparison between seasons 1982 and 2001', *Scandinavian Journal of Medicine and Science in Sports*, 13(6): 364–70.

Hagglund, M., Walden, M. and Ekstrand, J. (2005) 'Injury incidence and distribution in elite football – a prospective study of the Danish and the Swedish top divisions', *Scandinavian Journal of Medicine and Science in Sports*, 15(1): 21–8.

Hagglund, M., Walden, M. and Ekstrand, J. (2009) 'UEFA injury study: an injury audit of European Championships 2006 to 2008', *British Journal of Sports Medicine*, 43(7): 482–9.

Hawkins, R. D. and Fuller, C. W. (1996) 'Risk assessment in professional football: an examination of accidents and incidents in the 1994 World Cup finals', *British Journal of Sports Medicine*, 30(2): 165–70.

Hawkins, R. D. and Fuller, C. W. (1998) 'An examination of the frequency and severity of injuries and incidents at three levels of professional football', *British Journal of Sports Medicine*, 32(4): 326–32.

Hawkins, R. D. and Fuller, C. W. (1999) 'A prospective epidemiological study of injuries in four English professional football clubs', *British Journal of Sports Medicine*, 33(3): 196–203.

Hawkins, R. D., Hulse, M. A., Wilkinson, C., Hodson, A. and Gibson, M. (2001) 'The association football medical research programme: an audit of injuries in professional football', *British Journal of Sports Medicine*, 35(1): 43–7.

Hoskins, W. and Pollard, H. (2005) 'The management of hamstring injury part 1: issues in diagnosis', *Manual Therapy*, 10(2): 96–107.

Hoy, K., Lindblad, B. E., Terkelsen, C. J. and Helleland, H. E. (1992) 'European soccer injuries. A prospective epidemiologic and socioeconomic study', *American Journal of Sports Medicine*, 20(3): 318–22.

Jorgensen, U. (1984) 'Epidemiology of injuries in typical Scandinavian team sports', *British Journal of Sports Medicine*, 18(2): 59–63.

Junge, A., Dvorak, J. and Graf-Baumann, T. (2004a) 'Football injuries during the World Cup 2002', *American Journal of Sports Medicine*, 32(1): S23–7.

Junge, A., Dvorak, J. and Graf-Baumann, T. (2004b) 'Football injuries during FIFA tournaments and the Olympic Games, 1998–2001', *American Journal of Sports Medicine*, 32(1): S80–9.

Keller, C. S., Noyes, F. R. and Buncher C. R. (1987) 'The medical aspects of soccer injury epidemiology', *American Journal of Sports Medicine*, 15(3): 230–7.

Kellis, E., Katis, A. and Vrabas, I. S. (2006) 'Effects of an intermittent exercise fatigue protocol on biomechanics of soccer kick performance', *Scandinavian Journal of Medicine and Science in Sports*, 16(5): 334–44.

Lees, A. and Davies, T. (1988) 'The effects of fatigue on soccer kick biomechanics', *Journal of Sports Sciences*, 6: 156–7.

Lewin, G. (1989) 'The incidence of injury in an English professional soccer club during one competitive season', *Physiotherapy*, 75(10): 601–5.

Liberty Mutual Research Institute for Safety (1995) *Occupational Fatigue Research – Facing the Challenges Head On Quarterly Review*, Boston: Liberty Mutual Research Institute for Safety.

Lucci, S., Cortes, N., Van Lunen, B., Ringleb, S. and Onate, J. (2011) 'Knee and hip sagittal and transverse plane changes after two fatigue protocols', *Journal of Science and Medicine in Sport*, 14(5): 453–9.

Luthje, P., Nurmi, L., Kataja, M., Belt, E., Helenius, P., Kaukonen, J. P., Kiviluoto, H., Kokko, E., Lehtipuu, T. P., Lehtonen, A., Liukkonen, T., Myllyniemi, J., Rasilainen, P., Tolvanen, E., Virtanen, H. and Walldén, M. (1996) 'Epidemiology and traumatology of injuries in elite soccer: a prospective study in Finland', *Scandinavian Journal of Medicine and Science in Sports*, 16(3): 180–5.

McGregor, J. C. and Rae, A. (1995) 'A review of injuries to professional footballers in a premier football team (1990–93)', *Scottish Medical Journal*, 40(1): 16–18.

Mohr, M., Krustrup, P. and Bangsbo, J. (2003) 'Match performance of high-standard soccer players with special reference to development of fatigue', *Journal of Sports Sciences*, 21(7): 439–49.

Mohr, M., Krustrup, P., Nybo, L., Nielsen, J. J. and Bangsbo, J. (2004) 'Muscle temperature and sprint performance during soccer matches – beneficial effects of re-warm-up at half time', *Scandinavian Journal of Medicine and Science in Sports*, 14(3): 156–62.

Mohr, M., Krustrup, P. and Bangsbo, J. (2005) 'Fatigue is soccer: a brief review', *Journal of Sports Sciences*, 23(6): 593–9.

Moller, M. H., Oberg, B. E. and Gillquist, J. (1985) 'Stretching exercise and soccer: effect of stretching on range of motion in the lower extremity in connection with soccer training', *International Journal of Sports Medicine*, 6(1): 50–2.

Morgan, B. E. and Oberlander, M. A. (2001) 'An examination of injuries in Major League Soccer', *American Journal of Sports Medicine*, 29(4): 426–30.

Murphy, D., Connolly, D. and Beynnon, B. (2003) 'Risk factors for lower extremity injury: a review of the literature', *British Journal of Sports Medicine*, 37(1): 13–29.

Nicholas, C. W., Nuttall, F. E. and Williams, C. (2000) 'The Loughborough Intermittent Shuttle Test: a field test that simulates the activity pattern of soccer', *Journal of Sports Sciences*, 18(2): 97–104.

Nielsen, A. B. and Yde, J. (1989) 'Epidemiology and traumatology of injuries in soccer', *American Journal of Sports Medicine*, 17(6): 803–7.

Odetoyinbo, K., Wooster, B. and Lane, A. (2008) 'The effect of a succession of matches on the activity profiles of professional soccer players', in T. Reilly and F. Korkusuz (eds), *Science and Football VI*, Abingdon: Routledge, pp. 105–11.

Orchard, J. (2001) 'Intrinsic and extrinsic risk factors for muscle strains in Australian football', *American Journal of Sports Medicine*, 29(3): 300–3.

Ostenberg, A. and Roos, H. (2000) 'Injury risk factors in female European football. A prospective study of 123 players during one season', *Scandinavian Journal of Medicine and Science in Sports*, 10(5): 279–85.

Peterson, L., Junge, A., Chomiak, J., Baumann, T. G. and Dvorak, J. (2000) 'Incidence of football injuries and complaints in different age groups and skill-level groups', *American Journal of Sports Medicine*, 28(5): 51–7.

Pettrone, F. A. and Ricciardelli, E. (1987) 'Gymnastic injuries: the Virginia experience 1982–1983', *American Journal of Sports Medicine*, 15(1): 59–62.

Price, R. J., Hawkins, R. D., Hulse, M. A. and Hodson, A. (2004) 'The Football Association medical research programme: an audit of injuries in academy youth football', *British Journal of Sports Medicine*, 38(4): 466–71.

Rahnama, N., Reilly, T. and Lees, A. (2002) 'Injury risk associated with playing actions during competitive soccer', *British Journal of Sports Medicine*, 36(5): 354–9.

Rahnama, N., Reilly. T., Lees, A. and Graham-Smith, P. (2003) 'Muscle fatigue induced by exercise simulating the work-rate of competitive soccer', *Journal of Sports Sciences*, 21(3): 933–43.

Rahnama, N., Lees, A. and Reilly, T. (2005) 'Electromyography of selected lower-limb muscles fatigued by exercise at the intensity of soccer match-play', *Journal of Electromyography and Kinesiology*, 16(3): 257–63.

Reilly, T. and Thomas, V. (1976) 'A motion analysis of work-rate in different positional roles in professional football match-play', *Journal of Human Movement Studies*, 2: 87–97.

Reilly, T., Drust, B. and Clarke, N. (2008) 'Muscle fatigue during football match-play', *Sports Medicine*, 38(5): 357–67.

Renstrom, P. A. F. H. and Kannus, P. (2000) 'Prevention of injuries in endurance athletes', in R. J. Shephard and P.-O. Åstrand (eds), *Endurance in Sport*, Oxford: Blackwell Science Ltd., pp. 4–74.

Rey, E., Lago-Penas, C., Lago-Ballesteros, J., Casais, L. and Dellal, A. (2010) 'The effect of a congested fixture period on the activity of elite soccer players', *Biology of Sport*, 27(3): 181–5.

Roos, H., Lindberg, H., Gardsell, P., Lohmander, L. S. and Wingstrand, H. (1994) 'The prevalence of gonarthrosis and its relation to meniscectomy in former soccer players', *American Journal of Sports Medicine*, 22(2): 219–22.

Russell, M., Benton, D. and Kingsley, M. (2011) 'The effects of fatigue on soccer skills performed during a soccer match simulation', *International Journal of Sports Physiology and Performance*, 6(2): 221–33.

Sandelin, J., Santavirta, S. and Kiviluoto, O. (1985) 'Acute soccer injuries in Finland in 1980', *British Journal of Sports Medicine*, 19(1): 30–3.

Sanna, G. and O'Connor, K. M. (2008) 'Fatigue-related changes in stance leg mechanics during sidestep cutting maneuvers', *Clinical Biomechanics*, 23(7): 946–54.

Sheppard, C. and Hodson, A. (2006) 'Injury profiles in professional footballers', *SportEx Medicine*, 27: 6–9.

Small, K., McNaughton, L. R., Greig, M., Lohkamp, M. and Lovell, R. (2009) 'Soccer fatigue, sprinting and hamstring injury risk', *International Journal of Sports Medicine*, 30(8): 573–8.

Small, K., McNaughton, L., Greig, M. and Lovell, R. (2010) 'The effects of multidirectional soccer-specific fatigue on markers of hamstring injury risk', *Journal of Science and Medicine in Sport*, 13(1): 120–5.

Soderman, K., Pietila, T., Alfredson, H. and Werner, S. (2002) 'Anterior cruciate ligament injuries in young females playing soccer at senior levels', *Scandinavian Journal of Medicine and Science in Sports*, 12(2): 65–8.

Spencer, M., Lawrence, S., Rechichi, C., Bishop, D., Dawson, B. and Goodman, C. (2004) 'Time-motion analysis of elite feld hockey, with special reference to repeated-sprint activity', *Journal of Sports Sciences*, 22(9): 843–50.

Spencer, M., Bishop, D., Dawson, B. and Goodman, C. (2005) 'Physiological and metabolic responses of repeated-sprint activities: specific to field-based team sports', *Sports Medicine*, 35(12): 1025–45.

Spencer, M., Fitzsimons, M., Dawson, B., Bishop, D. and Goodman, C. (2006). 'Reliability of a repeated-sprint test for field-hockey', *Journal of Science and Medicine in Sport*, 9(1–2): 181–4.

van Mechelen, W., Hlobil, H. and Kemper, H. (1992) 'Incidence, severity, aetiology and prevention of sports injuries. A review of concepts', *Sports Medicine*, 14(2): 82–99.

Verrall, G. M., Slavotinek, J. P., Barnes, P. G., Fon, G. T. and Spriggins, A. J. (2001) 'Clinical risk factors for hamstring muscle strain injury: a prospective study with correlation of injury by magnetic resonance imaging', *British Journal of Sports Medicine*, 35(6): 435–40.

Woods, C., Hawkins, R., Hulse, M. and Hodson, A. (2002) 'The Football Association Medical Research Programme: an audit of injuries in professional football – analysis of preseason injuries', *British Journal of Sports Medicine*, 36(6): 436–41.

Woods, C., Hawkins, R., Hulse, M. and Hodson, A. (2003) 'The Football Association Medical Research Programme: an audit of injuries in professional football – an analysis of ankle sprains', *British Journal of Sports Medicine*, 37(3): 233–8.

Woods, C., Hawkins, R. D., Maltby, S., Hulse, M., Thomas, A. and Hodson, A. (2004) 'The Football Association Medical Research Programme: an audit of injuries in professional football – analysis of hamstring injuries', *British Journal of Sports Medicine*, 38(1): 36–41.

6

ENVIRONMENTAL FACTORS FOR FATIGUE AND INJURY IN ULTRA-ENDURANCE SPORTS

Beat Knechtle

UNIVERSITY OF ZURICH, ZURICH

Introduction

Ultra-endurance competitions are defined as events exceeding 6 hours in duration (Zaryski and Smith, 2005). Races in ultra-endurance can be mainly held in ultra-swimming such as the 'English Channel Crossing' (Eichenberger *et al.*, 2012a, 2012b; Fischer *et al.*, 2013), ultra-cycling such as the 'Race across America' (Hulton *et al.*, 2010; Knechtle *et al.*, 2005), ultra-running such as the 'Trans Europe Foot Race' (Schütz *et al.*, 2012) and the combination of triathlon such as ultra-triathlons (Knechtle *et al.*, 2011b; Lepers, 2008).

These longer events rely on long-term preparation, sufficient nutrition, accommodation of environmental stressors and psychological toughness (Knechtle *et al.*, 2011a, 2011c, 2012a, 2012b; Zaryski and Smith, 2005). A successful ultra-endurance performance is characterized by the ability to sustain a higher absolute speed for a given distance than other competitors (Zaryski and Smith, 2005). Training relies heavily on the athlete's tolerance to repetitive strain (Zaryski and Smith, 2005). For ultra-marathoners in 161 km ultra-marathons, finish times were found to have a significant negative association with training volume and were generally directly associated with body mass index (Hoffman and Fogard, 2011). For non-finishers, the primary reasons for dropping out were nausea and/or vomiting (23.0 per cent). Finishers compared with non-finishers were more likely to report blisters (40.1 per cent versus 17.3 per cent), muscle pain (36.5 per cent versus 20.1 per cent) and exhaustion (23.1 per cent versus 13.7 per cent) as adversely affecting race performance, but nausea and/or vomiting was similar between groups (36.8 per cent versus 39.6 per cent). Overall use of NSAIDs was high, and greater among finishers (60.5 per cent) than non-finishers (46.4 per cent).

While competing, ultra-endurance athletes are exposed to different environmental circumstances such as heat (Roth *et al.*, 2007), cold (Case *et al.*, 1995) and high altitude (Noakes, 2007) apart from the long duration of the race. There are well recognized effects of heat and hydration status on the cardiovascular and thermoregulatory systems in marathoners that can account for the decreased performance and increased sensation of effort that are experienced when competing in the heat (Maughan *et al.*, 2007). The aim of this chapter is to review the literature for environmental factors for fatigue and injury in ultra-endurance performances.

The effect of heat on ultra-endurance performance

The environment plays an important role during endurance activities. Ultra-endurance athletes such as 100 km ultra-runners, ultra-triathletes, and ultra-cyclists experience unique risks associated with their sports. Competitors in ultra-endurance races can be subjected to significant heat strain depending on environmental factors, dehydration and even exercise-associated hyponatremia (Knechtle *et al.*, 2011a; Rothenberg and Panagos, 2008). Elevated ambient temperatures have been shown to have a negative effect on ultra-endurance performance (Parise and Hoffman, 2011; Sparks *et al.*, 2005; Wegelin and Hoffman, 2011). In 161 km ultra-marathons, extreme heat impaired all runners' ability to perform, but faster runners were at a greater disadvantage compared to slower competitors because they completed a greater proportion of the race under hotter conditions (Parise and Hoffman, 2011). Warmer weather had a similar effect on finish rates for men and women. However, finish times were slower with advancing age, slower for women than men, and were less affected by warm weather for women than for men (Wegelin and Hoffman, 2011).

Hot environments result in a considerable heat stress, which is compounded by dehydration. The risk of heat illness during high intensity or endurance activities is substantially increased in hot and/or humid environments (Armstrong *et al.*, 2007). The amount of time needed to reach exercise-related exhaustion decreases with increasing temperature, humidity, and dehydration (Armstrong *et al.*, 2007). During increased environmental heat strain, an athlete must adjust for critical variables, such as temperature regulation, hydration status and electrolyte levels, as they can contribute to an impaired performance (Rothenberg and Panagos, 2008).

The effects of altered hydration status can influence athletes cognitively in addition to physically. This can even occur before the level of dehydration reaches a point where the performer's physical performance would normally be affected. Mild dehydration has been attributed to decreased performance without change in objective measurements (Rothenberg and Panagos, 2008). These deleterious effects are further exacerbated with increasing core temperatures > 40°C. For example, marathon performance is impaired in the heat, and a combination of high temperature and high humidity presents a major challenge to the elite marathon runner, who must sustain a high metabolic rate throughout the race. The optimum temperature for marathon performance is generally about 10–12°C (Maughan, 2010). Marathon races are performed over a broad range of environmental conditions. Hyperthermia is a primary challenge for runners in temperate and warm weather, but hypothermia can be a concern during cool-wet or cold conditions (Kenefick *et al.*, 2007). With respect to marathon encounters, heat stress increases both the finish-line medical encounter rate and the on-course drop-out rate, and seems to increase the incidence of exercise-associated hyponatremia and heat stroke (Roberts, 2007). For marathoners, the fact that climate can significantly limit temperature regulation and performance is evident from the direct relationship between heat casualties and wet bulb globe temperature, as well as the inverse relationship between record-setting race performances and ambient temperatures (Cheuvront and Haymes, 2001).

During exercise in the heat, the ensuing dehydration causes hyperthermia and the synergistic effects of both stressors reduce cardiac output and blood flow to muscle, skin, brain and possibly splanchnic tissues (González-Alonso, 2007). Galloway and Maughan (1997) demonstrated in a laboratory time trail where subjects cycled at ambient temperatures of 3.6 ± 0.3°C, 10.5 ± 0.5°C, 20.6 ± 0.2°C and 30.5 ± 0.2°C an effect of temperature on exercise capacity, which appeared to follow an inverted-U relationship. Time to exhaustion was considerably influenced by ambient temperatures: exercise duration was shortest at 30.5°C with 51.6 ± 3.7 minutes and longest at 10.5°C with 93.5 ± 6.2 minutes. The reasons for the impaired performance in heat are most probably high internal body temperatures causing fatigue during prolonged exercise in hot environments (González-Alonso *et al.*, 1999). To date, however, no study investigated the influence or drop-out race in ultra-endurance races due to extreme heat.

Another aspect of the heat in ultra-endurance performance is the higher prevalence of exercise-associated hyponatremia (Hoffman *et al.*, 2012; Lebus *et al.*, 2010). In the '161 km Western States Endurance Run' in the USA held in rather hot conditions, the prevalence of exercise-associated hyponatremia was reported to be at 30 per cent (Hoffman *et al.*, 2012) and 51 per cent (Lebus *et al.*, 2010). In the study of Lebus *et al.* (2010), the environmental temperature ranged from 12.2°C to 37.6°C. However, the duration of the ultra-endurance race might also increase the risk for exercise-associated hyponatremia. In a Triple Iron ultra-triathlon covering 11.4 km swimming, 540 km cycling and 124.4 km running, the prevalence of exercise-associated hyponatremia was at 26 per cent (Rüst *et al.*, 2012). Apart from heat and duration, cold might also increase the risk for exercise-associated hyponatremia. In ultra-endurance swimmers participating in the 'Marathon-Swim' in Lake Zurich, Switzerland, covering a distance of 26.4 km, two men (8 per cent) and four women (36 per cent) developed exercise-associated hyponatremia where one woman was symptomatic with plasma sodium (Na) of 127 mmol.L$_{-1}$ (Wagner *et al.*, 2012). Apart from the cold water, an increased fluid intake due to swallowing water in the lake might have occurred in these athletes. Generally, however, the prevalence of exercise-associated hyponatremia is not higher in ultra-endurance athletes (Knechtle *et al.*, 2011a).

The effect of cold on ultra-endurance performance

Exercising in the cold is not an attractive option for many athletes; however, defining what represents cold is difficult and is not standard for all events. If the exercise is prolonged and undertaken at a moderate intensity, environmental temperatures around 11°C can be an advantage. If the intensity is lower than this value and the individual does not generate sufficient metabolic heat to offset the effects imposed by the cold environment, then temperatures of 11°C can be detrimental to performance. Similarly, when the performance involves dynamic explosive contractions, then a cold ambient temperature can have a negative influence. Additional factors such as the exercising medium, air or water, and the anthropometric characteristics of the athlete will also make a difference to the strategies that can be adopted to offset any negative impact of a cold environment on performance (Nimmo, 2004).

Cold exposure facilitates body heat loss, which can reduce body core temperature, unless mitigated by enhanced heat conservation or an increased heat production (Young and Castellani, 2001). Both exercise and shivering may increase metabolic heat production, which may help offset body heat losses in the cold (Young and Castellani, 2001). Prolonged exhaustive exercise leading to energy substrate depletion may compromise maintenance of thermal balance in the cold simply by precluding continuation of further exercise and the associated thermogenesis (Young and Castellani, 2001). Participants in prolonged, physically demanding cold-weather activities are at risk for a condition called 'thermoregulatory fatigue'. During prolonged cold exposure, the increased gradient favouring body heat loss to the environment is opposed by physiological responses and clothing and behavioural strategies that conserve body heat stores to defend body temperature. The primary human physiological responses elicited by cold exposure are shivering and peripheral vasoconstriction. Shivering increases thermogenesis and replaces body heat losses, while peripheral vasoconstriction improves thermal insulation of the body and retards the rate of heat loss (Castellani *et al.*, 2010). In marathons, cold conditions increase the drop-out rate along the course and, if associated with wet conditions, also increase the encounter rate (Roberts, 2007). To date, however, no study investigated the influence or drop-out race in ultra-endurance races due to extreme cold.

Problems with the skeletal and locomotor system

Ultra-endurance athletes face many problems while competing. In ultra-endurance races such as ultra-marathons, the effect of endurance performance on problems of the locomotor system has been investigated. Scheer and Murray (2011) investigated in the 'Al Andalus Ultra Trail' in 2010, a 219 km, 5-day stage race in southern Spain in 69 ultra-marathoners the prevalence of medical problems. Of the 69 competitors, 39 runners were seen with a medical problem (56.5 per cent). There were a total of 99 clinical encounters. The most common reasons for consulting were foot blisters (33.3 per cent), followed by chafing (9.1 per cent). Lower limb musculoskeletal injuries accounted for 22.2 per cent, predominantly affecting the knee.

In a multi-stage race, the problems of the locomotor system seemed to appear in different time frames. Krabak *et al.* (2011) reported that medical illnesses were more likely on the first day of a seven-day, 250 km off-road ultra-marathon, whereas musculoskeletal and skin injuries were more likely on day three or four. Problems of the lower limbs seemed to be reduced with increased experience in runners. Hespanhol Junior *et al.* (2012) reported that running experience was associated with the absence of previous musculoskeletal running-related injuries.

Considering ultra-runners, overuse injuries of the lower limbs seem to be a major problem where injuries are typically associated with running. Problems with ankle and knee were the most frequent. Ankle injuries predominate in track races, whereas knee injuries are more common in road races (Bishop and Fallon, 1999; Fallon, 1996). In the 1,005 km ultra-marathon from Sydney to Melbourne 64 injuries were found in 32 runners (Fallon, 1996). The knee (31.3 per cent) and ankle (28.1 per cent) regions were most commonly injured. The most common single diagnosis was retropatellar pain syndrome, and Achilles tendinitis and medial tibial stress syndrome were the next most common injuries. Bishop and Fallon (1999) documented injuries during a 6-day track race in 17 competitors (16 men and 1 woman). A total of 36 injuries were recorded in 11 competitors. The ankle (36 per cent) and the knee (22 per cent) were the regions most frequently injured. The four most common diagnoses were: Achilles tendonitis (19 per cent); extensor digitorum longus tendonitis (14 per cent); retropatellar pain syndrome (14 per cent); and anterior compartment pain (11 per cent).

Nutritional aspects in ultra-endurance relating to finishing

Adequate nutrition during ultra-endurance performance seemed to be of utmost important for successful finishing (Knechtle *et al.*, 2011a, 2011c; Ranchordas, 2012). It has been shown that ultra-endurance races lead to a large energy deficit (Enqvist *et al.*, 2010; Knechtle *et al.*, 2005, 2008). A large energy deficit is caused by inadequate energy intake, possibly due to suppressed appetite and gastrointestinal problems (Enqvist *et al.*, 2010).

In ultra-endurance cyclists, nutrition during the race was associated with race time (Knechtle *et al.*, 2011c). Gastrointestinal distress is common during ultra-running. Stümpfle *et al.* (2011) compared finishers and non-finishers in a 161 km ultra-marathon regarding race diet. Completion of the race was related to greater fuel, fluid and sodium consumption rates. In another study on 161 km ultra-marathoners, Stümpfle *et al.* (in press) investigated 15 (10 male, 5 female) runners. Nine (8 male, 1 female) athletes experienced gastrointestinal distress including nausea (89 per cent), abdominal cramps (44 per cent) diarrhea (44 per cent), and vomiting (22 per cent). Fluid consumption rate was higher in runners without gastrointestinal distress compared to those with gastrointestinal distress. Runners without gastrointestinal distress consumed a higher percentage of fat compared to runners with gastrointestinal distress. Also, fat intake rate was higher in runners without gastrointestinal distress compared to runners with gastrointestinal distress. Overall, lower fluid and fat intake rates were evident in those developing gastrointestinal distress prior to the onset of symptoms.

Problems in the different endurance disciplines

As mentioned, ultra-endurance performances can be performed in swimming, cycling, running, and triathlon as the combination of these three disciplines. The influence of heat and/or cold on performance may be different in these different disciplines.

Swimming

Water temperature affects performance in ultra-endurance swimming. In the 26.4 km open-water ultra-swim 'Marathon Swim in Lake Zurich', swim time was negatively associated with water temperature in the top three swimmers (Eichenberger *et al.*, 2012b). In the 'English Channel Swim', athletes face temperatures between 15 and 18°C (Eichenberger *et al.*, 2012b) requiring a high body fat to resist heat loss (Acevedo *et al.*, 1997). It has been shown that a higher body fat enables ultra-endurance swimmers to stay longer in cold water (Keatinge *et al.*, 1969; Knechtle *et al.*, 2009).

Cycling

In ultra-endurance cycling, factors such as training (Knechtle *et al.*, 2011c, 2012a, 2012b) and nutrition (Knechtle *et al.*, 2011c) seemed of importance to successfully finish a race. In contrast, equipment and support during the race showed no association with race outcome (Knechtle *et al.*, 2011c). In addition, athletes with naps were highly significantly slower than athletes without naps (Knechtle *et al.*, 2012b). When cyclists preparing for ultra-endurance cycling races of different length were compared, the qualifiers in the longer race had greater intensity in training while the qualifiers in the shorter race relied more on training volume. Different strategies and types of training reflected the different demands of the races (Knechtle *et al.*, 2012a, 2012b).

Running

Ultra-marathons comprise any sporting event involving running longer than the traditional marathon length of 42.195 km (26.2 miles) (Millet and Millet, 2012). The repetitive strain of each foot stroke during an ultra-marathon may lead to considerable changes in the lower limb such as overuse injuries (Ferber *et al.*, 2009). In the Trans Europe Foot Race 2009, the diameter of the Achilles tendon bone lesions and subcutaneous oedema increased (Freund *et al.*, 2012). Finishers differed only regarding plantar aponeurosis and subcutaneous oedema from non-finishers in the Trans Europe Foot Race 2009 (Freund *et al.*, 2012).

Conclusions

Ultra-endurance athletes competing for hours or days face different problems while racing. While there is abundant literature for environmental related reasons for drop-outs in marathons, little is known about drop-outs in ultra-endurance races such as ultra-marathons due to extreme heat or extreme cold. Future studies need to investigate the effect of extreme heat and/or extreme cold on the performance and/or drop-out rate in ultra-endurance races.

References

Acevedo, E. O., Meyers, M. C., Hayman, M. and Haskin, J. (1997) 'Applying physiological principles and assessment techniques to swimming the English Channel. A case study', *Journal of Sports Medicine and Physical Fitness*, 37(1): 78–85.

Armstrong, L. E., Casa, D. J., Millard-Stafford, M., Moran, D. S., Pyne, S. W. and Roberts, W. O. (2007) 'American College of Sports Medicine position stand: exertional heat illness during training and competition', *Medicine and Science in Sports and Exercise*, 39(3): 556–72.

Bishop, G. W. and Fallon, K. E. (1999) 'Musculoskeletal injuries in a six-day track race: ultramarathoner's ankle', *Clinical Journal of Sport Medicine*, 9(4): 216–20.

Case, S., Evans, D., Tibbets, G., Case, S. and Miller, D. (1995) 'Dietary intakes of participants in the IditaSport Human Powered Ultra-marathon', *Alaska Medicine*, 37(1): 20–4.

Castellani, J. W., Sawka, M. N., de Groot, D. W. and Young, A. J. (2010) 'Cold thermoregulatory responses following exertional fatigue', *Frontiers in Bioscience (Scholar Edition)*, 2: 854–65.

Cheuvront, S. N. and Haymes, E. M. (2001) 'Thermoregulation and marathon running: biological and environmental influences', *Sports Medicine*, 31(10): 743–62.

Eichenberger, E., Knechtle, B., Knechtle, P., Rüst, C. A., Rosemann, T. and Lepers, R. (2012a) 'Best performances by men and women open-water swimmers during the 'English Channel Swim' from 1900 to 2010', *Journal of Sports Sciences*, 30(10): 1295–301.

Eichenberger, E., Knechtle, B., Knechtle, P., Rüst, C. A., Rosemann, T., Lepers, R. and Senn, O. (2012b) 'Sex difference in open-water ultra-swim performance in the longest freshwater lake swim in Europe', *Journal of Strength and Conditioning Research*, 27(5): 1362–9. doi: 10.1519/JSC.0b013e318265a3e9.

Enqvist, J. K., Mattsson, C. M., Johansson, P. H., Brink-Elfegoun, T., Bakkman, L. and Ekblom, B. T. (2010) 'Energy turnover during 24 hours and 6 days of adventure racing', *Journal of Sports Sciences*, 28(9): 947–55.

Fallon, K. E. (1996) 'Musculoskeletal injuries in the ultramarathon: the 1990 Westfield Sydney to Melbourne run', *British Journal of Sports Medicine*, 30(4): 319–23.

Ferber, R., Hreljac, A. and Kendall, K. D. (2009) 'Suspected mechanisms in the cause of overuse running injuries: a clinical review', *Sports Health*, 1(3): 242–6.

Fischer, G., Knechtle, B., Rüst, C. A. and Rosemann, T. (2013) 'Male swimmers cross the English Channel faster than female swimmers', *Scandinavian Journal of Medicine and Science in Sports*, 23(1): e48–55.

Freund, W., Weber, F., Billich, C. and Schuetz, U. H. (2012) 'The foot in multistage ultra-marathon runners: experience in a cohort study of 22 participants of the Trans Europe Footrace Project with mobile MRI', *BMJ Open*, 2(3): pii: e001118.

Galloway, S. D. and Maughan, R. J. (1997) 'Effects of ambient temperature on the capacity to perform prolonged cycle exercise in man', *Medicine and Science in Sports and Exercise*, 29(9): 1240–9.

González-Alonso, J. (2007) 'Hyperthermia impairs brain, heart and muscle function in exercising humans', *Sports Medicine*, 37(4–5): 371–3.

González-Alonso, J., Teller, C., Andersen, S. L., Jensen, F. B. Hyldig, T. and Nielsen, B. (1999) 'Influence of body temperature on the development of fatigue during prolonged exercise in the heat', *Journal of Applied Physiology*, 86(3): 1032–9.

Hespanhol Junior, L. C., Costa, L. O., Carvalho, A. C. and Lopes, A. D. (2012) 'A description of training characteristics and its association with previous musculoskeletal injuries in recreational runners: a cross-sectional study', *Revista Brasileira de Fisioterapia*, 16(1): 46–53.

Hoffman, M. D. and Fogard, K. (2011) 'Factors related to successful completion of a 161-km ultramarathon', *International Journal of Sports Physiology and Performance*, 6(1): 25–37.

Hoffman, M. D., Stuempfle, K. J., Rogers, I. R., Weschler, L. B. and Hew-Butler, T. (2012) 'Hyponatremia in the 2009 161-km Western States Endurance Run', *International Journal of Sports Physiology and Performance*, 7(1): 6–10.

Hulton, A. T., Lahart, I., Williams, K. L., Godfrey, R., Charlesworth, S., Wilson, M., Pedlar, C. and Whyte, G. (2010) 'Energy expenditure in the Race Across America (RAAM)', *International Journal of Sports Medicine*, 31(7): 463–7.

Keatinge, W. R., Prys-Roberts, C., Cooper, K. E., Honour, A. J. and Haight, J. (1969) 'Sudden failure of swimming in cold water', *British Medical Journal*, 22(5542): 480–3.

Kenefick, R. W., Cheuvront, S. N. and Sawka, M. N. (2007) 'Thermoregulatory function during the marathon', *Sports Medicine*, 37(4–5): 312–15.

Knechtle, B., Enggist, A. and Jehle, T. (2005) 'Energy turnover at the Race across America (RAAM) – a case report', *International Journal of Sports Medicine*, 26(6): 499–503.

Knechtle, B., Knechtle, P., Schück, R., Andonie, J. L. and Kohler, G. (2008) 'Effects of a Deca Iron Triathlon on body composition: a case study', *International Journal of Sports Medicine*, 29(4): 343–51.

Knechtle, B., Christinger, N., Kohler, G., Knechtle, P. and Rosemann, T. (2009) 'Swimming in ice cold water', *Irish Journal of Medical Science*, 178(4): 507–11.

Knechtle, B., Gnädinger, M., Knechtle, P., Imoberdorf, R., Kohler, G., Ballmer, P., Rosemann, T. and Senn, O. (2011a) 'Prevalence of exercise-associated hyponatremia in male ultraendurance athletes', *Clinical Journal of Sport Medicine*, 21(3): 226–32.

Knechtle, B., Knechtle, P. and Lepers, R. (2011b) 'Participation and performance trends in ultra-triathlons from 1985 to 2009', *Scandinavian Journal of Medicine and Science in Sports*, 21(6): e82–90.

Knechtle, B., Knechtle, P., Rüst, C. A., Rosemann, T. and Lepers, R. (2011c) 'Finishers and nonfinishers in the "Swiss Cycling Marathon" to qualify for the "Race Across America"', *Journal of Strength and Conditioning Research*, 25(12): 3257–63.

Knechtle, B., Wirth, A., Knechtle, P., Rüst, C. A. and Rosemann, T. (2012a) 'A comparison of ultra-endurance cyclists in a qualifying ultra-cycling race for Paris-Brest-Paris and Race Across America-Swiss cycling marathon', *Perceptual and Motor Skills*, 114(1): 96–110.

Knechtle, B., Wirth, A., Knechtle, P., Rüst, C. A., Rosemann, T. and Lepers, R. (2012b) 'No improvement in race performance by naps in male ultra-endurance cyclists in a 600-km ultra-cycling race', *Chinese Journal of Physiology*, 55(2):125–33.

Krabak, B. J., Waite, B. and Schiff, M. A. (2011) 'Study of injury and illness rates in multiday ultramarathon runners', *Medicine and Science in Sports and Exercise*, 43(12): 2314–20.

Lebus, D. K., Casazza, G. A., Hoffman, M. D. and Van Loan, M. D. (2010) 'Can changes in body mass and total body water accurately predict hyponatremia after a 161-km running race?', *Clinical Journal of Sport Medicine*, 20(3): 193–9.

Lepers, R. (2008) 'Analysis of Hawaii ironman performances in elite triathletes from 1981 to 2007', *Medicine and Science in Sports and Exercise*, 40(10): 1828–34.

Maughan, R. J. (2010) 'Distance running in hot environments: a thermal challenge to the elite runner', *Scandinavian Journal of Medicine and Science in Sports*, 20(3): S95–102.

Maughan, R. J., Watson, P. and Shirreffs, S. M. (2007) 'Heat and cold: what does the environment do to the marathon runner?', *Sports Medicine*, 37(4–5): 396–9.

Millet, G. P. and Millet, G. Y. (2012) 'Ultramarathon is an outstanding model for the study of adaptive responses to extreme load and stress', *BMC Medicine*, 10: 77.

Nimmo, M. (2004) 'Exercise in the cold', *Journal of Sports Sciences*, 22(10): 898–915.

Noakes, T. D. (2007) 'The limits of human endurance: what is the greatest endurance performance of all time? Which factors regulate performance at extreme altitude?', *Advances in Experimental Medicine and Biology*, 618: 255–76.

Parise, C. A. and Hoffman, M. D. (2011) 'Influence of temperature and performance level on pacing a 161 km trail ultramarathon', *International Journal of Sports Physiology and Performance*, 6(2): 243–51.

Ranchordas, M. K. (2012) 'Nutrition for adventure racing', *Sports Medicine*, 42(11): 915–27.

Roberts, W. O. (2007) 'Heat and cold: what does the environment do to marathon injury?', *Sports Medicine*, 37(4–5): 400–3.

Roth, H. J., Leithäuser, R. M., Doppelmayr, H., Doppelmayr, M., Finkernagel, H., von Duvillard, S. P., Korff, S., Katus, H. A., Giannitsis, E. and Beneke, R. (2007) 'Cardiospecificity of the 3rd generation cardiac troponin T assay during and after a 216 km ultra-endurance marathon run in Death Valley', *Clinical Research in Cardiology*, 96(6): 359–64.

Rothenberg, J. A. and Panagos, A. (2008) 'Musculoskeletal performance and hydration status', *Current Reviews in Musculoskeletal Medicine*, 1(2): 131–6.

Rüst, C. A., Knechtle, B., Knechtle, P. and Rosemann, T. (2012) 'Higher prevalence of exercise-associated hyponatremia in triple iron ultra-triathletes than reported for ironman triathletes', *Chinese Journal of Physiology*, 55(3): 147–55.

Scheer, B. V. and Murray, A. (2011) 'Al Andalus Ultra Trail: an observation of medical interventions during a 219-km, 5-day ultramarathon stage race', *Clinical Journal of Sport Medicine*, 21(5): 444–6.

Schütz, U.H., Schmidt-Trucksäss, A., Knechtle, B., Machann, J., Wiedelbach, H., Ehrhardt, M., Freund, W., Gröninger, S., Brunner, H., Schulze, I., Brambs, H. J. and Billich, C. (2012) 'The Transeurope Footrace Project: longitudinal data acquisition in a cluster randomized mobile MRI observational cohort study on 44 endurance runners at a 64-stage 4,486km transcontinental ultramarathon', *BMC Medicine*, 10: 78.

Sparks, S. A., Cable, N. T., Doran, D. A. and Maclaren, D. P. (2005) 'Influence of environmental temperature on duathlon performance', *Ergonomics*, 48(11–14): 1558–67.

Stümpfle, K. J., Hoffman, M. D., Weschler, L. B., Rogers, I. R. and Hew-Butler, T. (2011) 'Race diet of finishers and non-finishers in a 100 mile (161 km) mountain footrace', *Journal of the American College of Nutrition*, 30(6): 529–35.

Stümpfle, K. J., Hoffman, M. D, and Hew-Butler, T. (in press) 'Gastrointestinal distress in ultramarathoners is associated with race diet', *International Journal of Sport Nutrition and Exercise Metabolism*.

Wagner, S., Knechtle, B., Knechtle, P., Rüst, C. A. and Rosemann, T. (2012) 'Higher prevalence of exercise-associated hyponatremia in female than in male open-water ultra-endurance swimmers: the "Marathon-Swim" in Lake Zurich', *European Journal of Applied Physiology*, 112(3): 1095–106.

Wegelin, J. A. and Hoffman, M. D. (2011) 'Variables associated with odds of finishing and finish time in a 161-km ultramarathon', *European Journal of Applied Physiology*, 111(1): 145–53.

Young, A. J. and Castellani, J. W. (2001) 'Exertion-induced fatigue and thermoregulation in the cold', *Comparative Biochemistry and Physiology Part A: Molecular & Integrative Physiology*, 128(4): 769–76.

Zaryski, C. and Smith, D. J. (2005) 'Training principles and issues for ultra-endurance athletes', *Current Sports Medicine Reports*, 4(3): 165–70.

7

ENVIRONMENTAL FACTORS FOR FATIGUE AND INJURY IN BREATH-HOLD/ SCUBA DIVING

Jochen D. Schipke,[1] Lucia Donath,[2] Anne-Kathrin Brebeck[3]
and Sinclair Cleveland[2]

[1]UNIVERSITY HOSPITAL DUESSELDORF, DUESSELDORF
[2]HEINRICH-HEINE-UNIVERSITY, DUESSELDORF
[3]CARL-GUSTAV-CARUS UNIVERSITY, DRESDEN

Introduction

In 1942, the German pathologist Westenhöfer postulated an aquatic mode of life during an early stage of human evolution: the homo aquaticus (Westenhöfer, 1942). This idea was later supported by the British marine biologist Hardy (1960). Gradually adopting an upright posture would have been useful since it would free the hands to poke around and find food, while maybe also allowing the ape to wade into deeper water. Some suggest that a semi-aquatic past can also explain many modern human peculiarities (reduced body hair, increased subcutaneous fat, descended larynx and encephalization).

However, a 1987 symposium summarized the results as failing to support the idea that human ancestors were aquatic. But there was also some evidence that they may have swum and fed in inland lakes and rivers, with the result that modern humans can enjoy brief periods of time spent in the water (Reynolds, 1991).

The oldest archaeological evidence that would confirm human breath-hold diving dates back to at least 5400 BC. A Scandinavian Stone Age culture called Ertebølle (in some sources, 'Kjøkken-møddinger') lived along the coasts of Denmark and Southern Sweden, who are believed to have been a culture of shellfish-eating freedivers, as witnessed by large excavated kitchen middens (Association Internationale pour le Developpement de l'Apnee (AIDA), 2009). Much later, about 900 BC, the Ninive relief likely is the first presentation of a self-contained breathing apparatus used by Phoenician prisoners to escape from Assyrian soldiers by diving in the Tigris.

Historical accounts of breath-hold divers describe professional activities among the sponge divers of Greece, pearl divers in the Persian Gulf and India, and the seafood divers of southern Korea and Japan (Rahn and Yokoyama, 1965). More recently, freediving has gained considerable interest both for amateurs and for competitors. The latter apneists compete in different disciplines that are organized by AIDA.

Although recreational diving using self-contained underwater breathing apparatus has existed for some time, it has become one of the most widely embraced sports of the latter part of the twentieth century (Trevett *et al.*, 2010). Somewhat earlier in the twentieth century, Draeger in Germany released an oxygen rebreather in 1911 and produced an enriched air rebreather with a depth limit of 40 m in 1917. A few years later (1925), Yves Le Prieur released a very successful self-contained underwater breathing apparatus (scuba). In 1942, Hans Hass outfitted a research vessel for scuba expeditions and became the first person to dive in the Red Sea and on Australia's Great Barrier Reef using scuba (Hass, 1973). Only 1 year after that, Emile Gagnan and Jacques Cousteau completed the first commercially available open circuit scuba (= aqualung). Since then, recreational scuba diving has become one of the most rapidly growing tourism activities in the world (Davis, 1997). Interestingly, this document is concerned not with the environmental factors responsible for injury in breath-hold/scuba divers, but rather with the diving environment being injured by divers.

Aquatic environment

As man is not made to live in the water, we deal with some of its characteristics that make the environment water apparently different from the environment air.

Some water properties

One such property is density, which for water is about 800 times higher as for air (1,000 kg.m^{-3} versus 1.2 kg.m^{-3}). Other properties that cause alterations for the diver involve sound, vision and light.

Sound

Due to the high density of water, sound travels at a speed of about 1,500 m.s^{-1} (i.e. almost five times faster than in air, 330 m.s^{-1}). This difference does not directly cause injury to divers. However, the difference is inconvenient because it impedes directional hearing. With regard to that fact, the noise of a ship's engine cannot be easily located, necessitating a cautious ascent to the surface.

Vision

The human eye is adapted to the refractive index of air. After direct contact of the eye with water, the refraction is considerably changed, as cornea and water have quite similar refractive indices. Thus, the diver becomes hyperopic by about 44 diopters. Masks are employed to correct this ametropia. Owing to the air-filled space in front of the eyes, the refractive index of the interface between mask and water causes two effects: images seem magnified by about 33 per cent, and distances seem reduced by about 25 per cent. Thus a 3 m moray eel appears 4 m long, and the 4 m distance seems reduced to only 3 m. Owing to this distortion, beginners tend to get confused if they try to reach for an object.

Vision depends critically on the clarity of the water. Suspended particles can considerably impair vision. The occurrence of microorganisms depends on the season, and tributaries might import large amounts of silt. Not infrequently, silt out (i.e. a situation when visibility is rapidly reduced to functional zero) is initiated by divers making inappropriate use of their fins. Too forceful a motion whirls up silt, an endangering situation particularly in caves, wrecks or in still freshwater environments.

Light

As the diver descends, the water acts as a filter eliminating the red end of the visible spectrum of the sunlight entering the water, leaving only the greenish/bluish end of the spectrum at depths > 30 m. Depending on the depth and clarity of the water, eventually all sunlight is blocked, and the diver must rely on artificial light sources to see underwater.

Water in motion

With respect to their underwater mobility, divers can be regarded as plankton. Thus, water in motion presents hazards. Strong currents might create so much drag on the diver that progress upcurrent is severely restricted, transporting the diver away from the dive access point or the dive boat. In addition, in the open sea, vertical, waterfall-like currents can occur behind shallows. Surge, on the other hand, might carry the diver along and cause impact against the bottom terrain or underwater structures, causing injury. Waves will make tracing of an emerged diver difficult and impair orientation, and breathing on the surface. Breaking waves (surf) can, in addition, cause loss of or damage to the equipment.

Physiologic effects of water

Thermal conductivity – hypothermia

Water transfers heat almost 25 times more effectively than air, with the result that a diver will lose heat much more rapidly unless water is thermoneutral at about 32°C.

There is agreement that almost any level of cooling will substantially reduce muscle power (Drinkwater, 2008). Moreover, cold water is a predisposing factor for muscle cramps. The muscles most commonly affected are those in the sole of the foot, the calf and the thigh. This condition can cause injury if the diver is simultaneously coping with environmental problems such as white water, strong currents or tidal flows (Edmonds *et al.*, 2012). Yet, one study gives rise to some hope. A 6-hour total body immersion in cold water (18°C) did not affect the global contractile properties of leg muscles during static efforts (Coulange *et al.*, 2006).

Another aspect, however, needs mentioning: repeated dives over several days may produce long slow cooling and undetected hypothermia even in tropical water. This affects memory and the speed of reasoning and other cognitive functions, thus reducing a diver's effectiveness and possibly endangering him or her (Webb, 1975).

As thermoneutral water is rare to find, scuba divers create a personal environment to protect against cold. With decreasing ambient temperatures, insulating wetsuits cover more and more of the diver's body surface, using hoods, gloves, booties. In cold waters, wearing up to three layers of soft neoprene material is not uncommon. In even colder waters, drysuits become helpful to protect against hypothermia.

Hypothermia is the condition in which the body's temperature drops below that required for normal metabolism and body functions (e.g. muscle contraction). Once manual dexterity is impaired, correct handling of the equipment is no longer guaranteed. In addition, cognitive efficiency becomes reduced in cold water (Baddeley *et al.*, 1975).

Depending on the core temperature, three stages of hypothermia are defined. In stage one (core temperature drops by 1–2°C), the diver is unable to perform complex tasks, extremities such as hands become numb, and breathing becomes quick and shallow. If a diver starts shivering, then it is always a good idea to surface, in order to avert imminent injury. In stage two (core temperature drops by 2–4°C), the diver becomes disoriented or uncoordinated.

In stage three (core temperature drops below ~ 32°C), the body's metabolism is greatly reduced such that organs begin to fail. The diver is unable to coordinate movement or to speak. Organ failure eventually leads to cardiac arrest and death.

One aspect of heat loss is frequently forgotten. As the inspired air is cold and dry, heat will be lost during expiration by warming and humidifying the inspired air. This proportion of heat loss averages 10 per cent in the dry and warm atmosphere (Sullivan and Edmondson, 2008) and can increase up to 25 per cent depending on the ambient temperature (Cain *et al.*, 1990). In addition, in cold water air consumption can go up by as much as 29 per cent when diving (Dunford and Hayford, 1981).

Besides the elevated heat loss in cold water, another aspect that should be kept in mind is that both cold and pressure at depth seem to contribute to an adverse effect of even a single compressed-air dive on airway narrowing (i.e. on the pulmonary system) (Tetzlaff *et al.*, 2001). In a similar vein, cold was found to induce pulmonary oedema in both swimmers and scuba divers (Wilmshurst *et al.*, 1989). But although pulmonary oedema during swimming or scuba diving might exist, it seems to be extremely rare in healthy subjects (Pons *et al.*, 1995).

Immersion and buoyancy

According to Archimedes' principle, an upward buoyant force is exerted on a body immersed in a fluid. This force is equal to the weight of the fluid the body displaces. Because the density of water is close to the overall density of the human body, the body becomes nearly weightless.

After immersion, positive buoyancy acts on the blood within the vascular system. Thus, blood will be shifted from the extremities towards the thorax (Muth *et al.*, 2005). As one result, blood pressure in the thorax will increase, thereby expanding 'soft' blood vessels such as pulmonary capillaries, caval vein, and the cardiac atriae. Due to the atrial stretch, arrhythmia frequently develops while swimming and diving both with and without breathing apparatus (Itoh *et al.*, 2007; Jung and Stolle, 1981).

Due to pulmonary arterial or venous hypertension, immersion pulmonary oedema might also develop (Koehle *et al.*, 2005; Mahon, 2011). This condition with sudden onset in swimmers, apneists and scuba divers is suspected to be induced by the above hemodynamic changes and to be aggravated by cold water, although it does occur even with adequate thermal protection (Wester *et al.*, 2009) or in warmer waters (Schilling, 2010).

Submersion and diving response

If the human body is submersed, the face will of course also be exposed to water. The consequences of this difference in comparison to only immersion will now be discussed.

In 1870, Paul Bert observed that when ducks put their head under water, their heart rate decreased (Bert, 1870), a finding supported by later experiments on other diving birds, reptiles and diving mammals (Butler and Jones, 1997; Scholander, 1962; Wolf, 1964). In these animals, diving induces bradycardia and peripheral vasoconstriction, together with central blood pooling. As a result, the perfusion of vital organs can be maintained. By taking advantage of this oxygen sparing mechanism (Lemaitre *et al.*, 2009; Valic *et al.*, 2006; Wolf, 1964), diving birds and mammals are able to extend their dive times and consequently can also dive to greater depths (Butler and Jones, 1997). This reflex has also been recognized in humans (Andersson and Schagatay, 1998; Lindholm *et al.*, 1999; Wein *et al.*, 2007). Almost 40 years ago, Landsberg (1976) issued a warning: bradycardia during diving may be a physiological O_2 conserving reflex, or it may be the start of a pathophysiological asphyxial response.

In some studies, the term 'diving reflex' is used to mean bradycardia, whereas in others it is construed as involuntary apnea, peripheral vasoconstriction, increase in dermal resistance (Brown *et al.*, 2003; Schagatay *et al.*, 2007), glottal adduction/constriction (Dutschmann and Paton, 2002; Rozloznik *et al.*, 2009), bronchoconstriction (Mukhtar and Patrick, 1984) or splenic contraction (Hurford *et al.*, 1990; Palada *et al.*, 2007; Schagatay *et al.*, 2007). Consequently, the term 'diving response' has been introduced into the literature to account for these complex reactions.

The term diving reflex will be used here to signify a bradycardic reaction. Although always associated with the term 'diving', bradycardia can occur independently of water and/or cold to the face by solely holding the breath (i.e. arresting respiratory muscles) (Heindl *et al.*, 2004; Hong, 1987; Schaller, 2004; Schipke and Pelzer, 2001).

The effectiveness of this diving reflex – at least in some subjects – is astonishing, with heart rates dropping to 50 beats per minute (Perini *et al.*, 2008) or even 22 beats per minute (Ferrigno *et al.*, 1991). Furthermore, arrhythmia (Ferrigno *et al.*, 1991) and even cardioinhibitory syncope for breath-hold divers (Dzamonja *et al.*, 2010) are not infrequent. The incidence of arrhythmia seems to depend on the water temperature: among Korean Amas, it was 43 per cent in summer (27°C) and increased to 72 per cent in winter (10°C) (Hong *et al.*, 1967). Not surprisingly, during and shortly after breath-hold submersions in cold water, ectopic arrhythmias including premature atrial and junctional complexes, runs of supraventricular tachycardia, and premature ventricular complexes were detected. Recreational scuba diving reduces heart rate in experienced scuba divers (Brebeck *et al.*, 2011) likely due to both an increase in vagal activity and a decrease in cardiac sympathetic activity (Chouchou *et al.*, 2009).

A recent study underlines interindividual differences, describing the quite diverse responses of the human cardiovascular system to facial immersion and classifying them as nonreactive, paradoxical, reactive, or over-reactive (Baranova *et al.*, 2003). In the latter case, excessive diving bradycardia might become the cause of vagal sudden death in breath-hold divers (Alboni *et al.*, 2011; Wolf, 1964).

Blue orb syndrome

This syndrome is definitely not a physiologic reaction to the aquatic environment. Rather, it is a pathophysiologic reaction to the many differences between the environments above and below the surface of the water. After submersion, there is not much to hear and directional hearing is impaired. Colour vision is affected, because absorption tints the environment bluish. Poor visibility may also restrict vision. In addition, the mask narrows the field of vision. Finally, the near weightlessness underwater compromises the vestibular receptors that help maintain equilibrium. In such a situation, divers may experience a form of sensory deprivation that becomes aggravated if the diver loses contact with both the bottom and the surface of the water, leading to spatial disorientation. This problem might develop into agoraphobia and even panic (Campbell, 2009).

On the subject of 'panic': cases of the blue orb syndrome, of an unexpected and strong current, or of a failing regulator present complex environmental situations in which the last thing the diver can afford is to react with panic. Thus, the environment per se is not injurious, but only becomes injurious as a result of the diver's inappropriate reaction.

Personal environment – diving equipment

In order to reasonably stay in the adverse environment 'water', men have developed numerous pieces of equipment. To enable sharp underwater vision, special masks have been developed that also permit pressure equalization to the middle ear. For faster motion, a plethora of different fins has been developed. As a result, this fantastic example of bionics is provided in a wide variety of sizes, shapes and materials.

Various types of ambient pressure diving suits have been developed to prevent heat loss. (= protective work apparel). Dive skins are used in warm waters (> 25°C) to protect against stings, abrasion and sunburn but also against heat loss. Such suits, used by both breath-hold divers and scuba divers, are made from lycra or neoprene. In the range between 25 and 10°C, wetsuits and semi-drysuits are used to limit heat loss. Foamed neoprene – typically used for these suits – can only be made to a thickness of ≤ 10 mm before it becomes impractical to don and wear.

Drysuits are used at low water temperatures (–2°C–15°C). Seals at the neck and wrists prevent entry of water into the suit. Standard air-containing fabric undergarments beneath the suit insulate by maintaining pockets of air between the body and the cold water. In foamed neoprene drysuits the material itself contains insulating air. Both fabric and neoprene drysuits have advantages and disadvantages, creating endless discussions between their respective advocates.

For scuba diving, breathing air/gas is a must. Gases are contained in aluminium or steel bottles in sizes ranging from 7 to 15 L. With filling pressures up to 200 or 300 bar, it is evident that this part of the personal environment (i.e. the bottle with its valve) can become injurious if not properly maintained and checked. The compressors used to fill the bottles need meticulous maintenance to assure provision of the breathing gas free from humidity, dust, pollen, allergens and other microscopic particles. If the compressor is driven by a combustion engine, care must be taken not to take in exhaust gases containing poisonous CO.

Access to the pressurized air involves two stages. First, a regulator is used to reduce the in-bottle pressure to about 6–8 bar above the ambient pressure. The second stage – via a mouthpiece – delivers air at ambient pressure at the onset of the diver's inspiration. Malfunctioning regulators can injure the diver by either increasing respiratory work, delivering water in case of leaking, or rapidly discharging air thus reducing the air supply.

Many other devices have been constructed to keep the scuba divers uninjured. Among others, the dive watch informs about the elapsed dive time, the depth gauge informs about the present depth, the pressure gauge indicates the remaining air supply, and the compass helps to maintain orientation. Over the decades, a wide range of dive computers has been developed to inform, in particular, about the saturation with nitrogen in order to prevent from N_2 bubble-induced injury. And it should not be forgotten that a knife or scissors can be useful in case of entanglement.

When a dive suit is worn in colder waters, the suit will exert positive buoyancy. Then, weight belts are required to achieve neutral bouncy. With increasing depth, the neoprene in a wetsuit or drysuit will be compressed. The same is true for the air within a fabric or a neoprene drysuit. The result is that negative buoyancy develops. Buoyancy compensators are employed to prevent undesirable fin flapping for balancing. These devices contain a bladder, which helps to control buoyancy by adjusting the volume of air in the bladder.

Fatigue – exertion

Fatigue

Fatigue is defined as weariness usually caused by mental or physical overexertion (Humphre, 1968).

Leaving professional diving/technical diving or experimental deep diving with sometimes extremely extended safety stops aside, mental overexertion leading to fatigue can likely be excluded for both apneists and scuba divers. On the contrary, if the results of studies on patients watching fish in an aquarium can be translated to the underwater scenario, scuba diving ought to even reduce anxiety and/or sympathetic drive that can lead to mental overexertion (Barker *et al.*, 2004; Kidd and Kidd, 1999).

Nevertheless, an indirect connection might exist. Repeated diving with inadequate thermal protection may lead to an unwillingness to dive again or to disabling fatigue – states that are now known to be associated with being cold (Webb, 1975).

Another aspect of fatigue – namely feeling tired after a scuba dive using compressed air (Harris *et al.*, 2003) – depends on the N_2 partial pressure and will be addressed later.

Exertion

Prior to diving, the diver might be faced with considerable physical exertion, when heavy equipment needs to be transported at high temperatures and over longer distances. Exertion becomes even worse if the diver needs to climb steep gradients. Such situations might lead to fatigue, and it is conceivable that such fatigue might adversely influence the subsequent dive. As such, transporting relatively heavy equipment to and from the dive site does not seem to induce musculoskeletal injury causing low-back problems in healthy adults (Knaepen *et al.*, 2009). With the advent of scuba diving by children, that aspect deserves particular attention.

Physical exertion has played a role in a number of events during scuba diving. Between 1972 and 2005, 26 fatal accidents (9 per cent of 283) in Australia were ultimately triggered by overexertion (Lippmann, 2011). It is worth mentioning that the mean age of the scuba divers with exertion-related triggers was higher than with other triggers, such as those that were equipment-related, implying that the fitness to dive decreases with age.

In concert with the relatively high proportion of fatal accidents ascribable to overexertion, Di Fabio *et al.* (2012) tested the hypothesis that diving as an intense physical activity would be characterized by cerebral micro-vascular distress and thus be associated with an increased prevalence of developing headache. The fact that the hypothesis could not be confirmed suggests that scuba diving does not represent an overly intense physical activity.

The present authors do not share the concept of scuba diving per se as an intense physical activity. This is because in quite a few textbooks, a breathing gas consumption of only 20 L.min^{-1} is assumed for calculating the gas volume needed for the entire dive, corresponding to an O_2 consumption of about 0.8 L.min^{-1}. In occupational medicine, O_2 consumption up to 1.0 L.min^{-1} is regarded as 'easy work' (Zimmermann, 2012). If, on the other hand, heart rate correlates with O_2 consumption and metabolic demand (Green, 2011), then studies reporting decreases in heart rate while scuba diving (Chouchou *et al.*, 2009; Schipke and Pelzer, 2001) suggest that this activity cannot be regarded as particularly stressful. Moreover, diving has been catagorized as a 'mean' static and 'low' dynamic load (Maron and Mitchell, 1994). Thus, fatalities due to exertion during scuba diving are difficult to explain, unless one takes respiration and respiratory muscles into consideration.

The density of the respiratory gases increases in proportion to depth. At 40 m, for example, the density of air is increased by a factor of five, resulting in increased flow resistance, increased work of breathing, and decreased maximum breathing capacity (Lanphier and Camporesi, 1993). In addition, respiratory excursions can be impaired by the personal environment, such as malfunctional regulators or tight neoprene suits. If under these circumstances physical stress is exerted due to high diving speed, strong current or positive/negative buoyancy, then the depth and and rate of respiration will increase. After some time, the expiratory muscles will fatigue first due to the increased respiratory workload, which results in an increased functional residual capacity. In parallel, as CO_2 elimination is impaired, hypercapnia develops signalling dyspnea. In a vicious cycle, respiration is stimulated, which in turn intensifies overexertion of the expiratory muscles. The term 'essoufflement' (becoming out of breath) has been coined for this particular and threatening situation (see Klingmann and Tetzlaff, 2012). In consequence, training of the respiratory muscles has been recommended to improve swimming endurance at depth (Ray *et al.*, 2008; Wylegala *et al.*, 2007).

Whether or not scuba diving must be regarded as a physically demanding sport, a minimum fitness to dive is needed. Fitness can be assessed using bicycle ergometry, but because different muscle groups are employed on a bicycle and with the fins, a sophisticated fit to dive test has been developed to assess underwater swimming competence with scuba equipment and fins (Steinberg *et al.*, 2011).

Dysbarism

This term does not sound promising. In fact, it refers to medical conditions resulting from changes in ambient pressure. Various activities are associated with pressure changes. Breath-hold and scuba diving are the most frequently cited examples, but pressure changes also affect people who move in different altitudes or work in an environment with increased (caissons, hyperbaric chambers) or decreased (aeroplanes) pressure.

Pressure equals force per unit area applied in a direction perpendicular to the surface of an object. While the official SI unit is given in Pascal (1 Pa = 1 $N.m^{-2}$), a popular pressure unit in the context of diving is 'bar', which equals the pressure of a water column 10 m high. The air pressure at sea level is roughly 1 bar. Thus, if a diver is down to 10 m, the total pressure will equal 2 bar.

Direct effects of pressure on the human body are of no concern, as organic tissue is almost incompressible. A good example for that statement is the sperm whale, which blithely dives as deep as 3,000 m, which makes it the deepest diving mammal.

Pressure, on the one hand, has a considerable effect on gas-filled spaces. On the other hand, increased partial pressures of mixed gas can greatly contribute to injury by making the gases toxic.

Gas-filled spaces

For the gas-filled spaces in the body, the physical law of Boyle and Mariotte applies. This law states that the product of pressure and volume of a gas in a sealed container is constant. This means that a closed volume of 10 L gas in a balloon at sea level (1 bar) will be decreased to 5 L at an ambient pressure of 2 bar (i.e. the balloon's volume will be halved at a water depth of 10 m). If, on the other hand, a sealed balloon containing 5 L gas starts ascending from a depth of 10 m, its volume will have doubled at the surface, if it does not burst beforehand.

For a gas volume contained in a rigid, sealed space, a descent would lead to a relative negative pressure within that space, an example being the middle ear. If no care is taken to equilibrate, such a pressure difference can induce injury – in this case, barotrauma of the ear. Note, however, that it is not the pressure per se that is traumatizing, but the pressure gradient.

Such barotraumata can affect both breath-hold and scuba divers and they involve air-filled spaces both outside and inside the diver. Outside the diver, one thinks of goggles/masks and drysuits. Inside the diver, there are the sinuses in the head, and especially the middle ear and the lungs.

Increased partial pressures

Because other gases play no major role for recreational diving, only the effects of nitrogen and oxygen are addressed in the following.

Nitrogen

Saturation/desaturation in tissue. Nitrogen (N_2), being inert, is not metabolized, but can be dissolved in organic tissue. The amount of N_2 molecules dissolved in the tissue is governed by Henry's Law, which depends on the partial pressure of nitrogen (pN_2) and of the solubility coefficient of the various tissues: N_2 dissolves quickly in some tissues (blood, for example) and only slowly in others (fat, cartilage). Thus, the rate at which different portions of the body become saturated will vary. Saturation/desaturation with any gas develops exponentionally characterized by the half time.

For calculating simulations, up to 16 different compartments (tissues) are used, covering a range of half times from 4 to 635 minutes. As a rule of thumb, a tissue is completely saturated after about six times its half time. On a dive, N_2 will be stored in biological tissue during the descent, both in breath-hold and in scuba divers. In the latter, N_2 concentration will further increase during the bottom time. If during the ascent (i.e. during decompression) enough time is given, N_2 is eliminated from the various tissues. The process of desaturation lasts up to six times longer than saturation. Yet, desaturation half times of up to 1,280 minutes lay outside the range that can be explained with physiology (Sicko *et al.*, 2003).

If for some reason the time for desaturation is aborted, intra- and extravascular N_2 micro-bubbles can arise (Vann *et al.*, 2011), which are not transported towards the lungs to be exhaled, but remain in the tissue causing decompression sickness (DCS) (Lettnin, 1994), thereby affecting almost all compartments of the body.

Nitrogen narcosis. N_2 has another unpleasant characteristic: increased pressures make it a psychotropic substance (Bennett, 1969; Jennings, 1969) capable of impairing psychomotor capabilities, intellectual efficiency, concentration and short-term memory, as well as manual dexterity (Behnke *et al.*, 1935; Williamson *et al.*, 1989). At depths ≥ 30 m, 'rapture of the deep' may develop (Behnke *et al.*, 1935; Lettnin, 1994). This narcotic effect is a consequence of N_2-induced 'thickening' of the pre-synaptic membrane, which is suggested to be a consequence of N_2 dissolving at increased pressures in the lipid bilayer of cell membranes (Paton, 1975). If so, neurotransmitters can no longer be released into the synaptic cleft to be transmitted to the post-synaptic membrane and convey information.

Oxygen

Oxygen at increased pressures (hyperoxia) likely exerts toxic effects via oxidative stress, which is considered to be an imbalance between formation of O-radicals and antioxidative mechanisms. In cells subjected to hyperoxia, substantial amounts of reactive oxygen species (ROS) can be formed (Finne *et al.*, 2008; Kot *et al.*, 2003; Narkowicz *et al.*, 1993). One important ROS effect is the peroxidation of lipids with ensuing injury of the cell membranes and cell organelles (Janero, 1990; Pelaia *et al.*, 1995).

The authors of this article are confident that ROS – once formed in excess – will not much differentiate between cell types and will injure almost all of them. The reason why to date almost only the pulmonary system and the central nervous system have been reported as targets of injury might depend on the fact that the consequences to these systems are either easily assessed (lungs: spirometry) or become almost instantly apparent (CNS: seizure).

Injury due to dysbarism

Breath-hold diver

In 1932, the Japanese occupational scientist Teruoka became concerned about the occupational health of the amas, and studied the strenuous exertion and the hazards associated with their breath-hold diving for seafood to depths up to 20 m (Teruoka, 1932). Teruako was already aware that N_2 could have an adverse effect on these professional divers.

The number of Japanese and Korean amas and other divers from the Pacific region is likely decreasing. However, the number of spear fishers suffering accidents is on the rise, in particular during championships or using scooters. Finally, an increasing number of freedive athletes participate in championships, including some deep diving categories. In addition to this more 'professional' breath-hold diving, recreational breath-hold diving (including also snorkelling on the surface) has become one of the most widely embraced sports of the latter part of the twentieth century (Best Diving, 2012).

Breath-hold records are already very striking but they will surely be beaten in the near future. As a result, hypoxia, increased ambient pressure on the pulmonary gas volume, and increased gas partial pressures present major challenges (Lindholm and Lundgren, 2009). These three aspects of the subaquatic environment will now be addressed briefly, as they can readily injure the diver.

Hypoxia

This deleterious factor can lead to loss of consciousness. Hypoxia is not uncommon and is sometimes fatal in breath-hold divers. Competitors in the static apnea discipline hyperventilate before a dive attempt. This may lead to loss of motor control, but rarely to loss of consciousness (Lindholm and Lundgren, 2009). Likewise, hypoxia during ascent with resultant loss of motor control (Fitz-Clarke, 2006) and subsequent drowning is relatively common among spear fishermen (Landsberg, 1976).

The present world record in the 'static apnea' discipline is 11 minutes 35 seconds. With such hypoxic periods in mind, it is not surprising that in trained breath-hold divers a marker of brain damage (S100B) is increased. Apart from such acute hypoxic effects, long-term effects must be suspected that might even cumulate (Andersson *et al.*, 2009). On the other hand, repeated hypoxemia in elite breath-hold divers had no impact on performance of standard neuropsychological tasks (Ridgway and McFarland, 2006).

Pressure on gas volume

According to the Boyle-Mariotte Law, pulmonary gas volume decreases as ambient pressure increases. At the very most, total lung capacity (TLC) can be reduced to the residual volume (RV) (Schaefer *et al.*, 1968), because at RV alveolar collapse becomes possible (Fitz-Clarke, 2006; Steimle *et al.*, 2011). Using the ratio of TLC (6.0 L) to RV (1.5 L), TLC could be reduced by a factor of about four, which means that ambient pressure could be increased to about 4 bar at the most extreme. Thus, theoretically, dives to ~ 30 m would be feasible. However, the current world record in breath-hold deep diving (male, no limits) was set at 214 m (22.4 bar). Thus, TLC would roughly be decreased by a factor of 22 – to illustrate: from a 10 L bucket of water to a 0.5 L beaker of water.

As this is not compatible with physiology, other mechanisms must come into play, one being blood shift from the periphery into the thorax amounting to 1.0 L (Anthonisen, 1984; Schaefer *et al.*, 1968) and decreasing RV to 0.50 L. But there would still be a pressure gradient between ambient pressure and intrathoracic pressure. Because of the negative pressure within the lungs, pulmonary barotrauma (lung squeeze) in breath-hold deep divers is not uncommon (Kiyan *et al.*, 2001).

Hemoptysis is the visible consequence of pulmonary barotrauma, while any less severe damage might remain subclinical (Scherhag *et al.*, 2005). In contrast to breath-hold divers, scuba divers will not suffer from negative pressure pulmonary barotrauma while descending, as long as they breathe normally using the regulator.

During descent, both breath-hold divers and scuba divers are confronted with equalization (negative) pressure in the mask and the middle ear. Both manoeuvres are presumably easy for the healthy scuba diver. Nevertheless, the most common injury scuba divers experience is some form of barotrauma to the ear (Delphia, 1999). In severe cases, the tympanic membrane will rupture and acute vertigo can develop if cold water enters the middle ear.

The breath-hold deep diver cannot equalize his or her goggles and has not much air left in the mouth and throat to equalize the middle ear. Thus, glossopharyngeal exsufflation (sucking out air from the lungs) (Novalija *et al.*, 2007) has been developed to avoid barotrauma of the middle ear.

Gas partial pressure

After protracted controversy, it is only now accepted that decompression sickness (DCS) due to increased pN_2 might also affect breath-hold divers, although the first report dates back almost 45 years (Moretti, 1968). Some more recent case reports make clear that not only 'normal' breath-hold divers are severely affected (suffering cerebral DCS) (Gempp and Blatteau, 2006; Moon and Gray, 2010), but also professional divers (Tamaki *et al.*, 2010) and divers engaged in underwater hunting (Thorsen *et al.*, 2007). The large body of evidence on DCS in breath-hold divers has been summarized in three recent reviews (Fitz-Clarke, 2009; Lemaitre *et al.*, 2009; Schipke *et al.*, 2006).

Scuba diver

Pressure on gas volume

If a diver with a cold starts a dive, the narrow openings of the sinuses may become obstructed in the course of a longer lasting dive. In this case, air will expand during ascent but cannot escape. In the occluded sinuses, considerable pain will develop with increasing pressure within the sinus. Occlusion of the Eustachian tube bears the risk of an ear barotrauma. In contrast to ear barotrauma during descent, the injury to the ear drum is now the result of positive pressure within the middle ear.

In case of an emergency ascent, the scuba diver might suffer from positive pressure pulmonary barotrauma. During such an ascent, air tends to increase its volume in proportion to the decreasing ambient pressure. If the diver cannot or does not expire, intrathoracic pressure increases, likely overdistending and even rupturing the delicate alveoli.

Air from ruptured alveoli can enter the intrathoracic space and ascend within the thorax (gas in the supraclavicular region) to result in mediastinal and cutaneous (surgical) emphysema. Air may also enter the pleural cavity inducing pneumothorax. Finally, air can enter pulmonary veins, with the risk of being transported into the arterial system. The resulting arterial gas embolism (AGE) represents a massive hazard because of gas bubbles being transported to the central nervous system.

The danger of injuring the alveolar membranes should not be underestimated, as these membranes may rupture if they are subjected to even quite small pressure differences (e.g. when the ambient water pressure falls by about 0.1 bar below the intrapulmonary pressure, corresponding to an ascent of about 1 m towards the surface) (Edmonds and Thomas, 1972).

Air trapping

This situation occurs during ascent when small pulmonary areas become overinflated owing to narrowing or obstructing small bronchioli. Such obstructions might result from bronchial spasm, mucous congestion, common cold, bronchitis or smoking. Depending on the pressure difference, the alveolar membranes might rupture.

N_2 bubbles

Nitrogen bubbles are formed if this gas is not given enough time for duly release. Then, decompression sickness (DCS) might develop, also known as 'caisson workers disease', 'divers' disease' or 'the bends'. If DCS symptoms involve the skin, the musculoskeletal system or the lymphatic system, the sickness is termed type I DCS (simple). If symptoms involve other organs such as the inner ear or the CNS, the sickness is classified type II DCS (serious) (Golding *et al.*, 1960). Outcomes of type II DCS are usually worse than those of type I DCS. Because neurological symptoms can still develop after 'simple' DCS, today the classification is not very useful in diagnosis, as both have the same initial management.

Typically, N_2 bubbles within the blood will be transported to the lungs and will be filtered there. If shunt mechanisms come into play, bubbles may be transported to the arterial system (Ljubkovic *et al.*, 2011). In this context, a patent foramen ovale has been blamed, and therefore some authors have suggested that it should be closed (Billinger *et al.*, 2011), but others have rejected this suggestion (Gempp *et al.*, 2012). Alternatively, more 'conservative' dives have been the only recommendation (Klingmann *et al.*, 2012).

If, however, N_2 bubbles pass into the arterial system they might be transported to the CNS and occlude smaller arterial vessels. This N_2-related type of AGE can be just as injurious as pulmonary barotrauma-related AGE, causing ischemia and necrosis in the post-occlusive tissue. As a precise diagnosis cannot always be made, DCS and AGE are classified together as decompression illness (DCI).

N_2 toxicity

At greater depths, the increased pN_2 may induce narcosis, possibly decreasing some cognitive capacities (Brebeck *et al.*, 2011; Kiessling *et al.*, 1962) that will not necessarily become noticeable. At depths ≥ 40 m, the most dangerous effects of the 'rapture of the depth' impair decision-making ability and focus, judgement, and coordination. The syndrome may cause exhilaration, on the one hand, or extreme anxiety and depression, on the other. In serious cases, the diver may feel overconfident, disregarding normal safe diving practices (Lippmann and Mitchell, 2005). Thus, N_2 narcosis can cause serious, indirect injury if not reasonably terminated. In order to avoid the risk of narcotic N_2 actions, a maximum depth of 40 m is recommended for recreational scuba diving.

O_2 *toxicity*

Two different compartments are especially prone to oxidative stress-related injury: central nervous system (Paul Bert Effect) and pulmonary system (Lorrain Smith Effect).

Paul Bert Effect. As far as O_2 toxicity is concerned, the worst case scenario for the CNS is seizure (grand mal) (Lettnin, 1994; Smerz, 2004; Thalmann, 2007), which in conservative recreational diving ought to be extremely rare. However, with the advent of closed circuit rebreathing systems or with the usage of oxygen enriched air (nitrox), pO_2 values are readily increased even in recreational divers. Adverse conditions, such as exertion, cold, hypoglycemia, hypercapnia and dehydration facilitate the occurence of toxic O_2-related effects (Muth and Rademacher, 2006; Urban & Fischer (Hrsg.), 2003).

Lorrain Smith Effect. Prolonged and high O_2 concentrations can cause collapse of the alveoli in the lungs thereby reducing pulmonary volumes and conductances (Clark and Lambertsen, 1971). Symptoms of such injury are increased respiration rate, pulmonary pain, increased respiratory resistance and tightness in the chest (Gienow and Gienow, 2010; Muth and Rademacher, 2006; Smith, 1899).

On the other hand, O_2-induced injury seems to depend to a considerable extent on ambient pressure and dive time (van Ooij *et al.*, 2012). Yet, caution is advised as, in contrast to injury to the CNS, injury to the pulmonary system might accumulate (Carraway and Piantadosi, 1999; Shykoff, 2008).

Other oxidative stress-related injury. More recently, the focus has been concentrated on effects of oxidative stress on the vascular endothelium. Evidence is building up that even after a single air dive (Brubakk *et al.*, 2005) endothelial dysfunction of large arteries can develop (Madden *et al.*, 2010) that resembles that in patients with atherosclerosis. The dysfunction might accumulate and can persist (Obad *et al.*, 2010). The scuba diver, very likely, is not aware of this injury but might suffer from early or aggravated atherosclerosis late after abandoning scuba diving.

Data on diving fatalities

As a matter of fact, injuries and deaths are not uncommon in both types of diving. It will become clear that hard figures are not readily available, as many divers have a tendency to dissimulate, and for several other reasons, injuries and deaths often remain unreported.

Breath-hold diving fatalities

A recent series of 60 snorkelling deaths was compared to a previous series of 132 deaths. Interestingly, a change in the demographics was found. In the later series, divers were significantly older, and the proportion of women was higher. The three major causes of death were drowning (45 per cent), cardiac events (30 per cent) and hypoxia from hyperventilation and/or ascent producing drowning (20 per cent). Other causes included deaths from marine animals and trauma.

Tourists were over-represented in the drowning and cardiac groups. Contributors to their death were inexperience, medical and physical unfitness, equipment and environmental factors. Drowning usually occurred in situations with inadequate supervision, thus delaying rescue and resuscitation. In contrast, the cardiac events often happened in calm, still water, the deaths frequently being predictable from the divers' cardiovascular history.

The deaths in younger, fitter, experienced divers were more related to hypoxia after hyperventilation and breath-holding, often occurring during ascent and associated with spear fishing or underwater endurance attempts (Best Diving, 2012).

The entire hopelessness of providing sound statistics becomes apparent if one remembers that both the number of apneists and the number of annual fatalities are estimates. Thus, these numbers do not convey much information that could help prevent cases if their background (e.g. adverse aquatic environment or marine animals) were better known to the reader.

Data acquisition

As mentioned, data are sparse, contradictory and often not current. For some years now, Divers Alert Network (DAN) – the diving industry's largest association – has been dedicated to the safety of recreational divers. Among other activities, DAN operates a hotline. In 2007, roughly 2,500 calls came in at DAN regarding actual cases, roughly seven per day.

Barotrauma accounted for 347 cases. Within that category, middle ear barotrauma (61 per cent) constituted the major portion, while pulmonary barotrauma (15 per cent) was less frequent but likely more threatening.

As one result of operating the hotline, DAN publishes reports on breath-hold and scuba dive injuries (Divers Alert Network, 2008). In the more recent past, data on breath-hold and scuba dive fatalities have been collected for different areas in the world (e.g. for the Asia/Pacific area) (Divers Alert Network, 2012).

The data exhibit differences between breath-hold divers and scuba divers in terms of numbers and problems that have created the fatal situation. The four most important disabling agents in breath-hold diving were general health, blackout, boat strike and animals, together accounting for 88 per cent of the incidents in 2006. In comparison, the four leading disabling agents in scuba diving were asphyxia, arterial gas embolism, cardiac events and trauma, accounting for 93 per cent of the fatalities.

Is diving dangerous?

The largest number of dive-related fatalities has been reported for the USA/Canada, over the period of 10 years an average of 80 cases per annum. Compared with the Asia/Pacific area, the number of victims seems high, but the USA/Canada very likely have the largest estimated population of recreational divers in the world. The number of fatalities – at least for North America – is slowly declining.

The obvious question arises: Do these dive-related fatalities suggest that diving is dangerous? There is no firm answer for breath-hold diving and the situation is not very different for scuba diving (Gibb, 2012). And if one wants to start calculations, one quickly realizes not only the lack of clear-cut numbers, but also of clear-cut definitions. The first problem: Is somebody who last dived 3 years ago still counted as a diver? Thus, the worldwide numbers vary. One estimate in 2008 reported on 2,700,000 active recreational divers in the USA, 7,000,000 divers worldwide, and 500,000 more training every year (Levett and Millar, 2008). But what about drop-outs? The next question concerns the number of dives a diver makes per year. One estimate states 12 dives (Davison, 2007). If, on average, 80 divers die per annum, then 2.5 US divers would die per 1,000,000 dives, equal to 0.25 deaths per 100,000 dives. Similarly, a diving fatality occurs in one out of every 211,864 dives according to DAN (Denoble *et al.*, 2010). These rates seem somewhat low if compared to numbers from 'firm' sources, which vary from 0.8 to 1.6 per 100,000 dives (National Safety Council, 1989), 1.0 to 2.4 per 100,000 in Japan (Ikeda and Ashida, 2000), and 3 to 6 per 100,000 in Scotland (Trevett *et al.*, 2001). The relatively high rates in Scotland might, at least in part, be affected by the local environmental conditions (i.e. low water temperature, swell and current).

Whether these rates seem risky or not is a matter of personal opinion. For a more objective view, compare the above fatality rates with those of two other activities: one out of every 126,626 runners died of sudden cardiac arrest while running a marathon between 1975 and 2003 (National Safety Council, 2004) and one out of every 5,555 registered drivers in the US died in a car accident in 2008 (Census Bureau, 2008).

To further exemplify the difficulties associated with answering the question 'How safe is diving?', an additional measure, the individual risk per annum, is presented. The individual risk for recreational diving was 1:6,000, for motor vehicle accidents 1:6,493, and for jogging 1:7,700. The risks in these activities are of comparable magnitude (Denoble *et al.*, 2008). However, deaths during occupational exposures were often considerably lower: fatalities to employees with 1:125,000 by a factor of about 20 (Health and Security Excecutive, 2001).

Closing remarks

Breath-hold and scuba diving are fascinating activities that are subject to injuries and fatalities mediated mainly through the aquatic environment. Considering why divers suffer from injury and fatal injury, one comes to the understanding that for a responsible diver who is seeking training and is diving within his or her limits, the risks of diving are not abnormally high. One must remember that driving to the dive site bears nearly the same risk as scuba diving. Adherence to sound safety practices, good decision-making and properly preparing the personal diving environment will decrease the risk that the individual diver will become a victim.

An alternate view in closing: as both breath-hold diving and scuba diving find an increasing number of followers, injury to the environment through divers themselves might soon become alarming.

Some physics

Archimedes' principle. Any object, wholly or partially immersed in a liquid, is buoyed up by a force equal to the weight of the liquid displaced by the object.

Boyle – Mariotte. The product of the pressure and volume for a gas is a constant for a fixed amount of gas at a fixed temperature.

In mathematical terms:

$$P \bullet V = \text{constant}$$

where: P = pressure and V = volume.

Dalton. The total pressure of a mixture of ideal gases is equal to the sum of the partial pressures of the individual gases in the mixture. For example, air is a gas mixture and consists essentially of nitrogen (N_2: 78 per cent), oxygen (O_2: 21 per cent) and noble gases, in particular Argon (Ar: 1 per cent).

In mathematical terms:

$$p = pN_2 + pO_2 + pAr$$

where: p = total pressure of the gas mixture, pN_2 = partial pressure of nitrogen, pO_2 = partial pressure of oxygen, and pAr = partial pressure of argon.

Henry. The amount of a gas that will go into solution in a liquid is proportional to the partial pressure of that gas. If the partial pressure of a gas is twice as high, then on the average twice as many molecules will hit the liquid surface in a given time interval, and on the average twice as many will be captured and go into solution.

In mathematical terms:

$$C_{gas} = \alpha_{(temp,\ gas,\ liquid)} \times P_{gas}$$

where: C_{gas} = concentration of the gas in a liquid and $\alpha_{(temp,\ gas,\ liquid)}$ = solubility coefficient. α depends on the liquid's temperature, the type of gas, and the type of liquid.

References

Association Internationale pour le Developpement de l'Apnee (AIDA) (2009) *History of Freediving and Apnea*, available at: www.aidainternational.org/freediving/history (accessed 16 September 2012).

Alboni, P., Alboni, M. and Gianfranchi, L. (2011) 'Simultaneous occurrence of two independent vagal reflexes: a possible cause of vagal sudden death', *Heart*, 97(8): 623–5.

Andersson, J. P. and Schagatay, E. (1998) 'Arterial oxygen desaturation during apnea in humans', *Undersea and Hyperbaric Medicine*, 25(1): 21–5.

Andersson, J. P., Linér, M. H. and Jönsson, H. (2009) 'Increased serum levels of the brain damage marker S100B after apnea in trained breath-hold divers: a study including respiratory and cardiovascular observations', *Journal of Applied Physiology*, 107(3): 809–15.

Anthonisen, N. R. (1984) 'Physiology of diving respiration', in C. W. Shilling, C. B. Carlston and R. A. Mathias (eds), *The Physicians Guide to Diving Medicine*, New York: Plenum Press, pp. 71–85.

Baddeley, A. D., Cuccaro, W. J., Egstrom, G. H., Weltman, G. and Willis, M. A. (1975) 'Cognitive efficiency of divers working in cold water', *Human Factors*, 17(5): 446–54.

Baranova, T. L., Kovalenko, R. I., Molchanov, A. A., Sviridenko, M. V., Ianvareva, I. N. and Zhekalov, A. N. (2003) 'Mechanisms of human adaptation to hypoxia', *Russian Journal of Physiology*, 89(11): 1370–9.

Barker, S. B., Rasmussen, K. G. and Best, A. M. (2004) 'Effect of aquariums on electroconvulsive therapy patients', *Anthrozoös*, 16(3): 229–40.

Behnke, A. R., Thomson, R. M. and Motley, E. P. (1935) 'The psychologic effects from breathing air at 4 atmospheres pressure', *American Journal of Physiology*, 112: 554–8.

Bennett, P. B. (1969) 'Measurement and mechanisms of inert gas narcosis', *Journal of Occupational Medicine and Toxicology*, 11(5): 217–22.

Bert, P. (1870) *Physiologie de la respiration*, Paris: Bailliere.

Best Diving (2012) *Types of Diving and its Problems*, available at: www.best-diving.org/types-of-diving-and-its-problems/ (accessed 20 September 2012).

Billinger, M., Zbinden, R., Mordasini, R., Windecker, S., Schwerzmann, M., Meier, B. and Seiler, C. (2011) 'Patent foramen ovale closure in recreational divers: effect on decompression illness and ischaemic brain lesions during long-term follow-up', *Heart*, 97(23): 1932–7.

Brebeck, A., Muth, T., Koch, A., Kähler, W., Balestra, C., Schipke, J. and Deussen, A. (2011) 'Recreational scuba diving with enriched air nitrox: pulmonary injury?', *Proceedings of the 37th Annual Meeting of the European Underwater and Baromedical Society*, Gdansk: European Underwater and Baromedical Society.

Brown, C. M., Sanya, E. O. and Hilz, M. J. (2003) 'Effect of cold face stimulation on cerebral blood flow in humans', *Brain Resrearch Bulletin*, 61(1): 81–6.

Brubakk, A. O., Duplancic, D., Valic, Z. Palada, I., Obad, A., Bakovic, D., Wisloff, D. and Dujic, Z. (2005) 'A single air dive reduces arterial endothelial function in man', *Journal of Physiology*, 566(3): 901–6.

Butler, P. J. and Jones, D. R. (1997) 'Physiology of diving of birds and mammals', *Physiological Reviews*, 77(3): 837–99.

Cain, J. B., Livingstone, S. D., Nolan, R. W. and Keefe, A. A. (1990) 'Respiratory heat loss during work at various ambient temperatures', *Respiratory Physiololy*, 79(2): 145–50.

Campbell, E. (2009) *Panic Attacks and the Blue Orb Syndrome*, available at: www.scuba-doc.com/bluorb.htm (accessed 20 September 2012).

Carraway, M. S. and Piantadosi, C. A. (1999) 'Oxygen toxicity', *Respiratory Care Clinics*, 5(2): 265–95.

Census Bureau (2008) *Bureau of Economic Analysis*, available at: www.census.gov (accessed 30 September 2012).

Chouchou, F., Pichot, V., Garet, M., Barthélémy, J. C. and Roche, F. (2009) 'Dominance in cardiac parasympathetic activity during real recreational scuba diving', *European Journal of Applied Physiology*, 106(3): 345–52.

Clark, J. M. and Lambertsen, C. J. (1971) 'Pulmonary oxygen toxicity: a review', *Pharmacological Reviews*, 23(2): 37–133.

Coulange, M., Hug, F., Kipson, N., Robinet, C., Desruelle, A. V., Melin, B., Jimenez, C., Galland, F. and Jammes, Y. (2006) 'Consequences of prolonged total body immersion in cold water on muscle performance and EMG activity', *European Journal of Physiology*, 452(1): 91–101.

Davis, D. (1997) 'The development and nature of recreational scuba diving in Australia: a study in economics, environmental management and tourism', unpublished doctoral dissertation, The University of Queensland.

Davison, B. (2007) *How Many Divers Are There?*, available at: www.undercurrent.org/UCnow/dive_magazine/2007/HowManyDivers200705.html (accessed 10 September 2012).

Delphia, B. (1999) *Common Ear Injuries while Diving*, available at: www.diversalertnetwork.org/medical/articles/Common_%20Ear_Injuries_While_Diving (accessed 10 September 2012).

Denoble, P. J., Caruso, J. L., Dear, G. L., Pieper, C. F. and Vann, R. D. (2008) 'Common causes of open-circuit recreational diving fatalities', *Undersea and Hyperbaric Medicine*, 35(6): 393–406.

Denoble, P. J., Marroni, A. and Vann, R. D. (2010) 'Annual fatality rates and associated risk factors for recreational scuba diving', in R. D. Vann and M. A. Lang (eds), *Recreational Diving Fatalities Workshop Proceedings*, Durham, NC: Divers Alert Network, pp. 73–85.

Di Fabio, R., Vanacore, N., Davassi, C., Serrao, M. and Pierelli, F. (2012) 'Scuba diving is not associated with high prevalence of headache: a cross sectional study in men', *Headache*, 52(3): 385–92.

Divers Alert Network (2008) *Annual Diving Report*, available at: www.diversalertnetwork.org/medical/report/2008DANDivingReport.pdf (accessed 17 September 2012).

Divers Alert Network (2012) *Diving Fatalities Throughout the Asia-Pacific Region*, available at: www.danasiapacific.org/main/diving_safety/fatality_historical_data.php (accessed 17 September 2012).

Drinkwater, E. (2008) 'Effects of peripheral cooling on characteristics of local muscle', in F. Marino (ed.), *Thermoregulation and Human Performance. Physiological and Biological Aspects*, Basel: Karger, pp. 74–88.

Dunford, R. and Hayford. J. (1981) *Section 3: Diving Physiology*, National Oceanic and Atmospheric Administration, available at: www.jastra.com.pl/nurek/subsec34.htm (accessed 19 September 2012).

Dutschmann, M. and Paton, J. F. (2002) 'Influence of nasotrigeminal afferents on medullary respiratory neurones and upper airway patency', *European Journal of Physiology*, 444(1–2): 227–35.

Dzamonja, G., Tank, J., Heusser, K., Palada, I., Valic, Z., Bakovic, D., Obad, A., Ivancev, V., Breskovic, T., Diedrich, A., Luft, F. C., Dujic, Z. and Jordan, J. (2010) 'Glossopharyngeal insufflation induces cardio-inhibitory syncope in apnea divers', *Clinical Autonimic Research*, 20(6): 381–4.

Edmonds, C. and Thomas, R. L. (1972) 'Medical aspects of diving. Part 3', *Medical Journal of Australia*, 2: 1300–4.

Edmonds, C., Thomas, B., McKenzie, B. and Pennefather, J. (2012) *Diving Medicine for Scuba Divers: Chapter 27, Cold and Hypothermia*, available at: www.divingmedicine.info/Ch%2027%20SM10c.pdf (accessed 15 September 2012).

Ferrigno, M., Grassi, B., Ferretti, G., Costa, M., Marconi, C., Cerretelli, P. and Lundgren, C. (1991) 'Electrocardiogram during deep breath-hold dives by elite divers', *Undersea Biomedical Research*, 18(2): 81–91.

Finne, E. F., Olsvik, P. A., Berntssen, M. H., Hylland, K. and Tollefsen, K. E. (2008) 'The partial pressure of oxygen affects biomarkers of oxidative stress in cultured rainbow trout (Oncorhynchus mykiss) hepatocytes', *Toxicology in Vitro: An International Journal Published in Association with BIBRA*, 22(6): 1657–61.

Fitz-Clarke, J. R. (2006) 'Adverse events in competitive breath-hold diving', *Undersea and Hyperbaric Medicine*, 33(1): 55–62.

Fitz-Clarke, J. R. (2009) 'Risk of decompression sickness in extreme human breath-hold diving', *Undersea and Hyperbaric Medicine*, 36(2): 83–91.

Gempp, E. and Blatteau, J. E. (2006) 'Neurological disorders after repetitive breath-hold diving', *Aviation, Space, and Environmental Medicine*, 77(9): 971–3.

Gempp, E., Louge, P., Blatteau, J. E. and Hugon, M. (2012) 'Risks factors for recurrent neurological decompression sickness in recreational divers: a case-control study', *Journal of Sports Medicine and Physical Fitness*, 52(5): 530–6.

Gibb, N. (2012) *Is Scuba Diving Safe or Dangerous?*, available at: http://scuba.about.com/od/divemedicinesafety/p/Is-Scuba-Diving-Safe-Or-Dangerous.htm (accessed 15 September 2012).

Gienow, G. and Gienow, P. (2010) *Materia medica der urelemente Teil 3*, Berlin: epubli GmbH.

Golding, F. C., Griffiths, P., Hempleman, H. V., Paton, W. D. and Walder, D. N. (1960) 'Decompression sickness during construction of the Dartford Tunnel', *British Journal of Industrial Medicine*, 17(3): 167–80.

Green, J. A. (2011) 'The heart rate method for estimating metabolic rate: review and recommendations', *Comparative Biochemistry and Physiology, Part A*, 158(3): 287–304.

Hardy, A. (1960) 'Was man more aquatic in the past', *The New Scientist*, 7: 642–5.

Harris, R. J., Doolette, D. J., Wilkinson, D. C. and Williams, D. J. (2003) 'Measurement of fatigue following 18 msw dry chamber dives breathing air or enriched air nitrox', *Undersea and Hyperbaric Medicine*, 30(4): 285–91.

Hass, H. (1973) *Welt unter Wasser*, Wien: Fritz Molden Verlag.

Heindl, S., Struck, J., Wellhoner, P., Sayk, F. and Dodt, C. (2004) 'Effect of facial cooling and cold air inhalation on sympathetic nerve activity in men', *Respirotory Physiology and Neurobiology*, 142(1): 69–80.

Hong, S. K. (1987) 'Breath-hold bradycardia in man: an overview', in C. E. G. Lundgren and M. Ferrigno (eds), *The Physiology of Breath-hold Diving*, Bethesda, MD: Undersea and Hhyperbaric Medical Society, pp. 158–71.

Hong, S. K., Song, S. H., Kim, P. K. and Suh, C. S. (1967) 'Seasonal observations on the cardiac rhythm during diving in the Korean ama', *Journal of Applied Physiology*, 23(1): 18–22.

Health and Security Excecutive (2001) *Reducing Risk, Protecting People: HSE's Decision-making Process*, available at: www.hse.gov.uk/risk/theory/r2p2.pdf (accessed 19 September 2012).

Humphre, E. (1968) *The American Peoples Encyclopedia*, New York: Grolier Incorporated.

Hurford, W. E., Hong, S. K., Park, Y. S., Ahn, D. W., Shiraki, K., Mohri, M. and Zapol, W. M. (1990) 'Splenic contraction during breath-hold diving in the Korean ama', *Journal of Applied Physiology*, 69(3): 932–6.

Ikeda, T. and Ashida, H. (2000) *Is Recreational Diving Safe?*, Durham, NC: Undersea and Hyperbaric Medical Society.

Itoh, M., Fukuoka, Y., Kojima, S, Araki, H., Hotta, N., Sakamoto, T., Nishi, K. and Ogawa, H. (2007) 'Comparison of cardiovascular autonomic responses in elderly and young males during head-out water immersion', *American Journal of Cardiology*, 49(5): 241–50.

Janero, D. R. (1990) 'Malondialdehyde and thiobarbituric acid-reactivity as diagnostic indices of lipid peroxidation and peroxidative tissue injury', *Free Radical Biology and Medicine*, 9(6): 515–40.

Jennings, R. D. (1969) 'A behavioral approach to nitrogen narcosis', *Personality and Social Psychology Bulletin*, 69(3): 216–24.

Jung, K. and Stolle, W. (1981) 'Behavior of heart rate and incidence of arrhythmia in swimming and diving', *Biotelemetry Patient Monitoring*, 8(4): 228–39.

Kidd, A. H. and Kidd, R. M. (1999) 'Benefits, problems, and characteristics of home aquarium owners', *Psychological Reports*, 84(3): 998–1004.

Kiessling, R. J., Maag, J. and Clinton, H. (1962) 'Performance impairment as a function of nitrogen narcosis', *Journal of Applied Psychology*, 46(2): 91–5.

Kiyan, E., Aktas, S. and Toklu, A. S. (2001) 'Hemoptysis provoked by voluntary diaphragmatic contractions in breath-hold divers', *Chest*, 120(6): 2098–100.

Klingmann, C. and Tetzlaff, K. (2012) *Modern Diving Medicine: Pulmonary Over-dilation and Oedema*, Stuttgart: Gentner Verlag.

Klingmann, C., Rathmann, N., Hausmann, D., Bruckner, T. and Kern, R. (2012) 'Lower risk of decompression sickness after recommendation of conservative decompression practices in divers with and without vascular right-to-left shunt', *Diving Hyperbaric Medicine*, 42(3): 146–50.

Knaepen, K., Cumps, E., Zinzen, E. and Meeusen, R. (2009) 'Low-back problems in recreational self-contained underwater breathing apparatus divers: prevalence and specific risk factors', *Ergonomics*, 52(4): 461–73.

Koehle, M. S., Lepawsky, M. and McKenzie, D. C. (2005) 'Pulmonary oedema of immersion', *Sports Medicine*, 35(3): 183–90.

Kot, J., Sićko, Z. and Wozniak, M. (2003) 'Oxidative stress during oxygen tolerance test', *International Maritime Health*, 54(1–4): 117–26.

Landsberg, P. G. (1976) 'South African underwater diving accidents, 1969–1976', *South African Medical Journal*, 50(55): 2155–9.

Lanphier, E. H. and Camporesi, E. M. (1993) 'Respiration and exertion', in P. B. Bennett and D. H. Elliott (eds), *The Physiology and Medicine of Diving*, 4th edn, London: W. B. Saunders, pp. 77–120.

Lemaitre, F., Fahlman, A., Gardette, B. and Kohshi, K. (2009) 'Decompression sickness in breath-hold divers: a review', *Journal of Sports Science*, 27(14): 1519–34.

Lettnin, H. (1994) *Tauchen mit Mischgas (2. Auflage)*, Berlin: Springer-Verlag.

Levett, D. Z. and Millar, I. L. (2008) 'Bubble trouble: a review of diving physiology and disease', *Postgraduate Medical Journal*, 84(997): 571–8.

Lindholm, P. and Lundgren, C. E. (2009) 'The physiology and pathophysiology of human breath-hold diving', *Journal of Applied Physiology*, 106(1): 284–92.

Lindholm, P., Sundblad, P. and Linnarsson, D. (1999) 'Oxygen-conserving effects of apnea in exercising men', *Journal of Applied Physiology*, 87(7): 2122–7.

Lippmann, J. (2011) 'Diving deaths down under', *Proceedings of Recreational Diving Fatalities Workshop*, Durham, NC: Divers Alert Network, pp. 86–97.

Lippmann, J. and Mitchell, S. J. (2005) *Deeper into Diving*, 2nd edn, Victoria: J. L. Publications.

Ljubkovic, M., Dujic, Z., Møllerløkken, A., Bakovic, D., Obad, A., Breskovic, T. and Brubakk, A. O. (2011) 'Venous and arterial bubbles at rest after no-decompression air dives', *Medicine and Science in Sports Exercises*, 43(6): 990–5.

Madden, L. A., Chrismas, B. C., Mellor, D., Vince, R. V., Midgley, A. W., McNaughton, L. R., Atkin, S. L. and Laden, G. (2010) 'Endothelial function and stress response after simulated dives to 18 msw breathing air or oxygen', *Aviation, Space, and Environental Medicine*, 81(1): 41–5.

Mahon, R. T. (2011) 'Exploring the depths of immersion pulmonary edema', *Journal of Applied Physiology*, 110(3): 589–90.

Maron, B. J. and Mitchell, J. H. (1994) '26th Bethesda conference. Recommendations for determining eligibility for competition in athletes with cardiovascular abnormalities', *Journal of the American College of Cardiology*, 24(4): 845–99.

Moon, R. E. and Gray L. L. (2010) 'Breath-hold diving and cerebral decompression illness', *Undersea and Hyperbaric Medicine*, 37(1): 1–5.

Moretti, G. (1968) 'Decompression sickness as a consequence of repeated diving in apnea', *Annali di Medicina Navale*, 73(6): 509–22.

Mukhtar, M. R. and Patrick, J. M. (1984) 'Bronchoconstriction: a component of the "diving response" in man', *European Journal of Applied Physiology*, 53(2): 155–8.

Muth, C. M. and Rademacher, P. (2006) *Kompendium der Tauchmedizin 2*, Köln: Deutscher Ärzteverlag.

Muth, C. M., Ehrmann, U. and Radermacher, P. (2005) 'Physiological and clinical aspects of apnea diving', *Clinics in Chests Medicine*, 26(3): 381–94.

Narkowicz, C. K., Vial, J. H. and McCartney, P. W. (1993) 'Hyperbaric oxygen therapy increases free radical levels in the blood of humans', *Free Radical Research Community*, 19(2): 71–80.

National Safety Council (1989) *Injury Facts® S*, Itasca, IL: National Safety Council.

National Safety Council (2004) *Injury Facts® S*, Itasca, IL: National Safety Council.

Novalija, J. J., Lindholm, P. P., Loring, S. H., Diaz, E., Fox, J. A. and Ferrigno, M. M. (2007) 'Cardiovascular aspects of glossopharyngeal insufflation and exsufflation', *Undersea and Hyperbaric Medicine*, 34(6): 415–23.

Obad, A., Marinovic, J., Ljubkovic, M., Breskovic, T., Modun, D., Boban, M. and Dujic, Z. (2010) 'Successive deep dives impair endothelial function and enhance oxidative stress in man', *Clinical Physiology and Functional Imaging*, 30(6): 432–8.

Palada, I., Eterovic, D., Obad, A., Bakovic, D., Valic, Z., Ivancev, V., Lojpur, M., Shoemaker, J. K. and Dujic, Z. (2007) 'Spleen and cardiovascular function during short apneas in divers', *Journal of Applied Physiology*, 103(8): 1958–63.

Paton, W. (1975) 'Diver narcosis, from man to cell membrane', *Journal of the South Pacific Underwater Medicine Society*, 5(2): 20–22.

Pelaia, P., Rocco, M., De Blasi, R. A., Spadetta, G., Alampi, D., Araimo, F. S. and Nicolucci, S. (1995) 'Evaluation of lipidic peroxidation during hyperbaric oxygen therapy. Protective role of N-acetylcysteine', *Minerva Anestesiologica*, 61(4): 133–9.

Perini, R., Tironi, A., Gheza, A., Butti, F., Moia, C. and Ferretti, G. (2008) 'Heart rate and blood pressure time courses during prolonged dry apnoea in breath-hold divers', *European Journal of Applied Physiology*, 104(1): 1–7.

Pons, M., Blickenstorfer, D., Oechslin, E., Hold, G., Greminger, P., Franzeck, U. K. and Russi, E. W. (1995) 'Pulmonary oedema in healthy persons during scuba-diving and swimming', *European Respiratory Journal*, 8(5): 762–7.

Rahn, H. and Yokoyama, T. (1965) *Physiology of Breath-hold Diving and the Ama of Japan*, Washington, DC: National Research Council.

Ray, A. D., Pendergast, D. R. and Lundgren, C. E. (2008) 'Respiratory muscle training improves swimming endurance at depth', *Undersea and Hyperbaric Medicine*, 35(3): 185–96.

Reynolds, V. (1991) 'Cold and watery? Hot and dusty? Our ancestral environment and our ancestors themselves: an overview', in M. Roede, J. Wind, J. M. Patrick and V. Reynolds (eds), *The Aquatic Ape: Fact or Fiction?*, London: Souvenir Press, pp. 3–40.

Ridgway, L. and McFarland, K. (2006) 'Apnea diving: long-term neurocognitive sequelae of repeated hypoxemia', *The Clinical Neuropsychologist*, 20(1): 60–76.

Rozloznik, M., Paton, J. F. and Dutschmann, M. (2009) 'Repetitive paired stimulation of nasotrigeminal and peripheral chemoreceptor afferents cause progressive potentiation of the diving bradycardia', *American Journal of Physiology. Regulatory, Integrative and Comparative Physiology*, 296(1): R80–7.

Schaefer, K. E., Allison, R. D., Dougherty, J. H. Jr, Carey, C. R., Walker, R., Yost, F. and Parker, D. (1968) 'Pulmonary and circulatory adjustments determining the limits of depths in breath hold diving', *Science*, 162(3857): 1020–3.

Schagatay, E., Andersson, J. P. and Nielsen, B. (2007) 'Hematological response and diving response during apnea and apnea with face immersion', *European Journal of Applied Physiology*, 101(1): 125–32.

Schaller, B. (2004) 'Trigeminocardiac reflex. A clinical phenomenon or a new physiological entity?', *Journal of Neurology*, 251(6): 658–65.

Scherhag, A., Pfleger, S., Grosselfinger, R. and Borggrefe, M. (2005) 'Does competitive apnea diving have a long-term risk? Cardiopulmonary findings in breath-hold divers', *Clinical Journal of Sports Medicine*, 15(2): 95–7.

Schilling, U. M. (2010) 'Diving emergency – warm water induced pulmonary edema', *Caisson*, 25(4): 5–9.

Schipke, J. D. and Pelzer, M. (2001) 'Effect of immersion, submersion, and scuba diving on heart rate variability', *British Journal of Sports Medicine*, 35(3): 174–80.

Schipke J. D., Gams, E. and Kallweit, O. (2006) 'Decompression sickness following breath-hold diving', *Research in Sports Medicine*, 14(3): 163–78.

Scholander, P. F. (1962) *Physiological Adaptations to Diving in Animals and Man. The Harvey Lectures*, New York: Academic Press.

Shykoff, B. E. (2008) 'Pulmonary effects of submerged oxygen breathing in resting divers: repeated exposures to 140 kPa', *Undersea and Hyperbaric Medicine*, 35(2): 131–43.

Sicko, Z., Kot, J. and Doboszynski, T. (2003) 'The maximum tissue half time for nitrogen elimination from divers' body', *International Maritime Health*, 54(1–4): 108–16.

Smerz, R. W. (2004) 'Incidence of oxygen toxicity during the treatment of dysbarism', *Undersea and Hyperbaric Medicine*, 31(2): 199–202.

Smith, J. L. (1899) 'The pathological effects due to increase of oxygen tension in the air breathed', *The Journal of Physiology*, 24(1): 19–35.

Steimle, K. L., Mogensen, M. L., Karbing, D. S., Bernardino de la Serna, J. and Andreassen, S. (2011) 'A model of ventilation of the healthy human lung', *Computer Methods and Programs in Biomedicine*, 101(2): 144–55.

Steinberg, F., Dräger, T., Steegmanns, A., Dalecki, M., Röschmann, M. and Hoffmann, U. (2011) 'fit2dive – a field test for assessing the specific capability of underwater fin swimming with scuba', *International Journal of Performance Analysis in Sport*, 11(1): 197–208.

Sullivan, G. and Edmondson, C. (2008) 'Heat and temperature. Continuing education in anaesthesia', *Critical Care and Pain*, 8(3): 104–7.

Tamaki, H., Kohshi, K., Sajima, S., Takeyama, J., Nakamura, T., Ando, H. and Ishitake, T. (2010) 'Repetitive breath-hold diving causes serious brain injury', *Undersea and Hyperbaric Medicine*, 37(1): 7–11.

Tetzlaff, K., Friege, L., Koch, A., Heine, L., Neubauer, B., Struck, N. and Mutzbauer, T. S. (2001) 'Effects of ambient cold and depth on lung function in humans after a single scuba dive', *European Journal of Applied Physiology*, 85(1–2): 125–9.

Teruoka, G. (1932) 'Die Ama und ihre Arbeit', *Arbeitsphysiologie*, 5(3): 239–51.

Thalmann, E. D. (2007) *OXTOX: If You Dive Nitrox You Should Know about OXTOX*, available at: www.diversalertnetwork.org/medical/articles/OXTOX_If_You_Dive_Nitrox_You_Should_Know_About_OXTOX (accessed 20 September 2012).

Thorsen, H. C., Zubieta-Calleja, G. and Paulev, P. E. (2007) 'Decompression sickness following seawater hunting using underwater scooters', *Research in Sports Medicine*, 15(3): 225–39.

Trevett, A. J., Forbes, R., Rae, C. K., Sheehan, C., Ross, J., Watt, S. J. and Stephenson, R. (2001) 'Diving accidents in sports divers in Orkney waters', *Scottish Medical Journal*, 46(6): 176–7.

Trevett, A., Peck, D. and Forbes, R. (2010) 'The psychological impact of accidents on recreational divers: a prospective study', *Journal of Psychosomatic Research*, 68(3): 263–8.

Urban & Fischer (Hrsg.) (2003) *Roche Lexikon der Medizin, 5*, Auflage, München/Jena: Elsevier GmbH, Urban & Fischer Verlag.

Valic, Z., Palada, I., Bakovic, D., Valic, M., Mardesic-Brakus, S. and Dujic, Z. (2006) 'Muscle oxygen supply during cold face immersion in breath-hold divers and controls', *Aviation, Space, and Environental Medicine*, 77(12): 1224–9.

Vann, R. D., Butler, F. K., Mitchell, S. J. and Moon, R. E. (2011) 'Decompression illness', *Lancet*, 377(9760): 153–64.

van Ooij, P. J., van Hulst, R. A., Houtkooper, A., van der Weide, T. J. and Sterk, P. J. (2012) 'Lung function before and after oxygen diving: a randomized crossover study', *Undersea and Hyperbaric Medicine*, 39(3): 699–707.

Webb, P. (1975) 'Cold exposure', in P. B. Bennett and D. H. Elliott (eds), *The Physiology and Medicine of Diving and Compressed Air Work*, 2nd edn, London: Bailliers Tindall, pp. 285–306.

Wein, J., Andersson, J. P. and Erdeus, J. (2007) 'Cardiac and ventilatory responses to apneic exercise', *European Journal of Applied Physiology*, 100(6): 637–44.

Westenhöfer, M. (1942) *Der Eigenweg des Menschen*, Berlin: Mannstaedt & Co.

Wester, T. E., Cherry, A. D., Pollock, N. W., Freiberger, J. J., Natoli, M. J., Schinazi, E. A., Doar, P. O., Boso, A. E., Alford, E. L., Walker, A. J., Uguccioni, D. M., Kernagis, D. and Moon, R. E. (2009) 'Effects of head and body cooling on hemodynamics during immersed prone exercise at 1 ATA', *Journal of Applied Physiology*, 106(2): 691–700.

Williamson, A. M., Clarke, B. and Edmonds, C. W. (1989) 'The influence of diving variables on perceptual and cognitive functions in professional shallow-water (abalone) divers', *Environmental Research*, 50(1): 93–102.

Wilmshurst, P. T., Nuri, M., Crowther, A. and Webb-Peploe, M. M. (1989) 'Cold-induced pulmonary oedema in scuba divers and swimmers and subsequent development of hypertension', *Lancet*, 1(8629): 62–5.

Wolf, S. (1964) 'The bradycardia of the dive reflex – a possible mechanism of sudden death', *Transactions of the American Clinical and Climatological Association*, 76: 192–200.

Wylegala, J. A., Pendergast, D. R., Gosselin, L. E., Warkander, D. E. and Lundgren, C. E. (2007) 'Respiratory muscle training improves swimming endurance in divers', *European Journal of Applied Physiology*, 99(4): 393–404.

Zimmermann, J. (2012) 'Physical-physiological and technical causes of accidents in deep diving using compressed air,' *Caisson*, 2: 2–11.

8

BIOMECHANICAL AND PHYSIOLOGICAL STUDY ON ADAPTABILITY TO COLD ENVIRONMENT

Kazuhiko Watanabe

INSTITUTE OF SPORT AND HEALTH SCIENCE, HIGASHI-HIROSHIMA

Introduction

Human adaptation to the cold environment is mostly the concern of people who work or participate in sporting activities in such an environment. Our body temperature can be maintained in several ways to guarantee its optimum performance even in a cold environment. Good equipment is one of the best tools to protect our body from the cold environment. However, the use of heavy equipment sometimes diminishes human performance in exercise and sports. This chapter presents an experiment in cold environment. It also compares the heat insulation and physical performance provided by the winter outfit utilized in the Japanese Antarctic Research Expedition (JARE) and the outfit of the Greenland Eskimos. The comparison is performed through a special chamber with a temperature of $-40\,°C$. The adaptation of the peripheral parts of the body, such as the hand and fingers, to the cold weather is also discussed. The JARE outfit is suitable for physical activities, but its gloves require some improvements in heat insulation to cope with the severe cold. The experimental results and reports relating to cold adaptation are also provided. It is suggested that the clothing in cold environment should be chosen based on the demand of each individual's requirements and that standard clothing ensembles not be mandated for entire groups (Castellani *et al.*, 2006).

Method and procedure of the experiment

Experiment on heat insulation

Venue of the experiment

Low-temperature chamber: National Institute of Polar Research, Tokyo.

Subject

Four young, healthy males were requested to participate in the experiment (mean: age 21.5, height 172.0 cm, weight 63.90 kg, chest girth 89.2 cm; mean subcutaneous fat (mm): subscapula 6.2, upper arm 3.8, waist 6.8, navel 6.9).

Procedure of measurement

The subjects understood the purpose, contents, and method of the experiment and agreed to participate. The health conditions of the subjects were checked in a room with a temperature of 23.5°C. The wireless heart rate (HR) monitor and the cutaneous thermometer were set up (Figure 8.1).

The HR and temperature of the subjects were recorded at rest (the subjects sat on a chair). The subjects were carried by a caster as they sat on a chair to a chamber of − 40°C. The subjects were carried to prevent large muscle activity.

The temperature of the subjects was obtained every 3 minutes.

The subjects rested for 10 minutes in a room with a temperature of 23.5°C and were transferred to a − 40°C chamber for more rest. Afterward, the subjects performed 15 minutes of exercise on a bicycle (MONAK ergometer, 2.5 KP, 60 rs/min). The subjects were then asked to recover for 15 minutes in the chamber, after which the subjects were again carried by a caster from the cold chamber to the room with a temperature of 23.5°C. The vital statistics of the subjects during the recovery phase of 15 minutes were recorded.

Measurement equipment

The wireless HR monitor (SANEI Co. Ltd.) was operated in the 23.5°C room. The signal of the monitor was provided by an antenna connected by a wire from the cold chamber to the 23.5°C room. The thermometer (TAKARA Co. Ltd.) was also set in the 23.5°C room. The thermometer functioned through a digital signal.

Exercise tests

(a) Broad jump
(b) Side stepping
(c) Trunk flexibility: forward bending up to the ground level
(d) Trunk flexibility: backward bending with belly position
(e) Stepping
(f) Jump reaction time
(g) Back strength
(h) Sargent jump.

Each exercise test was performed after some practice.

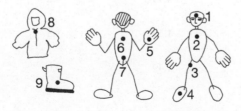

Figure 8.1 Position of the temperature measurement: (1) forehead; (2) breast (nipple level); (3) thigh; (4) instep; (5) hand (back); (6) back (subscapular level); (7) rectum; (8) overcoat (inside of breast level); (9) boot (inside of instep position).

Result and discussion

Features and size of the body of the subjects

The features and size of the body of the subjects are almost the same as those of ordinary Japanese people.

Weight and thickness of the outfits

Table 8.1 shows the weight and thickness of the JARE outfit and the outfit of the Eskimos. The JARE outfit includes a feather overcoat and feather trousers. The boots are especially made for D-type JARE. The boots of the Eskimos are made of the outer skin of seals and inner sheepskin. The JARE gloves are made of cotton and covered by calfskin. The Eskimo gloves are made of seal skin and arranged animal fur at the opening of the gloves. The same kind of underwear is utilized in JARE and by the Eskimos. They both utilize a cotton undershirt, men's long underpants, a long sweater made from grease woolen yarn, and a thin pair of nylon socks. The total weight of the JARE outfit is 5.63 kg, and the Eskimo outfit weighs 9.96 kg.

Comparison of thermal insulation

Figure 8.2a shows the result for the JARE outfit. The temperature obtained from the different parts of the body and HR are indicated in the figure. The vertical axis shows the temperature and HR. The horizontal axis shows the passage of time in the experiment. The room temperature and condition during the exercise on a bicycle ergometer in the − 40°C chamber are also indicated in the abovementioned figure. The temperature obtained from the 'core' parts of the body, including the breast (2), back (6), and rectum (7) was relatively stable during the experiment in the cold chamber. On the other hand, the temperature of the 'shell' parts

Table 8.1 Weight and thickness of the outfit of JARE and Eskimo

	Weight (kg)		Thickness (mm)	
	JARE	Eskimo	JARE	Eskimo
Gloves	0.15	0.35	2.0	6.0
Boots	2.15	2.38 (0.84 inner)	1.5	12.0 (6.0 inner)
Cost	0.98	4.15	4.2	4.0 (26.0 hair length)
Trousers	0.45	1.59	1.5	4.0 (34.0 hair length)
Underwear	1.47	1.49	3.0	6.0
Cap	0.32	–	4.0	4.0 (26.0 hair length)
Sole	–	–	53.0	17.0
Total	5.63	9.96	–	–

of the body, including the hand (5), thigh (3), and instep (4), decreased. The temperature obtained from the hand decreased to below 0°C. The JARE gloves should therefore be improved in terms of working performance and safety.

The 15-minute exercise increased the body temperature in the hand and thigh. However, the body temperature gradually decreased in the thigh and rapidly decreased in the hand after the 15-minute exercise.

Figure 8.2b shows the result for the Eskimo outfit. The temperature obtained from the different parts of the body and HR are indicated in the figure. The result is almost the same as the result for the JARE outfit. The clear difference between the two outfits is that in case of the Eskimo outfit, the body temperature obtained from the different parts of the body slightly decreased within 30 minutes after the subjects were moved to the cold (– 40°C) chamber from the warm (23.5°C) room. For example, the body temperature obtained from the hand was almost the same in the two conditions in the case of JARE: the body temperature decreased easily. However, the body temperature did not decrease to below 10°C in the cold chamber of – 40°C.

The temperature inside the JARE outfit, especially in the coat (8), exhibited a clear decrease in values compared with the Eskimo outfit. The outfit of the Eskimos has superior heat insulation compared with the JARE outfit. The effect of exercise on body temperature was also compared. The temperature in the hand and thigh clearly increased in the case of the Eskimo outfit and decreased after exercise. Overall, the temperature of the 'core' parts of the body showed minimal differences in the cold chamber; however, the 'shell' parts were easily affected by the cold environment.

Field test exercise with the JARE, Eskimo, and sports outfit

Sportswear produced a better result than the JARE and Eskimo outfits ($p < 0.01$) in the broad jump (a) test. The results for the JARE and Eskimo outfits were not statistically different. In general, no statistical difference was observed among these three outfits. These results suggest the superiority of the JARE and Eskimo outfits in terms of active movement. In the trunk flexibility test (d) (backward bending with belly position), the Eskimo outfit exhibited a less satisfactory performance on the average compared with the JARE outfit and sportswear.

Some studies on cold stress and adaptation

Numerous reports on cold stress and cold adaptation are available. Much interest has been devoted to the study of physiological response and adaptation. Some of the studies are as follows: Adams and Heberling (1958) showed the effect of cold stress during 3 weeks in an environment of 10°C. Livingstone (1976) stayed in Antarctica for 2 weeks to conduct an experiment. Chin *et al.* (1973) performed an experiment in a very cold condition. An animal (rat) was utilized to study the cold stress adaptation in a chamber with a temperature of – 20°C. The rat was placed in the chamber 3 hours per day for 3 weeks. The biochemical effects of cold stress on the rat were noted. Lange Andersen *et al.* (1963) compared the difference in the increment of body temperature and vasomotor reflex under the air temperature of 5°C between Eskimos and Caucasians.

Several studies on the effect of cold stress and the difference in body composition have also been conducted. The subjects in these studies were tested in water (Buskirk *et al.*, 1963; Kollias *et al.*, 1974; Mcadle *et al.*, 1984; Sloan and Keating, 1973).

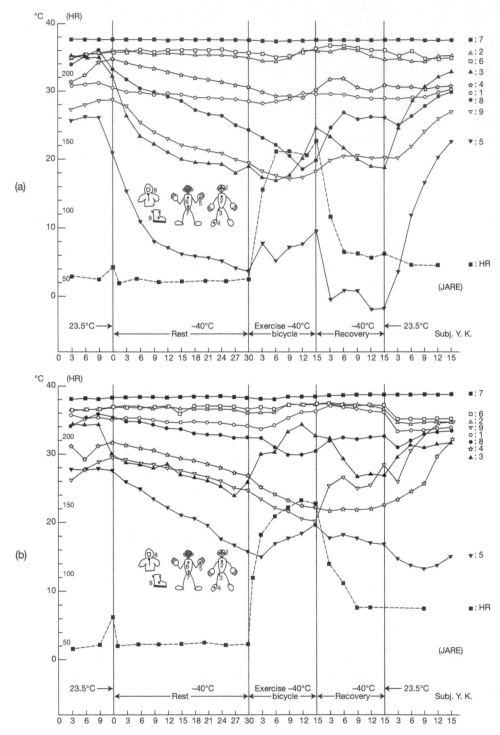

Figure 8.2 Monitoring of body temperature, outfit temperature and heart rate during the experiment in cold chamber: (a) JARE outfit; (b) Eskimo outfit.

The effect of cold stress on the body can now be monitored with a thermistor system or other similar equipment. Aside from laboratory tests or experiments, another practical way to evaluate the cold stress level is to conduct the evaluation in an actual condition.

The 'feeling' of cold stress to 'peripheral' body position

The 'feeling' of cold stress to 'peripheral' body position refers to the hand and its temperature monitored by a thermistor. The Borg scale (Borg, 1982) for perceived exertion was modified as the Rating of Perceived Cold Stress (RPCS). The term was translated into Japanese and utilized in this study to evaluate cold stress (Table 8.2).

The scale was originally set from 0 to 10 and above (*Maximal). For example, scale level 5 was described originally as 'Strong (or Heavy)'. The RPCS is described in Japanese as 'Feel Strong (or Feel Became Pain)'. Scale 7 in RPCS is 'Rather Pain'. Scale 10 in RPCS is 'Very Pain', and the scale of *Maximal is 'Can't Bear the Pain'.

Procedure of the experiment

Ten healthy young male volunteers (students) were requested to participate in the experiment as subjects. The subjects agreed to join the experiment. The hands of the subjects from the wrist joint to the fingers were soaked in water with a temperature of ± 0°C. The temperature of the fingers, palm, and back of the hand was monitored. The experiment lasted 20 minutes. The temperature from the five fingers was checked every 15 seconds.

Result and discussion

Figure 8.3 shows one of the typical results. The vertical axis indicates the RPCS and body temperature, and the horizontal axis indicates the duration of the experiment. The mean temperature obtained from the five fingers rapidly decreased to below 10°C just after the hand

Table 8.2 The RPCS (Rating of Perceived Cold Stress)

0	Nothing at all	全然感じない
0.5	Very very weak	ほとんど感じない
	(Just noticeable)	（わずかに感じ始める
1	Very weak	とても弱く感じる
2	Weak	弱く感じる
	(Light)	（弱い）
3	Moderate	中ぐらい
4	Somewhat strong	やや強く感じる
5	Strong	強く感じる
	(Heavy)	（きつい）痛みを感じ始める
6		
7	Very strong	かなり痛い
8		
9		
10	Very very strong	非常に痛い
	(Almost max)	（最大）
★	Maximal	耐えられない

Source: Modified from Borg (1982) for the peripheral part of body.

was soaked in the cold water. The average temperature of the fingers increased after 8 minutes of soaking by the vasodilatation action. The RPCS was at level 5, and the average temperature of the fingers was about 5°C at the end of the experiment. The strong relationship between RPCS and the average temperature of the fingers was statistically demonstrated except at the beginning when the hand was soaked in the cold water. The RPCS demonstrated relatively higher value at the beginning of being soaked in the cold water because water has a much higher thermal capacity than air, with the convective heat transfer coefficient being 70 times greater compared to air (Gagge and Gonzalez, 1996) and water has a thermal conductivity about 26 times greater than air. The heat loss by conduction is 26 times faster in water than in air, when all heat-transfer mechanisms are considered (radiation, conduction, convection, and evaporation). The body generally loses heat four times faster in water than it does in air of the same temperature (Wilmore and Costill, 2004). So the body temperature will very quickly drop in cold water. Swimming in a river, ocean or lake of cold water, or exercise in cold rainy weather can considerably lose body heat and cause the risk of hypothermia. In the case of long distance swimming in cold water, the benefit of adding clothing insulation to cover the active muscle areas is recommended (Wallingford *et al.*, 2000).

The test of hand manipulation with gloves in the cold chamber of − 50°C showed a statistical decrease in performance after 30 minutes in the chamber compared with the 24°C room. The reason for the decrease in work performance is attributed to the decrease in the temperature of the fingers. When the temperature of the hand was below 10°C, the subjects mentioned that they 'feel pain' in their hands (Watanabe, 1987). For safety, comfort and maintaining the skilled movement of the hand, external heat sources will be useful to keep the peripheral part of the body warm. Recently, a disposable chemical heat pack became popular. It is one of the practical ways of supplying an excellent source of warmth to cold fingers, hand, toes and the

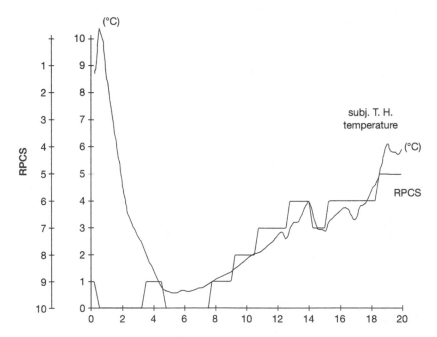

Figure 8.3 The record of temperature from fingers and RPCS (Rating of Perceived Cold Stress) during the hand soaked in cold water.

other parts of the body. However, it should be recommended that the best way is going inside for a warm-up break than staying in an extreme cold environment (Carlson, 2012).

Conclusion

The onset of pain and hand (finger) temperature are interesting issues. The onset of pain in the hand (finger) in an actual situation is one of the important warning signs for work performance and the safety of the body. We have to maintain our health by protecting our body from any cold environment to achieve the best performance in sports and exercise.

Adaptation to the cold environment can be achieved by training in the cold environment. However, proper equipment and outfits must be utilized to protect our body from the severe cold environment.

For prevention from the risk of hypothermia, coaches and athletes should be aware of the early symptoms; for example, feeling cold, shivering, pain of peripheral part of the body, apathy, social withdrawal. More clear hypothermia signs are confusion or sleepiness, slurred speech and a change in behaviour or appearance (Sallis and Chassay, 1999).

References

Adams, T. and Heberling, E. J. (1958) 'Human physiological responses to a standardized cold stress as modified physical fitness', *Journal of Applied Physiology*, 13(2): 226–30.

Borg, G. A. (1982) 'Psychophysical bases of perceived exertion', *Medicine and Science in Sports and Exercise*, 14(5): 377–81.

Buskirk, E., Thompson, R. H. and Whedon, D. G. (1963) 'Metabolic response to cold air in men and women in relation to total body fat content', *Journal of Applied Physiology*, 18(3): 603–12.

Carlson, M. J. (2012) 'Exercise in the cold', *ACSM's Health and Fitness Journal*, 16(1): 8–12.

Castellani, J. W., Young, A. J., Ducharme, M. B., Giesbrecht, G. G., Glickman, E. and Sallis, L. E. (2006) 'Prevention of cold injuries during exercise', *Medicine and Science in Sports and Exercise*, 38(11): 2012–29.

Chin, A. K., Seaman, R. and Kapileshwarker, M. (1973) 'Plasma catecholamine responses to exercise and cold adaptation', *Journal of Applied Physiology*, 34(4): 409–12.

Gagge, A. P. and Gonzalez, R. R. (1996) 'Mechanisms of heat exchange: biophysics and physiology', in M. J. Fregly and C. M. Blatteis (eds), *Handbook of Physiology: Environmental Physiology*, Bethesda, MD: American Physiological Society, pp. 45–84.

Kollias, J., Barlett, L., Bergsteinova, V., Skinner, J. S., Buskirk, E. R. and Nicholas, W. C. (1974) 'Metabolic and thermal response of women during cooling in water', *Journal of Applied Physiology*, 36(5): 577–80.

Lange Anderson, K., Hart, J. S., Hammel, H. T. and Sabean, H. B. (1963) 'Metabolic and thermal response of Eskimos during muscular exercise in cold', *Journal of Applied Physiology*, 18(3): 613–18.

Livingstone, S. D. (1976) 'Changes in cold induced vasodilatation during Arctic exercises', *Journal of Applied Physiology*, 40(3): 455–7.

Mcadle, W. D., Magel, J. R., Spina, R. J., Gergley, T. J. and Toner, M. M. (1984) 'Thermal adjustment to cold-water exposure in exercising men and women', *Journal of Applied Physiology*, 56(6): 1572–7.

Sallis, R. and Chassay, M. C. (1999) 'Recognizing and treating common cold-induced injury in outdoor sports', *Medicine and Science in Sports and Exercise*, 31(10): 1367–73.

Sloan, R. E. and Keating, W. R. (1973) 'Cooling rate of young people swimming in cold water', *Journal of Applied Physiology*, 35(3): 371–5.

Wallingford, R., Ducharme, M. B. and Pommier, E. (2000) 'Factors limiting cold-water swimming distance while wearing personal floatation devices', *European Journal of Applied Physiology*, 82(1–2): 24–9.

Watanabe, K. (1987) 'Cold environment and sport', *Japanese Journal of Sports Sciences*, 6(1): 10–16.

Wilmore, J. H. and Costill, D. L. (2004) 'Exercise in hot and cold environments: thermoregulation', in J. H. Wilmore and D. L. Costill (eds), *Physiology of Sport and Exercise*, 3rd edn, Champaign, IL: Human Kinetics, pp. 3–28.

SECTION 3

Environmental condition and sports performance

9

EFFECTS OF ENVIRONMENTAL CONDITIONS ON PERFORMANCE IN WINTER SPORTS

Martin Burtscher

UNIVERSITY OF INNSBRUCK, INNSBRUCK

Introduction

Winter sports continue to enjoy growing popularity. There are an estimated 200 million skiers and 70 million snowboarders in the world today (Langran, 2012). Additionally, there are millions of cross-country skiers, ski mountaineers or participants in one or more of the other numerous winter sports. The Olympic Winter Games encompass six different sports (biathlon, curling, ice hockey, skating, skiing and sled sports), with skiing consisting of six disciplines (alpine skiing, cross-country skiing, freestyle skiing, Nordic combined, ski jumping and snowboard) and skating (figure skating, speed skating, short track speed skating) and sled sports (bobsleigh, luge, skeleton) each consisting of three disciplines. The common characteristic of these sports is that they all are performed on snow or ice at low environmental temperatures. Whereas some sports are mostly performed indoors and at low altitude (e.g. skating, curling), others are typically performed outdoors and often at moderate (1,500–2,500 m) or even high (2,500–3,500 m) altitude (e.g. skiing, ski mountaineering, cross-country skiing). Both cold weather conditions and high-altitude hypoxia can affect exercise performance and health. Thus, the knowledge on physiological and pathophysiological responses to cold and/or high altitude are of utmost importance for diseased and healthy people as well.

Thermal regulation

Body temperature of human beings is regulated by the thermoregulatory centre in the hypothalamus at about 37°C; they are homeothermic. All tissues produce heat that helps to maintain body temperature. The resting metabolic rate (1.0 MET, ~ 3.5 $mlO_2.min^{-1}.kg^{-1}$, ~ 1 $kcal.kg^{-1}$) is sufficient to maintain body temperature under resting conditions at moderate ambient temperature (25–27°C = thermoneutral zone). However, external (e.g. warm environment, solar radiation) and internal (e.g. exercise) heat sources can contribute to body temperature and may challenge thermal regulation. Information to the regulatory centre is provided from central (hypothalamus, spinal cord) or peripheral (skin) thermoreceptors and cooling (e.g. peripheral vasodilation, evaporation) or heating (e.g. peripheral vasoconstriction, shivering) mechanisms are activated (Figure 9.1).

Whereas hot environments in summer add to the heat load arising from exercise, cold temperatures in winter time favour heat dissipation. Consequently, maintaining the balance between heat production and heat loss will be easier during exercise in winter. When the production of heat exceeds heat loss, body temperature rises, resulting in hyperthermia and when heat loss exceeds heat production the body temperature drops, causing hypothermia. Intense physical activity increases the energy expenditure by 10–20 times over resting condition and at least 75 per cent is degraded as heat. Without effective heat dissipation, even moderate exercise intensity would increase body temperature by ~ 1°C every 5–6 minutes (Nimmo, 2004). Beside ambient temperature, wind, humidity and radiant energy determine environmental or climatic heat stress. The overall effect of theses factors can be assessed by the Wet Bulb Globe Temperature (WBGT). Evaporation is the most effective mechanism to dissipate body heat, contributing about 80 per cent to total heat loss and to avoid the development of hyperthermia. One litre of sweat removes 580 kcal from the body. In contrast, the amount of metabolic heat production (e.g. due to shivering or exercise) is crucial at cold environmental temperature for the maintenance of body temperature and protecting from hypothermia.

Metabolic rate increases in cold environment due to enhanced muscle tone ('pre-shivering') and later by shivering up to four times of the resting metabolic equivalent (1 MET = 3.5 $mlO_2 min^{-1}.kg^{-1}$) (Toner and McArdle, 1988). Importantly, submaximal and maximal shivering and thus protection from hypothermia are related to the individual aerobic exercise capacity (Golden *et al.*, 1979). However, shivering also decreases muscular coordination and impairs performance. Whereas cool air seems to increase glucose metabolism, fat metabolism is rather enhanced in cold water. Other rapid physiological responses to counteract hypothermia are peripheral vasoconstriction and elevated thyroxin production. Vasoconstriction and reduced blood supply to the skin, increasing the body insulation, is stimulated by the sympathetic nervous

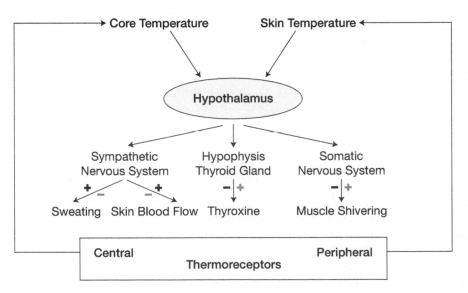

Figure 9.1 Thermoregulation in humans (+ means increase, − means decrease; black indicates warm environment, grey indicates cold environment).

system. The elevated thyroxin production increases general metabolic rate. Shivering becomes maximally at a core temperature of about 35°C followed by a suppression of shivering with a further decrease. All these mechanisms effectively support the maintenance of core temperature even with minimal clothing but may become insufficient with long exposure duration and/or wet and windy conditions. Heat loss is also relatively high at the sites of contracting muscles during exercise (Ainslie and Reilly, 2003). For example, low intensity exercise (30 per cent VO_2max) with minimal clothing (T-shirt and shorts) at an ambient temperature of 0°C and wind speed of 10 km.h^{-1}, core temperature may drop by more than 1°C per hour even in well-trained subjects (Burtscher *et al.*, 2012) Heat loss in water is 3–5 times faster than air because water is 25 times more conductive than air (Smith and Hames, 1962). Thus, protective clothing becomes extremely important in counteracting heat loss. Modern functional outdoor clothing helps to keep skin and clothing dry and to maintain insulating capacity and body temperature at various environmental temperatures and exercise intensities.

Cold and metabolic changes

Energy expenditure increases with decreasing ambient temperature. Of course, the energy requirements mainly depend on whether a drop in skin and core temperature is prevented by adequate clothing (Castellani *et al.*, 2006). Wearing normal clothing, energy expenditure was elevated by ~ 5 per cent even at 20°C when compared to 28°C (Warwick and Busby, 1990) and this increase may exceed 400 per cent during maximal shivering (Toner and McArdle, 1988). It has been demonstrated that muscles can sustain shivering for several hours using glucose, free fatty acids and lactate as substrates (Haman, 2006; Therminarias, 1992). Whereas cool air seems to increase glucose metabolism, fat metabolism is rather enhanced in cold water. The use of carbohydrates for shivering may severely affect these stores because this fuel represents only ~ 1 per cent of total energy stores (lipids ~ 95 per cent and proteins ~ 4 per cent) (Haman, 2006). Although shivering can be maintained for a prolonged time due to the use of different substrates and by changing muscle fibre recruitment it may deplete muscle glycogen stores and impair exercise performance.

Cold and the respiratory system

Ventilation at rest and during exercise is higher in cold conditions (i.e. − 2°C) compared to normal ambient temperatures. Because the ventilatory equivalent for oxygen remains almost unchanged, the increase in ventilation seems mainly due to the higher energy expenditure in the cold (Therminarias, 1992). Performing winter sports outdoors means breathing cold and dry air. Both coldness and dryness are considered to trigger respiratory symptoms or in the long term even respiratory disorders affecting health and performance. Cold air is dry air because of the low water content even when it is fully saturated. At rest, the inhaled air is almost fully conditioned to the body temperature and saturated with water vapour before reaching the lower airways. During intense exercise, however, minute ventilation is 20–30-fold increased above resting values (from 5–8 L.min^{-1} at rest to values higher than 150 L.min^{-1} in elite athletes). The airway epithelium is challenged by warming and saturating with water vapour of these very high breathing volumes, which will be completed, if at all, by the lower airways (Sue-Chu, 2012). The evaporative water loss causes cooling and dehydration of the airway surface, provoking the release of inflammatory mediators and bronchoconstriction (Anderson and Kippelen, 2008). Several cross-sectional studies suggested that repeated and prolonged hyper-ventilation of cold and dry air during winter sports activities can induce respiratory disorders

Table 9.1 Main (patho)physiological mechanisms resulting in reduced exercise performance in the cold

	Physiology/pathophysiology	*Performance impairment*
Respiratory system	Bronchoconstriction	Aerobic exercise
	Dyspnea	
	Oxygen desaturation	
Neuromuscular system	Contraction velocity	Force development
	Shivering	Coordination
	Glycogen depletion	Exercise intensity
Skin	Sensibility (e.g. fingers)	Dexterity

and affect performance in athletes (Pohjantahti *et al.*, 2005; Wilber *et al.*, 2000) (Table 9.1). These studies demonstrated the development of progressive obstructive airway obstruction and related ventilatory limitations. Interestingly, Olympic athletes treated with β2-agonists because of asthma have won more medals than their counterparts not taking this medication (Tsitsimpikou *et al.*, 2009). However, no ergogenic effects of β2-agonists were found in healthy subjects exercising at normal ambient temperature or in the cold (– 20°C) (Sporer *et al.*, 2008). Exercise-induced bronchoconstriction (EIB) due to cold exposure may also occur in healthy subjects but seems to be more common in athletes regularly training in the cold (Pohjantahti *et al.*, 2005). Healthy subjects seem to be much less sensitive to cold than those with asthma (O'Cain *et al.*, 1980). Even mild asthma is associated with decreased minute ventilation and maximal exercise performance (Pohjantahti *et al.*, 2005). Also, patients suffering from COPD experience EIB and performance decline when exercising in the cold, but loss in performance in those patients was rather due to the exercise dyspnea than diminished ventilation (Koskela *et al.*, 1998). Submaximal exercise duration was also decreased in heart failure patients (ejection fraction: 26 ± 4 per cent) in – 8 versus 20°C (– 21 per cent) but was increased in healthy volunteers (+ 20 per cent). Regional skin cooling resulting in increased sympathetic activity and arteriolar vasoconstriction, however, may be more important in COPD and cardiac patients than bronchoconstriction (Koskela *et al.*, 1998). The International Ski Federation recommends reasonable minimum temperature limits for the various alpine and Nordic skiing disciplines between – 16°C and – 20°C for adults and – 12°C for children (International Ski Federation, 2012). Individual medical advice should be provided to patients.

Cold and the cardiovascular system

Typically, cold exposure induces vasoconstriction of peripheral blood vessels resulting in elevation of central venous pressure, mean arterial pressure and cardiac output mostly associated with a decrease in heart rate (Rowell, 1983). Development of hyperthermia and the risk of dehydration are less likely to occur in cold than warm conditions. Dehydration when exercising in the heat is associated with a reduction in stroke volume, as well as a decline of blood flow to the working muscles resulting in impaired performance (Maughan *et al.*, 2007). These effects are largely prevented when exercising in a cold environment, thereby maintaining aerobic performance at high intensity provided there is no decrease in muscle temperature. However, cardiovascular adverse events in susceptible persons have been reported to occur more frequently at low outdoor temperature during the winter season (Marchant *et al.*, 1993). Several pathophysilogoical mechanisms may contribute to cold-related cardiovascular mortality and morbidity (e.g. non-favourable effects on endothelial function and blood pressure, on coagulation or blood lipids) (Hess *et al.*, 2009). Responses to cold exposure (i.e. systemic blood pressure) have been shown to be exaggerated in older individuals or subjects with coronary artery disease (Juneau *et al.*, 1989). This 'pressor response' explains the more frequent and severe angina attacks in these patients (Juneau *et al.*, 1989). Superficial skin cooling for 20 minutes has been demonstrated to augment systolic (but not diastolic) and mean blood pressure in older (~ 65 years) compared to younger (~ 25 years), subjects probably due to the higher central arterial stiffness in the older individuals (Hess *et al.*, 2009).

Cold and the neuromuscular system

Lowering muscle temperature below thermoneutral conditions reduces contraction velocity predominantly affecting dynamic exercises (Racinais and Oksa, 2010). This is explained by slower cross-bridges cycling leading to slower force development; however, without affecting the maximal isometric force development (De Ruiter and De Haan, 2000). Consequently, after muscle cooling movement velocity is reduced (Table 9.1). For example, Racinais and Oksa (2010) demonstrated that jump height decreases by almost 10 per cent per 1°C lowering of muscle temperature (between 34 and 29°C), and cycling at a high pedalling frequency was more affected than cycling at a low pedalling rate (Sargeant, 1987). Epidemiological data support the assumption that low muscle temperatures during downhill skiing might impair reaction times and fast movements, thereby not only diminishing skiing performance, but also increasing the risk of collisions and falling (Ruedl *et al.*, 2012).

Inorganic phosphate concentration and acidosis impact more negatively on contractile function and related muscle fatigue at low temperature compared to physiological temperature (Coupland *et al.*, 2001; Racinais and Oksa, 2010). Conduction velocity in both sensory and motor nerve fibres decrease with cooling. The Q10 (an indicator of temperature sensitivity per every 10°C change in tissue temperature) of the conduction velocity is about 1.4 and the decline vary between 1.1 and 2.4 m.s^{-1}.°C^{-1} (Denys, 1991).

Cold and endurance performance

Exercising at low intensity (~ 30 per cent VO$_2$max)

When exercising at low ambient temperatures, heat production may be too low to offset heat loss. Thus, adequate winter clothing is necessary to maintain core temperature at low exercise intensities; for instance, when walking at ~ 30 per cent VO$_2$max (~ 5 km.h^{-1}). In addition, wet winter clothing and wind reduce the insulating effect of clothing dramatically associated with an enhanced risk of hypothermia. When skin temperature drops below 25°C, a strong drive arises to walk or run faster to increase core temperature and thereby better tolerate the low skin temperature (Ainslie and Reilly, 2003; Weller *et al.*, 1997b). In the case of fatigue, however (e.g. due to exhaustion after prolonged exercise, low fitness, injury or illness), increasing exercise intensity is not possible, likely resulting in hypothermia without appropriate protection by clothing or shelter (Burtscher *et al.*, 2012).

Oxygen consumption during low-intensity exercise in the cold is enhanced in order to maintain core temperature. The additional energy may be met from increased utilization of carbohydrates (Weller *et al.*, 1997a, 1997b), at least partly originating from muscle glycogen stores (Jacobs *et al.*, 1985). This, again, may lead to accelerated depletion of those stores, resulting in reduced exercise performance especially at higher intensities. The increased use of glycogen is explained by the fact that elevated epinephrine concentrations favour muscle glycogenolysis but enhanced norepinephrine levels do not increase lipolysis due to the cold-induced decrease of blood flow to the adipose tissues (Weller *et al.*, 1997a, 1997b). Temperature of skeletal muscles may decrease with inadequate clothing during low-intensity exercise, resulting in decreased power output. Consequently, an earlier recruitment of additional motor units is necessary at low temperatures to sustain prolonged submaximal exercise, finally reducing maximal and submaximal endurance performances (Faulkner *et al.*, 1990).

Exercising at moderate intensity (~ 70 per cent VO$_2$max)

The risk of hypothermia remains low as long as relatively fit subjects (VO$_2$max > 40 ml/min/kg) are able to exercise at moderate intensities (i.e. 70 per cent VO$_2$max), even with minimal clothing (T-shirt and shorts) and at only moderate wind velocities (Burtscher *et al.*, 2012). Weller *et al.* (1997a, 1997b) showed that walking intensities of ~ 60 per cent VO$_2$max were sufficient to offset heat loss in cold and wet environments. Sustained exercise at the anaerobic threshold (~ 70 per cent VO$_2$max) was shown to be negatively affected by extreme cold temperatures (below − 20°C) (Faulkner *et al.*, 1990; Patton and Vogel, 1984). Patton and Vogel (1984), for example, demonstrated a ~ 40 per cent reduction in endurance performance after prolonged exposure to − 20°C compared to + 20°C. Several mechanisms may have contributed to the performance decline (e.g. respiratory symptoms, lowered muscle temperature accompanied by impaired contraction and movement velocity and/or frostbite and discomfort) (Nimmo, 2004) (Table 9.1). Studies systematically comparing endurance performance at different ambient temperatures wearing similar clothing revealed an optimal temperature range between + 3 and + 11°C (Galloway and Maughan, 1997; Parkin *et al.*, 1999). Using adequate clothing, rectal temperature will not drop at temperatures as low as − 10°C when exercising near to the individual anaerobic threshold (Layden *et al.*, 2002). Skin temperature at 10°C (Galloway and Maughan, 1997) and even at 0°C (Burtscher *et al.*, 2012) did not fall below 22°C and tissue damage is unlikely even when only wearing a T-shirt and shorts provided the use of gloves and cap. Exercising at temperatures below − 10°C oxygen consumption may increase associated with changes in mechanical efficiency of skeletal muscle (Layden *et al.*, 2002; Nimmo, 2004).

However, findings are equivocal and may strongly depend on the individual exercise intensity and clothing. Fuel utilization patterns seem not to be different at ambient temperatures above 0°C (Galloway and Maughan, 1997; Weller *et al.*, 1997a, 1997b). When temperature drops below 0°C, lipolysis is typically reduced, likely due to the diminished blood flow to adipose tissues (Layden *et al.*, 2002). Besides, uncoupling between the availability of free fatty acids and fat oxidation has also been suggested (Layden *et al.*, 2002). Glycogenolysis seems to be reduced at those low temperatures without changes in blood lactate concentration (Starkie *et al.*, 1999). Consequently, lactate production and removal may be diminished. This has to be taken into account during training in the cold because lower blood lactate concentration and lower heart rates may lead to underestimation of training intensity (Nimmo, 2004). Finally, hypohydration impairs endurance performance more in moderate temperature (20°C) compared to lower temperature (2°C) (Cheuvront *et al.*, 2005).

Exercising at high intensity (> 70 per cent VO$_2$max)

High-intensity exercise requires high minute ventilation and may therefore particularly challenge the respiratory system associated with bronchoconstriction and dyspnea affecting performance. Adequate warm-up exercises are important to reduce the development of these symptoms, especially at very low ambient temperatures. High-intensity exercises are typically interrupted by recovery periods with an increasing risk cooling down of working muscles. This not only increases the risk of injury during the subsequent high-intensity exercise, but also reduces muscle contraction velocity and performance as discussed above (Racinais and Oksa, 2010) (Table 9.1).

High-altitude and endurance performance

When ascending to high altitudes, aerobic exercise performance decreases upon ascent to altitude whereas anaerobic performance remains unchanged (Fulco *et al.*, 1998; McLellan *et al.*, 1990). With increasing altitude, the partial pressure of inspired oxygen (PiO$_2$) diminishes, leading to a drop in alveolar oxygen pressure (PAO$_2$) and arterial oxygen saturation (SaO$_2$). Also, maximal heart rate and cardiac output, and consequently oxygen delivery to skeletal muscle mitochondria, are reduced at high altitude. Because maximal oxygen extraction cannot compensate for this reduction, VO$_2$max inevitably decreases (see Fick Principle):

Fick Principle: VO$_2$ = Cardiac output × (Hb) × (SaO$_2$ – SvO$_2$)
VO$_2$: oxygen uptake; (Hb): haemoglobin concentration; SaO$_2$: arterial oxygen saturation; SvO$_2$: mixed venous oxygen.

Depending on various factors, especially the individual fitness level, a VO$_2$max decrease of about 1.5–3.5 per cent for every 300 m of additional increase above 1,500 m has been reported (Buskirk, 1966). During acute exposure to high altitude, endurance athletes in particular show rather small cardiorespiratory compensation and pronounced lactate production, resulting in a larger performance reduction as observed in sedentary subjects (Burtscher *et al.*, 2005; Ferretti *et al.*, 1997). It has been reported that well-trained athletes show a 35 per cent lower hypoxic ventilatory response (HVR) than non-athletes, resulting in a marked decline of aerobic performance in acute hypoxia (Byrne-Quinn *et al.*, 1971). This finding, however, has not been confirmed by other studies (Sheel *et al.*, 2006); but, more importantly, the HVR is a highly plastic response, increasing after a few days of exposure to hypoxia with a concomitant improved performance (Burtscher *et al.*, 2005).

The beneficial effects of hyperventilation on aerobic exercise performance, however, will be limited at high altitude by the increasing mechanical work of breathing and the related oxygen cost, and probably also by the associated respiratory alkalosis. Chin *et al.* (2007) suggested that respiratory alkalosis may impair O$_2$ kinetics and diminish oxygenation of skeletal muscle. With increasing exercise intensity, the oxygen costs of breathing also increases, amounting to 10–16 per cent of VO$_2$max at sea level (Dempsey *et al.*, 2003) and is additionally elevated by 35–40 per cent at intense exercise at altitude of about 3,000 m (Thoden *et al.*, 1969). It is not only the enhanced oxygen cost by the respiratory muscles that limit exercise performance, but also blood flow to exercising muscles and thus oxygen delivery are reduced. This may be caused by the fatigue of respiratory muscles and metaboreflexes from these muscles, which enhances sympathetic vasoconstriction of the exercising limb muscles (Sheel *et al.*, 2001).

Combined effects of high altitude and cold

Exercising in the mountainous areas in winter (and sometimes even in summer) is often challenged by exposure to cold and hypoxia (altitude) as well. There are several interactions between hypoxia and cold that may negatively affect exercise performance. For example, energy expenditure is increased in the cold and additionally in hypoxia (Butterfield, 1999; Toner and McArdle, 1988). On the other hand, hypoxia may delay the onset of vasoconstriction and shivering, and thus enhance the core cooling rate and the development of hypothermia (Johnston *et al.*, 1996). Minute ventilation increases in hypoxia in order to counteract arterial oxygen desaturation and decline in aerobic performance but is also associated with increased respiratory heat loss, likely contributing to the development of respiratory symptoms in the cold. Breathing cold air through the nose, however, may inhibit ventilation in normal subjects due to a diminished tidal volume associated with shortening of the duty cycle (Burgess and Whitelaw, 1988), resulting in relative hypoventilation, arterial oxygen desaturation and impairment of exercise performance at altitude. Both cold and hypoxia may mediate pulmonary hypertension and even pulmonary edema at high altitude (Giesbrecht, 1995). The increase in pulmonary arterial pressure is associated with reduced arterial oxygen saturation and oxygen delivery to skeletal muscles, again resulting in impaired aerobic exercise performance.

Cold exposures and high altitude: cross adaptation

Based on animal studies, it has been suggested that different environmental stimuli (i.e. cold and hypoxia) might elicit similar adaptive effects (LeBlanc, 1969). Both cold and hypoxia can stimulate sympathetic activation. Repeated exposures to one stimulus result in reduced sympathetic activation (habituation) to the other stimulus (cross-adaptive effect). Lunt *et al.* (2010) demonstrated that repeated short-term cold exposures resulted in reduced physiological strain (i.e. alteration in autonomic balance and reduced cardiorespiratory responses) during subsequent submaximal exercise in hypoxia. Such cross-adaptive effects may be favourable for certain susceptible subjects (e.g. patients suffering from cardiovascular diseases) exposed to acute hypoxia.

Preventive measures

Clothing

Beside avoidance of intense exercise in very severe cold conditions at low and high altitudes, the use of adequate clothing is the most effective measure to optimize performance and to prevent hypothermia in the cold. Layering of clothing helps to stay warm and dry in different conditions. Layers provide the opportunity to remove or add clothing, depending on the temperature, wind and physical activity. Generally, there are three main layers: wicking, insulating and weather protection layers. The wicking layer is worn next to the skin (underwear) and moves moisture away from the skin. It is typically made of synthetic material (e.g. polyester or silk). The following insulating layer (e.g. sweaters, sweatshirts, pullovers of wool or synthetic material) helps to stay warm and also wicks moisture away. The outer layer (protection layer; shells and pants) repels water from snow or rain and blocks the wind, but lets perspiration evaporate (waterproof and breathable). The combination of layers and types of clothing depends on the outdoor conditions and physical activity. Headwear and gloves or mittens are especially important since much of body heat escapes from the head and fingers, which are at particular risk for freezing. Helmets do not only protect from head injuries, but help also keep the head warm. Gloves should be made of waterproof and breathable fabrics and layering can be applied in extreme cold. The same is true for socks. Materials for headwear, gloves, mittens and socks include polyester, silk, wool, nylon and fleece. Finally, cold weather masks are also available (e.g. made of fleece) that help to keep the face dry and to humidify dry and cold inhaled air.

Nutrition

Winter sports activities may be associated with increased and specific energetic demands. Especially when exercising at relatively high intensity levels or competing in winter sports, athletes should carry foods and fluids for adequate fuelling to prevent glycogen depletion. Foods consumed during activities should include easily digestible, carbohydrate-rich sources, and fluids should be available as sweetened warm teas or sport drinks (Meyer *et al.*, 2011). Recovery may be negatively affected by altitude and cold as well. Thus, focusing on adequate recovery with optimal rehydration and filling of glycogen stores is of utmost importance. Proposed energy requirements during intense winter sports activities are: 6–10 g. kg^{-1}.d^{-1} of carbohydrates (Sjödin *et al.*, 1994), 1.0–1.9 g. kg^{-1}.d^{-1} of fat and 1.4–1.7 g. kg^{-1}.d^{-1} of proteins (Meyer *et al.*, 2011).

Acclimatization

During prolonged periods of cold exposure, a metabolic form of adaptation may occur. Typically, however, during repeated cold exposures, as practiced during winter sports activities, habituation occurs. Habituation is the most common pattern observed in acclimatization studies, requiring only brief intermittent cold exposures to be induced (Young *et al.*, 1986).

Habituation results in higher skin temperatures and a later onset of shivering associated with maintained manual dexterity and comfort. Acclimatization to high altitudes is of utmost importance to maintain aerobic performance and well-being. Typically submaximal, but not maximal, exercise performance improves even during short-term (~ 3 days) acclimatization to high altitude, mainly due to an increase in SaO$_2$ and haemoglobin concentration from increasing ventilation and decreasing plasma volume, respectively (Burtscher *et al.*, 2005). These improvements, however, seem to be even enhanced in well-trained individuals, partly compensating for the initial larger performance decrease. The acclimatization process is not completed after 3 days, but may take at least 1–2 weeks at moderate altitudes (Burtscher *et al.*, 2001).

References

Ainslie, P. N. and Reilly, T. (2003) 'Physiology of accidental hypothermia in the mountains: a forgotten story', *British Journal of Sports Medicine*, 37(6): 548–50.

Anderson, S. D. and Kippelen, P. (2008) 'Airway injury as a mechanism for exercise-induced bronchoconstriction in elite athletes', *The Journal of Allergy and Clinical Immunology*, 122(2): 225–35.

Burgess, K. R. and Whitelaw, W. A. (1988) 'Effects of nasal cold receptors on pattern of breathing', *Journal of Applied Physiology*, 64(1): 371–6.

Burtscher, M., Bachmann, O., Hatzl, T., Hotter, B., Likar, R., Philadelphy, M. and Nachbauer, W. (2001) 'Cardiopulmonary and metabolic responses in healthy elderly humans during a 1-week hiking programme at high altitude', *European Journal of Applied Physiology*, 84(5): 379–86.

Burtscher, M., Faulhaber, M., Flatz, M., Likar, R. and Nachbauer, W. (2005) 'Effects of short-term acclimatization to altitude (3,200 m) on aerobic and anaerobic exercise performance', *International Journal of Sports Medicine*, 27(8): 629–35.

Burtscher, M., Kofler, P., Gatterer, H., Faulhaber, M., Philippe, M., Fischer, K., Walther, R. and Herten, A. (2012) 'Effects of lightweight outdoor clothing on the prevention of hypothermia during low-intensity exercise in the cold', *Clinical Journal of Sport Medicine*, 22(6): 505–7.

Buskirk, E. R. (1966) 'Physiology and performance of track athletes at various altitudes in the United States and Peru', in R. F. Goddard (ed.), *The Effects of Altitude on Physical Performance*, Chicago: Athletic Institute, pp. 65–72.

Butterfield, G. E. (1999) 'Nutrient requirements at high altitude', *Clinics in Sports Medicine*, 18(3): 607–21.

Byrne-Quinn, E., Weil, J. V., Sodal, I. E., Filley, G. F. and Grover, R. F. (1971) 'Ventilatory control in the athlete', *Journal of Applied Physiology*, 30(1): 91–8.

Castellani, J. W., Young, A. J., Ducharme, M. B., Giesbrecht, G. G., Glickman, E. and Sallis, R. E. (2006) 'American College of Sports Medicine position stand: prevention of cold injuries during exercise', *Medicine and Science in Sports and Exercise*, 38(11): 2012–29.

Cheuvront, S. N., Carter, R. III, Castellani, J. W. and Sawka, M. N. (2005) 'Hypohydration impairs endurance exercise performance in temperate but not cold air', *Journal of Applied Physiology*, 99(5): 1972–6.

Chin, L. M., Leigh, R. J., Heigenhauser, G. J., Rossiter, H. B., Paterson, D. H. and Kowalchuk, J. M. (2007) 'Hyperventilation-induced hypocapnic alkalosis slows the adaptation of pulmonary O2 uptake during the transition to moderate-intensity exercise', *The Journal of Physiology*, 583(1): 351–64.

Coupland, M. E., Puchert, E. and Ranatunga, K. W. (2001) 'Temperature dependence of active tension in mammalian (rabbit psoas) muscle fibres: effect of inorganic phosphate', *The Journal of Physiology*, 536(3): 879–91.

De Ruiter, C. J. and De Haan, A. (2000) 'Temperature effect on the force/velocity relationship of the fresh and fatigued human adductor pollicis muscle', *European Journal of Physiology*, 440(1): 163–70.

Dempsey, J. A., Sheel, A. W., Haverkamp, H. C., Babcock, M. A. and Harms, C. A. (2003) 'The John Sutton Lecture: CSEP, 2002. Pulmonary system limitations to exercise in health', *Canadian Journal of Applied Physiology*, 28: S2–24.

Denys, E. (1991) 'AAEM Minimonograph # 14: the influence of temperature in clinical neurophysiology', *Muscle Nerve*, 14(9): 795–811.

Faulkner, J. A., Zerba, E. and Brooks, S. (1990) 'Muscle temperature of mammals: cooling impairs most functional properties', *The American Journal of Physiology*, 259(2): R259–65.

Ferretti, G., Moia, C., Thomet, J. M. and Kaiser, B. (1997) 'The decrease of maximal oxygen consumption during hypoxia in man: a mirror image of the oxygen equilibrium curve', *The Journal of Physiology*, 498(1): 231–7.

Fulco, C. S., Rock, P. B. and Cymerman, A. (1998) 'Maximal and submaximal exercise performance at altitude', *Aviation, Space, and Environmental Medicine*, 69(8): 793–801.

Galloway, S. D. and Maughan, R. J. (1997) 'Effects of ambient temperature on the capacity to perform prolonged cycle exercise in man', *Medicine and Science in Sports and Exercise*, 29(9): 1240–9.

Giesbrecht, G. G. (1995) 'The respiratory system in a cold environment', *Aviation, Space, and Environmental Medicine*, 66(9): 890–902.

Golden, F. St C., Hampton, I. F. G. and Smith, D. (1979) 'Cold tolerance in long distance swimmers', *The Journal of Physiology*, 290(2): P48–9.

Haman, F. (2006) 'Shivering in the cold: from mechanisms of fuel selection to survival', *Journal of Applied Physiology*, 100(5): 1702–8.

Hess, K. L., Wilson, T. E., Sauder, C. L., Gao, Z., Ray, C. A. and Monahan, K. D. (2009) 'Aging affects the cardiovascular responses to cold stress in humans', *Journal of Applied Physiology*, 107(4): 1076–82.

International Ski Federation (2012) *FIS Medical Guide 2012*, available at: www.fis-ski.com/uk/medical/medical.html (accessed 16 September 2012).

Jacobs, I., Romet, T. T. and Kerrigan-Brown, D. (1985) 'Muscle glycogen depletion during exercise at 9°C and 21°C', *European Journal of Physiology*, 54(1): 35–9.

Johnston, C. E., White, M. D., Wu, M., Bristow, G. K. and Giesbrecht, G. G. (1996) 'Eucapnic hypoxia lowers human cold thermoregulatory response thresholds and accelerates core cooling', *Journal of Applied Physiology*, 80(2): 422–9.

Juneau, M., Johnstone, M., Dempsey, E. and Waters, D. D. (1989) 'Exercise-induced myocardial ischemia in a cold environment. Effect of antianginal medications', *Circulation*, 79(5): 1015–20.

Koskela, H., Pihlajamäki, J., Pekkarinen, H. and Tukiainen, H. (1998) 'Effect of cold air on exercise capacity in COPD: increase or decrease?', *Chest*, 113(6): 1560–5.

Langran, M. (2012) *Snow Sports Injury Studies – What Are They All About?!*, available at: http://ski-injury.com/research (accessed 16 September 2012.

Layden, J. D., Patterson, M. J. and Nimmo, M. A. (2002) 'Effect of reduced ambient temperature on fat utilization during submaximal exercise', *Medicine and Science in Sports and Exercise*, 34(5): 774–99.

LeBlanc, J. (1969) Stress and interstress adaptation, *Federation Proceedings*, 28(3): 996–1000.

Lunt, H. C., Barwood, M. J., Corbett, J. and Tipton, M. J. (2010) '"Cross-adaptation": habituation to short repeated cold-water immersions affects the response to acute hypoxia in humans', *The Journal of Physiology*, 588(18): 3605–13.

McLellan, T. M., Kavanagh, M. F. and Jacobs, I. (1990) 'The effect of hypoxia on performance during 30 sec or 45 sec of supramaximal exercise', *European Journal of Physiology*, 60(2): 155–61.

Marchant, B., Ranjadayalan, K., Stevenson, R., Wilkinson, P. and Timmis, A. D. (1993) 'Circadian and seasonal factors in the pathogenesis of acute myocardial infarction: the influence of environmental temperature', *British Heart Journal*, 69(5): 385–7.

Maughan, R. J., Watson, P. and Shirreffs, S. M. (2007) 'Heat and cold. What does the environment do to the marathon runner?', *Sports Medicine*, 37(4–5): 396–9.

Meyer, N. L., Manore, M. M. and Helle, C. (2011) 'Nutrition for winter sports', *Journal of Sports Sciences*, 29(1): S127–36.

Nimmo, M. (2004) 'Exercise in the cold', *Journal of Sports Sciences*, 22(10): 898–916.

O'Cain, C. F., Dowling, N. B., Slutsky, A. S., Hensley, M. J., Strohl, K. P., McFadden E. R. Jr and Ingram R. H. (1980) 'Airway effects of respiratory heat loss in normal subjects', *Journal of Applied Physiology*, 49(5): 875–80.

Parkin, J. M., Carey, M. F., Zhao, S. and Febbraio, M. A. (1999) 'Effect of ambient temperature on human skeletal muscle metabolism during fatiguing submaximal exercise', *Journal of Applied Physiology*, 86(3): 902–8.

Patton, J. F. and Vogel, J. A. (1984) 'Effects of acute cold exposure on submaximal endurance performance', *Medicine and Science in Sports and Exercise*, 16(5): 494–7.

Pohjantahti, H., Laitinen, J. and Parkkari, J. (2005) 'Exercise-induced bronchospasm among healthy elite cross country skiers and non-athletic students', *Scandinavian Journal of Medicine and Science in Sports*, 15(5): 324–8.

Racinais, S. and Oksa, J. (2010) 'Temperature and neuromuscular function', *Scandinavian Journal of Medicine and Science in Sports*, 20(3): S1–18.

Rowell, L. B. (1983) 'Cardiovascular aspects of human thermoregulation', *Circulation Research*, 52(4): 367–79.

Ruedl, G., Fink, C., Schranz, A., Sommersacher, R., Nachbauer, W. and Burtscher, M. (2012) 'Impact of environmental factors on knee injuries in male and female recreational skiers', *Scandinavian Journal of Medicine and Science in Sports*, 22(2): 185–9.

Sargeant, A. J. (1987) 'Effect of muscle temperature on leg extension force and short-term power output in humans', *European Journal of Physiology*, 56(6): 693–8.

Sheel, A. W., Derchak, P. A., Morgan, B. J., Pegelow, D. F., Jacques, A. J. and Dempsey, J. A. (2001) 'Fatiguing inspiratory muscle work causes reflex reduction in resting leg blood flow in humans', *The Journal of Physiology*, 537(1): 277–89.

Sheel, A. W., Koehle, M. S., Guenette, J. A., Foster, G. E., Sporer, B. C., Diep, T. T. and McKenzie, D. C. (2006) 'Human ventilatory responsiveness to hypoxia is unrelated to maximal aerobic capacity', *Journal of Applied Physiology*, 100(4): 1204–9.

Sjödin, A. M., Andersson, A. B., Högberg, J. M. and Westerterp, K. R. (1994) 'Energy balance in cross-country skiers: a study using doubly labeled water', *Medicine and Science in Sports and Exercise*, 26(6): 720–4.

Smith, G. B. and Hames, E. F. (1962) 'Estimation of tolerance times for cold water immerson', *Aerospace Medicine*, 33: 834–40.

Sporer, B. C., Sheel, A. W. and McKenzie, D. C. (2008) 'Dose response of inhaled salbutamol on exercise performance and urine concentrations', *Medicine and Science in Sports and Exercise*, 40(1): 149–57.

Starkie, R. L., Hargreaves, M., Lambert, D. L., Proietto, J. and Febbraio, M. A. (1999) 'Effect of temperature on muscle metabolism during submaximal exercise in humans', *Experimental Physiology*, 84(4): 775–84.

Sue-Chu, M. (2012) 'Winter sports athletes: long-term effects of cold air exposure', *British Journal of Sports Medicine*, 46(6): 397–401.

Therminarias, A. (1992) 'Acute exposure to cold air and metabolic responses to exercise', *International Journal of Sports Medicine*, 13(1): S187–90.

Thoden, J. S., Dempsey, J. A., Reddan, W. G., Birnbaum, M. L., Forster, H. V., Grover, R. F. and Rankin, J. (1969) 'Ventilatory work during steady-state response to exercise', *Federation Proceedings*, 28(3): 1316–21.

Toner, M. M. and McArdle, W. D. (1988) 'Physiological adjustments of man to the cold', in K. B. Pandolf., M. N. Sawka and R. R. Gonzalez (eds), *Human Performance: Physiology and Environmental Medicine at Terrestrial Extremes*, Carmel, CA: Cooper Publishing Group, pp. 361–99.

Tsitsimpikou, C., Jamurtas, A., Fitch, K., Papalexis, P. and Tsarouhas, K. (2009) 'Medication use by athletes during the Athens 2004 Paralympic Games', *British Journal of Sports Medicine*, 43(13): 1062–6.

Warwick, P. M. and Busby, R. (1990) 'Influence of mild cold on 24 h energy expenditure in normally clothed adults', *The British Journal of Nutrition*, 63(3): 481–8.

Weller, A. S., Millard, C. E., Stroud, M. A., Greenhaff, P. L. and Macdonald, I. A. (1997a) 'Physiological responses to a cold, wet, and windy environment during prolonged intermittent walking', *The American Journal of Physiology*, 272(1/2): R226–33.

Weller, A. S., Millard, C. E., Stroud, M. A., Greenhaff, P. L. and Macdonald, I. A. (1997b) 'Physiological responses to cold stress during prolonged intermittent low- and high-intensity walking', *The American Journal of Physiology*, 272(6/2): R2025–33.

Wilber, R. L., Rundell, K. W., Szmedra, L., Jenkinson, D. M., Im, J. and Drake, S. D. (2000) 'Incidence of exercise-induced bronchospasm in Olympic winter sport athletes', *Medicine and Science in Sports and Exercise*, 32(4): 732–7.

Young, A. J., Muza, S. R., Sawka, M. N., Gonzalez, R. R. and Pandolf, K. B. (1986) 'Human thermoregulatory responses to cold air are altered by repeated cold water immersion', *Journal of Applied Physiology*, 60(5): 1542–8.

10

APPLIED ERGONOMICS OF CYCLING PERFORMANCE

Michael D. Kennedy and William N. Lampe

UNIVERSITY OF ALBERTA, ALBERTA

Introduction

Ergonomics 'attempts to best understand the interaction among humans and other elements of a system in order to optimize human well-being and overall system performance' (International Ergonomics Association Council, 2000). As this concept relates to sport, ergonomics is a useful way of examining how athletes interact with their environment whereby a systematic process of athlete-environment assessment and training serves to enhance performance. This has been previously defined as the 'mutual adjustment' of human and machine where the bicycle is the machine (de Groot *et al.*, 1994), although a more current perspective on cycling ergonomics would include the interaction of the cyclist on his or her bicycle and the bicycle-rider unit in the surrounding environment (Debraux *et al.*, 2011). Thus, this chapter will focus on the factors directly related to cycling velocity by exploring the relationship of the bicycle-rider unit with the external environment, and the factors that influence power output and are therefore indirectly related to cycling velocity by examining the bicycle-rider unit. This chapter will draw from road cycling and triathlon and focus on the three most typical cyclist positions: upright (hands on upper part or brake hoods of traditional road handlebar); drop (hands on bottom of traditional road handlebar); and time trial (elbows resting on pads on upper part of handler bar arms grasping 'aerobar') (see Figure 10.1).

Bicycle-rider unit in the environment

Models of resistance to determine cycling performance

The factor with the greatest influence on cycling velocity is the resistance to forward motion, including rolling resistance (necessary to overcome mechanical friction as well as wheel pneumatics and drive train friction) (Debraux *et al.*, 2011), aerodynamic drag force (displacement of air) and weight force (displacement on roads with non-horizontal gradients) (Iniguez-de-la-Torre and Iniguez, 2006). In accordance with Lamb (1995), air resistance is the major performance factor that impedes a cyclist's forward motion, especially at velocities greater than 13 km.h^{-1}. At such velocities, 70–90 per cent of the total resistive forces acting on the cyclist has been attributed to aerodynamic resistance (Chowdhury *et al.*, 2011; Defraeye *et al.*, 2010a). Thus, cyclists must employ technology and positioning on their bicycle in order to optimize aerodynamics and maintain the greatest average velocity (Foster *et al.*, 1994).

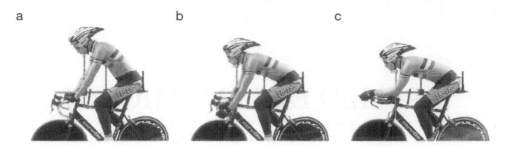

Figure 10.1 The three most typical cyclist positions during road and triathlon cycling: (a) upright position; (b) drop position; and (c) time trial position. (Reprinted from Journal of Biomechanics, Vol. 44/9, Defraeye, T., Blocken, B., Koninckx, E., Hespel, P., and Carmeliet, J., Computational fluid dynamics analysis of drag and convective heat transfer of individual body segments for different cyclist positions, Pages No. 1696, Copyright (2011), with permission from Elsevier.)

As the interaction of the bicycle-rider unit with the environment is the predominant factor influencing velocity, models to predict performance have focused on aerodynamic resistance or drag. This has been defined as pressure drag – the primary form of aerodynamic drag resulting from fore-aft air pressure differential formed during a cyclist's forward motion (Debraux *et al.*, 2011; Edwards and Byrnes, 2007). The simplest models use projected frontal area (A_p), coefficient of drag (C_D), and drag area (A_D), where C_D and $A_p = A_D$, to estimate the influence the aerodynamics has on velocity (Edwards and Byrnes, 2007). In this model, A_p is the composite of the size and observable shape or quality of that size and C_D is equated to the quality of streamlining (Edwards and Byrnes, 2007). The more accurate model to estimate aero drag (R_D) includes the factors of C_D and A_p as well as air density (ρ) and the velocity relative to the fluid (V_f^2), the fluid in this case being air, where:

$$R_D = 0.5 \times A_p \times C_D \times p \times V_f^2 \tag{1}$$

Although negligible relative to A_p and C_D, air density does have a significant influence on drag when at sea level compared to extreme altitude (decrease of 24 per cent from 0 m to 2,250 m above sea level) (Debraux *et al.*, 2011). The extension of this model to observable mechanical work, including the composite of aerodynamic resistance, rolling resistance while accounting for air speed, is described as:

$$W_C = a + R_D \times v^2 \tag{2}$$

where W_C is the mechanical work per given unit of distance, a is rolling resistance, R_D is aerodynamic resistance, and v^2 is the square of air speed (di Prampero, 2000).

Streamlining (C_D) has been described as 'viscous drag', or the friction between the boundary layer (of the skin, helmet, textiles, bicycle and wheels) and the environment (Defraeye *et al.*, 2011). Frontal area (A_p) has been described as 'form drag' or the drag due to the shape of the cyclist on his or her bicycle in the environment (Debraux *et al.*, 2011). Form drag is likely a more holistic way of looking at the mass/size of the cyclist because it accounts for forward pressure and the wake flow created. Finally, interference drag – the interaction of the cyclist on the drag coefficient of the bicycle, compared to the drag resistance created by the bicycle alone, without the rider – needs to be considered. In essence, interference drag accounts for the realistic drag acting on the bicycle and is an important consideration as it relates to aerodynamics in bicycle technology, where testing procedures should account for the reduction of total drag of the bicycle-rider unit in the development of bicycle aerodynamics.

Estimates of total drag area indicate that, regardless of cyclist position, the cyclist drag area accounts for about 64–72 per cent of total drag, and total drag can be reduced by 21 per cent (Chowdhury *et al.*, 2011) and 30 per cent (Defraeye *et al.*, 2010a) from upright to a time trial position. Methods to determine how drag area is calculated include 2D camera based models such as wind tunnel models and Computational Fluid Dynamic (CFD) models borrowing from the theories associated with the physics of fluid mechanics. The most rigorous example of a simple 2D method utilizes a two-camera (frontal and sagittal plane) motion capture system designed to estimate total drag from the frontal silhouette images (Chowdhury *et al.*, 2011). In this model, the direct determination of frontal surface area of a 'rider and bike' in a 2D frontal silhouette meets the requirement of analysing the bicycle-rider unit, an important component of the ergonomics of cycling performance. Furthermore, this set up is readily available in biomechanics and sport science laboratories and only requires a 2 m × 2 m area for analysis. Thus, in combination with the published predictive equation:

$$C_D = \frac{F_D}{1/2pV^2} \times A_p \qquad (3)$$

where C_D is the coefficient of drag and F_D, p, V and A are the drag force, air density, wind velocity and frontal area, respectively, this model can utilize the individual A_p for a cyclist and apply this A_p with F_D norms, p and V to determine individualized C_D. Normative data for F_D has been proposed by others (di Prampero, 2000) for both 'upright' and 'drop' positions and used with other values to provide a valid estimate of C_D.

Although the 2D camera-based models are valuable tools in determining aerodynamic drag, the wind tunnel likely remains the most valid way of doing so. Reference values for dynamic drag (defined as during pedalling, versus static drag where the pedals are in a fixed position parallel to ground) have been published, based on professional cyclists pedalling at 5.5 W.kg^{-1} in a wind tunnel (Garcia-Lopez *et al.*, 2008). In that project, the 'dynamic drag area' reference values were generated at a simulated velocity of 54 km.h^{-1} and revealed drag area estimates were 31 per cent greater cycling at 5.5 W.kg^{-1} compared to static drag area. This has significant implications regarding the utility of drag models and their applicability to real-world cycling performance. The limitations of wind tunnel to real-world estimates of total drag acting on the bicycle-rider system is also questionable when one considers the influence of sidewind. The influence of sidewind, although not widely studied, has been shown to have a significant braking effect (increased time of 2 minutes 44 seconds at a constant power output of 250 W over a 20 km TT) (Iniguez-de-la-Torre and Iniguez, 2006). Readers are referred to Iniguez-de-la-Torre and Iniguez (2006) for equations that provide estimates of how headwind, tailwind and sidewind affect forward motion.

Despite their widespread use in motor sports and swimming, it is only recently that computational fluid dynamic CFD models have been applied to cycling. The key benefit of the CFD model is that 'wake flow' created by the bicycle-rider unit and the resulting turbulence are accounted for, providing a more realistic representation of the composite (bicycle-rider) aerodynamic drag (Defraeye *et al.*, 2010a). CFD estimates of cyclist drag area indicate that CFD estimates of drag are 6–12 per cent greater than wind tunnel estimates, with the LES CFD model (LES one of two CFD computational methods) estimate being more realistic of actual wake flow compared to RAN CFD generated estimates (Defraeye *et al.*, 2010a). Differences have been ascribed to unaccounted interference drag (interaction of cyclist on bicycle drag) and viscous drag in the CFD model. In CFD models, interference drag cannot be separated from cyclist drag because it is a global estimate of wake flow. In the wind tunnel, it is possible to determine the interference drag by comparing drag of the bicycle-rider unit with those of the cyclist and the bicycle in isolation. Additionally, CFD models provide a more realistic estimate of viscous drag. As a result, cyclist drag values from CFD models are greater than those from wind tunnel tests and interference drag is accounted for in wind tunnel testing, providing a more accurate measure of cyclist drag (Defraeye *et al.*, 2010a).

Viscous drag

Although viscous drag accounts for a smaller portion of the total aerodynamic drag in cycling, it has important implications on cycling performance. Mathematically, viscous drag has been expressed as C_D, which is the ratio between aero drag and the product of dynamic pressure of the moving air and the projected frontal area (Debraux *et al.*, 2011). In simple terms, C_D depends mostly on the air velocity and the roughness of the surfaces (Debraux *et al.*, 2011) similar to CFD models, where viscous drag is measured by the boundary–layer interaction and is influenced by the relative speed of the rider and surrounding fluid and the rider's position on the bicycle (Defraeye *et al.*, 2010b). The influence of garment composition and qualities continues to be an emerging area of aerodynamic research, especially in regard to viscous drag (Chowdhury *et al.*, 2009). It is recognized that body position, fabric properties, garment construction and the fit of the garment all contribute to the overall drag, which, depending on the cyclist's speed, can significantly alter the turbulent flow created at the boundary-layer interface (Chowdhury *et al.*, 2009). As it relates to cycling garments, it appears that rougher fabrics produce less drag at low speeds (< 50 km.h^{-1}), whereas smoother fabrics produce less viscous drag at higher speeds, especially in the time trial position (Chowdhury, 2012). The aerodynamic effect of overshoes (stretch fabric socks put over cycling shoes) appears to be detrimental, producing a 2.5 W penalty to maintain the same velocity compared with uncovered tightly laced cycling shoes (Gibertini *et al.*, 2010).

Relationship between position and equipment on bicycle influencing drag

It has also become apparent that posture in combination with specific equipment (helmets and visors primarily) contribute to drag area, a finding with important implications to overall aerodynamic drag. Aero helmets generally reduce aerodynamic drag, although some studies have shown that at an individual level the lowest drag area is not achieved with an aero helmet (Garcia-Lopez *et al.*, 2008). Thus, the importance of how the aero helmet fits with the overall form (and subsequent form drag coefficient) is paramount to gaining the full benefit and thus the time trial position chosen should be the best combination of aero helmet – cyclist – bicycle resulting in the lowest drag area. To determine how the influence of aero helmets on the bicycle–rider unit actually differs, Barelle *et al.* (2010) utilized five different aero helmet shapes and three different head angles in a TT position to provide an updated analytical model of projected frontal area (A_p). The main outcome was that independent of body height and body mass (the key anthropometric measures utilized in the model), aero helmet configuration does influence A_p (Barelle *et al.*, 2010). Specifically, a normal or 'usual inclination' results in the lowest helmet specific drag resistance in a TT position with no difference in drag resistance between low and usual helmet positions when in an upright position (Chabroux *et al.*, 2008). Interestingly, venting also has a negligible effect on drag, which implies that vents do not affect viscous drag or the boundary-layer interaction significantly (Chabroux *et al.*, 2008).

Bicycle-rider unit

Considerations of factors indirectly affecting velocity

In both recreational and competitive cycling, the cyclist and the bicycle interact to form a functional unit. Ultimately, the ability of the cyclist to effectively apply propulsive forces to the pedals and the interaction of the bicycle-rider unit in the environment govern cycling performance.

With regards to cycling ergonomics, the points of contact between the cyclist and the bicycle – the handlebars, saddle, and pedals – and the cyclist's pedalling motion are of particular interest, as they determine how the internal work done by the cyclist is translated into motion on the bicycle. The cyclist produces power through the actions of the ankle, knee, and hip joints and of the upper body, which are transmitted through the hip joint (Broker and Gregor, 1994; Elmer *et al.*, 2011; Martin and Brown, 2009; van Ingen Schenau *et al.*, 1990). Through the shoe-pedal interface, this power is transferred to the drivetrain to propel the bicycle forward. As a rider's position on the bicycle dictates the boundaries of how their body – the lower extremities in particular – and specific joints are able to move, bicycle fit is an important factor in maximizing cycling performance. Thus, the following sections focus on how improved fit and posture improves power with secondary consideration of how posture influences drag.

Saddle-cyclist interface

The selection of an appropriate saddle position with relation to the pedals and bottom bracket is an important consideration for cycling comfort, power production, and mechanical efficiency. In manipulating the position of the saddle, the length and contraction velocity of the muscles of the lower limbs – specifically those that act at the hip, knee, and ankle – can be altered by changing the relative limb alignment. It has been suggested that the relative contribution of a muscle in producing a given movement is changed with changes in muscle length or contraction velocity (Sanderson and Amoroso, 2009). The influence of saddle height – the distance from the shoe-pedal interface to the top of the saddle – and seat tube angle – a function of the vertical and horizontal displacement of the saddle relative to the bottom bracket – on cycling ergonomics are discussed below.

Seat tube angle

Traditional racing bicycles are generally ridden with seat tube angles between 72 and 76°, while triathlon bicycles often have steeper seat tube angles of 76–78°. Experimentation with even steeper seat tube angles in an attempt to find more comfort, efficiency, and power production in an aerodynamic position has been reported, particularly in the triathlon community (Faria *et al.*, 2005; Heil *et al.*, 1995).

On a road bicycle with conventional handlebars, the range of seat tube angles that can be achieved practically does not appear to produce enough variation in the position of the cyclist on the bicycle to have a significant effect on pedalling efficiency or mechanics (Leirdal and Ettema, 2011). However, the use of aerobars makes a greater range of seat tube angles and cyclist positions possible and can have a significant influence on the cyclist's pedalling, producing physiological and biomechanical changes. The steepening of the seat tube angle towards vertical produces kinematic changes at the ankle and hip, with the mean hip angle increasing (the angle between the trunk and the thigh moves further towards 180°) during the pedal stroke, causing greater ankle plantar flexion (a larger angle between the shin and top of the foot). Knee angles are generally not influenced by the seat tube angle, nor is the range of motion of the ankle, knee, or hip (Heil *et al.*, 1995, 1997; Litka *et al.*, 2011).

The cardiorespiratory demands of cycling at submaximal intensities are also affected by the seat tube angle when using aerobars, thereby influencing cycling economy. Relatively steep seat tube angles (80–90°) have been found to reduce the cardiorespiratory demands (oxygen consumption (VO_2), heart rate (HR), and minute ventilation (V_E)) and Rating of Perceived Exertion (RPE) compared with more traditional seat tube angles (~ 70°), with all variables demonstrating negative relationships with seat tube angle. Likely of more significance to the overall cycling ergonomics is the lower metabolic cost associated with cycling at the same intensity with a steeper seat tube angle increase cycling economy, even before the aerodynamic benefits are taken into consideration (Heil *et al.*, 1995, 1997; Price and Donne, 1997). As an example of the practical importance of seat tube angle, the decrease in oxygen consumption and heart rate from a seat tube angle of 68–80° with an optimized saddle height was 3.7 $ml.kg^{-1}.min^{-1}$ in competitive male cyclists pedalling at 200 W (Price and Donne, 1997).

The range of seat tube angles that can be achieved with a conventional road bicycle and handlebars is small enough that the resulting seat tube angles and rider positions do not produce significant biomechanical, cardiorespiratory, or efficiency changes (Leirdal and Ettema, 2011). However, when using aerobars, adopting a steeper seat tube angle can alter pedalling kinematics, ultimately reducing the cardiorespiratory demands and increasing the cyclist's efficiency at the same work rate (Heil *et al.*, 1995, 1997; Litka *et al.*, 2011; Price and Donne, 1997). Thus, optimizing the seat tube angle is an important component of the bicycle-rider unit as it relates to ergonomics.

Saddle height

Saddle height – the distance from the pedal axle to the top of the saddle, with the pedal at its most distal position – interacts with the seat tube angle, influencing the cyclist's biomechanics, cardiorespiratory demands, and mechanical efficiency. During submaximal cycling over a range of seat tube angles (68–80°) and saddle heights (96–104 per cent of trochanteric length) in competitive male cyclists, a seat tube angle of 80° was found to have the lowest metabolic demands (VO_2) and greatest efficiency, and this angle combined with a saddle height of 100 per cent of trochanteric length elicited a lower HR response than the lower and higher saddle positions. Over a range of seat tube angles (68–80°), the cardiorespiratory demands were greater and efficiency was lower when the saddle height increased above 100 per cent of trochanteric length (Price and Donne, 1997). Similarly, a saddle height of 100 per cent of trochanteric length has been found to have lower metabolic costs than a height 5 per cent higher or lower (Nordeen-Snyder, 1977) or above 103 per cent of trochanteric length in recreational cyclists (Shennum and deVries, 1976). The kinematics of this excess saddle height above 100 per cent are increased ankle plantar flexion and lateral pelvic tilt (rocking on saddle) at the bottom of the pedal stroke to protect the knee from hyperextension (Nordeen-Snyder, 1977; Price and Donne, 1997). Overall, this increase in muscle activity at excessive saddle heights has higher cardiorespiratory demands at the same workload, reducing mechanical efficiency.

Interaction of saddle height and seat tube angle

The influence of saddle height and seat tube angle on oxygen consumption and gross efficiency during submaximal cycling are shown in Figures 10.2 and 10.3. To summarize the interaction

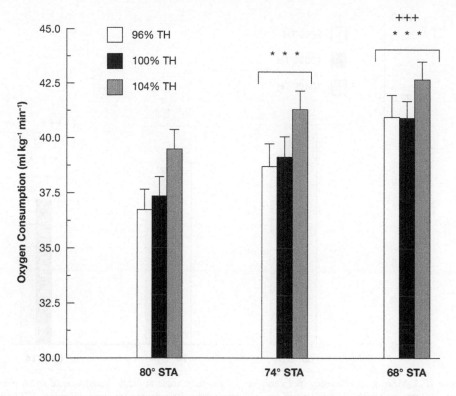

Figure 10.2 Mean oxygen consumption (ml.kg^{-1}.min^{-1}) versus seat tube angle at saddle heights equal to 96 per cent, 100 per cent, and 104 per cent of trochanteric height. Bars denote standard deviation. ***Denotes significantly different (P <0.001) from values at equivalent saddle heights at 80° seat tube angle. +++Denotes significantly different (P <0.001) from values at equivalent saddle heights at 74° seat tube angle. (Reprinted from Journal of Sports Sciences, Vol. 15/4, Price, D. and Donne, B., Effect of variation in seat tube angle at different seat heights on submaximal cycling performance in man, Pages No. 399, Copyright (1997), with permission from Elsevier.)

of saddle height and seat tube angle, both variables affect the cardiorespiratory response, pedalling biomechanics, and mechanical efficiency at submaximal efficiencies. A saddle position where saddle height and seat tube angle are both optimized should yield the greatest ergonomic benefit, while the combination of a saddle height that is too great and a seat tube angle that is too shallow is likely to be poorest ergonomically. Although steeper seat tube angles appear to be favorable compared with shallower seat tube angles, the upper limit of traditional road bicycle frames is generally under 80°, and cyclists generally adopt positions with seat tube angles between 72 and 76° (Faria *et al.*, 2005). It appears that a saddle height of ~ 100 per cent of trochanteric length is optimal in reducing cardiovascular demands and maintaining sound pedalling biomechanics during submaximal cycling. As the cardiovascular demands and biomechanical effects of a saddle height that is higher than optimal appear to be greater than those observed at saddle heights that are lower than optimal, the evidence would support there is a lesser ergonomic penalty associated with a saddle that is too low than those associated with a saddle that is too high (Nordeen-Snyder, 1977; Price and Donne, 1997).

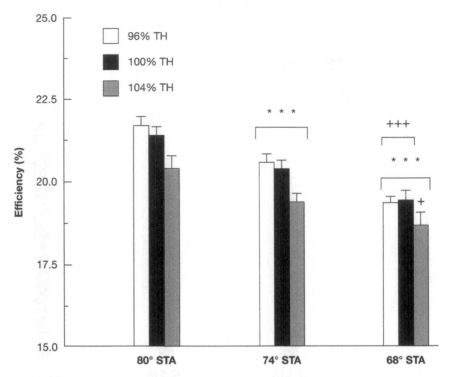

Figure 10.3 Mean gross efficiency (per cent) versus seat tube angle at saddle heights equal to 96 per cent, 100 per cent, and 104 per cent of trochanteric height. Bars denote standard deviation. ***Denotes significantly different (P<0.001) from values at equivalent saddle heights at 80° seat tube angle. +++Denotes significantly different (P<0.001) from values at equivalent saddle heights at 74° seat tube angle. (Reprinted from Journal of Sports Sciences, Vol. 15/4, Price, D. and Donne, B., Effect of variation in seat tube angle at different seat heights on submaximal cycling performance in man, Pages No. 399, Copyright (1997), with permission from Elsevier.)

Trunk angle

Within the limits imposed by the relative position of the saddle and handlebars, the cyclist is able to assume a variety of positions with his or her upper body by altering the placement of his or her hands on the handlebars and the angles of the upper body joints and torso. As well as affecting a cyclist's aerodynamics, the orientation of a cyclist's trunk influences upper body muscle activity, joint angles of the lower body, and possible thoracic dimensions, thereby having cardiorespiratory, neuromuscular, and biomechanical implications.

Cyclists often adopt an upright riding position in situations that favour high power output over aerodynamics, such as riding uphill and during performance test in laboratory settings (Jobson *et al.*, 2008). This is typically the 'upright' position (hands on the tops of the handlebars or on the brake hoods with the elbows relatively extended). In laboratory settings, riding in an upright position has been shown to have lower cardiorespiratory demands (oxygen consumption, heart rate and respiratory exchange ratio) compared with the more horizontal torso position assumed when riding in aerobars, and to elicit a lower VO_2 than riding in the drops of traditional handlebars, thereby increasing the rider's mechanical efficiency (Gnehm *et al.*, 1997). Similarly, riding a cycle ergometer in an upright position results in greater power production at the same submaximal cardiovascular demands (VO_2, HR, V_E, and RPE) than riding an ergometer in a 'time trial' position (Hubenig *et al.*, 2011; Jobson *et al.*, 2008) and a greater power output at VO_2max compared to riding in the 'drop' position (Welbergen and Clijsen, 1990). Thus, without accounting for the aerodynamic differences between torso positions, riding in an upright position is favorable in terms of the cardiovascular demands and mechanical efficiency, compared with riding in a more aerodynamic position, and is favorable when riding situations favour power production and mechanical efficiency over aerodynamics.

The changes in joint angles, muscle activity patterns, and power production profiles observed between riding in the 'upright', 'drop' and 'time trial' positions likely contribute to the differences in metabolic demands and mechanical efficiency associated with those cyclist positions (Hubenig *et al.*, 2011). Compared with the 'drop' position, and to a large extent the 'upright' position, the pedal stroke is altered when using a 'time trial' position in such a way that the resistive force applied to the pedal during the upstroke is greater and the propulsive force applied at the top of the pedal stroke is reduced. The application of greater propulsive force during the downstroke compensates for the larger counterproductive portions of the pedal stroke when using aerobars in the 'time trial' position (Dorel *et al.*, 2009). Hip flexion increases as the orientation of the trunk moves towards horizontal, altering the length of the muscles crossing the hip and knee joints and altering their operating point on the force-velocity and force-length curves (Dorel *et al.*, 2009; Gnehm *et al.*, 1997; Welbergen and Clijsen, 1990). Additionally, the activation of the hip extensor (*gluteus maximus*) and flexor (*rectus femoris*) and the knee extensors (*vastus lateralis* and *medialis*) is delayed until later in the pedal cycle as the trunk orientation becomes more horizontal (Dorel *et al.*, 2009). These changes during the pedal cycle between the 'upright', 'drop' and 'time trial' positions likely contribute to the metabolic and efficiency discrepancies between them.

Pedal cycle and cadence

In optimizing cycling performance, it is important to maximize the translation of the energetic costs into mechanical work. The path along which the pedals are able to travel in relation to the bottom bracket is fixed, and is a function of the bicycle cranks. The variables that can be manipulated to determine the cyclist's application of force to the pedals are crank length, pedalling cadence, and pedalling technique.

While gross efficiency – the total metabolic rate, including muscle work rate, for a given external work rate – is an important factor in cycling performance and is generally believed to be related to good technique, force effectiveness and dead centre are better measures of pedal cycle and often used to assess pedalling technique. Force effectiveness is the ratio between the force directed at 90° to the crank arm and the total resultant force applied to the pedal. Although the mechanical constraints of the bicycle-rider system necessitate considerable radial forces to be produced for an effective and powerful crank cycle (Kautz and Hull, 1993), forces directed other than perpendicular to the crank arm do not contribute to the work rate, and the energy cost associated with such force production is considered wasted (Leirdal and Ettema, 2011). The dead centre is the ratio of the minimum power to average power output during the pedal stroke (Leirdal and Ettema, 2011), essentially providing a measure of the cyclist's consistency in applying power to the pedals throughout the pedal cycle.

Pedal cadence has been shown to be negatively related to all three measures of efficiency mentioned above. Force effectiveness is greater at lower than at higher cadences, and this relationship extends to ranges well below and above self-selected cadences of well-trained cyclists in laboratory settings (~ 95 rpm) (Leirdal and Ettema, 2011) and racing situations among professional cyclists (~ 70 rpm during ascents, ~ 90 rpm during flat races and time trials) (Lucia *et al.*, 2001). This relationship has been observed for a range of cadences from 60 to 105 rpm during submaximal cycling (Candotti *et al.*, 2007) (60–105); (Loras *et al.*, 2009) (60–100); (Sanderson, 1991) (60–100). Recently, the dead centre has been shown to have a similar relationship with pedalling cadence during submaximal cycling (Leirdal and Ettema, 2011), suggesting that the power output profile during the pedal cycle is more uniform at lower than at higher cadences. Gross cycling efficiency shows the same trend as the indexes of pedalling efficiency, with lower cadences being more economical than higher cadences during submaximal cycling (Chavarren and Calbet, 1999).

It should be noted that the most economical cadence may differ at different workloads – the cadence associated with the highest economy increases as the work rate increases (Foss and Hallen, 2004; Hansen and Sjogaard, 2007; Samozino *et al.*, 2006), and much of the research uses relatively low workloads. However, the most efficient cadence is still likely lower than the self-selected preferred cadence of most cyclists. For example, the most economical cadence at 50 W and 350 W were found to be 60 and 80 rpm (Foss and Hallen, 2004), and 50 and 80 rpm at 100 W and 300 W (Coast and Welch, 1985) in elite cyclists. Cadences of 50–60 rpm are less than typical self-selected cadences of professional and well-trained cyclists, whereas a cadence of 80 rpm is likely at the low end of, but still within, the range of cadences adopted by such cyclists (Lucia *et al.*, 2001). At higher power outputs, the negative effect of high pedalling rates on gross efficiency is diminished because the metabolic cost of pedalling at a high cadence relative to the total metabolic cost of pedalling is reduced (Chavarren and Calbet, 1999).

Considering the short length of the bouts of cycling used in many investigations (most no longer than 6 minutes), the applicability of their findings to real-world cycling performance is limited (Brisswalter *et al.*, 2000). In research using longer cycling protocols, the data suggest that the most economical cadence during the first minute's cycling may be lower than that during prolonged periods. For example, the most efficient cadence between the 3rd and 6th minute of exercise was found to be ~ 70 rpm, and had increased to ~ 85 rpm from the 25th to 28th minute in trained cyclists. Cyclists' self-selected cadences were ~ 80 rpm and ~ 83 rpm during the same periods, suggesting that self-selected cadence is greater than the cadence that is most efficient at the onset of exercise but not different during prolonged cycling, due to an increase in the most efficient pedalling rate (Brisswalter *et al.*, 2000).

The lower muscular force per pedal stroke required at higher pedalling cadences would be metabolically favorable during longer bouts of cycling, reducing the development of muscular fatigue and the cyclist's ratings of perceived exertion (Lollgen *et al.*, 1980; Lucia *et al.*, 2001). In addition, there may be hemodynamic and neuromuscular benefits to adopting higher cadences that are more relevant during prolonged exercise (Gotshall *et al.*, 1996; Lucia *et al.*, 2001, 2004; Takaishi *et al.*, 1996), shifting the most economical cadence upwards as exercise duration increases. Evidence indicates that these hemodynamic benefits across a range of cadences often adopted by cyclists (70–110 rpm) include increased heart rate, stroke volume, cardiac output, and blood pressure concomitant with lower vascular resistance (Gotshall *et al.*, 1996). These benefits are suggested to be mediated through the skeletal muscle pump, which may be more effective in increasing blood flow and venous return at higher cadences (Gotshall *et al.*, 1996; Lucia *et al.*, 2001, 2004; Takaishi *et al.*, 1996).

Practical applications and conclusions

In Jeunkendrup and Martin's review entitled 'Improving Cycling Performance: How Should We Spend Our Time and Money' (Jeukendrup and Martin, 2001) they state that training is the overarching factor in cycling performance; however, they also state that 'relatively small changes in body position can have a large effect' as well. This contention is supported by evidence presented throughout this chapter with the underlying theme that maximizing power (rider) over a given distance (environment) with the least drag (bicycle-rider unit in environment) is the ultimate application of ergonomics for cycling performance.

References

Barelle, C., Chabroux, V. and Favier, D. (2010) 'Modeling of the time trial cyclist projected frontal area incorporating anthropometric, postural and helmet characteristics', *Sports Engineering*, 12(4): 199–206.

Brisswalter, J., Hausswirth, C., Smith, D., Vercruyssen, F. and Vallier, J. M. (2000) 'Energetically optimal cadence vs. freely-chosen cadence during cycling: effect of exercise duration', *International Journal of Sports Medicine*, 21(1): 60–4.

Broker, J. P. and Gregor, R. J. (1994) 'Mechanical energy management in cycling: source relations and energy expenditure', *Medicine and Science in Sports and Exercise*, 26(1): 64–74.

Candotti, C. T., Ribeiro, J., Soares, D. P., De Oliveira, A. R., Loss, J. F. and Guimaraes, A. C. (2007) 'Effective force and economy of triathletes and cyclists', *Sports Biomechanics*, 6(1): 31–43.

Chabroux, V., Barelle, C. and Favier, D. (2008) 'Aerodynamics of time trial bicycle helmets', in M. Estivalet and P. Brisson (eds), *The Engineering of Sport 7*, Paris: Springer, pp. 401–10.

Chavarren, J. and Calbet, J. A. (1999) 'Cycling efficiency and pedalling frequency in road cyclists', *European Journal of Applied Physiology and Occupational Physiology*, 80(6): 555–63.

Chowdhury, H. (2012) 'Aerodynamic design of sports garments,' in J. C. Lerner (ed.), *Applied Aerodynamics*, Croatia: InTech, pp. 21–40.

Chowdhury, H., Alam, F., Mainwaring, D., Subic, A., Tate, M., Forster, D. and Eyto-Ferre, J. (2009) 'Design and methodology for evaluating aerodynamic characteristics of sports textiles', *Sports Technology*, 2(3–4): 81–6.

Chowdhury, H., Alam, F. and Mainwaring, D. (2011) 'A full scale bicycle aerodynamics testing methodology', *Procedia Engineering*, 13: 94–9.

Coast, J. R. and Welch, H. G. (1985) 'Linear increase in optimal pedal rate with increased power output in cycle ergometry', *European Journal of Applied Physiology and Occupational Physiology*, 53(4): 339–42.

Debraux, P., Grappe, F., Manolova, A. V. and Bertucci, W. (2011) 'Aerodynamic drag in cycling: methods of assessment', *Sports Biomechanics*, 10(3): 197–218.

Defraeye, T., Blocken, B., Koninckx, E., Hespel, P. and Carmeliet, J. (2010a) 'Aerodynamic study of different cyclist positions: CFD analysis and full-scale wind-tunnel tests', *Journal of Biomechanics*, 43(7): 1262–8.

Defraeye, T., Blocken, B., Koninckx, E., Hespel, P. and Carmeliet, J. (2010b) 'Computational fluid dynamics analysis of cyclist aerodynamics: performance of different turbulence-modelling and boundary-layer modelling approaches', *Journal of Biomechanics*, 43(12): 2281–7.

Defraeye, T., Blocken, B., Koninckx, E., Hespel, P. and Carmeliet, J. (2011) 'Computational fluid dynamics analysis of drag and convective heat transfer of individual body segments for different cyclist positions', *Journal of Biomechanics*, 44(9): 1695–701.

de Groot, G., Welbergen, E., Clijsen, L., Clarijs, J., Cabri, J. and Antonis, J. (1994) 'Power, muscular work, and external forces in cycling', *Ergonomics*, 37(1): 31–42.

di Prampero, P. E. (2000) 'Cycling on Earth, in space, on the Moon', *European Journal of Applied Physiology*, 82(5): 345–60.

Dorel, S., Couturier, A. and Hug, F. (2009) 'Influence of different racing positions on mechanical and electromyographic patterns during pedalling', *Scandinavian Journal of Medicine and Science in Sports*, 19(1): 44–54.

Edwards, A. G. and Byrnes, W. C. F. (2007) 'Aerodynamic characteristics as determinants of the drafting effect in cycling', *Medicine and Science in Sports and Exercise*, 39(1): 170–6.

Elmer, S. J., Barratt, P. R., Korff, T. and Martin, J. C. (2011) 'Joint-specific power production during submaximal and maximal cycling', *Medicine and Science in Sports and Exercise*, 43(10): 1940–7.

Faria, E. W., Parker, D. L. and Faria, I. E. (2005) 'The science of cycling: factors affecting performance – part 2', *Sports Medicine*, 35(4): 313–37.

Foss, O. and Hallen, J. (2004) 'The most economical cadence increases with increasing workload', *European Journal of Applied Physiology*, 92(4–5): 443–51.

Foster, C., Schrager, M., Snyder, A. C. and Thompson, N. N. (1994) 'Pacing strategy and athletic performance', *Sports Medicine*, 17(2): 77–85.

Garcia-Lopez, J., Rodriguez-Marroyo, J. A., Juneau, C. E., Peleteiro, J., Martinez, A. C. and Villa, J. G. (2008) 'Reference values and improvement of aerodynamic drag in professional cyclists', *Journal of Sports Sciences*, 26(3): 277–86.

Gibertini, G., Grassi, D., Macchi, C. and De Bortoli, G. (2010) 'Cycling shoe aerodynamics', *Sports Engineering*, 12(3): 155–61.

Gnehm, P., Reichenbach, S., Altpeter, E., Widmer, H. and Hoppeler, H. (1997) 'Influence of different racing positions on metabolic cost in elite cyclists', *Medicine and Science in Sports and Exercise*, 29(6): 818–23.

Gotshall, R. W., Bauer, T. A. and Fahrner, S. L. (1996) 'Cycling cadence alters exercise hemodynamics', *International Journal of Sports Medicine*, 17(1): 17–21.

Hansen, E. A. and Sjogaard, G. (2007) 'Relationship between efficiency and pedal rate in cycling: significance of internal power and muscle fibre type composition', *Scandinavian Journal of Medicine and Science in Sports*, 17(4): 408–14.

Heil, D. P., Wilcox, A. R. and Quinn, C. M. (1995) 'Cardiorespiratory responses to seat-tube angle variation during steady-state cycling', *Medicine and Science in Sports and Exercise*, 27(5): 730–5.

Heil, D. P., Derrick, T. R. and Whittlesey, S. (1997) 'The relationship between preferred and optimal positioning during submaximal cycle ergometry', *European Journal of Applied Physiology and Occupational Physiology*, 75(2): 160–5.

Hubenig, L. R., Game, A. B. and Kennedy, M. D. (2011) 'Effect of different bicycle body positions on power output in aerobically trained females', *Research in Sports Medicine*, 19(4): 245–58.

Iniguez-de-la-Torre, I. and Iniguez, J. (2006) 'Cycling and wind: does sidewind brake?', *European Journal of Physics*, 27(1): 71.

International Ergonomics Association Council (2000) *Definition of Ergonomics*, available at: www.iea.cc/01_what/What%20is%20Ergonomics.html (accessed 31 September 2012.

Jeukendrup, A. E. and Martin, J. (2001) 'Improving cycling performance: how should we spend our time and money?', *Sports Medicine*, 31(7): 559–69.

Jobson, S. A., Nevill, A. M., George, S. R., Jeukendrup, A. E. and Passfield, L. (2008) 'Influence of body position when considering the ecological validity of laboratory time-trial cycling performance', *Journal of Sports Sciences*, 26(12): 1269–78.

Kautz, S. A. and Hull, M. L. (1993) 'A theoretical basis for interpreting the force applied to the pedal in cycling', *Journal of Biomechanics*, 26(2): 155–65.

Lamb, D. R. (1995) *Basic Principles for Improving Sport Performance*, Columbus, OH: Gatorade Sport Science Institute.

Leirdal, S. and Ettema, G. (2011) 'Pedaling technique and energy cost in cycling', *Medicine and Science in Sports and Exercise*, 43(4): 701–5.

Litka, K. L., LaRoche, D. P., Cook, S. B. and Quinn, T. J. (2011) 'Effects of seat tube angle manipulation on cardiorespiratory response and frontal area in female cyclists', *Medicine and Science in Sports and Exercise*, 43(5/1): S88–9.

Lollgen, H., Graham, T. and Sjogaard, G. (1980) 'Muscle metabolites, force, and perceived exertion bicycling at varying pedal rates', *Medicine and Science in Sports and Exercise*, 12(5): 345–51.

Loras, H., Ettema, G. and Leirdal, S. (2009) 'The muscle force component in pedaling retains constant direction across pedaling rates', *Journal Applied Biomechanics*, 25(1): 85–92.

Lucia, A., Hoyos, J. and Chicharro, J. L. (2001) 'Preferred pedalling cadence in professional cycling', *Medicine and Science in Sports and Exercise*, 33(8): 1361–6.

Lucia, A., San Juan, A. F., Montilla, M., CaNete, S., Santalla, A., Earnest, C. and Perez, M. (2004) 'In professional road cyclists, low pedaling cadences are less efficient', *Medicine and Science in Sports and Exercise*, 36(6): 1048–54.

Martin, J. C. and Brown, N. A. (2009) 'Joint-specific power production and fatigue during maximal cycling', *Journal of Biomechanics*, 42(4): 474–9.

Nordeen-Snyder, K. S. (1977) 'The effect of bicycle seat height variation upon oxygen consumption and lower limb kinematics', *Medicine and Science in Sports*, 9(2): 113–17.

Price, D. and Donne, B. (1997) 'Effect of variation in seat tube angle at different seat heights on submaximal cycling performance in man', *Journal of Sports Sciences*, 15(4): 395–402.

Samozino, P., Horvais, N. and Hintzy, F. (2006) 'Interactions between cadence and power output effects on mechanical efficiency during sub maximal cycling exercises', *European Journal of Applied Physiology*, 97(1): 133–9.

Sanderson, D. J. (1991) 'The influence of cadence and power output on the biomechanics of force application during steady-rate cycling in competitive and recreational cyclists', *Journal of Sports Sciences*, 9(2): 191–203.

Sanderson, D. J. and Amoroso, A. T. (2009) 'The influence of seat height on the mechanical function of the triceps surae muscles during steady-rate cycling', *Journal of Electromyography and Kinesiology*, 19(6): e465–71.

Shennum, P. L. and deVries, H. A. (1976) 'The effect of saddle height on oxygen consumption during bicycle ergometer work', *Medicine and Science in Sports*, 8(2): 119–21.

Takaishi, T., Yasuda, Y., Ono, T. and Moritani, T. (1996) 'Optimal pedalling rate estimated from neuromuscular fatigue for cyclists', *Medicine and Science in Sports and Exercise*, 28(12): 1492–7.

van Ingen Schenau, G. J., van Woensel, W. W., Boots, P. J., Snackers, R. W. and de Groot, G. (1990) 'Determination and interpretation of mechanical power in human movement: application to ergometer cycling', *European Journal of Applied Physiology and Occupational Physiology*, 61(1–2): 11–19.

Welbergen, E. and Clijsen, L. P. (1990) 'The influence of body position on maximal performance in cycling', *European Journal of Applied Physiology and Occupational Physiology*, 61(1–2): 138–42.

11

EFFECTS OF ENVIRONMENTAL CONDITIONS ON COMPETITIVE SWIMMING PERFORMANCE

Joshua Guggenheimer, Kasey Young and Dennis Caine

UNIVERSITY OF NORTH DAKOTA, GRAND FORKS

Introduction

The role of ergonomics in sport is complex: not only do we strive to enhance the comfort and safety of the competing individual, but the approach of ergonomics is also to understand the relationship one has with the task they are trying to perform, while at the same time acknowledging the equipment and environment with which they work (Reilly, 2010). Whether working in a scientific or leisure setting, closer examination into the environmental factors affecting injury and performance may lead the reader to reconsider the prescription of swimming by making small, albeit important environmental changes in the equipment used, practice techniques employed, or even to the swimming pool itself.

There are over 250,000 high school and 20,000 college students who participate in competitive swimming in the United States (U.S. Bureau of the Census, 2011). The Centers for Disease Control (CDC) estimates approximately 360 million patrons visit aquatic facilities annually (Centers for Disease Control, 2003) and with the high participation in competitive swimming, the proper operation of aquatic facilities is essential for maintaining water and air quality while minimizing the risk of disease transmission. Pool and spa operators must have a working knowledge of pool operations to comply with state standards, which in some cases have as much as a 50 percent greater water clarity requirement than currently in force for most municipal drinking water (Williams, 2006).

The purpose of this chapter is to examine the impact of environmental conditions on competitive swimming performance. Specifically, we strive to examine the influence of equipment, hydrodynamic influences, technique, and water quality on corresponding injury and performance throughout the sport of competitive swimming.

Equipment and apparel

Many advances have been made to swimming equipment over the previous years. The primary purpose of these advances has been twofold: to enhance performance and to increase the safety of the participant. For example, the use of a wetsuit in water has been shown to increase buoyancy (Cordain and Kopriva, 1991), thus decreasing surface drag and increasing swimming speed. Furthermore, the added buoyancy allows the swimmer to preferentially exert energy for propulsion, rather than focusing on maintenance of a horizontal position. The use of a wetsuit has been shown to have physiological implications as well, by mitigating the decrease in core temperature frequently experienced when swimming in cold water. Some argue that the use of a wetsuit may also have more direct effects on swimming performance by increasing stroke rate and correspondingly swimming speed (Hue *et al.*, 2003). The use of a wetsuit therefore appears to have significant benefits for athletes with limited swimming skill, such as triathletes.

Similar performance adaptations have been found using technical swimsuits. In one case, these performance enhancements were so dramatic that full-body, polyurethane swimsuits have been banned by the Federation Internationale de Natation following 43 broken records at the 2009 World Championship in Rome (O'Conner and Vozenilek, 2011). Despite records frequently being broken in the sport of swimming, 43 records at one meet was unprecedented, leading to a thorough investigation of the results posted in Rome. Close scrutiny of the 2009 performances led to the understanding that the abrupt increases in performance were caused not by physiological or societal changes, but rather by equipment enhancements, as evidenced by the fact that every new record was set by an individual wearing the full-body technical swimsuit. Such technical suits have been credited with enhancing performance via three means: increased buoyancy, decreased surface drag and increased body compression, all of which would in turn positively impact performance (O'Conner and Vozenilek, 2011). Such dramatic changes resulted in the prohibition of such technical suits, due to the fact that they were considered a form of 'artificial enhancement' similar to doping.

The modification of equipment has also been conducted in the training arena. Equipment such as parachutes has been used to overload the neuromuscular system while swimming, while the use of hand paddles to enhance propulsion has been employed as a means of augmenting training performance (Telles *et al.*, 2011). Pull buoys are also commonly utilized in the pool in order to enhance buoyancy of the legs, allowing the swimmer to focus on upper-body stroke mechanics (Pichon *et al.*, 1995). Despite the use of equipment to modify training adaptations, there are few data available regarding the translation of such adaptations to competitive scenarios and risk prevention. Regardless of data, the use of overload and its converse, potentiation, is common in many sports, and will likely be the continued focus of many equipment manufacturers in the future.

A well-accepted and frequently used equipment modification in swimming is the silicone swim cap (Hue and Galy, 2012). The introduction of the swim cap was primarily based upon the desire to reduce drag and increase hygiene, although there are secondary effects relating to heat regulation when swimming in non-regulation-temperature waters. Due to the high heat transfer coefficient of water (Hue and Galy, 2012) and the high vascularity of the scalp, having one's head submerged in extreme water temperatures may have significant implications on the thermoregulatory capacity of an individual. The use of equipment to facilitate adequate thermoregulation has received much attention in the realm of adolescent athletics due to the fact that prepubescent children are less effective at regulating core temperature due to the increased surface area-to-mass ratio (Kenney *et al.*, 2012). Thus, the use of swim caps, while influential in decreasing drag, may have the additive benefit of maintaining core temperature in colder water temperatures.

Perhaps more pertinent to the concept of ergonomics is the notion of equipment modification as a means of enhancing participant safety. Eye goggles are one type of equipment commonly used in swimming in order enhance participant safety. Specifically, safety is enhanced by the use of eye goggles in two respects: by enhancing visual quality, and by reducing the eye discomfort and corneal staining (Wu *et al.*, 2011), in addition to the obvious protection necessary to guard against the flailing limbs of the competitors in adjacent lanes. The need for visual feedback during a swimming event is apparent to anyone who has spent time in the pool; rather than swimming with the eyes closed and running the risk of veering out of one's lane, goggles are utilized in order to allow the swimmer to 'watch' the lines underwater, therefore providing guidance to the opposing wall and back.

The use of event-specific equipment is commonplace throughout sport. Swimming, although fairly minimalist in comparison to others sports (e.g. hockey), is not bereft of equipment needs. Competitive swimmers employ the use of streamlining swim caps, skin-tight bathing suits, and low-profile goggles, all with the intent of minimizing drag and maximizing buoyancy. Even the recreational swimmer commonly employs some, if not most, of this equipment to ensure comfort and safety when swimming laps at the pool. Despite the relatively low-profile equipment used in the sport of swimming, the function these few items provide is invaluable to the competitive athlete and recreational swimmer alike.

Hydrodynamics

Swimming performance is affected by many environmental conditions specific to the medium surrounding the swimmer. In most cases, when an individual is swimming through water, he or she is subject to a variety of forces, each of which affects performance in different ways (Benjanuvatra *et al.*, 2002). These hydrodynamic forces play a significant role in the movement of, and ability to perform a given task in, the water. Hydrodynamic forces can be loosely categorized into two groups: resistive forces and propulsive forces. As each of the names suggests, resistive forces are those forces acting 'against' the individual, thus inhibiting his or her progress, whereas propulsive forces are those forces acting 'with' the individual. Each of these respective forces may be more easily understood when broken down into their respective components: resistive forces are comprised of drag and buoyancy, whereas propulsive forces are comprised of the physiological (e.g. body length, mass, and surface area) and biomechanical (e.g. swimming technique, swimming style, stroke length) output of the individual swimmer (Kjendlie *et al.*, 2004b).

Resistive forces

As illustrated by de Koning *et al.* (2011) the force of drag (F_{drag}) is equal to:

$$F_{drag} = \frac{1}{2} \left(p C_d A v_2 \right) \qquad (1)$$

where p is the density of the water, C_d is the drag coefficient, A is the frontal area exposed to the medium, and v is the velocity of the body. Figure 11.1 illustrates the various forces acting upon an individual as he or she swims through the water.

Further complicating the complex interaction between drag and swimming performance is the differentiation of passive and active drag, which can be defined as resistive forces during a static position and resistive forces during actual swimming, respectively (Havriluk, 2007). Considering the above equation and the added complexity of static and passive drag, it becomes clear that discussion of drag alone could warrant an entire chapter. However, for the purpose of this text, discussion of drag will be kept relatively simplistic in the context of just one of many factors affected by environmental ergonomics in the swimming pool. If one were to

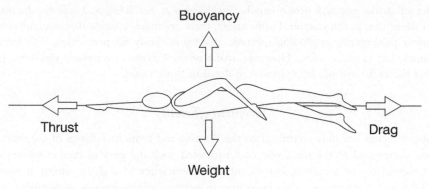

Figure 11.1 Forces acting upon a swimming body.

rearrange the above equation, it becomes clear that there is an inverse relationship between the area of exposure and the drag coefficient (Havriluk, 2005). Drag is thus influenced by a plethora of factors; some of which are environmental – such as water density, which is most often manipulated by changing water temperature – while others are anthropometric in nature, such as body length and body density. Despite the complexity of drag in fluid environments, in the context of swimming performance the primary principle is relatively simplistic: a reduction in drag will result in an increased swimming velocity, thereby theoretically enhancing performance (Kjendlie *et al.*, 2004b).

Bouyancy is best explained by considering Archimedes' principal in which an object is buoyed relative to the amount of fluid it displaces. In other words, the more fluid displaced, the greater the buoyancy of the immersed body. Therefore, a submerged passive body in the water will be subject to the competing forces of buoyancy and weight (Kjendlie *et al.*, 2004a). Theoretically, one would want to maximize buoyancy in order to limit drag, thereby increasing swimming velocity, assuming that is the goal. Buoyancy, unlike active and passive drag, is primarily determined by anthropometric parameters; that is to say body density. One's body density is determined by the cumulative composition of fat-free mass (muscle, bone, etc.) and fat mass. Intuitively, the less dense the individual (i.e. the greater proportion of fat mass), the more buoyant he or she will be. Although one's percentage body fat will not change in an acute sense, it can change significantly over time, and therefore may play a significant role in the buoyancy – and therefore drag – of a given individual. Additional factors affecting buoyancy in the water include the volume of air in one's lungs. As might be expected, the inhalation of air results in a temporary decrease in the overall density of the system and therefore increases the buoyancy of the individual. Considering this transient change in the overall density of the body, it should become clear that with each inhalation and corresponding exhalation, one is manipulating one's buoyancy and, by default, one's drag.

Propulsive forces

Acting in opposition to resistive forces are those forces responsible for propulsion. As anyone that has swam before can attest to, there are a plethora of factors that contribute to one's ability to propel oneself through the water. These factors include biomechanical motor patterns; that is to say the sequence of biomechanical events leading to a swimming stroke (e.g. the combination of shoulder flexion, plantar flexion, etc. leading to a swim stroke) as well as the product of stroke rate and stroke length (Psycharakis *et al.*, 2008) and will be discussed in greater detail later in this chapter. Furthermore, there are many additional physiological factors that affect performance, including substrate utilization, body fat percentage, and breathing mechanics, just to name a few. However, many of these factors are outside the scope of this text and therefore will not be addressed in detail in this chapter.

Movement efficiency

The above factors not only contribute to the resistive and propulsive forces of the individual, but also correspond to the metabolic cost associated with the performance of swimming as well. Oftentimes, the metabolic cost or metabolic efficiency of a given activity is measured using kilojoules per kilogram, thus providing an estimate of the amount of metabolic energy required to transport a body a specific unit of distance (Capelli *et al.*, 1998). Energy cost is typically assessed using oxygen consumption (VO_2) and speed of movement. Thus, the movement efficiency of a given stroke may be determined by not only the intensity (e.g. submaximal versus maximal-intensity) of the activity performed, but also the type of stroke performed (e.g. front crawl versus backstroke).

In the context of environmental ergonomics, consideration must be given to factors influencing an individual's safety as well as those affecting performance. Maximizing safety while at the same time maximizing performance should be a primary goal for athletes and coaches alike. In a mechanical sense, efficiency can be thought of as minimizing extraneous or unnecessary movements; this efficiency is most often accomplished by minimizing drag by adopting a streamlined position in the water (Naemi and Sanders, 2008). Consider again the swimmer from Figure 11.1: by elongating his or her body and adopting a streamlined position, he or she is minimizing the opposing drag, which corresponds to an increased metabolic efficiency. Now picture the same individual flexed at the wrists and plantar flexed at the ankles; what effect would these changes have on the amount of drag acting against the individual? Similarly, what effect would these changes have on the metabolic cost associated with such a change in drag?

Efficiency is a term that is often used to mean many different things, but when used in the context of swimming ergonomics it refers to the concept of minimizing metabolic cost for a given activity while maintaining velocity (Naemi and Sanders, 2008). Thus, the less energy required to propel one through the water, the more efficient one becomes. Efficiency is thus strongly correlated to economy, which can be interpreted to mean the 'fluidity' of the movement as influenced by the unnecessary movements alluded to above.

Training and technique

The vast majority of swimming-related literature pertains to the training and techniques employed by swimmers. In order to positively manipulate swimming performance, attention is usually given to one of two primary considerations: technique (i.e. the motor organization based upon coordination of temporal patterns of the arms, legs, and body) and training (i.e. enhancing physiological performance). Manipulation of these overarching parameters in turn will affect several performance-related characteristics of the swimmer, including the time spent in each of the phases (e.g. glide, catch, pull, push), the speed at which he or she is propelled, and the fatigue resulting from such performances (see Figure 11.2).

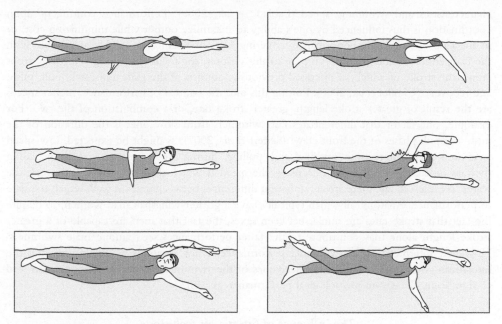

Figure 11.2 Swimming phases of the freestyle swim stroke.

Swimming technique

Much work has been done in an attempt to qualitatively analyze fatigue-related changes in swimming technique. As a result, there is a significant amount of data pertaining to competitive swimming and swimming to exhaustion, which conclusively indicates changes in swimming technique with fatigue. However, there is little consensus on the extent to which each specific parameter is affected; these inconsistencies stem in part from the different classification systems used to characterize stroke technique. In the most basic sense, stroke rate (frequency) and stroke length are used; the interaction of the two determining speed (Alberty *et al.*, 2008). This simplistic view allows one to examine stroke characteristics from a purist perspective as it relates to speed. Thus, an increase or decrease in speed must be caused by an increase or decrease in stroke rate or stroke length, respectively.

For a more detailed examination of swimming technique, however, the stroke itself may be broken into its respective components. For the front crawl, the stroke can be broken into four phases: glide and catch, pull, push, and recovery (Chollet *et al.*, 2000). The contribution of each of these phases, however, will vary greatly depending on the experience of the swimmer, the pace of the performance, and ergonomic factors such as water temperature and equipment. Adding to the complex understanding of the swim stroke is the consideration of underwater propulsion, which is affected by both 'pumping' and whiplash effects, the former creating an accelerating low-pressure mass of water along the swimmer's body surface, while the latter generates a vortex, both of which contribute to lift-based propulsion (Collard and Oboeuf, 2009). Despite the proven effectiveness of underwater propulsion, it is given little attention in the literature due to the fact that much of the time is spent above water in order to breathe effectively.

Regardless of the stroke being performed, arm-leg coordination is of paramount importance to the overall performance of the individual, which in turn is affected by individual characteristics and swimming speed (Leblanc *et al.*, 2009). Performance contingent upon coordination is thus influenced by one's ability to maximize output while minimizing cost; or in the case of swimming performance, covering a given distance as quickly as possible with the least effort possible. For the purpose of this chapter, the focus has been given to the front crawl, the stroke of which, as discussed previously, consists of the glide and catch, pull, push, and recovery (Chollet *et al.*, 2000). Putting this into the context of performance, higher speeds are the result of greater stroke length, greater stroke rate, or a combination of the two. For example, one factor that differentiates fast swimmers from slow ones is the duration of the push and pull phases of the front crawl (Seifert *et al.*, 2007); as might be expected, low-speed swimmers spend more time 'pushing' and 'pulling' during the swim stroke, thus decreasing the rate of stroke, which in turn decreases the speed at which they are propelled through the water. Needless to say, there are also inherent differences between sexes as well, which translate to performance. Anatomically, men typically have a greater wingspan than women; so despite the fact that stroke rates are similar between sexes, the fact that men are capable of a greater stroke length alone may contribute to the faster performances seen among male swimmers. However, interpretation of swimming performance is not as simple as just interpreting the inter-limb coordination and stroke mechanics of the swimmer; proper training can also lead to significant changes in physiological performance as well.

The influence of fatigue on technique

As mentioned previously, swimming performance is greatly influenced by both coordination and physiological parameters alike, both of which factor in to the overall health and safety of the participant. Factors such as aerobic capacity, cardiorespiratory function, and muscular strength all play significant roles in physiological function and the corresponding swimming performance. Aerobic capacity in turn can be assessed using individual performances, constant-load tests, and incremental tests (Palayo *et al.*, 2007). Each of these tests provides valuable insight into the aerobic performance of an individual, but they must be interpreted with caution, as individual responses to exercise vary greatly from person to person. Furthermore, the individualized physiological response will also be influenced by mechanical and psychological contributions, making it difficult to make generalizations about the training techniques best employed for optimum performance.

Optimizing training intensity in swimming requires careful assessment of many physio-logical parameters. Blood lactate concentration and heart rate are two of the more commonly examined characteristics and can provide valuable insight to the physiological responses during prolonged and intermittent swimming performances (Keskinen *et al.*, 2007). Blood lactate, although not a direct indication of metabolic output, is a strong indicator of anaerobic performance, with higher levels of blood lactate corresponding to higher reliance upon quicker means of producing andenosine triphosphate (ATP), such as rapid glycolysis. Regardless of the length of swimming performance, a significant amount of ATP is also derived from aerobic metabolism, which is typically limited by cardiac output (the product of stroke volume and heart rate), and measured using oxygen consumption (VO_2). Obviously, the amount of oxygen consumed and the cardiac parameters corresponding to such consumption are subject to a variety of influential factors: race length, racing speed, technique, physical characteristics, etc. (Lavoie and Montpetit, 1986).

Of particular interest to swimming ergonomics is the concept of fatigue, as it will greatly impact the technique and performance of the swimmer, and by association, the health and safety. There are many compensatory techniques that are used by swimmers in order to minimize the effect of fatigue. Recall that the performance goal in swimming is typically contingent upon maximizing speed, which is a product of the stroke length and stroke rate (Alberty *et al.*, 2008). Swimming speed is thus maintained by increasing one of the afore-mentioned parameters in order to negate a decrease in its counterpart. In order to illustrate this point, consider the high-speed swimmer who has a longer stroke than his or her slower counterpart. This elongated stroke allows one to take fewer strokes, placing a decreased metabolic demand on the system, the net result of which is a decrease in the resultant fatigue experienced by the swimmer. However, in most cases the faster swimmer not only exhibits greater stroke length, but a consistent stroke rate as well; thus leading to a significantly faster swimming speed (Seifert *et al.*, 2007) with subjectively similar levels of fatigue.

As in all sports, the training and technique used in swimming has great influence on the outcome expected. Physical characteristics often drive the length of one's stroke, whereas biomechanical factors such as the temporal and mechanical inter-limb coordination frequently dictate the rate of stroke performed. The interaction of stroke rate and length not only dictate swimming speed, but the metabolic demands related to such performance as well. Fatigue has long been acknowledged as a complex and multifactorial phenomenon, the point of which is clearly illustrated when analysing the technique and training patterns used in competitive swimming.

Factors affecting water quality

Water quality is affected by pH, disinfectant level (free chlorine in chlorinated pools), and temperature, and if any of the three are not maintained correctly the decreasing water quality can affect patron comfort and health. In a chemically balanced pool, the pH level is considered the most important variable because of its influence on the effectiveness of chlorine used to disinfect chlorinated aquatic venues. The typical state health code in the United States requires the pH level to be maintained between 7.0 and 8.0 (Williams, 2006), and pools with low pH can experience damage to the heating elements and water circulation components, and can contribute to the irritation of patrons' skin and eyes. A venue that has high pH can also experience patron eye and skin irritation, but more importantly high pH decreases the effectiveness of chlorine used to disinfect pools (Centers for Disease Control, 2010b) thus increasing the risk of disease transmission and contributing to an overall decrease in water quality.

Free chlorine levels in pools vary from state to state, with the accepted minimum amount of free chlorine being 1.0 ppm, while the maximum can be higher than 5 ppm in many state health codes (Ford, 2009). Chlorine is most effective for disinfecting pools when the pH of the water is 7.0 (Williams, 2006) and water temperature is maintained at 77°F or higher (Centers for Disease Control, 2010a). The free chlorine is consumed when it reacts with inorganic or organic compounds introduced into the water in the form of urine or sweat, or from contaminates in the environment around the facility. The introduction of these compounds decreases the free chlorine available and creates disinfection by products (DBPs) that can cause irritation to swimmers' eyes, skin, and lungs, and increases the risk of recreational water illness (RWIs) such as Cryptosporidium.

Water quality and health

Maintaining optimal water quality in aquatic facilities requires the facility to have trained and certified operators on staff and checking the water on regular intervals to ensure compliance with state recreational water codes. However, data from 120,975 pool inspections in four states found that 10.7 percent of pools had pH violations, 8.9 percent had disinfectant level violations and 12.5 percent had other water chemistry violations (Centers for Disease Control, 2010a). These results were similar to 22,131 pool inspections conducted in 2002, where 38.7 percent of inspections found water chemistry violations (Centers for Disease Control, 2003). Violations of pH and disinfectant levels are considered important because improper maintenance of water chemistry increases the chance of RWIs, and water chemistry violations have been associated with positive microbiologic test results that result in pool closures (Hadjichristodoulou *et al.*, 2006).

Operators who are trying to maintain chemical ranges during heavy use of a facility face a difficult task. Weng and Blatchley (2011) found that when free chlorine levels were monitored during a national swimming competition, the water chemistry was significantly affected during the event. When intense bather loads (150–200 swimmers) were present in the pool, a rapid drop in free chlorine was observed and DBPs ($CNCHCL_2$ and CH_3NgCL_2) increased by a factor of 2–3 during the competition. The amount of total nitrogen a swimmer contributes to a pool has been rarely studied even though the creation of DBPs is directly influenced by the amount of nitrogen contributed by these swimmers. Weng and Blatchley (2011) estimated that each swimmer contributes 0.56–1.20 g of urea per person, and Keuten *et al.* (2012) notes that 0.56–1.20 g of urea would correspond with a total nitrogen (TN) contribution of 260–560 mg TN per person without showering prior to entering the water compared to 70 mg TN per person with a pre-swim shower. By reducing the nitrogen contribution to pool water by patrons, the facility requires less chlorine to be consumed and thus reduces the formation of DBPs that can cause discomfort to swimmers in the form of eye and skin irritants, as well as the development of respiratory-related conditions and the transmission of RWIs.

Air quality and health

Recently the effects of air quality (as it relates to water quality) on patron health have been given increased attention, with numerous studies warning about the health risk of swimming pool attendance and competitive swimmers (Aggazzotti *et al.*, 1998; Fiks *et al.*, 2012; Uyan *et al.*, 2009). Although swimming is recommended for children with asthma, because of the warm humid environment, results of studies on young swimmers with asthma have been mixed and need to be studied more (Uyan *et al.*, 2009). In elite swimmers, Langdeau *et al.* (2000) found that 29.3 percent have higher airway hyperactivity then sedentary individuals the same age, and other studies have found that swimmers have higher bronchial hyperactivity then non-swimmers (Helenius and Haahtela, 2000). One area of increasing concern is the effects of DBPs such as Trihalomethanes (THMs) on swimmers' respiratory health, with some studies finding THMs to be located in the alveolar breath, blood (Aggazzotti *et al.*, 1998), and urine of swimmers (Caro and Gallego, 2007) after only 1 hour of swimming.

Water temperature

The ideal water temperature at aquatic facilities varies depending on the type of programming conducted and can fluctuate greatly depending on the type of activity being conducted. USA swimming requires that the water temperature for competitive events be maintained between 77 and 82.4°F, with air temperature no lower than 76°F. Studies involving competitive swimmers in water temperatures above 80.6°F have found increased water temperatures can influence the performance of swimmers by increasing core body temperature (Holmer and

Bergh, 1974; Macaluso *et al.*, 2011), increasing the sweat rate, lowering urine volumes (Macaluso *et al.*, 2011), and increasing heart rate (Mougios and Deligiannis, 1993). While the ideal temperature for performance recorded by Macaluso *et al.* (2011) is 80.6°F, studies on the effects of water cooler than 80.6°F have demonstrated that cooler water decreases both heart rate and lactate levels in well-trained competitive swimmers (Loupos *et al.*, 2008).

Injury in competitive swimming

A tenet of ergonomics is that the work (sport) environment will not harm the individual; hence, safety is an overriding criterion (Reilly, 2010). Since the injured athlete is unable to perform at full capacity and loses fitness when not able to train, evidence-based injury prevention becomes paramount. A look at injury, therefore, is important in providing an important perspective of the outcome of the interaction between the swimmer and the swimming environment. Top-level competitive swimmers train on average 20–30 hours a week. In addition to water-based training, competitive swimmers are also exposed to weight training regimens that are designed to increase muscular strength and endurance (Kammer *et al.*, 1999). A key problem with high-intensity aerobic and strength-training programmes is the risk of injury, particularly repetitive strain injury.

Injury epidemiology in swimming is concerned with quantifying injury occurrence with respect to who is affected by injury, where and when injuries occur, and what is their outcome for the purpose of explaining how and why injuries occur and identifying strategies to control and prevent them. The study of the distribution of varying rates of injuries (i.e. who, when, where, what) is referred to as descriptive epidemiology, and the study of the determinants of an exhibited distribution of varying rates of injury (i.e. why and how) is referred to as analytical epidemiology (Caine *et al.*, 2006).

The incidence and distribution of injury

An important foundation in understanding and preventing injury in competitive swimming is first to quantify the nature and extent of injury. Table 11.1 summarizes studies that report injury rates for competitive swimmers (Bak *et al.*, 1989; Chase *et al.*, in press; Garrick and Requa, 1978; Graham and Bruce, 1977; Grimmer, 1996; Junge *et al.*, 2009; Kennedy *et al.*, 1978; Knobloch *et al.*, 2008; Lanese *et al.*, 1990; McFarland and Wasik, 1996; Mountjoy *et al.*, 2010; Mutoh *et al.*, 1988; Richardson, 1999; Wolf *et al.*, 2009). Most of these studies reported clinical incidence rates (i.e. number of injuries divided by number of participants), ranging from 2.2 to 194.7 injuries per 100 participants. Unfortunately, these rates are difficult to compare because they do not account for the varying exposure of swimmers to the risk of injury. Other factors that may compromise meaningful comparison of study results include variation in competitive and training levels of swimmers studies, the retrospective design used in most studies (i.e. recall bias), and variability in injury definition, and thus the way injury rates were derived across studies.

Determination of exposure-based injury rates is essential for meaningful comparison of studies and as an objective basis for the analysis of injury risk factors and preventive measures. As shown in Table 11.1, only a handful of studies reported exposure-based injury rates. One recent study reported that competition injury incidence rates were lower than for 15-year average rates for both males and females in all other NCAA sports (Chase *et al.*, in press; Hootman *et al.*, 2007). However, practice injury rates were relatively high in comparison to

Table 11.1 Comparison of injury rates

Authors	Year	Study design	Method	Gender	Level	No. of swimmers	No. of injuries	Rate per 100 athletes*	Rate per 1,000 AEs	Rate per 1,000 hours
Graham and Bruce	1977	R	Q	78F	C	78	8	10.2		
Garrick and Requa	1978	R	IR	77M; 82F	HS	159	8	5		
Kennedy et al.	1978	R	S		I	35	43	122.9		
		R	Q		NS	2,496	261	10.5		
Mutoh et al.	1988	R	Q	10F; 9M	E/N	19	37	194.7		
Bak et al.	1989	R	Q		NS	268	100	37.3		
Lanese et al.	1990	P	IR	21F 36M	C	57	29	50.9		
Grimmer	1996	R	Q	193F/159M	N	352	16	4.5		
McFarland and Wasik	1996	R	S	68F	C	68	56	82.4	1.05	
Richardson	1999	R	S		A	1,500	886	59.1		
Knobloch et al.	2008	P			E	341				0.39
Wolf et al.	2009	R	IR	44M 50F	C	94	166	176.6	M = 4.00 F = 3.78	
*Junge et al.	2009	P	IR	M/F	I	23	1046	2.2		
*Mountjoy et al.	2010	P	IR	M/F	I	1,502	43	M = 2.2; F = 3.5		
Chase et al.	in press	P	IR	16M 18F	C	34	31	91.2	M = 5.33 F = 6.5 5.55	3.04

Level: A = Age Group; C = Collegiate; E = Elite; HS = High School; N = National; I = International; NS = Not Specified.
Study Design: R = Retrospective; P = Prospective; L = Longitudinal.
Methods: Q = Questionnaire; S = Survey; IR = Injury Report; E = Examination.
Gender: M = Male; F = Female.
* International competitions.

other NCAA sport practice rates, likely reflecting the highly repetitive nature of training for competitive swimming.

A summary of the distribution of injury by anatomical location is provided in Table 11.2 (Chase *et al.*, in press; Grimmer, 1996; Kennedy *et al.*, 1978; McFarland and Wasik, 1996; Mutoh *et al.*, 1988; Richardson, 1999; Wolf *et al.*, 2009). This research indicates that the body part most affected by injury in competitive swimming is the shoulder, ranging from 3 to 55 percent of all injuries, followed by the back (16–37 percent) then knee (5–28 percent).

Several studies have focused on the occurrence of injuries involving specific body parts. A summary of these studies is provided in Table 11.3 and described below. An important shortcoming of most of these retrospective studies was that they depended on surveys, therefore rendering them subject to recall bias.

Anatomical location

Determination of body parts most affected by injury is important because it alerts health-care professionals to anatomical locations in need of special attention during musculoskeletal screening and it provides researchers with a focus for the establishment of preventive measures. The finding that shoulder injuries are most common in competitive swimming is not surprising given the repetitive overhead movement required in swimming. In all swimming strokes, the swimmer uses large moment arm forces to reach forward and drag the water (Sein *et al.*, 2010).

The most frequently diagnosed shoulder injury is known as 'swimmer's shoulder', which is an impingement syndrome that occurs when either the supraspinatus muscle tendon, biceps brachii tendon or both become compressed by the acromion of the scapula, making shoulder motion extremely painful and making swimming almost impossible (Johnson *et al.*, 1987). In one study, 91 percent (73/80) of elite swimmers aged 13–25 years reported shoulder pain, and 69 percent of those examined with MRI (36/52) had supraspinatus tendinopathy (Sein *et al.*, 2010). Bak and Fauno (1997) performed complete physician examinations on 36 swimmers with a history of shoulder injuries and found that 12 swimmers were classified as having a primary impingement and 25 swimmers were classified as having a secondary impingement. In a recent study of 236 female swimmers, ages 8–77 years, 48 (20.3 percent) swimmers had shoulder pain and disability. Other shoulder injuries that can affect a swimmer include directional instability, glenohumerallabral injuries, brachial plexus injuries, acromioclavicular joint pain, arthritis and rotator cuff injuries (McMaster, 1999).

Knee injuries account for 5–28 percent of all swimming injuries (Table 11.2). Four studies have looked specifically at knee injuries (Hahn and Foldspang, 1998; Rovere and Nichols, 1985; Stulberg *et al.*, 1980; Vizsolyi *et al.*, 1987). Perhaps the most common injury involving the swimmer's knee is 'breaststroker's knee' (Fowler and Regan, 1986). Clinically, 'breaststroker's knee' occurs when the swimmer's knee is placed in a maximal valgus position, causing a medial collateral ligament sprain (Fowler and Regan, 1986). Other injuries to the knee that were identified include patellar dislocation, general joint effusion, meniscus injuries, and medial synovitis (Fowler and Regan, 1986).

Stulberg *et al.* (1980) found that of 23 breaststroke swimmers surveyed, 10 identified a history of knee injury relating to swimming. Further examination found 18 swimmers with tenderness over the medial facet of the patella, and five of them also had pain over the medial collateral ligament (Stulberg *et al.*, 1980). Vizsolyi *et al.* (1987) found that 53 percent of the 391 swimmers in their study had a history of knee pain and 46 percent of the swimmers experienced most of the pain during the first part of their kick.

Table 11.2 A per cent distribution of injuries by anatomical location

Authors	Year	Study design	No. of athletes	No. of injuries	Head/neck	Shoulder	Arm/hand	Thigh/adductor	Knee	Ankle/foot	Back	Other
Kennedy et al.	1978	R	35	43		37			28	19		16
Mutoh et al.	1988	R	2,496	261		31			26.8	32.5		9.7
Grimmer	1996	R	19	37	3	31.3	3		20	5.6	37.1	0.5
			352	16		47	5.8	5.8	23.5		17.4	
McFarland and Wasik	1996	L	68	56	7	55	4	5	11		18	
Richardson	1999	R	1,500	886	26	3	18		5		3	13
Wolf et al.	2009	R	94	176		31.2[a]				32	21.6[b]	
Mountjoy et al.	2010	P	1,502	43		20.9	20.9[c]		6.9		11.6	
Chase et al.	in press	P	34	31	3.2	38.7		6.5	12.9	12.9	16.1	9.7

Study Design: R = Retrospective; P = Prospective; L = Longitudinal.
a, includes upper arm injuries; b, includes neck injuries; c, includes wrist.

Table 11.3 Injury rates to specific anatomical locations

Authors	Year	Study design	Method	Specific location	Gender	Level	No. of swimmers	No. of injuries	% of athletes injured	Rate per 100 athletes
Dominguez	1978	XC/R	E	Shoulder	133F 130M	A	263	90		34.2
Richardson et al.	1980	XC/R	Q/E	Shoulder	83F 54M	N	137	58		42.3
McMaster and Troup	1993	R	S	Shoulder		A/E/N	1262		10-26	
Burchfield et al.	1994	R	Q	Shoulder	54F 46M	NS	100	29		29
Stocker et al.	1995	R	Q	Shoulder		C/M	927	445		48
Bak and Fauno	1997	XC/R	Q/E	Shoulder	22F 14M	N	36	49		136.1
McMaster	1999	R	Q	Shoulder	13F 27M	N	40	23		57.5
Stulberg et al.	1980	XC	E	Knee	14F 9M	A/E	23	18		78.3
Rovere and Nichols	1985	R	S	Knee	17F 19M	A/C	36	27		75
Vizsolyi et al.	1987	R	S	Knee	216F 175M	A	391	209		53.5
Hahn and Foldspang	1998	R	Q	Knee		C	53	33		62.3
Loosli and Quick	1992	R	Q	Thigh/Adductor	16F 14M	C	30	10		33.3
Grote et al.	2004	R	S	Thigh/Adductor	98F 198M	C/N	296		21.5-42.7	
Soler and Calderon	2000	XC	E	Back		N	176	18		10.2

Level: A = Age Group Swimmers; N = National Swimmers; C = Collegiate Swimmers; O = Olympic Swimmers; E = Elite Swimmers; M = Masters Swimmers; NS = Not Specified.
Study Design: Q = Retrospective; P = Prospective; XC = Cross Sectional.
Methods: Q = Questionnaire; S = Survey; IR = Injury Report; E = Exam.

As shown in Table 11.2, thigh and adductor muscle strains have been reported to account for about 5 percent of all injuries sustained in competitive swimming (Grimmer, 1996; McFarland and Wasik, 1996). Two studies (as shown in Table 11.3) have reported the frequency of thigh/adductor injuries. Loosli and Quick (1992) found that 10 of 30 Division I swimmers had a history of or a present thigh injury. Their questionnaire indicated that the most common thigh injuries were defined as adductor magnus and/or brevis strains (Loosli and Quick, 1992). Grote *et al.* (2004) found that of the 296 swimmers who mainly participated in breaststroke ($n = 130$), individual medley ($n = 80$), or neither ($n = 86$), breaststroke swimmers had a greater adductor strain prevalence than either of the two other groups (Grote *et al.*, 2004).

Back injuries account for 11.0–37.1 percent of all injuries sustained as a result of participating in competitive swimming (see Table 11.2). Major back injuries, such as spondylolysis and spondylolisthesis, can significantly compromise the swimmer's ability to practice or compete and may also require corrective surgery (Kammer *et al.*, 1999). Soler and Calderon (2000) found the prevalence rate of spondolysis to be 10.23 percent among 176 swimmers. Capaci *et al.* (2002) reported that 33.3 per cent of butterfly swimmers and 22.2 percent of breaststroke swimmers experienced low back pain. A relatively high prevalence of intervertebral disk degeneration has also been reported among advanced competitive swimmers (Hangai *et al.*, 2009; Kaneoka *et al.*, 2007).

Environmental location

There is a lack of research reporting on the environmental location of competitive swimming injuries. Swimming injuries not only occur in the swimming pool, but in dry land training and other associated venues as well. Richardson (1999) found that of the 886 injuries reported, 42 percent occurred in the water, 22 percent occurred on the pool deck, while the rest occurred on the periphery of the pool. McFarland and Wasik (1996) found that of the 125 injuries sustained by 68 swimmers between the years 1984 and 1991, 45 percent were swimming-related (both practice and competition), and 44 percent were related to cross-training. They also found that injury rates related to cross-training were very similar to injury rates obtained in swimming (1.07 injuries per 1,000 exposures compared to 1.05 injuries per 1,000 exposures, respectively).

Onset and severity of injury

Not surprisingly, the majority of competitive swimming injuries are overuse injuries. Knobloch *et al.* (2008) reported rates of 0.22 overuse injuries and 0.17 acute injuries among elite swimmers. Similarly, Chase *et al.* (in press) reported that overuse injuries accounted for 58.1 percent of injuries in their study of collegiate swimmers. Shoulder impingement was the most common overuse injury in this study.

Time loss associated with injury is of great concern in swimming because the swimmers lose rather than gain fitness. Richardson *et al.* (1980) found that of the 58 swimmers who complained of shoulder pain during the physician-based examination, 43 swimmers had to reduce their daily swimming yardage and 21 were forced to stop training altogether. Stocker *et al.* (1995) found that 47 percent of 532 collegiate swimmers and 48 percent of 395 master swimmers had a history of shoulder pain that lasted three or more weeks, and that it was severe enough to force the swimmer to change his or her swimming routine or stop swimming altogether. The South Australian Branch of Sports Medicine found that 75 percent of the total injuries sustained by 352 national swimmers were classified as minor injuries that did not restrict the swimmer from participating in competitions and practices, and 12.5 were considered major injuries, requiring the swimmer to leave the competition and not finish (Grimmer, 1996).

Grote *et al.* (2004) found that swimmers with thigh injuries missed, on average, 7–12 practices each season depending on their stroke preference. They also found that breaststroke swimmers were more likely to miss practice because of adductor pain (42.7 percent) and missed an average of 11.5 practices a season. Wolf *et al.* (2009) reported 33–41 percent of injuries resulted in missed time. Chase *et al.* (in press) reported the 41.9 per cent of injuries required more than seven days' time loss before return to full practice.

Etiology of injury

The epidemiological approach to sports injuries is rooted in the assumption that swimming injuries do not happen purely by chance, so an important part of swimming injury epidemiology is the identification of factors that contribute to the occurrence of injury. Risk factors may be classified as intrinsic or extrinsic. Intrinsic factors are individual biological and psychosocial characteristics predisposing a person to the outcome of injury, such as previous injury, flexibility or life stress. Once the athlete is 'predisposed', extrinsic or 'enabling' factors may facilitate manifestation of injury (Meeuwisse, 1994). Extrinsic risk factors are factors that have an impact on the sport participant 'from without', and include such factors as coach's qualifications, exposure time and equipment.

Intrinsic risk factors

Sallis *et al.* (2001) found that female swimmers were more likely to sustain an injury than male swimmers (47.08 percent compared to 12.37 percent, $p < 0.0001$). The study also reported gender differences in specific injuries related to anatomical location. Female swimmers were more likely to sustain injuries to the shoulder (21.05 percent versus 6.55 percent, $p < 0.01$) and knee (5.85 percent versus 1.45 percent, $p < 0.01$) compared to their male counterparts. In contrast, Wolf *et al.* (2009) reported a higher but non-significant rate of injuries for male swimmers.

In a study comparing swimmers aged 8–77 years with and without shoulder pain or disability, Tate *et al.* (2012) found differences in two or more age groups included a higher incidence of previous traumatic injury, and reduced participation in another sport ($p < 0.05$). They also found reduced shoulder flexion, weakness of the middle trapezius and internal rotation, shorter pectoralis minor and latissimus, and decreased core endurance in symptomatic females in single varying age groups ($p < 0.05$).

Chase *et al.* (in press) also found history of any injury (IRR = 2.86, 95 percent CI = 1.23, 6.64) and history of injury to the same anatomical location (IRR = 1.67, 95 percent CI = 1.21, 2.31) to be associated with an increased injury rate in adjusted multivariate analyses.

Extrinsic risk factors

In a study comparing swimmers aged 8–77 years with and without shoulder pain or disability, Tate *et al.* (2012) found differences in two or more age groups that included greater swimming exposure and reduced participation in another sport ($p < 0.05$). Knobloch *et al.* (2008) reported that swimming more than four times per week was associated with a higher risk for knee (RR = 2.1) and shoulder (RR = 4.0) injuries. The prevalence of shoulder injury may also relate to the swimmer's competitive and training levels. Based on their study of 993 competitive swimmers representing three competitive levels (national aged group, senior elite development group, and US national swimming team), McMaster and Troup (1993) reported that the US national team swimmers had the highest percentage of shoulder injuries (26 percent) compared to both the national aged level (10 percent) and the senior elite level (13 percent) swimmers. The US national team also had the highest percentage of shoulder injury history among the three groups (McMaster and Troup, 1993). However, these differences were not tested statistically.

Prevention of injury

Once the analytical evidence points to an association between certain risk factors and injury, thereby establishing a degree of predictability for those participants who are likely to sustain injury, the next step in epidemiologic research is to seek ways to prevent or reduce the occurrence of such injury. Testing the suggested preventive measure to determine its effectiveness is an important aspect of the analytical epidemiologic process and fulfills the ultimate goal of epidemiology – that is, prevention. Ideally, the effectiveness of injury prevention measures should be tested prior to recommending their general implementation.

Unfortunately, there has been no controlled research designed to determine the effectiveness of injury prevention measures on reducing injury rates in competitive swimming. This finding is surprising given the popularity of competitive swimming and the common occurrence of overuse injuries in this sport, particularly those injuries that affect the shoulder and may cause significant loss of training and potential long-term disability. In the absence of intervention research, suggestions for injury prevention that appear in the research reviewed include the importance of pre-season history and musculoskeletal screening, with appropriate follow-up physical therapy and adjustments to training, particularly with regards to shoulder injuries. Adjustments to the repetitive nature of training through individualized and cross-training also seems appropriate.

Conclusion

Review of the previous topics should provide a clear illustration of the complexity of sport ergonomics and its application in the realm of swimming. The impact of one's environment is significant and is likely to influence one's performance and safety, and perhaps more importantly one's enjoyment. The adoption of new technique may increase enjoyment while at the same time decrease the prevalence of injury. Similarly, changing the pool pH may decrease the likelihood of transmitting a foreign bacterial body, but will likely affect the density of the water, thereby influencing drag. Whether out for a leisurely set of laps or fine-tuning one's stroke for an upcoming race, it should be clear that the environmental factors influencing swimming ergonomics are many, and proper consideration of such factors may greatly influence the enjoyment, safety, and functionality of one's daily swim.

References

Aggazzotti, G., Fantuzzi, G., Righi, E. and Predieri, G. (1998) 'Blood and breath analysis as biological indicators of exposure to trihalomethanes in indoor swimming pools', *The Science of the Total Environment*, 217(1–2): 155–63.

Alberty, M., Potdevin, F., Dekerle, J., Pelayo, P., Gorce, P. and Sidney, M. (2008) 'Changes in swimming technique during time to exhaustion at freely chosen and controlled stroke rates', *Journal of Sports Sciences*, 26(11): 1191–200.

Bak, K. B. and Fauno, P. (1997) 'Clinical finding in competitive swimmers with shoulder pain', *American Journal of Sports Medicine*, 25(2): 254–60.

Bak, K., Bue, P. and Olsson, G. (1989) 'Injury patterns in Danish competitive swimming', *Ugeskrift for Laeger*, 151(45): 2982–4.

Benjanuvatra, N., Dawson, G., Blanksby, B. A. and Elliott, B. C. (2002) 'Comparison of buoyancy, passive and active net drag forces between Fastskin and standard swimsuits', *Journal of Science and Medicine in Sport*, 5(2): 115–23.

Burchfield, D., Cofield, S. and Cofield, R. (1994) 'Shoulder pain in competitive, age group swimmers', *Medicine and Sport Science*, 39: 218–25.

Caine, D., Caine, C. and Maffulli, N. (2006) 'Incidence and distribution of pediatric sport-related injuries', *Clinical Journal of Sport Medicine*, 16(6): 501–14.

Capaci, I., Ozcaldiran, B. and Durmaz, B. (2002) 'Musculoskeletal pain in elite competitive male swimmers', *The Pain Clinic*, 14(3): 229–34.

Capelli, C., Pendergast, D. and Termin, B. (1998) 'Energetics of swimming at maximal speeds in humans', *European Journal of Applied Physiology*, 78(5): 385–93.

Caro, J. and Gallego, M. (2007) 'Assessment of exposure of workers and swimmers to trihalomethanes in an indoor swimming pool', *Environment Science Technology*, 41(13): 4793–8.

Centers for Disease Control (2003) 'Surveillance data from swimming pool inspections: selected states and counties, United States, May–September 2002', *MMWR*, 52(2): 513–16.

Centers for Disease Control (2010a) 'Violations identified from routine swimming pool inspections: selected states and counties, United States, 2008', *MMWR*, 59(19): 582–7.

Centers for Disease Control (2010b) *Fecal Incident Response Recommendations for Pool Staff*, available at: www.cdc.gov/healthyswimming (accessed 15 August 2012).

Chase, K., Caine, D., Goodwin, B. J., Whitehead, J. and Romanick, R. (in press) 'A prospective study of injury affecting competitive collegiate swimmers', *Research in Sports Medicine*.

Chollet, D., Chalies, S. and Chatard, J. (2000) 'A new index of coordination for the crawl: description and usefulness', *International Journal of Sports Medicine*, 21(1): 54–9.

Collard, L. and Oboeuf, A. (2009) 'Comparison of expert and nonexpert swimmers' opinions about value, potency, and activity of four standart swimming strokes and underwater undulatory swimming', *Percept Motor Skills*, 108(2): 491–8.

Cordain, L. and Kopriva, R. (1991) 'Wetsuits, body density and swimming performance', *British Journal of Sports Medicine*, 25(1): 31–3.

de Koning, J. J., Foster, C., Lucia, A., Bobbert, M. F., Hettinga, F. J. and Porcari, J. P. (2011) 'Using modeling to understand how athletes in different disciplines solve the same problem: swimming versus running versus speed skating', *International Journal of Sports Physiology and Performance*, 6(2): 276–80.

Dominguez, R. H. (1978) 'Shoulder pain in age group swimming', in B. Erickson and B. Furberg (eds), *Swimming Medicine IV*, Baltimore: University Park Press, pp. 105–9.

Fiks, L. N., Albuquerque, A. P., Dias, L., Fernandes, C. R. and Carvalho, C. R. (2012) 'Occurrence of asthma symptoms and of airflow obstruction in amateur swimmers between 8 and 17 years of age', *Jornal Brasileiro de Pneumologia*, 38(1): 24–32.

Ford, R. (2009) *Pool and Spa Operator Handbook*, Colorado Springs, CO: National Swimming Pool Foundation.

Fowler, P. J. and Regan, W. D. (1986) 'Swimming injuries of the knee, foot, and ankle, elbow, and back', *Clinics in Sports Medicine*, 5(1): 139–48.

Garrick, J. G. and Requa, R. K. (1978) 'Injuries in high school sports', *Pediatrics*, 61(3): 465–9.

Graham, G. P. and Bruce, P. J. (1977) 'Survey of intercollegiate athletic injuries to women', *Research Quarterly*, 48(1): 217–20.

Grimmer, K. (1996) *Injury Surveillance of South Australian Sporting Participants*, Sports Medicine Australia-South Australian Branch 1996, available at: www.smasa.asn.au/resources/downloads/injury_surveillance2.pdf (accessed 27 March 2007).

Grote, K., Lincoln, T. L. and Gamble, J. G. (2004) 'Hip adductor injury in competitive swimming', *American Journal of Sports Medicine*, 32(1): 44–52.

Hadjichristodoulou, C., Mouchtouri, V., Vousoureli, A., Konstantinidis, A., Petrikos, P., Velonakis, E., Boufa, P. and Kremastinou, J. (2006) 'Waterborne diseases prevention: evaluation of inspection scoring system for water sites according to water microbiological tests during the Athens 2004 pre-Olympic and Olympic period', *Journal of Epidemiology and Community Health*, 60(10): 829–35.

Hahn, T. and Foldspang, A. (1998) 'Prevalent knee pain and sport', *Scandinavian Journal of Social Medicine*, 26(1): 44–52.

Hangai, M., Kaneoka, K., Hinotsu, S., Shimizu, K., Okubo, Y., Miyakawa, S., Mukai, N., Sakane, M. and Ochiai, N. (2009) 'Lumbar intervertebral disk degeneration in athletes', *American Journal of Sports Medicine*, 37(1): 149–55.

Havriluk, R. (2005) 'Performance level differences in swimming: a meta-analysis of passive drag force', *Research Quarterly for Exercise and Sport*, 76(2): 112–18.

Havriluk, R. (2007) 'Variability in measurement of swimming forces: a meta-analysis of passive and active drag', *Research Quarterly for Exercise and Sport*, 78(2): 32–9.

Helenius, I. and Haahtela, T. (2000) 'Allergy and asthma in elite summer sport athletes', *Journal of Allergy and Clinical Immunology*, 106(3): 444–52.

Holmer, I. and Bergh, U. (1974) 'Metabolic response to swimming in water at varying temperatures', *Journal of Applied Physiology*, 37(5): 702–5.

Hootman, J. M., Dick, R. and Agel, J. (2007) 'Epidemiology of collegiate injuries for 15 sports: summary and recommendations for injury prevention initiatives', *Journal of Athletic Training*, 42(2): 311–19.

Hue, O. and Galy, O. (2012) 'The effect of a silicone swim cap on swimming performance in tropical conditions in pre-adolescents', *Journal of Sports Science and Medicine*, 11: 156–61.

Hue, O., Benavente, H. and Chollet, D. (2003) 'The effect of wet suit use by traithletes: an anlaysis of the different phases of arm movement', *Journal of Sports Sciences*, 21(12): 1025–30.

Johnson, J. E., Sim, F. H. and Scott, S. G. (1987) 'Musculoskeletal injuries in competitive swimmers', *Mayo Clinic Proceedings*, 62(4): 289–304.

Junge, A., Engebretsen, L., Mountjoy, M. L., Alonso, J. M., Renström, P. A., Aubry, M. J. and Dvorak, J. (2009) 'Sports injuries during the Summer Olympic Games 2008', *American Journal of Sports Medicine*, 37(11): 2165–72.

Kammer, C. S., Young, C. C. and Niedfeldt, M. W. (1999) 'Swimming injuries and illnesses', *The Physician and Sports Medicine*, 27(4): 51–60.

Kaneoka, K., Shimizu, K., Hangai, M., Okuwaki, T., Mamizuka, N., Sakane, M. and Ochiai, N. (2007) 'Lumbar intervertebral disk degeneration in elite competitive swimmers: a case control study', *American Journal of Sports Medicine*, 35(8): 1341–45.

Kennedy, J. C., Hawkins, R. and Kissoff, W. B. (1978) 'Orthopaedic manifestations of swimming', *American Journal of Sports Medicine*, 6(6): 309–22.

Kenney, W., Wilmore, J. and Costill, D. (2012) *Physiology of Sport and Exercise*, 5th edn, Champaign, IL: Human Kinetics.

Keskinen, O., Keskinen, K. and Mero, A. (2007) 'Effect of pool length on blood lactate, heart rate, and velocity in swimming', *International Journal of Sports Medicine*, 28(5): 407–13.

Keuten, M. G., Schets, F. M., Schijven, J. F., Verberk, J. Q. and van Dijk, J. C. (2012) 'Definition and quantification of initial anthropogenic pollutant release in swimming pools', *Water Research*, 46(11): 3682–92.

Kjendlie, P. L., Ingjer, F., Stallman, R. K. and Stray-Gundersen, J. (2004a) 'Factors affecting swimming economy in children and adults', *European Journal of Applied Physiology*, 93(1–2): 65–74.

Kjendlie, P. L., Stallman, R. K. and Stray-Gundersen, J. (2004b) 'Passive and active floating torque during swimming', *European Journal of Applied Physiology*, 93(1–2): 75–81.

Knobloch, K., Yoon, U., Kraemer, R. and Vogt, P. M. (2008) '200–400m breaststroke event dominate among knee overuse injuries in elite swimming', *Sportverletz Sportschaden*, 22(4): 213–19.

Lanese, R. R., Strauss, R. H., Leizman, D. J. and Rotondi, A. M. (1990) 'Injury and disability in matched men's and women's intercollegiate sports', *American Journal of Public Health*, 80(12): 1459–62.

Langdeau, J. B., Turcotte, H., Bowie, D. M., Jobin, J., Desgagne, P. and Boulet, L. P. (2000) 'Airway hyperresponsiveness in elite athletes', *American Journal of Respiritory and Critical Care Medicine*, 161(5): 1479–84.

Lavoie, J. and Montpetit, R. (1986) 'Applied physiology of swimming', *Sports Medicine*, 3(3): 165–89.

Leblanc, H., Seifert, L. and Chollet, D. (2009) 'Arm-leg coordination in recreational and competitive breaststroke swimmers', *Journal of Science and Medicine in Sport*, 12(3): 352–6.

Loosli, A. R. and Quick, J. (1992) 'Thigh strains in competitive swimming', *Journal of Sports Rehabilitation*, 1: 49–53.

Loupos, D. L., Tsalis, G., Papadopoulos, A., Mathas G. and Mougios, A. (2008) 'Physiological and biochemical responses to competitive swimming in cold water', *The Open Sports Medicine Journal*, 2: 34–7.

Macaluso, F., Felice, V. D., Boscaino, G., Bonsignore, T., Stampone, T., Farina, F. and Morici, G. (2011) 'Effects of three different water temperatures on dehydration in competitive swimmers', *Science and Sports*, 26: 265–71.

McFarland, E. G. and Wasik, M. (1996) 'Injuries in female collegiate swimmers due to swimming and cross training', *Clinical Journal of Sport Medicine*, 6(3): 178–82.

McMaster, W. C. (1999) 'Shoulder injuries in competitive swimmers', *Clinics in Sports Medicine*, 18(2): 349–59.

McMaster, W. C. and Troup, J. (1993) 'A survey of interfering should pain in United States competitive swimmers', *American Journal of Sports Medicine*, 21(1): 67–70.

Meeuwisse, W. (1994) 'Assessing causation in sport injury: a multifactorial model', *Clinical Journal of Sport Medicine*, 4(3): 166–70.

Mougios, V. and Deligiannis, A. (1993) 'Effect of water temperature on performance, lactate production and heart rate at swimming of maximal and submaximal intensity', *Journal of Sprots Medicine and Physical Fitness*, 33(1): 27–33.

Mountjoy, M., Junge, A., Alonso, J. M., Engebretsen, L., Dragan, I., Gerrard, D., Kouidri, M., Luebs, E., Shahpar, F. M. and Dvorak, J. (2010) 'Sports injuries and illnesses in the 2009 FINA World Aquatics Championships', *British Journal of Sports Medicine*, 44(7): 522–7.

Mutoh, Y., Takamoto, M. and Miyashita, M. (1988) 'Chronic injuries of elite competitive swimmers, divers, water polo players, and synchronized swimmers', in B. Ungerechts, K.Wilke and K. Reischle (eds), *Swimming Science V*, Champaign, IL: Human Kinetics, pp. 333–7.

Naemi, R. and Sanders, R. (2008) 'A "hydrokinematic" method of measuring the glide efficiency of a human swimmer', *Journal of Biomechanical Engineering*, 130(6): 1–9.

O'Conner, L. and Vozenilek, J. (2011) 'Is it the athlete of the equipment? An analysis of the top swim performances from 1990 to 2010', *Journal of Strength and Conditioning Research*, 25(12): 3239–41.

Palayo, P., Alberty, M., Sidney, M., Potdevin, F. and Dekerle J. (2007) 'Aerobic potential, stroke parameters, and coordination in swimming front-crawl performance', *International Journal of Sports Physiology and Performance*, 2(4): 347–59.

Pichon, F., Chatard, J. C., Martin, A. and Cometti, G. (1995) 'Electrical stimulation and swimming performance', *Medicine and Science in Sports and Exercise*, 27(12): 1671–6.

Psycharakis, S. G., Cooke, C. B., Paradisis, G. P., O'Hara, J. and Phillips, G. (2008) 'Analysis of selected kinematic and physiological performance detriments during incremental testing in elite swimmers', *Journal of Strength and Conditioning Research*, 22(3): 951–7.

Reilly, T. (2010) *Ergonomics in Sport and Physical Activity*, 1st edn, Champaign, IL: Human Kinetics.

Richardson, A. B. (1999) 'Injuries in competitive swimming', *Clinics in Sports Medicine*, 18(2): 287–91.

Richardson, A. B., Jobe, F. W. and Collins, H. R. (1980) 'The shoulder in competitive swimming', *American Journal of Sports Medicine*, 8(3): 159–63.

Rovere, G. D. and Nichols, A. W. (1985) 'Frequency, associated factors, and treatment of breaststroker's knee in competitive swimmers', *American Journal of Sports Medicine*, 13(2): 99–104.

Sallis, R. E., Jones, K., Sunshine, S., Smith, G. and Simon, L. (2001) 'Comparing sports injuries in men and women', *International Journal of Sports Medicine*, 22(6): 420–3.

Seifert, L., Chollet, D. and Chatard, C. (2007) 'Kinematic changes during a 100-m front crawl: effects of performance level and gender', *Medicine and Science in Sports and Exercise*, 39(10): 1784–93.

Sein, M. L., Walton, J., Linklater, J., Appleyard, R., Kirkbride, B., Kuah, D. and Murrell, G. A. (2010) 'Shoulder pain in elite swimmers: primarily due to swim volume-induced supraspinatus tendinopathy', *British Journal of Sports Medicine*, 44(2): 105–13.

Soler, T. and Calderon, C. (2000) 'The prevalence of spondylolysis in the Spanish elite athlete', *American Journal of Sports Medicine*, 28(1): 57–62.

Stocker, D., Pink, M. and Jobe, F. W. (1995) 'Comparison of shoulder injury in collegiate and master's level swimmers', *Clinical Journal of Sport Medicine*, 5(1): 4–8.

Stulberg, S. D., Shulman, K., Stuart, S. and Culp, P. (1980) 'Breaststroker's knee: pathology, etiology, and treatment', *Clinical Journal of Sports Medicine*, 5(3): 4–8.

Tate, A., Turner, G. N., Knab, S. E., Jorgensen, C., Strittmatter, A. and Michener, L. A. (2012) 'Risk factors associated with shoulder pain and disability across the lifespan of competitive swimmers', *Journal of Athletic Training*, 47(2): 149–58.

Telles, T., Barbosa, A. C., Campos, M. H. and Junior, O. A. (2011) 'Effect of hand paddles and parachute on the index of coordination of competitive crawl-strokers', *Journal of Sports Sciences*, 29(4): 431–8.

U.S. Bureau of the Census (2011) *Statistical Abstract of the United States: 2011*, Washington, DC: U.S. Bureau of the Census.

Uyan, Z. S., Carraro, S., Piacentini, G. and Baraldi, E. (2009) 'Swimming pool, respiratory health, and childhood asthma: should we change our beliefs?', *Pediatric Pulmonology*, 44(1): 31–7.

Vizsolyi, P., Taunton, J., Robertson, G., Filsinger, L. and Shannon, H. S. (1987) 'Breaststroker's knee: an analysis of epidemiological and biomechanical factors', *American Journal of Sports Medicine*, 15(1): 63–71.

Weng, S. and Blatchley, E. R. (2011) 'Disinfection by-products dynamics in a chlorinated, indoor swimming pool under conditions of heavy use: national swimming competition', *Water Research*, 45(16): 5241–8.

Williams, K. (2006) *The Aquatic Facility Operators Manual*, Hoffman Estates: NRPA Aquatic Section.

Wolf, B. R., Ebinger, A. E., Lawler. M. P. and Britton, C. L. (2009) 'Injury patterns in Division I collegiate swimming', *American Journal of Sports Medicine*, 37(10): 2037–42.

Wu, Y. T., Tran, J., Truong, M., Harmis, N., Zhu, H. and Stapleton, F. (2011) 'Do swimming goggles limit microbial contamination of contact lenses?', *Optometry and Vision Science*, 88(4): 456–60.

12

THE EFFECTS OF ENVIRONMENTAL CONDITION ON PERFORMANCE IN SOCCER

Billy Sperlich and Dennis-Peter Born

UNIVERSITY OF WUPPERTAL, WUPPERTAL

Soccer is one of the world's most popular team sports and is performed in all four seasons on most continents, in varying climatic and atmospheric conditions. When soccer games are held during extreme environmental conditions, such as in the heat, in the cold or at altitude, proper preconditioning and precautions are vital for the success and health of the players. The aim of this chapter is to provide the following: (1) an overview of the physiological and mental aspects; and (2) practical recommendations for players, coaches and supporting staff to cope with these special environmental aspects.

Playing soccer in the heat

During repeated muscle contraction, the human body transfers 20–25 per cent of metabolic energy into mechanical locomotion from which most energy is converted into heat (Nadel, 1988) and dissipated from the body via convection, conduction, radiation and evaporation to avoid hyperthermia (i.e. elevated body temperature due to impaired thermoregulation).

In healthy humans, the body temperature is maintained at approximately 37 ± 0.5°C, with lower temperatures in the morning that increase throughout the day. Core temperature is the temperature of the deep tissues of the body, in contrast to the temperatures of peripheral tissues, such as the skin, and is maintained at a fairly constant temperature to ensure that crucial enzymatic biochemical processes perform properly.

Of the four heat transfer pathways, evaporation from the skin (i.e. cooling of the skin, as illustrated in Figure 12.1) and the respiratory tract are the most effective mechanisms for heat dissipation during exercise (Gavin, 2003). By sweat vaporization, even during intense exercise, the core temperature is elevated by no more than 2–3°C (Maughan *et al.*, 2010). However, in hot conditions (> 30°C), heat dissipation does not match the metabolic heat production, which results in an elevated core temperature. In soccer, when playing in hot conditions, core temperatures may rise to 39–40°C (Shirreffs *et al.*, 2006). As a main physiological response to regulate core temperature, heart rate and vasodilatation of skin vessels increase to improve skin perfusion and evaporative heat transfer mechanisms in hot environments (Rowell, 1983).

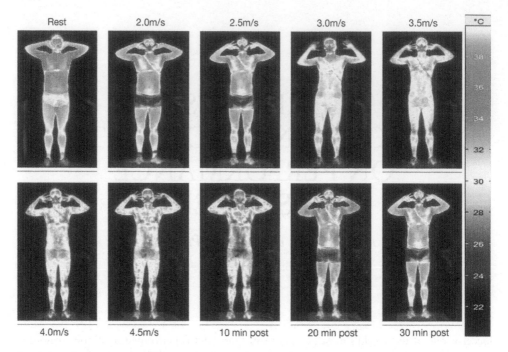

Figure 12.1 Skin temperature of a soccer player during and 30 minutes after incremental testing to exhaustion (ambient conditions: 23°C; 55 per cent humidity). Skin temperature decreases with increasing treadmill velocity due to evaporative sweating to maintain core temperature.

Additionally, blood lactate concentrations and the rate of muscle glycogen depletion are higher due to heat stress (Jentjens *et al.*, 2002). In soccer, depleted muscle glycogen stores were measured at the end of a match and were associated with continuing fatigue (Krustrup *et al.*, 2006). Because hyperthermia induces a more pronounced depletion of glycogen stores, limited substrate availability might be one reason for impaired soccer performance in the heat.

It has been shown that exercising in the heat reduces central neural drive with higher ratings of perceived effort (Nielsen and Nybo, 2003) due to interference with cerebral neurotransmitters (Nybo, 2010). Therefore, peripheral and central factors contribute to fatigue when exercising in the heat (Periard *et al.*, 2011). Consequently, soccer performance may be limited due to the following: (1) increased plasma epinephrine concentrations and greater perceived exertion (Parkin *et al.*, 1999); and (2) impaired cognitive function such as attention, visual-motor tracking, short-term memory and decision-making (Racinais *et al.*, 2008).

Effects of heat on performance

A small increase in muscle temperature is beneficial for various exercise tasks. Increased muscle temperature ($\sim 2°C$) resulting from warm-up routines improves repeated sprint ability (Mohr *et al.*, 2004) and power output during single (Falk *et al.*, 1998) and repeated sprints (Girard *et al.*, 2013). However, during prolonged endurance exercise, the time to exhaustion is impaired at 20°C and 30°C when compared to 10°C (Galloway and Maughan, 1997). In conclusion, the optimal body temperature and environmental conditions are dependent on the type and duration of the exercise. While warm temperatures of 25–35°C seem to be optimal for explosive motor tasks, cooler conditions ($\sim 10°C$) are beneficial for prolonged endurance activities.

Unfortunately, soccer exhibits both prolonged 10–13 km running at 70 per cent peak oxygen uptake (VO$_2$peak), including 2.5 km at high-intensity velocity, and maximal explosive efforts (Bangsbo *et al.*, 2006; Di Salvo *et al.*, 2007; Stølen *et al.*, 2005). However, when playing soccer in the heat (31–36°C), the total distance and number of sprints decrease, especially at the end of a game (Mohr *et al.*, 2010; Ozgunen *et al.*, 2010). Repeated vertical jumping heights after a soccer game are also reduced (Mohr and Krustrup, 2012). In a non-specific soccer test design, hyperthermia impaired attention, visual-motor tracking, short-term memory and decision-making (Racinais *et al.*, 2008).

Many of the negative effects of hyperthermia on performance may become more obvious as a result of dehydration (Mohr and Krustrup, 2012). Fluid loss during exercise reduces cutaneous and muscle blood flow, thereby hampering heat dissipation and the availability of nutrients and oxygen (Nielsen *et al.*, 1981) and accelerating the onset of fatigue. Moderate dehydration also induces headache, exhaustion, sickness and dizziness (Wenger, 1988) and causes detrimental effects on soccer performance (Shirreffs *et al.*, 2006), including repeated 20-second runs (Maxwell *et al.*, 1999). For example, a 1.5–2.0 per cent loss of body fluid impairs 1,500–10,000 m performance by 3–6 per cent (Armstrong *et al.*, 1985). However, vertical jumping and sprinting (50–400 m) appeared to be unaffected by moderate dehydration (Maughan, 2003; Watson *et al.*, 2005).

In conclusion, heat exposure does not seem to affect single maximal power exercises but exhibits detrimental effects on repeated explosive muscle contractions, prolonged endurance exercises, cognitive functions and soccer-specific performance.

Heat acclimatization

Long-term exposure to heat stress results in several acute adaptations, including more effective regulation of core temperature and improved exercise performance in the heat (Taylor, 2000). Several physiological and neuronal adaptations to heat stress are described that, together, improve body temperature regulation: (1) early onset of sweating; (2) elevated sweat rate (Taylor, 2000); (3) decreased core temperature at a given exercise intensity; (4) decreased concentration of electrolytes in sweat (Sawka and Montain, 2000); (5) increased plasma volume (Armstrong, 2000); (6) lower heart rate during exercise (Armstrong, 2000); and (7) increased skin vasodilatation (Cheung and McLellan, 1998; Chinevere *et al.*, 2008; Magalhaes Fde *et al.*, 2006).

The time course of the most important acclimatization adaptations to heat are summarized in Table 12.1. The onset of adaptations to heat stress occurs within a few days (Lind and Bass, 1963); however, athletes should acclimatize to heat within 1–2 weeks when exercising each day for 50–70 minutes at 50–60 per cent of their individual VO$_2$ peak (Wendt *et al.*, 2007). Interestingly, the adaptations to heat may still be evident three weeks after returning to a colder environment (Pichan *et al.*, 1985).

Table 12.1 The time course of the most important acclimatization responses to heat

Time course	Acclimatization response	Reference
3–6 days	↑ plasma volume; ↓ in heart rate	(Armstrong and Dziados, 1986; Wendt *et al.*, 2007)
5–10 days	↓ electrolyte concentration	(Armstrong, 2000)
7–14 days	↑ skin vasodilation, sweat sensitivity and sweat rate	(Armstrong, 2000)

Counteracting heat

Several modifications to pre-exercise routines, such as modified clothing, warm-up and pre-cooling, help athletes cope with hot environmental conditions.

In general, each layer of clothing impairs the heat transfer from the skin by its isolative properties (Gavin, 2003). Team-sports athletes often wear an additional layer of tight clothes under their regular uniform, thereby hindering heat transfer mechanisms. In the heat, soccer players may benefit from: (1) minimizing the amount of clothing worn; and (2) wearing loose-fitting synthetic textiles (Gavin, 2003) with bright colours (Nielsen, 1990) to reduce radiation of the sun (Pascoe *et al.*, 1994) and facilitate evaporative and convective mechanisms (Gavin, 2003).

Previous research has shown beneficial effects of cooling the body before and during competition (Booth *et al.*, 2001; Drust *et al.*, 2000; Price and Mather, 2004; Young *et al.*, 1987), with the highest effects on endurance performance and only slight improvements for (intermittent) sprinting performance. Cold drinks, cooling packs and vests have been shown to be beneficial for reducing heat stress (Wegmann *et al.*, 2012). In soccer, 20 minutes of pre-cooling with a vest has been shown to be effective when applied before the game and for 10 minutes during the half-time break (Price *et al.*, 2009).

Rehydration and nutrition when playing soccer in the heat

In professional soccer, the sweat loss during a match performed at 6–8°C was reported to be 1.68 ± 0.4 L (Maughan *et al.*, 2007). The sweat loss at 31–33°C may average 1.5–3.0 L (Mustafa and Mahmoud, 1979; Shirreffs *et al.*, 2005) and could peak at 4.4 L (Aragón-Vargas *et al.*, 2009). These data emphasize the necessity to compensate for fluid loss during the game and at the half-time break. The loss of 1 kg of body mass due to exercise and heat-induced dehydration should be replaced by 1.5 L of fluid (Shirreffs *et al.*, 1996). However, this recommendation is subject to remarkable inter-individual variability. For practical purposes, a pale colour of urine may serve as a sign for adequate (re-)hydration (Shirreffs and Maughan, 1998).

Based on previous research, a sports drink to improve soccer performance should feature the following: (1) 500–700 mg.L^{-1} of sodium to guarantee fluid absorption (Sawka *et al.*, 2007); (2) 7.5 per cent carbohydrates (Currell *et al.*, 2009); and (3) pleasant taste and cold temperature (Passe, 2001). In general, for activities lasting 60–90 minutes, an intake of 0.7g.kg^{-1}.h^{-1} carbohydrates is recommended (Kreider *et al.*, 2010).

Recommendations for playing soccer in the heat

Based on the aforementioned findings, the following recommendations can be provided to players and coaches to counteract heat stress:

1   Heat exposure and dehydration do not appear to affect single power tasks but have detrimental effects on repeated sprint and jumping exercises, prolonged endurance exercise, cognitive functions and soccer-specific performance.
2   Heat-acclimatized athletes experience greater fluid loss due to improved sweating; the elevated risk of dehydration emphasizes the need for additional fluid intake.
3   The loss of 1 kg of body mass due to dehydration should be replaced by 1.5 L of fluid. Pale rather than dark urine colour may serve as a practical indicator of (re-)hydration.
4   A sport drink should contain 500–700 mg.L^{-1} of sodium and 0.7 g.kg^{-1}.h^{-1} carbohydrates.

5   Players should be allowed 1–2 weeks of heat acclimatization in the target climate zone, via training camps under conditions with similar temperature conditions or by training with extra clothing or general exposure to heat (e.g. sauna).

6   When playing in the heat, extra clothing underneath the normal sports dress should be avoided.

7   The use of bright-coloured and loose-fitting jerseys instead of dark and tight clothing is recommended.

8   Cooling before a game and during the half-time break with cold drinks, cooling packs and cooling vests helps to improve heat storage capacity and enhances performance.

Playing soccer in the cold

Thermoregulation in the cold

When exposed to cold, cutaneous receptors sense the skin temperature, and the sympathetic nervous system provokes vasoconstriction in the peripheral limbs. This vasoconstriction reduces heat transfer to the upper skin layers but also reduces the heat loss by decreasing the temperature gradient between the skin and the ambient air. The increase in blood volume within the central organs stimulates urine production (Lennquist *et al.*, 1974; Wallenberg and Granberg, 1976), cold-induced dehydration and has the same negative effects on performance as hyperthermic conditions. Finally, cold-mediated vasoconstriction impairs oxygen transport to the working muscles and reduces their mechanical efficiency (Nimmo, 2004).

Cold-induced vasoconstriction is not uniformly distributed in the periphery. To prevent significant heat loss and to protect the vital organs from cold injuries, the shift in blood volume is more pronounced in the feet, toes, hands and fingers but is less evident in the head (Werner and Reents, 1980). Cold-induced vasoconstriction increases the blood pressure within the arterial system and enhances venous return, leading to elevated stroke volume (Rowell, 1983) and decreased heart rate at a given exercise intensity (Hanna *et al.*, 1975; Layden *et al.*, 2002; Weller *et al.*, 1997).

Exercise-induced hyperventilation in the cold stresses the respiratory organs. Inhaled cold air dries the upper respiratory mucosa and facilitates upper-respiratory tract infections (Giesbrecht, 1995; Ritzel, 1961; Sabiston and Livingstone, 1973; Walsh *et al.*, 2002), asthma-like symptoms (Heir and Oseid, 1994; Sue-Chu *et al.*, 1996) and cold-induced dehydration (Noakes, 2002).

The fluid loss in soccer is reported to average 1.2 L at 25°C and 1.0 L at 10°C (Rehrer and Burke, 1996). Because dehydration in the cold has the same detrimental effects on performance as in the heat (Freund and Sawka, 1996), measurements of body mass, as indicators of fluid loss, are also recommended in the cold to avoid dehydration.

Effects of cold conditions on performance

There is no generalized consensus on the ideal temperature for performance. When the ambient temperatures decrease to – 10°C, oxygen consumption and lipid oxidation are slightly reduced (Layden *et al.*, 2002; Quirion *et al.*, 1989), with an increased rate of carbohydrate oxidation (Armstrong, 2000; Pitsiladis and Maughan, 1999). The exposure to cold reduces the time to exhaustion (Galloway and Maughan, 1997), which may be due to vasoconstriction with impaired oxygen delivery (Doubt, 1991) and extraction (Shiojiri *et al.*, 1997), along with decelerated enzymatic processes.

The cold reduces the velocity of nerve impulses and diminishes muscle spindle sensitivity, which causes maximum muscle contraction to decrease by 3 per cent per 1°C reduction of muscle temperature (Reilly and Waterhouse, 2005). Therefore, the temperature of the peripheral receptors, nerve endings and nerves have a more crucial impact on motor control than the temperature of the central organs or the core temperature (Heus *et al.*, 1995).

Adaptation to and preparing for a cold environment

Scientific findings regarding acclimatization responses to cold are sparse. There is evidence that athletes appear to acclimatize to cold environmental conditions during autumn and winter due to daily exposure to cold (Baum *et al.*, 1976). Improved cold tolerance was characterized by a delayed onset of shivering and a reduced sensation of discomfort during exposure to cold due to vasoconstriction, with decreases in the peripheral blood flow (Baum *et al.*, 1976). Repeated cold–water immersion as an artificial inducer of cold stress appears to increase the activity of the sympathetic nervous system, the resting norepinephrine concentration and vasoconstriction (Launay *et al.*, 2002; O'Brien *et al.*, 2000; Young *et al.*, 1986).

Soccer games take place under various environmental conditions, including temperatures $\leq 0°C$ (Reilly, 2007); therefore, the key aspects of playing soccer, such as sprinting, jumping and prolonged running, might be impaired in the cold. However, with the application of adequate warm-up strategies and proper clothing, motion analysis in the cold revealed no detrimental effects on soccer performance (Carling *et al.*, 2011).

When exercising in windless conditions (0°C), it is recommended to wear the amount of clothing that keeps a resting athlete comfortable at 21°C (Gavin, 2003). Because wind speed impacts heat loss, tight-fitting clothing should be worn to maximize insulating properties without hindering the normal movement pattern.

Practical applications for players exposed to cold environments

Based on the findings in the previous section, the following recommendations can be provided to players and coaches for coping with cold environments:

1   Adequate warm-up strategies and clothing counteract the detrimental effects on soccer performance in the cold.
2   Regular exposure to the cold appears to delay the onset of shivering, reduces the sensation of discomfort and improves cold tolerance.
3   In the cold, clothing should be fitted tightly and worn in multiple layers.
4   Because exposure to the cold induces dehydration, changes in body mass should be monitored to ensure adequate rehydration.

Playing soccer at low and moderate altitudes

Soccer teams playing in international tournaments, such as the World Cups held in Mexico and South Africa, may be used to playing at low or moderate altitudes, which forces teams to cope with the special atmospheric, physiological and mental conditions associated with lowered oxygen partial pressure (pO_2).

Based on the physiological and mental responses to the different levels of altitude, five 'altitude zones' from near sea level to extreme altitude (see Table 12.2) have been consensually defined (Bartsch *et al.*, 2008a, 2008b).

Table 12.2 Definitions of different 'altitude zones'

Level of altitude (m)	Term	Side effects
0–500	Near sea level	–
500–2,000	Low altitude	Minimal decrease in aerobic performance
2,000–3,000	Moderate altitude	Increasing risk of altitude sickness; acclimatization to hypoxic exposure becomes important
3,000–5,500	High altitude	Mountain sickness becomes a relevant issue
> 5,500	Extreme altitude	Weakening increases

Source: Modified from Bartsch *et al.* (2008b).

Because most soccer games are played at sea level or at low and moderate altitudes, the chapter will focus on these two 'altitude zones'. However, matches in South America may also take place at high altitudes (e.g. at the Hernando Siles Stadium in La Paz, Bolivia located at ~ 3,600 m). In 2007, a 'high-altitude debate' occurred when the international football governing body (FIFA) banned international events at > 2,500 m. FIFA justified the rule with potential health concerns and the benefits of the altitude-adjusted home playing teams. This regulation implied that Bolivia, Colombia and Ecuador were prohibited from holding qualification events for the FIFA World Cup in their cities. After numerous discussions and expert conventions, FIFA suspended the ban 1 year later after an official protest from the South American governing body for soccer.

Hypoxia (i.e. breathing air with a lower pO_2 than at sea level) leads to several acute and chronic responses that need to be considered when: (1) conditioning lowland soccer teams for events at altitude (pre-acclimatization strategies); (2) participating in events at altitudes (acclimatization); and (3) conditioning acclimatized teams for events at sea level. For coaches and supporting staff, numerous combinations of hypoxic strategies need to be discussed and planned to encourage optimal conditioning.

An analysis of more than 1,000 matches revealed that soccer teams that consistently play and train at high altitude won more games against teams from sea-level locations (McSharry, 2007). Numerous reasons need to be considered for the decreased performance of players from sea-level locations at higher altitudes: limited mental and physiological adaptations due to stress associated with altitude, impairment in endurance performance, sleep and appetite. Finally, the less dense air at altitude compared to sea level alters the aerodynamic properties of the ball and impairs technical and tactical qualities.

Acute and chronic responses to altitude

With increasing hypoxia, arterial haemoglobin saturation (S_aO_2) decreases; however, this decrease is subject to great inter-individual variance. The decline in S_aO_2 mediates all following acute responses and acclimatization processes. Hyperventilation (Daniels and Oldridge, 1970) and increased resting and submaximal heart rates are the two most commonly experienced responses to low and moderate altitudes. Both responses increase oxygen availability to working tissues. Single sprint performance up to 400 m is not necessarily negatively affected by hypoxia (Figure 12.2); however, when sprints last longer (> 400 m) or are repeated, performance compared with sea-level performance decreases. The mechanisms of fatigue associated with hypoxia have not entirely been investigated so far; however, slower phosphate synthesis (Haseler *et al.*, 1999) in hypoxia may be one reason for more rapid onset of fatigue at altitude.

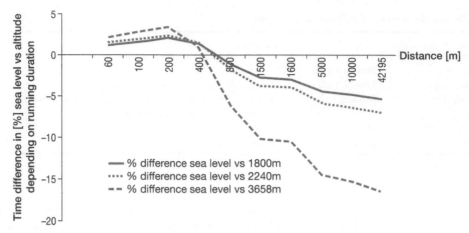

Figure 12.2 Per cent differences in running times for various distances at sea level compared with running times at 1,800, 2,240 and 3,645 m elevation. (The figure is summarized from previously published data by Noakes (2003).)

Soccer incorporates intermittent loads from high to lower intensities, provoking rapid changes in oxygen uptake during training and matches that average 70–80 per cent VO$_2$peak (Helgerud *et al.*, 2001). The distance covered by a player during a match is approximately 10–12 km (Stølen *et al.*, 2005), with 2–3 km at a velocity of > 15 km.h^{-1} and 600 m at a velocity of > 20 km.h^{-1} (Iaia *et al.*, 2009). This match analysis emphasizes the aerobic and anaerobic energy provisions and high oxygen demands, and explains the direct negative consequences on physical and mental performance when soccer is played during hypoxia.

As a rule of thumb, the VO$_2$peak, which is considered to be one of the most important key variables related to endurance performance (Åstrand and Rodahl, 1986; Hoff and Helgerud, 2004), may decrease by approximately 1 per cent per 100 m of altitude gain above 1,500 m, with great inter-individual differences (Levine *et al.*, 2008).

Other main acute responses when lower barometric pressure is sensed are summarized in Table 12.3. For further detailed information, readers are directed to previous reviews on the topic (Gore *et al.*, 2008; Mazzeo, 2008; Millet *et al.*, 2010). Most of the present acute and chronic responses have not been evaluated in team players because strategically planned hypoxic interventions are rare and are scientifically difficult to standardize.

In the past, numerous strategies for combining hypoxic training methods have been developed and evaluated especially for improving performance in endurance athletes at sea level or for acclimatization purposes (Millet *et al.*, 2010). Currently, athletes execute various forms of hypoxic training methods, such as 'live high-train high', 'live high-train low' and intermittent hypoxic exposure procedures (Millet *et al.*, 2010). These strategies are performed either in natural environments or in chambers and tents with artificial manipulation of pO$_2$. The duration of hypoxic intervention, the level of pO$_2$, the mechanisms and the performance outcomes from hypoxic interventions are highly debated by coaches, athletes and scientists, and have not been fully evaluated in soccer.

The effects of hypoxic training (2–8 weeks) for increasing the VO$_2$peak at sea level have been thoroughly investigated, with improvements in the range of 4.1 ± 3.8 per cent in trained and 10.0 ± 4.3 per cent in untrained individuals (Hoppeler *et al.* 2008). Other training methods, such as high-intensity interval training, elevate VO$_2$peak to the same magnitude (8.5–10.2 per cent) but with less technical, infrastructural and financial effort (Helgerud *et al.*, 2001, 2007;

Table 12.3 Summary of the main acute and chronic responses to low and moderate altitudes

Time of response	Variable	Reference
Acute	↑ sympathetic nervous system	(Hansen and Sander, 2003; Mazzeo and Reeves, 2003; Mazzeo et al., 1991, 1995)
	↑ resting and submax HR	(Grover et al., 1986; Wolfel et al., 1991)
	Slight ↓ stroke volume	
	↑ diuresis ⇒↓ plasma and blood volume	(Hildebrandt et al., 2000; Sawka et al., 2000)
	Hyperventilation at rest and exercise ⇒↑ respiratory water loss	(Wagner et al., 1986)
	↑ EPO; ↑ % reticulocytes	(Berglund, 1992; Sawka et al., 2000)
	↓ VO$_{2max}$	(Grover et al., 1986; Levine and Stray-Gundersen, 1992; Levine et al., 2008; Lundby et al., 2006)
	↑ levels of blood lactate	(Terrados et al., 1988)
	↓ quality of sleep	(Barash et al., 2001; Luks et al., 1998; West, 2003)
	↓ appetite	(Armstrong, 2006)
Chronic response	↓ cardiac output and normalized resting HR ↑ submax HR	(Mazzeo, 2008)
	↑ haemoglobin mass; ↓ blood volume; ↑ haematocrit; ↑ haemoglobin	(Millet et al., 2010; Sawka et al., 2000)
	↓ VO$_2$max	(Grover et al., 1986; Levine and Stray-Gundersen, 1992; Levine et al., 2008; Lundby et al., 2006)
	↑ mitochondrial density; capillarization; oxidative enzymes	(Wolski et al., 1996)
	↑ buffer capacity	(Mizuno et al., 1990; Saltin et al., 1995)
	↓ muscle mass	(Reilly and Waterhouse, 2005)
	↑ glycolytic and ↓ fat metabolism	(Beidleman et al., 2002; Brooks et al., 1992)

Sperlich *et al.*, 2011). Nevertheless, the effects of supplementing endurance training with hypoxic training methods in soccer have not been investigated.

For endurance athletes, the main objective in using hypoxic training is to improve performance at sea level. This may not necessarily be the main objective for a soccer team because of the following: (1) training time before and during the season is limited for training camps; and (2) the same improvements in endurance training may be achieved through other training methods. However, teams playing at sea level can be forced to play at low and moderate altitudes due to qualification matches and championship tournaments; therefore, they need to prepare for conditions at low and moderate altitudes. Teams that constantly play at low or moderate altitude may need to prepare for sea-level matches. The question for soccer teams may not be how to improve endurance performance via hypoxic training; rather, the question might involve which type of preparation would be optimal for success at low and moderate altitudes.

Intermittent hypoxia

Intermittent hypoxic exposure has been defined as an exposure to hypoxia lasting from seconds to hours that is repeated over several days to weeks (Millet *et al.*, 2010). The most important practical question to answer is 'How long, how often, how frequent and at what dose (i.e. level of pO_2) should the "hypoxic treatment" be administered?'. Due to the great variety of individual responses, this question is difficult to answer. As Gore *et al.* (2008) have concluded from previous work (Sawka *et al.*, 2000), during the initial phase of hypoxic exposure, increased S_aO_2 may be a consequence of ventilatory acclimatization processes. Consequently, preparation strategies enhancing ventilatory acclimatization are of practical relevance but of short duration.

The general outcomes of intermittent hypoxic exposure for endurance activities may be the following: (1) increase in hematological parameters for 90 minutes (3 days.wk^{-1} for 3 wk) (Rodriguez *et al.*, 2000); (2) increased EPO level (3 h.d^{-1}, 5 days.wk^{-1} over 4 wk (Abellan *et al.*, 2005) and altered erythropoiesis (4 h in a hypobaric chamber at 58.9 kPa) (Savourey *et al.*, 2004); and (3) enhanced ventilatory acclimatization (Ricart *et al.*, 2000). However, the effects on performance variables are subject to discussion (Millet *et al.*, 2010).

Intermittent hypoxic training or 'live low-train high' strategy

To avoid costly travel to altitude sites with hypoxia-induced side effects (see Tables 12.2 and 12.3), hypoxic exposure at sea level has been utilized by endurance athletes. In the past, this concept has been titled 'live low-train high'. This concept is either executed under genuine conditions by daily travel to and from training sites at altitude or by artificial hypoxic exposure provided by climatic chambers that extract oxygen or add nitrogen to the air. Two major concerns about this strategy have been brought forward previously (Millet *et al.*, 2010): (1) the time of hypoxic exposure may not be sufficient to mediate hematological responses and improve O_2 transportation; and (2) from a practical point of view, depending on the duration of hypoxic exposure, training intensity cannot be maintained due to reduced VO_2peak during hypoxia.

When exercise and intermittent hypoxia are combined, the VO_2peak may not increase because of a low overall hypoxic 'dose'; however, improvements in performance may occur when high-intensity work is added to the training stress due to mitochondrial adaptations and improved buffering regulation. For detailed information, we refer to previous work (Millet *et al.*, 2010). The application of intermittent hypoxic exposure in short- and long-term situations is likely to be impractical in soccer because most responses are temporary.

'Live high-train low' concept

One issue when exercising at low and especially at moderate and high altitudes is controlling training intensity. The lower pO_2 leads to several consequences for conditioning: (1) biomarkers, such as heart rate or blood lactate concentration, exhibit different responses in hypoxic conditions; (2) due to hypoxia, training intensity needs to be reduced; and (3) long-term hypoxic exposure may impair muscle mass, quality of sleep and appetite. To avoid most of these side effects, the 'live high-train low' concept has been favoured by many coaches and athletes.

The potential benefits that might derive from this concept include the following: (1) elevated levels of erythropoietin (Dehnert *et al.*, 2002; Levine and Stray-Gundersen, 1997); (2) improved exercise economy (Gore *et al.*, 2007; Saunders *et al.*, 2004); (3) increased buffer capacity (Gore *et al.*, 2001); and (4) increased aerobic and anaerobic performance (Hoppeler *et al.*, 2008; Levine and Stray-Gundersen, 1997; Millet *et al.*, 2010).

To the best of our knowledge, no soccer-specific studies have implemented the 'live high-train low' concept with high standardization. However, a comprehensive overview by Millet *et al.* (2010) recommends an optimal altitude of 2,200–2,500 m for a duration of 3–4 weeks. Based on their findings, the hypoxic dose should be administered for as long as possible (e.g. 22 $h.d^{-1}$, with a minimum 'dosage' of 12 $h.d^{-1}$).

Based on previous unpublished findings (Figure 12.3), it may be interesting to mention that more frequent exposure to hypoxia may result in a faster acclimatization, as evidenced by the resting heart rate. In endurance runners, a series of hypoxic training camps resulted in a faster decline in resting heart rate over time.

Technical adaptations

By reducing the barometric pressure, the physical properties of aerodynamics when kicking or throwing a ball are different at high altitudes compared with sea level (Levine *et al.*, 2008). Based on the lower barometric pressure and consequently lower air density, the ball will perform with the following characteristics: (1) accelerate and move faster; (2) travel farther; and (3) rotate less. The change in the ball activities is both tactically and technically important. Teams that are not adapted to the new atmospheric conditions should consider the new 'physics' by emphasizing technical drills when arriving at altitude. For more detailed information on this topic, the reader is directed to previous work (Levine *et al.*, 2008).

Practical recommendations

In the past, a reasonable debate on the ideal time to arrive at altitude before a competition has led to numerous recommendations. Time courses for acclimatization may vary from 48 hours to weeks. These recommendations have been mostly based on personal investigations, individual

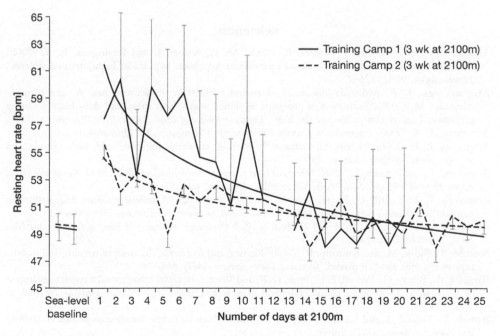

Figure 12.3 Resting heart rate of endurance athletes at sea level during two 3-week exposures to 2,100 m altitude. The camps were separated by 12 weeks of sea-level training.

success and scientific evidence in endurance athletes. Based on previous consensus (Bartsch *et al.*, 2008b) and recommendations (Gore *et al.*, 2008; Millet *et al.*, 2010) for soccer, the following basic preparation strategies have been recommended:

1   A player's health status, including iron levels, should be constantly checked to ascertain the benefits derived from hypoxic exposure.
2   For 'boosting' performance in soccer, other methods, such as high-intensity intervals, may provide greater performance effects, and are cheaper and more applicable for soccer players than hypoxic interventions.
3   Basic measurements of S_aO_2 and resting heart rate may be appropriate for checking an individual's acclimatization progress. Values close to sea-level baseline indicate good acclimatization.
4   For teams playing at low altitude, a brief acclimatization phase of 5 days is preferable.
5   Sea-level teams preparing to play at moderate altitude should acclimate for 7–14 days at the altitude of the match.
6   Sea-level teams preparing to play at high altitude should acclimate > 14 days at the altitude of the match.
7   Exposure to artificial altitude for 1–16 $h.d^{-1}$ for 10–14 days before a match may support faster acclimatization at low and moderate altitudes.
8   When arriving at low and moderate altitudes, training should focus on low-intensity activities, such as technical and tactical drills. The intensity and duration of the workload should thereby gradually increase.
9   Additional hydration and sufficient nutrition should be checked (Armstrong, 2006).
10 Extra recovery time should be administered between training sessions, especially when sleep quality is impaired.

References

Abellan, R., Remacha, A. F., Ventura, R., Sarda, M. P., Segura, J. and Rodriguez, F. A. (2005) 'Hematologic response to four weeks of intermittent hypobaric hypoxia in highly trained athletes', *Haematologica*, 90(1): 126–7.

Aragón-Vargas, L. F., Moncada-Jiménez, J., Hernández-Elizondo, J., Barrenechea, A. and Monge-Alvarado, M. (2009) 'Evaluation of pre-game hydration status, heat stress, and fluid balance during professional soccer competition in the heat', *European Journal of Sport Science*, 9(5): 269–76.

Armstrong, L. E. (2000) *Performing in Extreme Environments*, Champaign, IL: Human Kinetics.

Armstrong, L. E. (2006) 'Nutritional strategies for football: counteracting heat, cold, high altitude, and jet lag', *Journal of Sports Sciences*, 24(7): 723–40.

Armstrong, L. and Dziados, J. (1986) 'Effects of heat exposure on exercising adult', in D. Bernhardt (ed.), *Sports Physical Therapy*, New York: Churchill Livingstone, pp. 197–216.

Armstrong, L. E., Costill, D. L. and Fink, W. J. (1985) 'Influence of diuretic-induced dehydration on competitive running performance', *Medicine and Science in Sports and Exercise*, 17(4): 456–61.

Åstrand, P.-O. and Rodahl, K. (1986) *Textbook of Work Physiology: Physiological Bases of Exercise*, 3rd edn, New York: McGraw-Hill.

Bangsbo, J., Mohr, M. and Krustrup, P. (2006) 'Physical and metabolic demands of training and match-play in the elite football player', *Journal of Sports Sciences*, 24(7): 665–74.

Barash, I. A., Beatty, C., Powell, F. L., Prisk, G. K. and West, J. B. (2001) 'Nocturnal oxygen enrichment of room air at 3,800 meter altitude improves sleep architecture', *High Altitude Medicine and Biology*, 2(4): 525–33.

Bartsch, P., Dvorak, J. and Saltin, B. (2008a) 'Football at high altitude', *Scandinavian Journal of Medicine and Science in Sports*, 18(1): Siii–iv.

Bartsch, P., Saltin, B. and Dvorak, J. (2008b) 'Consensus statement on playing football at different altitude', *Scandinavian Journal of Medicine and Science in Sports*, 18(1): 96–9.

Baum, E., Bruck, K. and Schwennicke, H. P. (1976) 'Adaptive modifications in the thermoregulatory system of long-distance runners', *Journal of Applied Physiology*, 40(3): 404–10.

Beidleman, B. A., Rock, P. B., Muza, S. R., Fulco, C. S., Gibson, L. L., Kamimori, G. H. and Cymerman, A. (2002) 'Substrate oxidation is altered in women during exercise upon acute altitude exposure', *Medicine and Science in Sports and Exercise*, 34(3): 430–7.

Berglund, B. (1992) 'High-altitude training. Aspects of haematological adaptation', *Sports Medicine*, 14(5): 289–303.

Booth, J., Wilsmore, B. R., Macdonald, A. D., Zeyl, A., Mcghee, S., Calvert, D., Marino, F. E., Storlien, L. H. and Taylor, N. A. (2001) 'Whole-body pre-cooling does not alter human muscle metabolism during sub-maximal exercise in the heat', *European Journal of Applied Physiology*, 84(8): 587–90.

Brooks, G. A., Wolfel, E. E., Groves, B. M., Bender, P. R., Butterfield, G. E., Cymerman, A., Mazzeo, R. S., Sutton, J. R., Wolfe, R. R. and Reeves, J. T. (1992) 'Muscle accounts for glucose disposal but not blood lactate appearance during exercise after acclimatization to 4,300 m', *Journal of Applied Physiology*, 72(6): 2435–45.

Carling, C., Dupont, G. and Le Gall, F. (2011) 'The effect of a cold environment on physical activity profiles in elite soccer match-play', *International Journal of Sports Medicine*, 32(7): 542–5.

Cheung, S. S. and McLellan, T. M. (1998) 'Heat acclimation, aerobic fitness, and hydration effects on tolerance during uncompensable heat stress', *Journal of Applied Physiology*, 84(5): 1731–9.

Chinevere, T. D., Kenefick, R. W., Cheuvront, S. N., Lukaski, H. C. and Sawka, M. N. (2008) 'Effect of heat acclimation on sweat minerals', *Medicine and Science in Sports and Exercise*, 40(5): 886–91.

Currell, K., Conway, S. and Jeukendrup, A. E. (2009) 'Carbohydrate ingestion improves performance of a new reliable test of soccer performance', *International Journal of Sport Nutrition and Exercise Metabolism*, 19(1): 34–46.

Daniels, J. and Oldridge, N. (1970) 'The effects of alternate exposure to altitude and sea level on world-class middle-distance runners', *Medicine and Science in Sports*, 2(3): 107–12.

Dehnert, C., Hutler, M., Liu, Y., Menold, E., Netzer, C., Schick, R., Kubanek, B., Lehmann, M., Boning, D. and Steinacker, J. M. (2002) 'Erythropoiesis and performance after two weeks of living high and training low in well trained triathletes', *International Journal of Sports Medicine*, 23(8): 561–6.

Di Salvo, V., Baron, R., Tschan, H., Calderon Montero, F. J., Bachl, N. and Pigozzi, F. (2007) 'Performance characteristics according to playing position in elite soccer', *International Journal of Sports Medicine*, 28(3): 222–7.

Doubt, T. J. (1991) 'Physiology of exercise in the cold', *Sports Medicine*, 11(6): 367–81.

Drust, B., Cable, N. T. and Reilly, T. (2000) 'Investigation of the effects of the pre-cooling on the physiological responses to soccer-specific intermittent exercise', *European Journal of Applied Physiology*, 81(1–2): 11–17.

Falk, B., Radom-Isaac, S., Hoffmann, J. R., Wang, Y., Yarom, Y., Magazanik, A. and Weinstein, Y. (1998) 'The effect of heat exposure on performance of and recovery from high-intensity, intermittent exercise', *International Journal of Sports Medicine*, 19(1): 1–6.

Freund, B. J. and Sawka, M. N. (1996) 'Influence of cold stress on human fluid balance', in B. M. Marriot and S. J. Carlson (eds), *Nutrient Requirements for Work in Cold and High Altitude Environments*, Washington, DC: National Academy of Science Press, pp. 161–79.

Galloway, S. D. and Maughan, R. J. (1997) 'Effects of ambient temperature on the capacity to perform prolonged cycle exercise in man', *Medicine and Science in Sports and Exercise*, 29(9): 1240–9.

Gavin, T. P. (2003) 'Clothing and thermoregulation during exercise', *Sports Medicine*, 33(13): 941–7.

Giesbrecht, G. G. (1995) 'The respiratory system in a cold environment', *Aviation, Space, and Environmental Medicine*, 66(9): 890–902.

Girard, O., Bishop, D. J. and Racinais, S. (2013) 'Hot conditions improve power output during repeated cycling sprints without modifying neuromuscular fatigue characteristics', *European Journal of Applied Physiology*, 113(2): 359–69.

Gore, C. J., Hahn, A. G., Aughey, R. J., Martin, D. T., Ashenden, M. J., Clark, S. A., Garnham, A. P., Roberts, A. D., Slater, G. J. and Mckenna, M. J. (2001) 'Live high:train low increases muscle buffer capacity and submaximal cycling efficiency', *Acta Physiologica Scandinavica*, 173(3): 275–86.

Gore, C. J., Clark, S. A. and Saunders, P. U. (2007) 'Nonhematological mechanisms of improved sea-level performance after hypoxic exposure', *Medicine and Science in Sports and Exercise*, 39(9): 1600–9.

Gore, C. J., McSharry, P. E., Hewitt, A. J. and Saunders, P. U. (2008) 'Preparation for football competition at moderate to high altitude', *Scandinavian Journal of Medicine and Science in Sports*, 18(1): 85–95.

Grover, R. F., Weil, J. V. and Reeves, J. T. (1986) 'Cardiovascular adaptation to exercise at high altitude', *Exercise and Sport Sciences Reviews*, 14: 269–302.

Hanna, J. N., McN, H. P. and Sinclair, J. D. (1975) 'Human cardiorespiratory responses to acute cold exposure', *Clinical and Experimental Pharmacology and Physiology*, 2(3): 229–38.

Hansen, J. and Sander, M. (2003) 'Sympathetic neural overactivity in healthy humans after prolonged exposure to hypobaric hypoxia', *The Journal of Physiology*, 546(3): 921–9.

Haseler, L. J., Hogan, M. C. and Richardson, R. S. (1999) 'Skeletal muscle phosphocreatine recovery in exercise-trained humans is dependent on O_2 availability', *Journal of Applied Physiology*, 86(6): 2013–8.

Heir, T. and Oseid, S. (1994) 'Self-reported asthma and exercise induced symptoms in high level competitve cross-country skiers', *Scandinavian Journal of Medicine and Science in Sports*, 4(2): 128–33.

Helgerud, J., Engen, L. C., Wisloff, U. and Hoff, J. (2001) 'Aerobic endurance training improves soccer performance', *Medicine and Science in Sports and Exercise*, 33(11): 1925–31.

Helgerud, J., Hoydal, K., Wang, E., Karlsen, T., Berg, P., Bjerkaas, M., Simonsen, T., Helgesen, C., Hjorth, N., Bach, R. and Hoff, J. (2007) 'Aerobic high-intensity intervals improve VO_2max more than moderate training', *Medicine and Science in Sports and Exercise*, 39(4): 665–71.

Heus, R., Daanen, H. A. and Havenith, G. (1995) 'Physiological criteria for functioning of hands in the cold: a review', *Applied Ergonomics*, 26(1): 5–13.

Hildebrandt, W., Ottenbacher, A., Schuster, M., Swenson, E. R. and Bartsch, P. (2000) 'Diuretic effect of hypoxia, hypocapnia, and hyperpnea in humans: relation to hormones and O_2 chemosensitivity', *Journal of Applied Physiology*, 88(2): 599–610.

Hoff, J. and Helgerud, J. (2004) 'Endurance and strength training for soccer players: physiological considerations', *Sports Medicine*, 34(3): 165–80.

Hoppeler, H., Klossner, S. and Vogt, M. (2008) 'Training in hypoxia and its effects on skeletal muscle tissue', *Scandinavian Journal of Medicine and Science in Sports*, 18(1): S38–49.

Iaia, F. M., Rampinini, E. and Bangsbo, J. (2009) 'High-intensity training in football', *International Journal of Sports Physiology and Performance*, 4(3): 291–306.

Jentjens, R. L., Wagenmakers, A. J. and Jeukendrup, A. E. (2002) 'Heat stress increases muscle glycogen use but reduces the oxidation of ingested carbohydrates during exercise', *Journal of Applied Physiology*, 92(4): 1562–72.

Kreider, R. B., Wilborn, C. D., Taylor, L., Campbell, B., Almada, A. L., Collins, R., Cooke, M., Earnest, C. P., Greenwood, M., Kalman, D. S., Kerksick, C. M., Kleiner, S. M., Leutholtz, B., Lopez, H., Lowery, L. M., Mendel, R., Smith, A., Spano, M., Wildman, R., Willoughby, D. S., Ziegenfuss, T. N. and Antonio, J. (2010) 'ISSN exercise & sport nutrition review: research & recommendations', *Journal of the International Society of Sports Nutrition*, 7: 7.

Krustrup, P., Mohr, M., Steensberg, A., Bencke, J., Kjaer, M. and Bangsbo, J. (2006) 'Muscle and blood metabolites during a soccer game: implications for sprint performance', *Medicine and Science in Sports and Exercise*, 38(6): 1165–74.

Launay, J. C., Besnard, Y., Guinet, A., Hanniquet, A. M., Bittel, J. and Savourey, G. (2002) 'Thermoregulation in the cold after physical training at different ambient air temperatures', *Canadian Journal of Physiology and Pharmacology*, 80(9): 857–64.

Layden, J. D., Patterson, M. J. and Nimmo, M. A. (2002) 'Effects of reduced ambient temperature on fat utilization during submaximal exercise', *Medicine and Science in Sports and Exercise*, 34(5): 774–9.

Lennquist, S., Granberg, P. O. and Wedin, B. (1974) 'Fluid balance and physical work capacity in humans exposed to cold', *Archives of Environmental Health*, 29(5): 241–9.

Levine, B. D. and Stray-Gundersen, J. (1992) 'A practical approach to altitude training: where to live and train for optimal performance enhancement', *International Journal of Sports Medicine*, 13(1): S209–12.

Levine, B. D. and Stray-Gundersen, J. (1997) '"Living high-training low": effect of moderate-altitude acclimatization with low-altitude training on performance', *Journal of Applied Physiology*, 83(1): 102–12.

Levine, B. D., Stray-Gundersen, J. and Mehta, R. D. (2008) 'Effect of altitude on football performance', *Scandinavian Journal of Medicine and Science in Sports*, 18(1): S76–84.

Lind, A. R. and Bass, D. E. (1963) 'Optimal exposure time for development of acclimatization to heat', *Federation Proceedings*, 22: 704–8.

Luks, A. M., Van Melick, H., Batarse, R. R., Powell, F. L., Grant, I. and West, J. B. (1998) 'Room oxygen enrichment improves sleep and subsequent day-time performance at high altitude', *Respiration Physiology*, 113(3): 247–58.

Lundby, C., Sander, M., Van Hall, G., Saltin, B. and Calbet, J. A. (2006) 'Maximal exercise and muscle oxygen extraction in acclimatizing lowlanders and high altitude natives', *The Journal of Physiology*, 573(2): 535–47.

McSharry, P. E. (2007) 'Effect of altitude on physiological performance: a statistical analysis using results of international football games', *British Medical Journal*, 335(7633): 1278–81.

Magalhaes Fde, C., Machado-Moreira, C. A., Vimieiro-Gomes, A. C., Silami-Garcia, E., Lima, N. R. and Rodrigues, L. O. (2006) 'Possible biphasic sweating response during short-term heat acclimation protocol for tropical natives', *Journal of Physiological Anthropology*, 25(3): 215–19.

Maughan, R. J. (2003) 'Impact of mild dehydration on wellness and on exercise performance', *European Journal of Clinical Nutrition*, 57(2): S19–23.

Maughan, R. J., Watson, P., Evans, G. H., Broad, N. and Shirreffs, S. M. (2007) 'Water balance and salt losses in competitive football', *International Journal of Sport Nutrition and Exercise Metabolism*, 17(6): 583–94.

Maughan, R. J., Shirreffs, S. M., Ozgunen, K. T., Kurdak, S. S., Ersoz, G., Binnet, M. S. and Dvorak, J. (2010) 'Living, training and playing in the heat: challenges to the football player and strategies for coping with environmental extremes', *Scandinavian Journal of Medicine and Science in Sports*, 20(3): 117–24.

Maxwell, N. S., Gardner, F. and Nimmo, M. A. (1999) 'Intermittent running: muscle metabolism in the heat and effect of hypohydration', *Medicine and Science in Sports and Exercise*, 31(5): 675–83.

Mazzeo, R. S. (2008) 'Physiological responses to exercise at altitude: an update', *Sports Medicine*, 38(1): 1–8.

Mazzeo, R. S. and Reeves, J. T. (2003) 'Adrenergic contribution during acclimatization to high altitude: perspectives from Pikes Peak', *Exercise and Sport Sciences Reviews*, 31(1): 13–18.

Mazzeo, R. S., Bender, P. R., Brooks, G. A., Butterfield, G. E., Groves, B. M., Sutton, J. R., Wolfel, E. E. and Reeves, J. T. (1991) 'Arterial catecholamine responses during exercise with acute and chronic high-altitude exposure', *American Journal of Physiology*, 261(4/1): E419–24.

Mazzeo, R. S., Brooks, G. A., Butterfield, G. E., Podolin, D. A., Wolfel, E. E. and Reeves, J. T. (1995) 'Acclimatization to high altitude increase muscle sympathetic activity both at rest and during exercise', *American Journal of Physiology*, 269(1/2): R201–7.

Millet, G. P., Roels, B., Schmitt, L., Woorons, X. and Richalet, J. P. (2010) 'Combining hypoxic methods for peak performance', *Sports Medicine*, 40(1): 1–25.

Mizuno, M., Juel, C., Bro-Rasmussen, T., Mygind, E., Schibye, B., Rasmussen, B. and Saltin, B. (1990) 'Limb skeletal muscle adaptation in athletes after training at altitude', *Journal of Applied Physiology*, 68(2): 496–502.

Mohr, M. and Krustrup, P. (2012) 'Heat stress impairs repeated jump ability after competitive elite soccer games', *Journal of Strength and Conditioning Research*, doi:10.1519/JSC.0b013e31825c3266.

Mohr, M., Krustrup, P., Nybo, L., Nielsen, J. J. and Bangsbo, J. (2004) 'Muscle temperature and sprint performance during soccer matches – beneficial effect of re-warm-up at half-time', *Scandinavian Journal of Medicine and Science in Sports*, 14(3): 156–62.

Mohr, M., Mujika, I., Santisteban, J., Randers, M. B., Bischoff, R., Solano, R., Hewitt, A., Zubillaga, A., Peltola, E. and Krustrup, P. (2010) 'Examination of fatigue development in elite soccer in a hot environment: a multi-experimental approach', *Scandinavian Journal of Medicine and Science in Sports*, 20(3): S125–32.

Mustafa, K. Y. and Mahmoud, N. E. (1979) 'Evaporative water loss in African soccer players', *Journal of Sports Medicine and Physical Fitness*, 19(2): 181–3.

Nadel, E. R. (1988) 'Temperature regulation and prolonged exercise', in D. R. Lamb and R. Murray (eds), *Perspectives in Exercise Science and Sports Medicine. Vol. 1, Prolonged Exercise*, Indianapolis, IN: Benchmark, pp. 125–52.

Nielsen, B. (1990) 'Solar heat load: heat balance during exercise in clothed subjects', *European Journal of Applied Physiology and Occupational Physiology*, 60(6): 452–6.

Nielsen, B. and Nybo, L. (2003) 'Cerebral changes during exercise in the heat', *Sports Medicine*, 33(1): 1–11.

Nielsen, B., Kubica, R., Bonnesen, A., Rasmussen, I. B., Stoklosa, J. and Wilk, B. (1981) 'Physical work capacity after dehydration and hyperthermia: a comparison of the effect of exercise versus passive heat and sauna and diuretic dehydration', *Scandinavian Journal of Sports Science*, 3: 2–10.

Nimmo, M. (2004) 'Exercise in the cold', *Journal of Sports Sciences*, 22(10): 898–915; discussion 915–6.

Noakes, T. D. (2002) 'Exercise and the cold', in T. Reilly and J. Greeves (eds), *Advances in Sport, Leisure and Ergonomics*, London: Routledge, pp. 13–31.

Noakes, T. D. (2003) *Lore of Running*, Champaign, IL: Human Kinetics.

Nybo, L. (2010) 'Cycling in the heat: performance perspectives and cerebral challenges', *Scandinavian Journal of Medicine and Science in Sports*, 20(3): S71–9.

O'Brien, C., Young, A. J., Lee, D. T., Shitzer, A., Sawka, M. N. and Pandolf, K. B. (2000) 'Role of core temperature as a stimulus for cold acclimation during repeated immersion in 20 degrees C water', *Journal of Applied Physiology*, 89(1): 242–50.

Ozgunen, K. T., Kurdak, S. S., Maughan, R. J., Zeren, C., Korkmaz, S., Yazici, Z., Ersoz, G., Shirreffs, S. M., Binnet, M. S. and Dvorak, J. (2010) 'Effect of hot environmental conditions on physical activity patterns and temperature response of football players', *Scandinavian Journal of Medicine and Science in Sports*, 20(3): S140–7.

Parkin, J. M., Carey, M. F., Zhao, S. and Febbraio, M. A. (1999) 'Effect of ambient temperature on human skeletal muscle metabolism during fatiguing submaximal exercise', *Journal of Applied Physiology*, 86(3): 902–8.

Pascoe, D. D., Shanley, L. A. and Smith, E. W. (1994) 'Clothing and exercise. I: biophysics of heat transfer between the individual, clothing and environment', *Sports Medicine*, 18(1): 38–54.

Passe, D. (2001) 'Physiological and psychological determinants of fluid intake', in R. J. Maughan and R. Murray (eds), *Sports Drink*, Boca Raton, FL: CRC Press, pp. 45–88.

Periard, J. D., Caillaud, C. and Thompson, M. W. (2011) 'Central and peripheral fatigue during passive and exercise-induced hyperthermia', *Medicine and Science in Sports and Exercise*, 43(9): 1657–65.

Pichan, G., Sridharan, K., Swamy, Y. V., Joseph, S. and Gautam, R. K. (1985) 'Physiological acclimatization to heat after a spell of cold conditioning in tropical subjects', *Aviation, Space, and Environmental Medicine*, 56(5): 436–40.

Pitsiladis, Y. P. and Maughan, R. J. (1999) 'The effects of exercise and diet manipulation on the capacity to perform prolonged exercise in the heat and in the cold in trained humans', *The Journal of Physiology*, 517 (3): 919–30.

Price, M. J. and Mather, M. I. (2004) 'Comparison of lower- vs. upper-body cooling during arm exercise in hot conditions', *Aviation, Space, and Environmental Medicine*, 75(3): 220–6.

Price, M. J., Boyd, C. and Goosey-Tolfrey, V. L. (2009) 'The physiological effects of pre-event and midevent cooling during intermittent running in the heat in elite female soccer players', *Applied Physiology, Nutrition, and Metabolism*, 34(5): 942–9.

Quirion, A., Laurencelle, L., Paulin, L., Therminarias, A., Brisson, G. R., Audet, A., Dulac, S. and Vogelaere, P. (1989) 'Metabolic and hormonal responses during exercise at 20 degrees, 0 degrees and −20 degrees C', *International Journal of Biometeorology*, 33(4): 227–32.

Racinais, S., Gaoua, N. and Grantham, J. (2008) 'Hyperthermia impairs short-term memory and peripheral motor drive transmission', *The Journal of Physiology*, 586(19): 4751–62.

Rehrer, N. J. and Burke, L. M. (1996) 'Sweat losses during various sports', *Australian Journal of Nutrition and Dietetics*, 53(4): S13–16.

Reilly, T. (2007) *The Science of Training – Soccer : A Scientific Approach to Developing Strength, Speed and Endurance*, London: Routledge.

Reilly, T. and Waterhouse, J. M. (2005) *Sport Exercise and Environmental Physiology*, Edinburgh: Churchill Livingstone.

Ricart, A., Casas, H., Casas, M., Pages, T., Palacios, L., Rama, R., Rodriguez, F. A., Viscor, G. and Ventura, J. L. (2000) 'Acclimatization near home? Early respiratory changes after short-term intermittent exposure to simulated altitude', *Wilderness and Environmental Medicine*, 11(2): 84–8.

Ritzel, G. (1961) 'Critical evaluation of vitamin C as a prophylactic and therapeutic agent in colds', *Helvetica MedicaActa*, 28: 63–8.

Rodriguez, F. A., Ventura, J. L., Casas, M., Casas, H., Pages, T., Rama, R., Ricart, A., Palacios, L. and Viscor, G. (2000) 'Erythropoietin acute reaction and haematological adaptations to short, intermittent hypobaric hypoxia', *European Journal of Applied Physiology*, 82(3): 170–7.

Rowell, L. B. (1983) 'Cardiovascular aspects of human thermoregulation', *Circulation Research*, 52(4): 367–79.

Sabiston, B. H. and Livingstone, S. D. (1973) *Investigation of Health Problems Related to Canadian Northern Military Operations*, Toronto: Defence and Civil Institute of Environmental Medicine.

Saltin, B., Kim, C. K., Terrados, N., Larsen, H., Svedenhag, J. and Rolf, C. J. (1995) 'Morphology, enzyme activities and buffer capacity in leg muscles of Kenyan and Scandinavian runners', *Scandinavian Journal of Medicine and Science in Sports*, 5(4): 222–30.

Saunders, P. U., Telford, R. D., Pyne, D. B., Cunningham, R. B., Gore, C. J., Hahn, A. G. and Hawley, J. A. (2004) 'Improved running economy in elite runners after 20 days of simulated moderate-altitude exposure', *Journal of Applied Physiology*, 96(3): 931–7.

Savourey, G., Launay, J. C., Besnard, Y., Guinet, A., Bourrilhon, C., Cabane, D., Martin, S., Caravel, J. P., Pequignot, J. M. and Cottet-Emard, J. M. (2004) 'Control of erythropoiesis after high altitude acclimatization', *European Journal of Applied Physiology*, 93(1–2): 47–56.

Sawka, M. N. and Montain, S. J. (2000) 'Fluid and electrolyte supplementation for exercise heat stress', *American Journal of Clinical Nutrition*, 72(2): S564–72.

Sawka, M. N., Convertino, V. A., Eichner, E. R., Schnieder, S. M. and Young, A. J. (2000) 'Blood volume: importance and adaptations to exercise training, environmental stresses, and trauma/sickness', *Medicine and Science in Sports and Exercise*, 32(2): 332–48.

Sawka, M. N., Burke, L. M., Eichner, E. R., Maughan, R. J., Montain, S. J. and Stachenfeld, N. S. (2007) 'American College of Sports Medicine position stand. Exercise and fluid replacement', *Medicine and Science in Sports and Exercise*, 39(2): 377–90.

Shiojiri, T., Shibasaki, M., Aoki, K., Kondo, N. and Koga, S. (1997) 'Effects of reduced muscle temperature on the oxygen uptake kinetics at the start of exercise', *Acta Physiologica Scandinavica*, 159(4): 327–33.

Shirreffs, S. M. and Maughan, R. J. (1998) 'Urine osmolality and conductivity as indices of hydration status in athletes in the heat', *Medicine and Science in Sports and Exercise*, 30(11): 1598–602.

Shirreffs, S. M., Taylor, A. J., Leiper, J. B. and Maughan, R. J. (1996) 'Post-exercise rehydration in man: effects of volume consumed and drink sodium content', *Medicine and Science in Sports and Exercise*, 28(10): 1260–71.

Shirreffs, S. M., Aragon-Vargas, L. F., Chamorro, M., Maughan, R. J., Serratosa, L. and Zachwieja, J. J. (2005) 'The sweating response of elite professional soccer players to training in the heat', *International Journal of Sports Medicine*, 26(2): 90–5.

Shirreffs, S. M., Sawka, M. N. and Stone, M. (2006) 'Water and electrolyte needs for football training and match-play', *Journal of Sports Sciences*, 24(7): 699–707.

Sperlich, B., De Marees, M., Koehler, K., Linville, J., Holmberg, H. C. and Mester, J. (2011) 'Effects of 5 weeks of high-intensity interval training vs. volume training in 14-year-old soccer players', *Journal of Strength and Conditioning Research*, 25(5): 1271–8.

Stølen, T., Chamari, K., Castagna, C. and Wisloff, U. (2005) 'Physiology of soccer: an update', *Sports Medicine*, 35(6): 501–36.

Sue-Chu, M., Larsson, L. and Bjermer, L. (1996) 'Prevalence of asthma in young cross-country skiers in central Scandinavia: differences between Norway and Sweden', *Respiratory Medicine*, 90(2): 99–105.

Taylor, N. (2000) 'Principles and practices of heat adaptation', *Journal of the Human – Environment System*, 4(1): 11–22.

Terrados, N., Melichna, J., Sylven, C., Jansson, E. and Kaijser, L. (1988) 'Effects of training at simulated altitude on performance and muscle metabolic capacity in competitive road cyclists', *European Journal of Applied Physiology and Occupational Physiology*, 57(2): 203–9.

Wagner, P. D., Gale, G. E., Moon, R. E., Torre-Bueno, J. R., Stolp, B. W. and Saltzman, H. A. (1986) 'Pulmonary gas exchange in humans exercising at sea level and simulated altitude', *Journal of Applied Physiology*, 61(1): 260–70.

Wallenberg, L. R. and Granberg, P. O. (1976) 'Is cold diuresis a pressure diuresis?', in R. J. Shephard and S. Itah (eds), *Circumpolar Health*, Toronto: University of Toronto Press, pp. 49–55.

Walsh, N. P., Bishop, N. C., Blackwell, J., Wierzbicki, S. G. and Montague, J. C. (2002) 'Salivary IgA response to prolonged exercise in a cold environment in trained cyclists ', *Medicine and Science in Sports and Exercise*, 34(10): 1632–7.

Watson, G., Judelson, D. A., Armstrong, L. E., Yeargin, S. W., Casa, D. J. and Maresh, C. M. (2005) 'Influence of diuretic-induced dehydration on competitive sprint and power performance', *Medicine and Science in Sports and Exercise*, 37(7): 1168–74.

Wegmann, M., Faude, O., Poppendieck, W., Hecksteden, A., Frohlich, M. and Meyer, T. (2012) 'Pre-cooling and sports performance: a meta-analytical review', *Sports Medicine*, 42(7): 545–64.

Weller, A. S., Millard, C. E., Stroud, M. A., Greenhaff, P. L. and Macdonald, I. A. (1997) 'Physiological responses to a cold, wet, and windy environment during prolonged intermittent walking', *American Journal of Physiology*, 272(1/2): R226–33.

Wendt, D., Van Loon, L. J. and Lichtenbelt, W. D. (2007) 'Thermoregulation during exercise in the heat: strategies for maintaining health and performance', *Sports Medicine*, 37(8): 669–82.

Wenger, C. B. (1988) 'Human heat acclimatization', in K. B. Pandolf., M. N. Sawka and R. R. Gonzalez (eds), *Human Performance Physiology and Environmental Medicine at Terrestrial Extremes*, Indianapolis, IN: Benchmark, pp. 153–97.

Werner, J. and Reents, T. (1980) 'A contribution to the topography of temperature regulation in man', *European Journal of Applied Physiology and Occupational Physiology*, 45(1): 87–94.

West, J. B. (2003) 'Improving oxygenation at high altitude: acclimatization and O_2 enrichment', *High Altitude Medicine and Biology*, 4(3): 389–98.

Wolfel, E. E., Groves, B. M., Brooks, G. A., Butterfield, G. E., Mazzeo, R. S., Moore, L. G., Sutton, J. R., Bender, P. R., Dahms, T. E., Mccullough, R. E. Huang, S.-Y., Sun, S. F., Crover, R. G., Hultgren, H. N. and Reeves, J. T. (1991) 'Oxygen transport during steady-state submaximal exercise in chronic hypoxia', *Journal of Applied Physiology*, 70(3): 1129–36.

Wolski, L. A., Mckenzie, D. C. and Wenger, H. A. (1996) 'Altitude training for improvements in sea level performance. Is the scientific evidence of benefit?', *Sports Medicine*, 22(4): 251–63.

Young, A. J., Muza, S. R., Sawka, M. N., Gonzalez, R. R. and Pandolf, K. B. (1986) 'Human thermoregulatory responses to cold air are altered by repeated cold water immersion', *Journal of Applied Physiology*, 60(5): 1542–8.

Young, A. J., Sawka, M. N., Epstein, Y., Decristofano, B. and Pandolf, K. B. (1987) 'Cooling different body surfaces during upper and lower body exercise', *Journal of Applied Physiology*, 63(3): 1218–23.

SECTION 4

Effects of load weight on body posture and performance

13

EFFECT OF BACKPACK TYPES AND LOADS ON CHILDREN'S MEDIOLATERAL SPINAL POSTURE DURING STAIR WALKING

Youlian Hong,[1] Daniel Tik-Pui Fong[2] and Jing Xian Li[3,4]

[1]CHENGDU SPORTS UNIVERSITY, CHENGDU
[2]CHINESE UNIVERSITY OF HONG KONG, HONG KONG
[3]SHANGHAI UNIVERSITY OF SPORT, SHANGHAI
[4]UNIVERSITY OF OTTAWA, OTTAWA

Introduction

Heavy backpacks have raised extensive discussion among children, parents and health-care professionals about their potential to cause shoulder and back pain and even spine deformity (Mackenzie *et al.*, 2003). The weight of school bags in terms of the percentage of body weight of children has been reported as 17.7 per cent in the United States (Pascoe *et al.*, 1997), 20 per cent in Italy (Negrini and Carabalona, 2002) and 20 per cent in Hong Kong (Hong Kong Society for Child Health and Development, 1988). The heavy loads caused spinal symptoms (Johnson *et al.*, 1995), back pain (Sheir-Neiss *et al.*, 2003), fatigue (Negrini and Carabalona, 2002), breathing restriction (Lai and Jones, 2001) and even acute injuries (Wiersema *et al.*, 2003).

Numerous studies were conducted to demonstrate the biomechanics effect of load carriage. In level overground walking and walking on a treadmill, a load of 15 per cent body weight or more in a double-strap backpack significantly introduced forward trunk lean (Hong and Cheung, 2003), prolonged blood pressure recovery time (Hong and Bruggemann, 2000), increased oxygen update and energy expenditure (Hong *et al.*, 2000), increased breathing frequency (Li *et al.*, 2003) and increased trapeizius muscle activity and fatigue (Hong *et al.*, 2008). In standing, the heavy load also altered the posture in healthy subjects (Chansirinukor *et al.*, 2001), and even introduced imbalance in medial-lateral direction in girls with adolescent idiopathic scoliosis (Chow *et al.*, 2006). Beside the load, the carrying method also affected the body posture. Kinoshita (1985) found that an asymmetrical carrying method caused more spine tilt in level walking, while Troussier *et al.* (1994) found that it was a risk factor of lower back pain. Pascoe *et al.* (1997) also found that an asymmetrical school bag carrying method, represented by a single-strap backpack and a shoulder-supported athletic bag, significantly increased lateral spine deviation during level walking.

In Hong Kong, schools and living places are often multistorey buildings, and thus walking on stairs is a common daily functional activity. Previous studies showed that stair walking and level walking are two different kinds of gait (Loy and Voloshin, 1991; McFadyen and Winter, 1998). Since one has to propagate one's body forward and also upward or downward in stair walking, doing so with a heavy school bag may result in increased dynamic loading on the human body. Hong *et al.* (2003) found that a load of 10 per cent of body weight or more significantly introduced forward spine lean during stair ascending. Moreover, greater spine motion in the sagittal plane was observed when the subjects carried a single-strap shoulder-supported athletic bag, which represented an asymmetrical carrying method. In kinetics, Hong and Li (2005) found increased peak plantar force during stair descending with a load of 10 per cent of body weight in an athletic bag. However, there is little study reporting the spine biomechanics in the frontal plane during stair walking.

It is believed that stair walking, especially stair ascending, is a highly physically demanding task compared to level walking. The effect of load carriage and carrying method may impose a greater challenge to the spine, and thus may lead to a higher risk of spinal symptoms. This study reported the effect of load carriage and school bag design on spine posture during stair walking in children.

Materials and methods

Thirteen male children (aged 12.2 ± 1.0 years; body mass 47.1 ± 9.7 kg; body height 159.7 ± 9.7 cm) participated in this study. The test took place at a 33-step staircase at the audience seat of the university sport field. All participants were free of injury on the testing day, and had no history of injury that may have caused them to have abnormal gait or difficulties in walking on stairs. Consent forms from participants and parents were collected before the test. Participants were required to dress in black, tight T-shirts and shorts, with six reflective skin markers attached at the positions of left and right shoulders, hips and toes. The black dressing and the reflective markers were to facilitate the automatic video image digitization when analysing the video data in motion analysis software.

Each participant performed stair ascending and descending with different loads in school bags, with a different design in each trial. They started at the bottom of the 33-step staircase, walked up to the top and then walked down to the bottom at their natural cadence three times. A total of eight trials from a combination of four different loads in two different school bag designs were performed by each participant in a random sequence. The four load conditions equaled 0, 10, 15 and 20 per cent of the participant's body weight. Percentage weight instead of absolute weight was used in order to achieve normalization across participants. The required weight was prepared by filling the school bag with objects that students usually bring to school, such as books, pencil box, drawing materials, PE T-shirt and shoes. The two types of school bag included a single-strap athletic bag and a double-strap backpack. In trials with the single-strap athletic bag, the school bag was placed on the left, with the strap placed on the right shoulder – this represented an asymmetrical carrying method (Figure 13.1a), with the left as the loading side and the right as the supporting side. In trials with the double-strap backpack, the fillings in the school bag were arranged in a symmetrical way and the two straps were placed on both shoulders – this represented a symmetrical carrying method (Figure 13.1b).

A video camera (JVC DVL9800, Japan) was positioned at the bottom of the staircase, viewing upwards, to record the spine movement in the frontal plane with 50 Hz filming rate and 1/250 s shutter speed. The camera zoom level was adjusted to have a full-picture view when the participant stepped on the middle of the staircase for one complete gait cycle (from the 15th

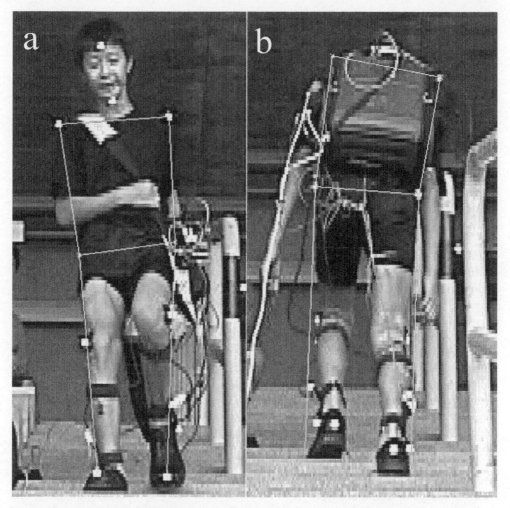

Figure 13.1 The two carrying methods investigated in this study: (a) asymmetrical carrying method with a single-strap athletic bag, with the school bag placed on the left (loading side) and the school bag strap on the right shoulder (supporting side); and (b) symmetrical carrying method with a double-strap backpack.

to the 17th step). The films were captured and saved on a computer. Video data of one complete gait cycle was trimmed during every ascending and descending trial. The video data were digitized by a motion analysis system (Ariel Performance Analysis System, USA). The spine was defined by the line joining the midpoint between the shoulders and the midpoint between the hip, and the spine posture was defined as the angle between the spine and the initial vertical position of each participant. The maximum spine tilting angle to the left and to the right, and the range of the spine tilting angle, were averaged over the participants at each load and each school bag design for stairs ascending and descending.

For both stairs ascending and descending, two-way multivariate analysis of variance (bag type × load) with repeated measures (MANOVA) was applied on the dependent variables to see significant effects by bag type and load. If interactive effect was found, stratified analysis of variance (ANOVA) was conducted to demonstrate the load effect on each bag type (for all parameters), and the bag type effect on each load (for range of spine motion only), with Tukey pairwise comparisons conducted between 0 per cent load to other loads. If not, ANOVA on each main effect was conducted. To further demonstrate the symmetry of spine posture, independent t-tests were conducted between the maximum tilting angle to the left and to the right for each bag type and load. Independent t-tests were also conducted among stairs ascending and descending in every pair of parameters. Statistical significance was set at 95 per cent level of confidence.

Results

Table 13.1 shows the mean and standard deviation of the spine posture parameters, including the maximum spine tilting angle to the left, the maximum spine tilting angle to the right and the range of the spine tilting angle at each load with each school bag type in stairs ascending and descending, respectively. MANOVA showed significant interactive (bag type × load) effect (Wilk's lambda = 0.664, $F = 2.646$, $p = 0.023$). Therefore, stratified ANOVA was conducted.

In ascending stairs, ANOVA showed that significant difference was found in maximum tilting angle to the left and also to the right for a single-strap athletic bag ($p < 0.05$). Tukey pairwise comparisons showed that the maximum tilting angle to the left, or the loading side, was significantly reduced from 3.0° to 1.5° when the load was increased from 0 to 20 per cent of body weight ($p < 0.05$). The maximum tilting angle to the right, or the supporting side, significantly increased from 6.9° to 8.3° when the load was increased from 0 to 15 per cent of body weight ($p < 0.05$), and further to 8.6° when the load was increased from 0 to 20 per cent of body weight ($p < 0.05$). No significant difference was found for the maximum spine tilting angles for a double-strap backpack, and also the range of spine motion for both school bags. For a single-strap school bag, independent t-tests showed significant difference between tilting angles to the left (loading side) and to the right (supporting side) when the load reached 15 and 20 per cent of body weight ($p < 0.05$).

In descending stairs, the tilting angles and the range of spine motions were, in general, smaller than that during ascending stair. ANOVA showed no significant difference among different loads and school bag type.

Independent t-tests showed that significant differences were found between each pair of parameters among stairs ascending and descending, except the spine tilting angle to the left with a 15 and 20 per cent load in a single-strap athletic bag.

Discussion

The range of spine motion did not differ among loads in both single-strap athletic bag and double-strap backpack in both stairs ascending and descending. However, in each load × carrying method combination, it was found to be greater during stairs ascending. The range was about 4.5–7.2° during stairs descending, and it was almost doubled to 9.9–11.9° in stairs ascending. The range of motion did not differ among the two school bag designs in all loads. For a double-strap backpack, which represented a symmetrical carrying method, the spine tilting angles to the left and to the right did not differ among each other and among loads in both stairs ascending and descending. However, it was significantly increased from 1.9–2.8° in stairs descending to 5.3–6.5° in stairs ascending. These findings suggested that the spine motion was, in general, much larger during stairs ascending than in stairs descending. Load effect was not significant. Moreover, the similar spine tilting angles to the left and to the right

Table 13.1 Maximum and range of spine tilting angles for single- and double-strap school bag

Load (% body weight)	Single-strap athletic bag			Double-strap backpack			Range of spine motion (degree)		
	Max angle – left (degree)	Max angle – right (degree)	Statistical difference	Max angle – left (degree)	Max angle – right (degree)	Statistical difference	Single-strap athletic bag	Double-strap backpack	Statistical difference
Stairs ascending									
0	#3.0 (2.1)	#6.9 (3.5)	–	#5.5 (2.1)	#5.9 (2.2)	–	#9.9 (2.7)	#11.4 (2.7)	–
10	#4.0 (2.1)	#6.1 (3.8)	–	#5.4 (2.1)	#6.5 (3.1)	–	#10.1 (3.8)	#11.9 (2.7)	–
15	2.7 (3.4)	#*8.3 (4.4)	$p < 0.05$	#5.4 (2.0)	#5.3 (1.8)	–	#11.0 (4.1)	#10.7 (2.5)	–
20	*1.5 (3.2)	#*8.6 (3.1)	$p < 0.05$	#5.4 (1.6)	#5.7 (2.5)	–	#10.1 (2.0)	#11.1 (1.9)	–
Stairs descending									
0	#1.5 (1.8)	#3.6 (1.9)	$p < 0.05$	#1.9 (1.6)	#2.6 (1.7)	–	#5.1 (1.5)	#4.5 (1.3)	–
10	#1.1 (1.9)	#4.6 (2.1)	$p < 0.05$	#2.7 (0.9)	#2.1 (1.6)	–	#5.7 (2.1)	#4.8 (1.3)	–
15	2.1 (2.4)	4.2 (2.4)	$p < 0.05$	#2.5 (1.3)	#2.2 (1.4)	–	#6.3 (1.9)	#4.7 (1.4)	–
20	2.5 (2.6)	4.7 (2.7)	$p < 0.05$	#2.6 (1.0)	#2.8 (2.1)	–	#7.2 (2.6)	#5.4 (1.3)	–

Standard deviation in brackets.
Significant difference between stair ascending and descending, $p < 0.05$.
* Significant difference with 0% load condition, $p < 0.05$.

with a double-strap backpack suggested that such a carrying method is symmetrical in the human frontal plane.

In stairs ascending with a single-strap athletic bag, there was a trend of shift of spine tilt to the support side (right) when the load increased. The spine tilt to the left was significantly reduced when the load was 20 per cent ($p < 0.05$), and that to the right was significantly increased when the load was 15 and 20 per cent ($p < 0.05$). The spine was tilted to the support side for 8.3 and 8.6° when the load was 15 and 20 per cent, respectively. The spine became asymmetrical as the spine tilting angle to the right was larger than that to the left when the load was 15 and 20 per cent ($p < 0.05$). In stairs descending, significant differences were found between the tilting angle to the left and to the right in each load ($p < 0.05$). In general, the tilting angles during stairs ascending were higher, except that to the left when the load was 15 and 20 per cent, as the spine was more tilted to the support side (right).

In level walking, Pascoe *et al.* (1997) studied the effect on lateral spine tilt in 10 subjects (aged 11–13 years) carrying different school bags with a load of 17.6 per cent of body weight. They reported that the lateral spine tilt was much greater in an asymmetrical carrying method than in a symmetrical carrying method. In walking without load carriage, the lateral spine tilt was 1.9°. In carrying the load in a two-strap backpack, the lateral spine tilt was about 2.1° and did not significantly differ. However, when the load was put in a one-strap backpack or a one-strap athletic bag, the lateral spine tilt was significantly increased to 8.5 and 8.3°, respectively. In stair walking, Hong *et al.* (2003) found that load carriage in an asymmetrical school bag caused more spine sagittal motion. In kinetics, significant increase of peak plantar force was found when the load was 10 per cent of body weight in an asymmetrical load carrying method during stairs ascending; however, such significant increase was found when the load reached 15 per cent of body weight in a symmetrical load carrying method (Hong and Li, 2005).

In this study, significant spine tilt was observed in both stairs ascending and descending with a load in a single-strap athletic bag. Moreover, the range of spine motion was 9.9–11.9° during stairs ascending, which was greater than that in level walking (8.5°) as reported by Pascoe *et al.* (1997). The results with the findings in previous studies together suggested that an asymmetrical carrying method imposed greater stress to the spine, especially in stairs ascending when the load was 15 per cent of body weight or above. Stair walking is different from level walking in the nature of the locomotion. In level walking, a person stays in the same horizontal level, thus he or she only propagates his or her body, or centre of gravity, in a forward direction. In stair walking, a person needs to propagate his or her body forward and also upward or downward. In doing this, he or she has to bend his or her legs to raise or lower one side of the body to land on the next step. This introduces greater spine motion when compared to level walking. The fact was more significant when there was a heavy load (> 15 per cent of body weight) in an asymmetrical carrying method.

The spine tilt was to the supported side (the side with the school bag strap on the shoulder) instead of the loading side. This is the human adaptation to minimize the disturbance of balance and stability of the body centre of mass. When a single-strap athletic bag is loaded on the left, the centre of gravity of the person plus the school bag shifts to the left. This introduces posture instability, thus the person has to tilt the body to the right in order to shift the centre of gravity back to the middle of the supporting base, which is between both feet. Doing so in a prolonged period requires repetitive activation of spine stabilizing muscles. This may lead to muscle pain, lower back pain and chronic injuries, thus further study on spine stabilizing muscle activity and fatigue is suggested.

Conclusion

This study suggested that the spine posture was not altered when stair walking with a double-strap backpack. However, significant spine tilt to the support side was observed with a single-strap athletic bag. The spine tilt was much more significant when the load was 15 per cent of body weight or above. It is concluded that a symmetrical backpack or an asymmetrical single-strap athletic bag with a load not exceeding 10 per cent should be recommended for school children in order to avoid spine posture alteration during stair walking. Further study in muscle activity is suggested.

References

Chansirinukor, W., Wilson, D., Grimmer, K. and Dansie, B. (2001) 'Effects of backpacks on students: measurement of cervical and shoulder posture', *Australian Journal of Physiotherapy*, 47(2): 110–16.

Chow, D. H., Kwok, M. L., Cheng, J. C., Lao, M. L., Holmes, A. D., Au-Yang, A., Yao, F. Y. and Wong, M. S. (2006) 'The effect of backpack weight on the standing posture and balance of schoolgirls with adolescent idiopathic scoliosis and normal controls', *Gait and Posture*, 24(2): 173–81.

Hong, Y. and Brueggemann, G. (2000) 'Changes of gait pattern in 10-year-old boys with increasing loads when walking on a treadmill', *Gait and Posture*, 11(3): 245–59.

Hong, Y. and Cheung, C. K. (2003) 'Gait and posture responses to backpack load during level walking in children', *Gait and Posture*, 17(1): 28–33.

Hong, Y. and Li, J. X. (2005) 'Influence of load and carrying methods on gait phase and ground reactions in children's stair walking', *Gait and Posture*, 22(1): 63–8.

Hong, Y., Li, J. X., Wong, A. S. K. and Robinson, P. D. (2000) 'Effects of loads carriage on heart rate, blood pressure and energy expenditure in children', *Ergonomics*, 43(6): 717–27.

Hong, Y., Lau, T. C. and Li, J. X. (2003) 'Effects of loads and carrying methods of school bags on movement kinematics of children during stair walking', *Research in Sports Medicine*, 11(1): 33–49.

Hong, Y., Li, J. X. and Fong, D. T. P. (2008) 'Effect of prolonged walking with backpack loads on trunk muscle activity and fatigue in children', *Journal of Electromyography and Kinesiology*, 18(6): 990–6.

Hong Kong Society for Child Health and Development (1998) *The Weight of School Bags and its Relation to Spinal Deformity*, Hong Kong: The Department of Orthopaedic Surgery, University of Hong Kong.

Johnson, R. F., Knapik, J. J. and Merullo, D. J. (1995) 'Symptoms during load carrying: effects of mass and load distribution during a 20-km road march', *Perceptual and Motor Skills*, 81(1): 331–8.

Kinoshita, H. (1985) 'Effects of different loads and carrying systems on selected biomechanical parameters describing walking gait', *Ergonomics*, 28(9): 1347–62.

Lai, J. P. and Jones, A. Y. (2001) 'The effect of shoulder-girdle loading by a school bag on lung volumes in Chinese primary school children', *Early Human Development*, 62(1): 79–86.

Li, J. X., Hong, Y. and Robinson, P. D. (2003) 'The effect of load carriage on movement kinematics and respiratory parameters in children during walking', *European Journal of Applied Physiology*, 90(1–2): 35–43.

Loy, D. J. and Voloshin, A. S. (1991) 'Biomechanics of stair walking and jumping', *Journal of Sports Science*, 9(2): 137–49.

McFadyen, B. J. and Winter, D. A. (1998) 'An integrated biomechanical analysis of normal stair ascent and descent', *Journal of Biomechanics*, 21(9): 733–44.

Mackenzie, W. G., Sampath, J. S., Kruse, R. W. and Sheir-Neiss, G. J. (2003) 'Backpacks in children', *Clinical Orthopaedics and Related Research*, 409: 78–84.

Negrini, S. and Carabalona, R. (2002) 'Backpacks on! Schoolchildren's perceptions of load, associations with back pain and factors determining the load', *Spine*, 27(2): 187–95.

Pascoe, D. D., Pascoe, D. E., Wang, Y. T., Shim, D. M. and Kim, C. K. (1997) 'Influence of carrying book bags on gait cycle and posture of youths', *Ergonomics*, 40(6): 631–41.

Sheir-Neiss, G. I., Kruse, R. W., Rahman, T., Jacobson, L. P. and Pelli, J. A. (2003) 'The association of backpack use and back pain in adolescents', *Spine*, 28(9): 922–30.

Troussier, B., Davoine, P., de Gaudemaris, R., Fauconnier, J. and Phelip, X. (1994) 'Back pain in school children: a study among 1178 pupils', *Scandinavian Journal of Rehabilitation Medicine*, 26(3): 143–6.

Wiersema, B. M., Wall, E. J. and Foad, S. L. (2003) 'Acute backpack injuries in children', *Pediatrics*, 111(1): 163–6.

14

THE EFFECT OF UNILATERAL LOAD CARRIAGE ON THE MUSCLE ACTIVITIES OF THE TRUNK AND LOWER LIMB OF YOUNG HEALTHY MALES DURING GAIT

Liam Corrigan and Jing Xian Li

UNIVERSITY OF OTTAWA, OTTAWA

Introduction

Load carrying with backpack, side packs, and front packs have been found to alter the gait, posture, trunk and lower limb biomechanics, and muscle activities of the human body (Cook and Neumann, 1987; Knapik *et al.*, 1996; Motmans *et al.*, 2006; Smith *et al.*, 2006). Many studies indicate that the more drastic and perhaps the more injury prone method of load carriage is unilateral (side pack) carrying (DeVita *et al.*, 1991; Fowler *et al.*, 2006; Motmans *et al.*, 2006). Sports such as golf, football, soccer, baseball and ice hockey all require the recreational athlete to carry his or her equipment to the field of play. The hockey bag, when full of equipment, is large in volume and weight. Its weight is considerably more than the bags of other sports. A recent survey, conducted by our research team, of 33 participants at the University of Ottawa's Sports Complex arena showed that male and female university-aged students between 19 and 23 years (20.63 ± 1.53 years) carry a hockey bag of average 18.77 (± 5.13) per cent of body weight (BW) over one shoulder and walk distances of average 641.67 (± 687.67) m. In the same survey, the maximum weight of a hockey bag recorded was by a 21-year-old male goaltender, with a weight that equaled 33.29 per cent of his total body weight (Corrigan *et al.*, 2010).

Unilateral load carriage is commonly found in ice hockey players carrying their equipment. It is also found that during play in hockey, participants perform repetitive or continuous forward trunk flexion. This particular movement, in addition to the chronic and repetitive forward flexion with load carriage, may lead to injury involving the spinal column (Baranto *et al.*, 2009; Mountain, 2002). Biomechanical studies of unilateral load carriage typically use loads of up to 20 per cent of one's body weight (Crosbie *et al.*, 1994; DeVita *et al.*, 1991; Fowler *et al.*, 2006; Gillette *et al.*, 2010; Lee and Li, in press; Motmans *et al.*, 2006). However, muscle activity of the trunk and the lower limb during walking while unilaterally carrying a load more than 20 per cent of the carrier's body weight is unknown. Therefore, a comprehensive study on temporospatial, kinematics and muscle activities of the trunk and lower limb during walking with a hockey bag of different weight will add to our understanding on the impact of unilateral load carrying on the biomechanical responses. The purpose of the study was to investigate the trunk and lower limb muscle activity during heavy unilateral load carriage. It was hypothesized that the muscle activity of the trunk and lower limb would be increased and muscle activity would be higher in the non-carrying side.

Methodology

Hockey bag

One standard Reebok hockey bag (0.11 m^3) was used in this study. Insulation was placed in the hockey bag to allow for a full volume and metal weights were positioned into the hockey bag to account for the load weight of 10 per cent, 20 per cent and 30 per cent of the subject's body weight. The insulation and metal weights allowed for an equal distribution of weight and to limit any shifting or movement of the weights during walking (see Figures 14.1 and 14.2)

Walking path

The walking path was located in a laboratory and had smooth rubber flooring. It was 8 m in length and was surrounded by infrared motion analysis cameras. In the middle of the 8 m pathway were four force plates, placed in a staggered position. The flooring in the laboratory was made flush with the force plates.

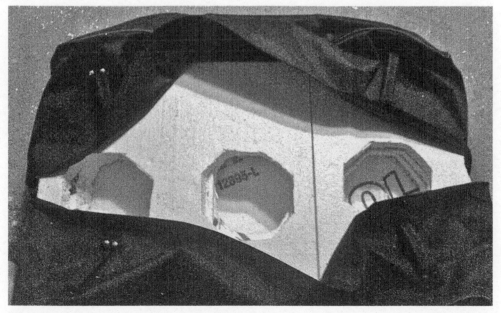

Figure 14.1 The hockey bag is shown above with styrofoam and designated sections along the centre for the placement of metal weights.

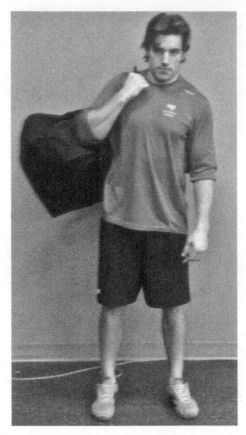

Figure 14.2 A display of the style (posterior-lateral) during hockey bag carriage.

Instrumentation

The instruments used to capture temporospatial kinematic data included 10 infrared, high speed, optical cameras with the Vicon Motion Analysis System, recording at 100 Hz (Vicon MX-13, Oxford Metrics, Oxford, UK). The Vicon cameras were set up around the walking path either from mounted tripods or hung from the ceiling. Four force plates were used to aid in the detection of foot contact (two models 9286AA, Kistler Instruments Corp, Winterhur, Switzerland; two models FP 4060-08, Bertec Corporation, Columbus, OH). The force plates were positioned in a way that mocks a regular walking pattern. A 16-channel EMG system (DS-B04, Bagnoli™-16 Desktop EMG system, DelsysInc., Boston, MA) was used to record muscle activity in 16 muscles at 1,000 Hz. The sensors were applied with double-sided tape and placed on the muscle belly of the muscle being recorded. The analogue data coming from the EMG sensors were then synchronized with the temporospatial data through a VICON acquisition board.

Participants

The participants were composed of 15 male hockey players (23.40 ± 2.63 years) with an average of 16.56 ± 4.92 years of ice hockey experience and therefore hockey bag carriage experience. The average body mass index (BMI) of the participants was 24.97 kg.m^{-2} and no participant was in an obese weight range. All but one of the participants carried the bag on their dominant right shoulder. For the one participant who carried his bag on his dominant left, the left gait cycle and left muscles were used for analysis and pooled in with the right of the others. It is in this way that the 'right' muscles will be defined as the carrying side.

Data collection

The participants were asked to come to the biomechanics lab at the University of Ottawa campus once for data collection. The details of the research and the experiment procedures were explained to each participant before reading and signing a consent form approved by the University of Ottawa Health Sciences and Science Research Ethics Board. A questionnaire regarding the subject's experience with hockey bag load carriage was completed at this time. Participants wore their own gym shorts and gym shirt with regular running shoes.

Participants were encouraged to warm up on a stationary bicycle and stretch before executing the trials in the experiment. For EMG sensor placement, the skin overlying the following muscle bellies (left and right) were shaven and cleaned with alcohol wipes: *erector spinae* (ES) (located at the level of the L4-L5 interspace and 2 cm away from the midline), *rectus abdominis* (RA) (located on the belly of the muscle just below the umbillicus), *rectus femoris* (RF), *vastus medialis* (VM), *biceps femoris* (BF), *semitendinosus* (ST), *medial gastrocnemius* (GAS) and *gluteus maximus* (GM), with the reference electrode placed on the skin overlying the left olecranon. Retro-reflective markers were attached via double-sided tape to the anatomical landmarks of the toe, heel, lateral and medial malleoli of both feet. These markers provided enough data to determine temporospatial parameters such as stride length, stride width, and double and single support time.

The participants performed 3–5 practice trials of walking and walking with the load for each condition in an effort to maintain a normal gait unaffected by the increased attention. The participants were asked to carry the hockey bag over their self-chosen, dominant shoulder in a manner that they would carry their own hockey bag and to walk the 8 m through the testing area. The walking speed of the participants was self-determined and at a natural pace. Motion was captured by 10 VICON MX-13 cameras during four trials of each condition of 0 per cent of BW (no load), 10 per cent of BW, 20 per cent of BW and 30 per cent of BW. The total number of trials was 16. The condition order for each participant was randomly selected from one of the scenarios in a Latin Square design.

Data processing

Movement was analysed for one gait cycle. Data were expressed as a percentage of the dominant side gait cycle. Foot contact was identified visually while inspecting the labelled markers of the heel, toe, and malleoli on VICON Nexus software (v1.3) and through force plate data signals. Measurements included stride length (right heel to right heel), stride width (max distance within the gait cycle between left medial malleolus to right medial malleolus), single leg support (left foot off to left foot on and right foot off to right foot on) and double support phase (right foot on to left foot off and left foot on to right foot off). These measurements were made through formulas on SMART Analyzer (BTS Software, Italy).

The EMG data were rectified using the temporal mean, filtered using a single, low-pass Butterworth filter to smoothen the data and then processed with a cut of frequency of 4 Hz. The filtered EMG data were then normalized to 100 per cent of the gait cycle and plotted as a percentage of the peak amplitude in the average of the control condition. This was done to give representations of peak magnitude of EMG in the 10, 20 and 30 per cent of BW condition in comparison to normal walking. It has also been shown that for dynamic testing such as running, cycling and walking, using a control condition similar to the testing protocols would be more appropriate (Benoit *et al.*, 2003; Mirka, 1991). As a result, data for the peak EMG activity are shown as a percentage of normal walking. Integrated EMG (iEMG) was also examined. The iEMG were calculated using the normalized EMG with the following formula:

$$\text{area} = \sum (X_{i+1} - x_i) \star 1/2[f(x_{i+1}) + f(x_i)] \tag{1}$$

where 'x_i' represents an initial percentage value in the gait cycle and 'x_{i+1}' represents the following percentage value. The '$f(x)$' are the y-values or the normalized peak EMG value for the given 'x' coordinate. The formula is an adaption of the sum of: area = base × height/2.

Statistical analysis

A two-way repeated measures analysis of variance (two-way repeated measures ANOVA) was used to examine the differences between the repeated factor of hockey bag load weight (four levels: no load, load of 10 per cent of BW, load of 20 per cent of BW and load of 30 per cent of BW) and muscle side (left and right). When significance was found, a Bonferroni Post-Hoc test was performed using repeated measures of t-tests for load, and independent t-tests were used for examining any differences of the measurements between left and right muscles. The probability of error in all tests is presented with a p-value of < 0.05. All analyses were performed using the statistical software package SPSS 20.0 for Mac (SPSS Inc., Chicago, IL).

Results

All measurements and results are expressed as a mean with standard error (SE).

Temporospatial variables

The carrying side is defined as the right side, while the non-carrying side is defined as the left in this study. No differences were observed between left and right gait cycle in the study. As a result, only the right gait cycle was used for analysis. The stride length had shown to decrease as the load increased, with significance in the 30 per cent of BW condition when compared to all other conditions ($p = 0.048$). The stride width had shown to increase as load increased, with significance in the 30 per cent of BW condition when compared to all other conditions ($p = 0.044$). Finally, the double support increased and single support decreased as load weight was increased, with the largest significant difference being from the control to 30 per cent of BW ($p < 0.001$) (Table 14.1).

Peak magnitude of EMG and iEMG

The results of the peak EMG and the iEMG are illustrated in Figure 14.3. Carrying a load of 10 per cent of BW did not result in any significant change in peak EMG and iEMG in the measured muscles. The peak EMG of the right RA increased by 1.35 times in 20 per cent of BW load condition and 1.86 times in 30 per cent of BW condition compared to no load condition, with significance taking place for the 30 per cent of BW against all other load

Table 14.1 Mean and standard error of the tempospatial variables during walking with a unilateral hockey bag

Load (% of BW)	Stride length (m)	p-value	Stride width (cm)	p-value	Single support (% of a gait cycle)	p-value	Double support (% of a gait cycle)	p-value
0	1.51 ± 0.03	–	10.6 ± 0.5		73.8 ± 0.9	–	26.2 ± 0.9	–
10	1.46 ± 0.03	0.211	11.2 ± 0.7	1.000	72.3 ± 1.1★	0.026	27.7 ± 1.1★	0.026
20	1.45 ± 0.03	0.117	13.1 ± 0.9	0.053	70.5 ± 0.8★	0.001	29.5 ± 0.8★	0.001
30	1.39 ± 0.03★	0.002	16.3 ± 1.1★	< 0.001	68.9 ± 0.8★	< 0.001	31.1 ± 0.8★	< 0.001

Measurements are compared against the control condition of no load.
★ $p < 0.05$, versus 0% BW load condition.

conditions ($p = 0.026$). Similar increases were found in the right RA for the iEMG, being significantly greater in the 30 per cent of BW load compared to all other conditions ($p = 0.013$). No significant increases in peak EMG and iEMG were discovered in the left RA.

The right VM was significantly higher in peak EMG for the 30 per cent of BW condition (2.08 ± 0.27) when compared to all other conditions ($p = 0.031$). The iEMG for the same muscle showed similar significant results, with the 30 per cent of BW condition (81.801 ± 11.246) larger than all the other conditions ($p = 0.005$). No significant increases in peak EMG and iEMG were discovered in the left VM.

No significant increases occurred in peak or iEMG for either the left or right RF and the left or right BF against the no load condition.

The ST peak activity increased in both the right (1, 1.11, 1.329, 2.024) and left (1, 1.777, 2.979, 3.894) with load increase, but differed significantly only in the right ST when comparing the 30 per cent of BW to the 10 per cent of BW load ($p = 0.032$) in the peak EMG and in the left iEMG when looking at the 30 per cent of BW to the control ($p = 0.042$).

The GAS also increased for the right (1, 1.484, 1.762, 2.782) and left (1, 1.331, 1.856, 2.903) for peak EMG and for the right (53.637, 76.27, 90.86, 129.30) and left (45.376, 65.605, 91.998, 151.9) for iEMG. In the right for both peak and iEMG, significance occurs from 30 per cent of BW to the control ($p = 0.03$) and 20 per cent of BW to the control ($p = 0.013$). The left GAS shows significance from 30 per cent of BW to control, 10 per cent of BW and 20 per cent of BW ($p = 0.046$) and at the 20 per cent of BW to control, 10 per cent of BW, and 30 per cent of BW ($p = 0.046$).

The ES and GM showed no significant increases in either right or left muscles.

The muscle activity between the left and right side at each load condition showed differences. The muscles on the left side were more active than the right side during walking and carrying a load compared to no load carrying. Significance takes place at peak EMG of the RF in the 20 per cent of BW ($p = 0.022$) and the 30 per cent of BW ($p = 0.041$), both showing to have larger peak EMG in the left. Significance in the iEMG for the same muscle was not found. The ST also showed significance at the 30 per cent of BW condition for both the peak and iEMG ($p = 0.044$). Again, more activity occurred for the left muscle.

Discussion

The current study examined the effect of variations in mass of hockey bag load carriage on the stride length, stride width, support time and the muscle activities of the trunk and lower

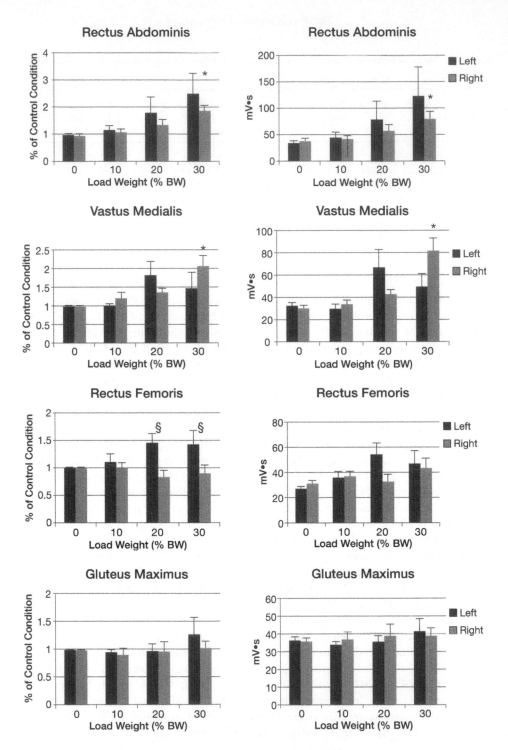

Figure 14.3 The changes in peak EMG (charts on the left) and iEMG (charts on the right) of the muscles on the right and left side of the body during walking at different load condition. Data were normalized to the values obtained at no load condition (0 per cent of BW) of the left and right muscles, respectively. (★ $p < 0.05$ versus 0 per cent of BW load condition; §, $p < 0.05$, left side muscle versus right side muscles.)

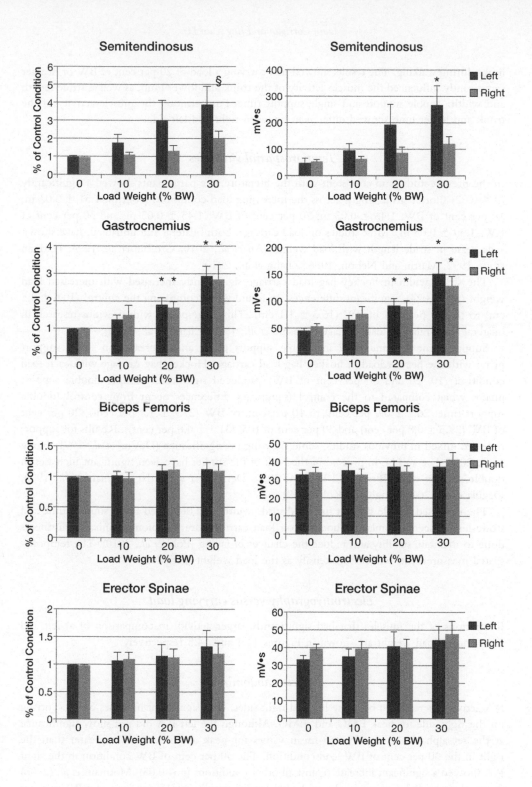

limbs during walking. The results showed that carrying a load of 20 per cent of BW or heavier significantly influenced the muscle activity of the trunk and lower limb, as well as stride length and width, double support and single support time. Furthermore, the muscle activity of the trunk and lower limb showed differences between right and left side.

Temporospatial variables

In the present study, and consistent with the literature, the participants showed a significantly ($p < 0.02$) shorter stride length across the increasing load conditions (control: 1.51 ± 0.03 m; 10 per cent of BW: 1.46 ± 0.03 m; 20 per cent of BW: 1.45 ± 0.03 m; and 30 per cent of BW: 1.39 ± 0.03 m). Most studies on load carriage, both bilateral and unilateral, have shown a decrease in stride length with load weight (An *et al.*, 2010; Crosbie *et al.*, 1994; Harman *et al.*, 1992; Martin and Nelson, 1986; Zhang *et al.*, 2010).

The stride width in hockey bag load carriage significantly increased with increased load weight ($p = 0.024$). Significant differences are found when comparing the control (10.6 ± 0.5 cm) to the 30 per cent of BW (16.3 ± 1.1 cm). This corresponds with previous research in bilateral and unilateral load carriage (Crosbie *et al.*, 1994; Zhang *et al.*, 2010).

Support time had increased in double support phase and decreased in single support phase with the heavier load in hockey bag load carriage. Hockey bag carriage with each load condition (10, 20 and 30 per cent of BW) produced significantly longer double support phases when compared to the control (significant differences occur from control (double support time: 26.2 ± 0.9 per cent) to 10 per cent of BW (27.7 ± 1.1 per cent), 20 per cent of BW (29.5 ± 0.8 per cent) and 30 per cent of BW (31.1 ± 0.8 per cent)). Results for support time are mixed in previous studies, some showing no significance (DeVita *et al.*, 1991; Hong *et al.*, 2008; Lee and Li, in press), but the bulk of the studies have seen significant increases in double support time (Birrell and Haslam, 2010; Demura *et al.*, 2010; Harman *et al.*, 1992; Özgüla *et al.*, 2011; Singh and Koh, 2009).

The increased double support time and stride width, and decreased single support time and stride length seen in unilateral hockey bag load carriage, are the biomechanical adjustments done to maintain stability and reduce the chances of falling (Pohl *et al.*, 2010). The temporospatial measurements tended to intensify as the load weight increased.

Electromyography versus carrying load

Illustrations of the muscles that had significantly larger activity in comparison of a) left and right and b) load weight are shown in Figures 14.4 and 14.5 respectively.

Rectus abdominis

RA activity increased in both the left and right sides, with significant increases only occurring on the right side for peak EMG and iEMG. Although the left RA did not show significance at the set alpha level of 0.05, the mean values for peak and iEMG were greater than the right in the 30 per cent of BW load condition. The 30 per cent of BW condition in the right RA showed a significant increase against all other conditions ($p < 0.05$). Motmans *et al.* (2006) found that the RA activity in the unilateral loaded condition (15 per cent of BW) was not significantly different than the control condition (no load). There are several explanations as to why the RA activity was significantly larger in the present study compared to being insignificant in Motmans' study on unilateral load carriage. First, it may have been because of the mass of the load. Motmans used 15 per cent of BW, whereas the present study found significance at the 30 per cent of BW load. Second, Motmans examined the participants in static standing. In the present study, the participants are walking forward, usually associated with a forward lean in load carriage studies (Simpson *et al.*, 2011). Lastly, the position of the load may play a factor. In Motmans' study, participants had the bag over the shoulder and across the body, positioned directly on the hip. The present study had the hockey bag in the more posterior position, much like a backpack. In the bilateral backpack studies, the RA muscles show significant increases to compensate for the tension placed on the anterior muscles as the result of a posterior load (Al-Khabbaz *et al.*, 2006; Motmans *et al.*, 2006).

Erector spinae

No significant changes occurred in the left or right ES as a result of increasing load in hockey bag unilateral load carriage. Similar findings are found in bilateral studies; the ES has no significant increase (Cook and Neumann, 1987) and in some cases are significantly lower than the control (Bobet and Norman, 1984; Motmans *et al.*, 2006). Again, this may reflect the positioning of the hockey bag load. In its posterior-lateral location on the subjects, the hockey bag is akin to many backpacks.

Gluteus maximus

Much like the ES, the GM showed no significant increase at any of the loaded conditions. Little evidence in previous studies exists on the EMG activity of the *gluteus maximus*. The insignificant results for this muscle suggest that, much like the erector spinae, active hip extension via the GM is not an integral part of hockey bag load carriage.

Knee flexors (biceps femoris and semitendinosus)

Increased load weight resulted in large increases in muscle activities of both sides of the ST (30 per cent of BW; LST: 3.89 ± 0.98 and RST: 2.02 ± 0.38) and little change to the BF (30 per cent of BW; LBF: 1.12 ± 0.12 and RBF: 1.10 ± 0.12). Due to small changes in the BF and large variation around the mean in the ST, significance was only found in iEMG of the left ST (significant when comparing the 30 per cent of BW condition to the control, $p = 0.042$) and in the right ST for the 30 per cent of BW load against the 10 per cent of BW. The high measurements for the ST peak and iEMG are unknown. Possible causes may be cross-talk with underlying muscles or poor connectivity of the EMG sensor to the skin (Mirka, 1991).

Recent research in bilateral load carriage reveals that heightened muscle activity may be present in the hamstrings (Simpson *et al.*, 2011). However, past studies have concluded that there is no significance in the hamstring muscle activities during walking with load carrying (Harman *et al.*, 1992; Knapik *et al.*, 1996).

Gastrocnemius

Significant increases in peak EMG and iEMG occurred in both GAS and at the 20 and 30 per cent of BW load increments. This result parallels with the literature. Simpson *et al.* (2011) collected data for the medial gastrocnemius and found that the iEMG of this muscle significantly increased when participants carried the 20 per cent BW, 30 per cent BW, and 40 per cent BW loads compared to 0 per cent BW. It has been well documented in the bilateral studies that peak EMG of the GAS increases (Harman *et al.*, 1992; Norman, 1979), but no studies on the muscle activity of the gastrocnemius could be found for unilateral load carriage.

Knee extensors (rectus femoris and vastus medialis)

The RF on the right and left sides showed no significant change in peak EMG or iEMG. The VM muscles of both sides increased in peak EMG and iEMG, with significance found only in the right VM when compared to the control (30 per cent of BW for peak EMG ($p = 0.008$), 20 per cent of BW ($p = 0.005$) and 10 per cent of BW ($p = 0.002$) for iEMG). Like the ST of the hamstrings, the VM showed some inconsistence among participants in terms of the muscle activation patterning. In this case, it could have been from cross-talk with the RF.

Ghori and Luckwill (1985) noticed significant muscle prolongation in the unloaded side of the *vastus lateralis* when they studied the effects of unilateral loading. In a bilateral load carriage study, Simpson *et al.* (2011) revealed significant peak activation in the *vastus lateralis* with increasing load. Other studies have shown mixed results, either no significance (Harman *et al.*, 1992) or significant increase (Norman, 1979).

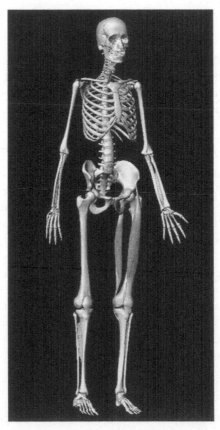

Figure 14.4 Left muscles that significantly increased when compared to the right of the same muscle. Significant increases occurred in the left RF and the left ST.

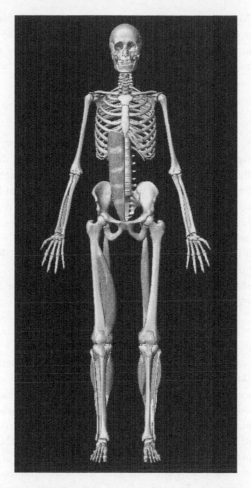

Figure 14.5 Muscles that significantly increased in activity with an increased load weight in hockey bag load carriage. Muscles are: right RA, right VM, right and left ST, and right and left GAS.

Electromyography versus carrying side

A summary of the muscles that had significantly larger muscle activity when compared to its corresponding contralateral muscle during load carriage is shown in Figure 14.4. In the present study, significantly greater peak EMG and iEMG for the left sides of the RF and ST compared to the right side at the 30 per cent of BW load condition occur ($p < 0.05$). Also, increased peak EMG, although not significant, was found to be greater in the left when compared to the right of all muscles, excluding the VM for the 30 per cent load condition. Similarly, the literature in unilateral load carriage shows significant differences between right and left, and carrying and non-carrying muscles. Increases in the peak EMG of the left, non-carrying side have occurred for the *vastus lateralis, semimembranosus, gluteus medius, rectus abdominis* and *erector spinae* in unilateral load carriage examination (Cook and Neumann, 1987; Ghori and Luckwill, 1985; Motmans *et al.*, 2006). The findings of increased activity of the *rectus abdominis* and no change of the *erector spinae* are similar to many bilateral studies studying the same muscles

(Knapik *et al.*, 1996; Motmans *et al.*, 2006; Simpson *et al.*, 2011). It is also noted that the increases in the muscles of the carrying side are representative of many unilateral load carriage studies (Motmans *et al.*, 2006; Smith *et al.*, 2006). It is suggested by the researchers that the posterior-lateral position of the hockey bag in load carriage creates the results to be similar to the both types of load carriage.

Limitations

Limitations in this study include the make-up of the hockey bag load. Styrofoam was used to generate the hockey bag's true volume. For many hockey players, this may be unnatural as the hockey bag normally contains flexible equipment that can bend around the carrier's trunk. The hockey bag has non-adjustable straps, positioning the two sizes of hockey bags at different places on the participants. The non-adjustable straps also limit the researchers to control for the position between participants. However, the non-adjustable straps are characteristic of the hockey bags on the market.

Walking on smooth laboratory flooring also poses as a limitation. Realistically, carriers are walking over gravel, bumps and sometimes snow and ice.

Limitations of the EMG set-up and lying over skin can change the activity recorded by the device. Cross-talk may be possible with underlying muscles.

Conclusion

The study reveals that hockey bag load carriage may be different than unilateral and bilateral load carriage. The hockey bag is carried over one shoulder, as seen in a unilateral style. But the hockey bag is placed more posterior than the athletic duffle bags studied in unilateral studies, which is carried lying over the hip. In this way, the muscle activity of carrying a hockey bag is also similar to that of bilateral backpack carrying. Carrying a hockey bag with 20 per cent of BW and 30 per cent of BW significantly increased the muscle activity in the *rectus abdomininis* and *vastus medialis* of right side and *gastrocnemius* and *semitendinosus* of the both left and right sides. The muscle activity in the *rectus femoris* and *semitendinosus* between left and right was significantly different. The left sides of these muscle activities were greater when compared to the right.

It is recommended that young hockey players alternate the shoulder they use during hockey bag load carriage to avoid asymmetrical muscle fatigue. If possible, hockey players should limit the amount of excess weight they may have in their hockey bag. Hockey players should also choose bags that stay close to the body's centre of mass to avoid excessive rotation around the hip and trunk and have adjustable straps. Future research should investigate the influences of posterior-lateral load carriage on joint biomechanics of the trunk and lower limb, and how the gait and posture of young hockey players may be affected by the heavy loads applied after walking for relatively long distances and on different surfaces.

References

Al-Khabbaz, Y. S., Shimada, T. and Hasegawa, M. (2008) 'The effect of backpack heaviness on trunk-lower extremity muscle activities and trunk posture', *Gait and Posture*, 28(2): 297–302.

An, D. H., Yoon, J. Y., Yoo, W. G. and Kim, K. M. (2010) 'Comparisons of the gait parameters of young Korean women carrying a single-strap bag', *Nursing and Health Sciences*, 12(1): 87–93.

Baranto, A., Hellström, M., Cederlund, C. G., Nyman, R. and Swärd, L. (2009) 'Back pain and MRI changes in the thoraco-lumbar spine of top athletes in four different sports: a 15-year follow-up study', *Knee Surgery, Sports Traumatology, Arthroscopy*, 17(9): 1125–34.

Benoit, D. L., Lamontagne, M., Cerulli, G. and Liti, A. (2003) 'The clinical significance of electromyography normalisation techniques in subjects with anterior cruciate ligament injury during treadmill walking', *Gait and Posture*, 18(2): 56–63.

Birrell, S. A. and Haslam, R. A. (2010) 'The effect of load distribution within military load carriage systems on the kinetics of human gait', *Applied Ergonomics*, 41(4): 585–90.

Bobet, J. and Norman, R. W. (1984) 'Effects of load placement on back muscle activity in load carriage', *European Journal of Applied Physiology*, 53(1): 71–5.

Cook, T. M. and Neumann, D. (1987) 'The effects of load placement on the EMG activity of the low back muscles during load carrying by men and women', *Ergonomics*, 30(10): 1413–23.

Corrigan, L., Law, N. H. and Law, N. Y. (2010) *The Hockey Bag Survey*, Ottawa: University of Ottawa.

Crosbie, J., Flynn, W. and Rutter, L. (1994) 'Effect of side load carriage on the kinematics of gait', *Gait and Posture*, 2(2): 103–8.

Demura, T., Demura, S. I. and Shin, S. (2010) 'Comparison of gait properties during level walking and stair ascent and descent with varying loads', *Health*, 2(12): 1372–6.

DeVita, P., Hong, D. and Hamill, J. (1991) 'Effects of asymmetric load carrying on the biomechanics of walking', *Journal of Biomechanics*, 24(12): 1119–29.

Fowler, N. E., Rodacki, A. L. and Rodacki, C. D. (2006) 'Changes in stature and spine kinematics during a loaded walking task', *Gait and Posture*, 23(2): 133–41.

Ghori, G. M. and Luckwill, R. G. (1985) 'Responses of the lower limb to load carrying in walking man', *European Journal of Applied Physiology*, 54(2): 145–50.

Gillette, J. C., Stevermer, C. A., Miller, R. H., Meardon, S. A. and Schwab, C. V. (2010) 'The effects of age and type of carrying task on lower extremity kinematics', *Ergonomics*, 53(3): 355–64.

Harman, E., Han, K. H., Frykman, P., Johnson, M., Russell, F and Rosenstein, M. (1992) 'The effects on gait timing, kinetics, and muscle activity of various loads carried on the back', *Medicine and Science in Sports and Exercise*, 24(5): S129.

Hong, Y., Li, J. X. and Fong, D. T. (2008) ' Effect of prolonged walking with backpack loads on trunk muscle activity and fatigue in children', *Journal of Electromyography and Kinesiology*, 18(6): 990–6.

Knapik, J., Harman, E. and Reynolds, K. (1996) 'Load carriage using packs: a review of physiological, biomechanical and medical aspects', *Applied Ergonomics*, 27(3): 207–16.

Lee, S. and Li, J. X. (in press) 'Effects of high-heeled shoes and asymmetrical load carriage on lower extremity kinematics during walking in young women', *Journal of the American Podiatric Medical Association*.

Martin, P. E. and Nelson, R. C. (1986) 'The effect of carried loads on the walking patterns of men and women', *Ergonomics*, 29(10): 1191–202.

Mirka, G. A. (1991) 'The quantification of EMG normalization error', *Ergonomics*, 34(3): 343–52.

Motmans, R. R., Tomlow, S. and Vissers, D. (2006) 'Trunk muscle activity in different modes of carrying schoolbags', *Ergonomics*, 49(2): 127–38.

Mountain, M. (2002) *Muscle Imbalance in Hockey Players Contributes to Back Pain*, available at: http://hockeytrainingpro.com/wordpress/2009/11/muscle-imbalance-in-hockey-players-contributes-to-back-pain/ (accessed 1 May 2011).

Norman, R. W. (1979) 'The utility of combining EMG and mechanical work rate data in load carriage studies', *Proceedings of the 4th Congress of the international Society of Electrophysiological Kinesiology*, Boston, MA: International Society of Electrophysiological Kinesiology, pp. 148–9.

Özgüla, B., Akalanb, E., Kuchimovc, S., Uygurd, F., Temellie, Y. and Polata, M. G. (2011) 'During asymmetrical backpack loading: Is unloaded side of body segments truly unloaded?', *Journal of Biomechanics*, 44(1): S1–21.

Pohl, M. B., Lloyd, C. and Ferber, R. (2010) 'Can the reliability of three-dimensional running kinematics be imporved using functional joint methodology?', *Gait and Posture*, 32(4): 559–63.

Simpson, K. M., Munro, B. J. and Steele, J. R. (2011) 'Backpack load affects lower limb muscle activity patterns of female hikers during prolonged load carriage', *Journal of Electromyography and Kinesiology*, 21(5): 782–8.

Singh, T. and Koh, M. (2009) 'Effects of backpack load position on spatiotemporal parameters and trunk forward lean', *Gait and Posture*, 29(1): 49–53.

Smith, B., Ashton, K. M., Bohl, D., Clark, R. C., Metheny, J. B. and Klassen, S. (2006) 'Influence of carrying a backpack on pelvic tilt, rotation, and obliquity in female college students', *Gait and Posture*, 23(3): 263–7.

Zhang, X. I., Ye, M. and Wang, C. (2010) 'Effect of unilateral load carriage on postures and gait symmetry in ground reaction force during walking', *Computer Methods in Biomechanics and Biomedical Engineering*, 13(3): 339–44.

15

DIFFERENCES IN PHYSIOLOGY, BIOMECHANICS AND MOTOR CONTROL OF WALKING WITH BACKPACK LOADS BETWEEN CHILDREN AND ADULTS

Tarkeshwar Singh[1,2] and Michael Koh[3]

[1]CLEVELAND CLINIC, CLEVELAND
[2]PENNSYLVANIA STATE UNIVERSITY, PENNSYLVANIA
[3]REPUBLIC POLYTECHNIC, SINGAPORE

Introduction

Backpacks are used for many purposes, such as recreational hiking, industrial applications, load carriage by military soldiers and most importantly by children to carry books to and from schools. Children who are still in their developmental phase are the ones who are most likely to be affected by prolonged usage of heavy backpacks. Backpack-related medical injuries involving tissue damage under the straps, lower and upper back problems, neck pain and limb injuries have been reported (Grimmer and Williams, 2000; Negrini *et al.*, 1999; Puckree *et al.*, 2004; Whittfield *et al.*, 2005). Hence, numerous research groups have focused their attention on analysing the effects of backpack load carriage on gait, postural stability and its long-term impact on the musculoskeletal system (reviewed in Knapik *et al.*, 1996, 2004).

Some of the most commonly reported injuries due to backpacks are: (1) foot blisters caused by heavy loads due to the increasing pressure on the skin and causing more movement between the foot and shoes through higher propulsive and breaking forces (Kinoshita, 1985; Knapik *et al.*, 1996); (2) stress fractures; (3) knee pain due to the high forces and moments generated at the knee joint under loaded conditions; (4) low-back injuries because of heavier loads leading to changes in trunk angles that can put excessive strain on the back muscles (Harman *et al.*, 1992); (5) rucksack palsy caused by shoulder straps of backpacks that can cause a traction injury of the nerve roots of the upper brachial plexus; and (6) postural changes caused by a reduction in the amount of available motion for pelvic obliquity and rotation in loaded conditions. The postural changes may also lead to permanent postural deviations after long-term carriage (Smith *et al.*, 2006).

Given the plethora of evidence on the detrimental effects of backpack load carriage, there are many potential parameters that could be investigated. Some of these effects have been described in detail in the other three chapters in this section of the book. For the purpose of this chapter, we will focus our attention on the comparisons of some biomechanical, physiological and motor control parameters of load carriage between children and adults. Our specific research has focused on the spatio-temporal parameters (defined later) and shock transmission from inferior to superior segments during load carriage. We will present the results from our studies and discuss them along with the results obtained from other studies on children and adults.

The effects of backpack loads on gait biomechanics

Our research has focused on two biomechanical aspects of gait with heavy backpack loads: the roles of spatio-temporal parameters (Singh and Koh, 2009a) and the roles of pelvic and trunk movement in attenuating shock transmission from the ankle all the way up to the head (Singh and Koh, 2009b). Most of the prior research that had looked at these gait parameters had focused on adults, and not much was known about children. Our studies were done on primary school children. In this section, we will first provide a theoretical framework on these parameters and what they mean for gait. Then, we will contrast our results with those obtained in previous studies to compare the differences between adults and children.

Experimental methods of our study

Seventeen primary school boys aged 8–12 years completed the study. The mean age, height and weight of the remaining 15 participants were 10.01 (± 1.31) years, 136.40 (± 10.08) cm and 31.83 (± 7.13) kg, respectively. Informed consent and participation assent was obtained from the parents and participants as mandated by the Research and Graduate Review Committee of the Academic Group of Physical Education and Sports Science (PESS), Nanyang Technological University, Singapore. All experimental procedures were done indoors at the Sports Biomechanics Laboratory. A belt-driven instrumented H-P Cosmos Gaitway® treadmill with Kistler force plates was used for the study (see Figure 15.1). The incline of the treadmill was set to 0°. A synchronized digital six-camera (Motion Analysis Corporation (MAC), Santa Rosa, CA) optical motion analysis system was used to capture motion.

The walking protocol involved walking at self-selected speeds under different load conditions on the treadmill. The participants walked on the treadmill for 6 minutes, at the end of which kinematic and spatio-temporal data were collected. The gait data were collected during the last 10 seconds of the sixth minute. One stride cycle was chosen at random from the 10 seconds of collected data to obtain the kinematic and kinetic parameters. The means of the spatio-temporal parameters over the 10 seconds of data collection were reported. The same process was repeated for the loaded conditions. Participants carried backpack loads of 10, 15 and 20 per cent of their body weight (BW) loads. Spatio-temporal gait parameters such as velocity, cadence and stride length were normalized (Stansfield *et al.*, 2003).

To calculate the shock transmission ratio (TR), the time series of vertical acceleration (a_i) of the joints, including ankle, knee, pelvis, trunk and head, were calculated using the following equation (Ratcliffe and Holt, 1997):

$$a_i = (Z_{i+1} - 2Z_i + Z_{i-1})/\Delta t^2 \tag{1}$$

where Z_i is the vertical displacement of the marker on the body segment at the timeframe i. Δt was 0.0167 seconds. i is an instant in time during the gait cycle and varies from 1 to 100. The acceleration due to heel contact travels sequentially from the lower body joints to upper

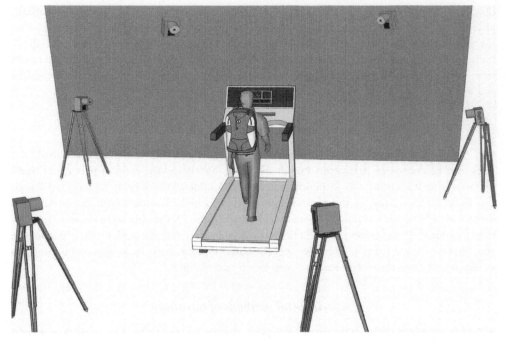

Figure 15.1 Experimental set-up for our experiment. Gait kinematics was measured using a six-camera motion analysis system. We used the modified Helen Mayes marker system. Spatio-temporal parameters and ground reaction forces were obtained from a belt-driven instrumented Gaitway treadmill.

body joints. The temporal sequential order of the occurrence of the acceleration peaks of the five segments were recorded following heel strike. For each trial, the first peak acceleration following heel strike of the most inferior segment (the ankle) was recorded. The next temporal occurrence of the peak acceleration of a more superior segment was then recorded. Only positive peak acceleration values were considered. The shock TR between the ankle and the head for each trial were computed by cumulatively multiplying the shock transmission values from the ankle to head (see Figure 15.2). The shock TR was calculated using the formula:

$$TR = U_{max}/L_{max} \tag{2}$$

where L_{max} is the positive peak acceleration of the inferior joint and U_{max} is the next temporal positive peak acceleration of the more superior joint.

Changes in spatio-temporal and kinematic parameters during load carriage

Spatio-temporal parameters are often described by the changes within a complete *gait cycle*. They are often used to assess gait development in children and to identify potential disorders. The analysis of these parameters, in addition to evaluating aspects of pathological gait, also assists in quantifying post-surgical improvement (Sorsdahl *et al.*, 2008; Stolze *et al.*, 1998). A gait cycle is defined as the time interval between two successive recurrences of the same event of the same limb (e.g. right heel strike to the next right heel strike). Some typical spatio-temporal parameters are velocity (or speed), cadence (or step frequency, SF), step length

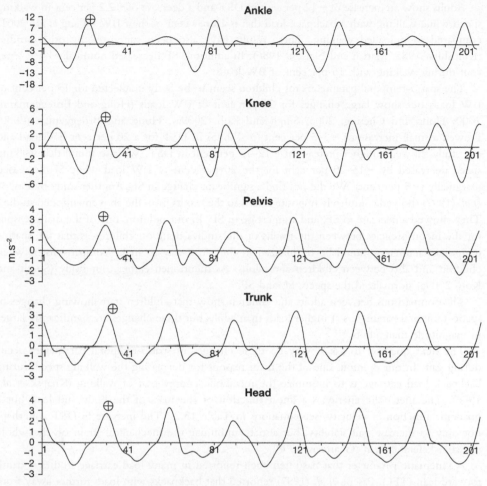

Figure 15.2 Vertical acceleration time series immediately following heel strike showing peak accelerations (m.s^{-2}) for a representative participant. The symbol, +, is the temporal occurrence of the peak vertical acceleration and occurs later in time for a more superior segment than an inferior segment.

(or stride length, SL); single stance time (percentage of time one leg is in contact with the floor during a gait cycle, SST); and double support time (percentage of time both legs are in contact with the floor during a gait cycle, DST).

Backpack loads increase the height of the combined centre of mass (COM) of the body and backpack system and thereby induce instability for standing as well as walking conditions. DST has been used as a measure of gait stability in the sagittal plane (Charteris, 1998; Hong and Brueggemann, 2000; McGraw et al., 2000). Walking velocity has also been associated with gait stability and it has been suggested that a lower walking velocity is a consequence of induced gait instability due to higher COM (Dingwell and Marin, 2006; England and Granata, 2007). Other parameters that have been reported to change during load carriage are stride length (SL, cm) and stride frequency (SF, steps per minute). It should be noted that the walking speed is a product of SL and SF.

Adults show an increase of ~ 12 per cent in DST and a decrease of ~ 2.2 per cent in walking speed while walking with a backpack load that is 15 per cent of their BW (Wang *et al.*, 2001) compared to unloaded walking. These results have also been supported by other studies (Kinoshita, 1985; Martin and Nelson, 1986). In addition, SF decreased nominally by ~ 1 per cent during walking with 15 per cent of BW loads.

The spatio-temporal parameters for children seem to be fairly unaffected for 15 per cent of BW loads but show large changes for 20 per cent of BW loads (Hong and Brueggemann, 2000; Hong and Cheung, 2003; Singh and Koh, 2009a). Hong and Brueggeman (2000) showed a small increase of ~ 3–5 per cent ($p < 0.05$) in DST for a 20 per cent BW load and our study showed a higher increase of ~ 12–15 per cent in DST. We also found that walking speed decreased by ~ 15–20 per cent for the 20 per cent of BW load while SF decreased marginally (~ 5 per cent). We did not find a significant change in SL. Another study by Pascoe *et al.* (1997) showed completely opposite results to the results from the abovementioned studies. They showed a decrease in SF, and an increase in SL. In our opinion, one of the main reasons for the inconsistencies between the results of the studies done on children is that the spatio-temporal parameters should be normalized in the same way to make comparisons between children and also between children and adults. As mentioned earlier, our study (Singh and Koh, 2009a) normalized the speed, SL and SF.

The comparisons between adults and children show that children start showing changes in spatio-temporal parameters at higher loads than adults but these changes are significantly larger in magnitude than adults.

The next question to ask is why do these changes in spatio-temporal parameters occur during gait. In our opinion, one of the main reasons for decreasing the walking speed during backpack load carriage is to minimize the metabolic energy cost of walking (Knapik *et al.*, 1996). The metabolic energy is a linear function of the mass of the body and load but a quadratic function of velocity (see equations in Table 15.2). The increase in DST is perhaps not only to increase gait stability, but also to minimize the mechanical strain on the whole musculoskeletal system (Charteris, 1998).

A kinematic parameter that has often been reported in many load carriage studies is trunk forward lean (TFL). Pascoe *et al.* (1997) reported that backpacks with loads further away from the COM of the body in the sagittal plane induced a higher TFL than backpacks with loads closer to the COM of the body. Contrary to expectations, for trained soldiers, significant TFL occurs at higher loads compared to untrained individuals. Goh *et al.* (1998) showed that significant TFL occurred in soldiers for loads only as high as 30 per cent of BW. Studies done on children have reported that a load of 20 per cent of BW induces a significant increase in the TFL (Hong and Cheung, 2003; Singh and Koh, 2009a). Our study showed that TFL increases for both static as well as dynamic conditions, and the increase is larger for dynamic conditions. For dynamic conditions, TFL increased significantly for loads > 15 per cent of BW.

In particular, we used the inverted pendulum model of gait (Cavagna *et al.*, 1977) and the concept of extrapolated COM (Hof *et al.*, 2005), also referred to as XCOM. The inverted pendulum model simplifies dynamics of COM movement during single support phase (see Figure 15.3). The point mass of the inverted pendulum corresponds to the body COM, and the pivot corresponds to the ankle joint of the support leg. Using the concepts of inverted pendulum and XCOM, we showed that a higher TFL for dynamic conditions could be an additional mechanism employed by the central nervous system (CNS) to provide gait stability under dynamic conditions. The higher TFL for > 15 per cent of BW load conditions indicate

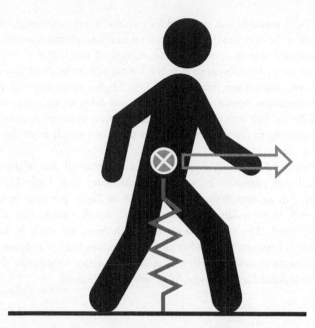

Figure 15.3 A simple inverted pendulum (plus a leg spring) of gait produces a ground reaction force (GRF) pattern that is a close approximation of the GRF observed during walking in humans. This model has been extensively used in gait research over the last three decades.

that loads higher than 15 per cent load may result in a significantly higher trunk forward lean than unloaded conditions for two possible reasons. The first could be to bring the combined COM (body + backpack) over the BOS and second to move the combined COM inferiorly closer to the walking surface to make the whole system more stable. That may explain why soldiers who are trained to maintain high walking speeds with heavy backpack loads tend to bend their trunks more than untrained people. Of course, we are not advocating that people walk with higher TFL with backpack loads, as it may also have harmful consequences. We are suggesting that the TFL during load carriage is perhaps a reflection of economizing stability against excessive strain on the lower back muscles.

Changes in trunk and pelvic coordination during load carriage

When analysing locomotion, the human body can be divided into two subsystems: (1) the upper part – head and trunk; and (2) the lower part of the body – the lower limbs (Cappozzo, 1981). The latter supports and transports the former. The pattern of motion of the lower limbs is to minimize mechanical energy exchange between the two subsystems (Saunders *et al.*, 1953). Large forces are produced during gait at the lower extremity joints due to muscle contractions and impacts with the ground (Ratcliffe and Holt, 1997). Previous backpack studies have shown that increases in muscle-mediated stiffness maintains a constant vertical excursion of the COM under loaded conditions and this stiffness thereby limits increases in metabolic cost that would otherwise have occurred if the COM would travel through a greater vertical range of motion (Holt *et al.*, 2003).

However, stiffer systems facilitate the transmission of forces between segments through elastic energy storage between the distal and proximal segment. This is, of course, not desirable.

Cappozzo *et al.* (1978) reasoned that the need for minimal energy exchange could be to protect sensory organs such as the eyes and the brain from excessive mechanical stimulus. Pelvis rotation could play an important role in controlling the amount of shock that is transmitted from the lower subsystem to the upper subsystem as pelvis rotation provides flexibility or stiffness to the link between the two subsystems (see Figure 15.4). Higher flexibility will reduce superiorly directed shock transmission because pelvis rotation can assist in absorbing part of the shock (LaFiandra *et al.*, 2003). For backpack load carriage, pelvic rotation is reduced (Smith *et al.*, 2006) and could possibly facilitate transmission of impulsive shock from the lower subsystem to the upper subsystem.

Our results (Singh and Koh, 2009b) showed that a substantial part of the shock absorption took place at the lower extremity between the ankle-knee (see Table 15.1) and the knee-pelvis area, resulting in an overall shock transmission of 25–36 per cent from from the ankle to the head. Overall, these results are consistent with another study that was performed on adults (Holt *et al.*, 2005). The more noteworthy result from our study is that there were no significant differences between the loaded and baseline (no load) conditions, indicating that there are locomotion mechanisms in place to attenuate inferior to superior shock transmission through the musculoskeletal system even in 10-year-old children.

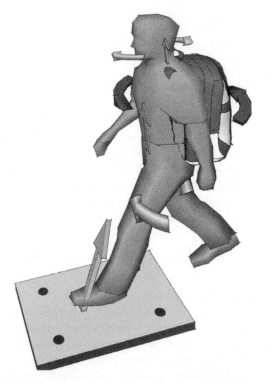

Figure 15.4 An illustration of the counter rotation in the transverse plane between adjacent segments facilitates attenuation of shock transmission from the inferior to superior segments. In the figure, the lower limb is rotating clockwise; the pelvis and trunks are rotating counterclockwise; and the head is rotating clockwise during the stance phase of the left leg. The counter rotation facilitates attenuation of the shock as it travels superiorly.

Table 15.1 The means of the shock transmission ratio (TR) between the ankle-knee, knee-pelvis, pelvis-trunk and trunk-head for the different load conditions

	Ankle-Knee	Knee-Pelvis	Pelvis-Trunk	Trunk-Head	Ankle-Head
0% of BW	0.44 ± 0.28	0.82 ± 0.3	1.03 ± 0.21	0.82 ± 0.11	0.27 ± 0.1
10% of BW	0.49 ± 0.22	0.69 ± 0.29	1.11 ± 0.27	0.94 ± 0.16	0.33 ± 0.13
15% of BW	0.41 ± 0.12	0.8 ± 0.32	1.06 ± 0.31	0.85 ± 0.17	0.27 ± 0.08
20% of BW	0.39 ± 0.17	0.72 ± 0.31	1.13 ± 0.27	0.86 ± 0.19	0.23 ± 0.09

Values are reported as mean ± SD.
Source: Singh and Koh (2009b).

Physiology of backpack load carriage

A study published in 2005 compared the differences in metabolic energy expenditure between Nepalese porters and African women (Bastien *et al.*, 2005a). Previously, it has been shown that African women carry loads of up to 60 per cent of their BW more economically than army recruits carrying equivalent loads in backpacks (Maloiy *et al.*, 1986). The mechanical work, required in maintaining the motion of the common COM of the body and load, decreases with load in the African women, and this decrease is a result of a greater conservation of mechanical energy resulting from a transfer of energy during each step, back and forth between gravitational potential energy and kinetic energy of the COM (Heglund *et al.*, 1995). This strategy is utilized more effectively by the Nepalese porters who routinely carry about 100–200 per cent of the BW load up the treacherous slopes of the Himalayas with a gait that is economically more efficient than the African women.

There are two main questions that need to be asked to address issues of energy consumption with backpack load carriage. The first question is: Why should energy efficiency be an important, if not critical, issue for backpack load carriage for children? Unlike the porters and recreational hikers who spend hours with a heavy backpack load on a regular basis, school-going children only have to walk, on average, 7–10 minutes a day (Negrini and Negrini, 2007). The second issue that could be raised is: Would a little bit of energy expenditure per day not be useful for children since societies across the globe are adopting more and more sedentary lifestyles?

The answers to both these questions are complicated and inextricably linked with the relationships between the biomechanics and physiology of load carriage. Before we look into these two issues in greater detail, let us understand how energy efficiency is measured during load carriage. Typically, VO_2max test has been used to measure energy consumption during walking and running. VO_2 is the measure of the peak volume of oxygen (VO_2) one can consume and use in a minute. It is measured in $ml.kg^{-1}.min^{-1}$ and is relative to one's body weight. There are other accepted methods as well, such as heart rate, electromyography (EMG), pulmonary ventilation (Quesada *et al.*, 2000) and mechanical work (Burdett *et al.*, 1983; Pigrrynowsi *et al.*, 1981): (1) mechanical work done on the COM per kg BW per second is calculated by integration of the ground reaction forces (GRF, measured by force platforms, see Figure 15.4); (2) total body segmental work per kg BW per second is calculated from individual body segment energies measured by motion analysis; and (3) the sum of the normalized absolute moment impulses per second acting on the joints of the lower extremities calculated from both force and motion data.

Returning to the two questions that we asked earlier, could the short duration of heavy backpack load carriage serve as a form of aerobic exercise instead of being detrimental to the health of children? To answer this question, let us first look into the metabolic costs associated with walking with backpack loads.

A lot of studies have attempted to determine the metabolic cost of walking with backpack loads. Two of the most widely used equations (for a detailed review, cf. Epstein *et al.*, 1987; Knapik *et al.*, 1996; Pandolf *et al.*, 1977) are shown in Table 15.2. Some other studies have reported that for adults metabolic cost is fairly constant below 20 per cent of BW (Charteris *et al.*, 1989; Quesada *et al.*, 2000) but that is not true for children, as they show an increase in metabolic costs over 10 per cent of BW load (Hong *et al.*, 2000), as well as changes in respiratory parameters (Li *et al.*, 2003). A few studies have also shown that the metabolic cost of walking with heavy backpack loads is not constant, and increases with the duration of walking even at relatively low intensities (Epstein *et al.*, 1988; Patton *et al.*, 1991). These studies argue that prolonged load carriage leads to a reduction in mechanical efficiency due to altered locomotion biomechanics, as the subject adjusts to the weight and discomfort due to the increased pressure from the straps of the pack. Therefore, it can be said that the longer one walks, the more stress backpacks exert on our physiological system.

Load placement is also an important consideration in minimizing metabolic cost (Kinoshita, 1985; Legg and Mahanty, 1985; Legg *et al.*, 1992; Lloyd and Cooke, 2000; Stuempfle *et al.*, 2004). Locating the load as close as possible to the COM of the body also appears to result in lowest energy costs (Malhotra and Gupta, 1965). It has also been argued that distributing the loads over the body minimizes the metabolic cost. Packing heavy items high in the backpack may be the most energy efficient method of carrying a load on the back (Stuempfle *et al.*, 2004). A load carriage system that allows the load to be distributed between the back and front of the trunk is more appropriate for carrying relatively heavy loads than a system that loads the back only (Kinoshita, 1985; Lloyd and Cooke, 2000). It is also advisable that light loads be carried on backpacks rather than shoulders (Legg *et al.*, 1992) or very low on the waist.

Another key determinant of metabolic cost is walking speed. Many studies have shown that while walking unloaded, there is an optimal speed where the energy cost per unit distance travelled is minimized (Cotes and Meade, 1960; Zarrugh *et al.*, 1974). A study showed that the gross metabolic power increases curvilinearly with speed (as a quadratic function, see equations in Table 15.2) and is directly proportional to the load at any speed (Bastien *et al.*, 2005b). For all loaded conditions, the gross metabolic energy cost (J.kg^{-1}.m^{-1}) presents a U-shaped curve with a minimum at around 1.3 m.s^{-1} (see Figure 15.5). In addition, the optimal speed for net cost minimization is around 1.06 m.s^{-1} and is independent of load. However, these values are for adults. Since children are not necessarily scaled down versions of adults, care must be taken in considering the appropriate approach to normalize the data suitably before suggesting a recommended optimal walking speed for children.

Table 15.2 The equations for predicting the energy cost of locomotion with backpack loads

---

Equation 1: (Pandolf *et al.*, 1977)

$$M_W = (1.5 \times BW) + 2.0 \times (BW + L) \times (^L/_{BW})^2 + T \times (BW + L) \times \{(1.5 \times V^2) + (0.35 \times V \times G)\}$$

Equation 2: (Epstein *et al.*, 1987)

$$M_T = M_W - 0.5 \times \{1 - (0.01 \times L)\} \times \{M_W - (1.5 \times L) - 850\}$$

Where M_W is metabolic cost of walking (watts); M_T is metabolic cost of running (watts); BW = body mass (kg); L = load mass (kg); T = terrain coefficient and is higher for softer roads; V = velocity of walking; and G = slope or grade (%). An increase in gradient increases the metabolic cost significantly.

Source: Liu (2007).

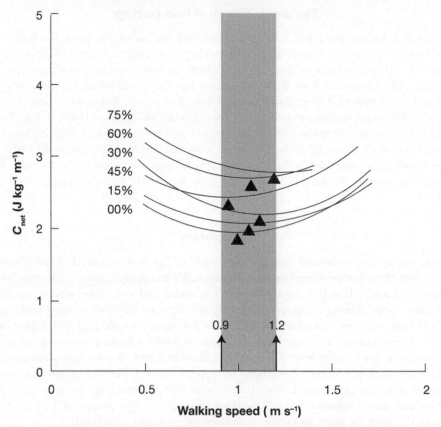

Figure 15.5 Optimal speed as a function of walking speed and load. The mass-specific net cost of locomotion (C_{net}; J.kg^{-1}.m^{-1}) is presented as a function of the walking speed and load. Lines are the second-order polynomial fit through all of the data points for each loading condition, as noted in the figure. Upward triangles indicate the optimal speed for each loading condition; the grey area shows the speed range in which the optimal speed is included for all loading conditions from 0 to 75 per cent of BW. (Figure obtained from Bastien *et al.* (2005b) and reprinted by permission from Springer.)

In our opinion, the main physiological concern with backpack load carriage for children is not the metabolic cost, but the mechanical cost that is associated with backpack load carriages (Holewijn, 1990; Pierrynowski *et al.*, 1981). In fact, since joint moments are direct measures of muscle force, a direct relationship between metabolic energy consumption and joint moments may exist (Burdett *et al.*, 1983). Additionally, joint moments have been shown to increase, at the hip and the ankle, as a quadratic function with walking speeds (Lelas *et al.*, 2003). The role of higher joint moments in contributing to overuse injuries or knee pain is not entirely known, but it could be argued that subjecting the joints to large joint moments on a daily basis may not be the best thing to do for children.

To conclude, we think that children carrying loads above the recommended limit of 15 per cent of BW should do so only for short durations to minimize injury risk to the lower limbs and back. It is also recommended for children to walk at or below the optimal speed. Whereas walking slower than the optimal speed may result in higher metabolic costs, it would have less of a deleterious impact on the joints. Walking at speeds faster than the optimal speed should certainly be avoided.

The motor control of load carriage

Not much is known about the motor control of load carriage except for a dissertation study done by Ou *et al.* (2010). The study used a force plate to measure the centre of pressure (COP) trajectory and goniometers to measure the changes in spine curvature during a 30-second standing trial. The results from this study suggest that the spinal postural control gets better with age and is better for 15 year olds compared to 11 year olds. The authors used ideas from fractional Brownian motion, namely the Hurst exponent (discussed in detail in Lai, 2004) to characterize the short-term and long-term control processes associated with backpack load carriage. The study showed that the sway range, sway velocity and randomness of COP motion were significantly higher when the loads were placed high on the back. Additionally, it was shown that carrying the load in front of the body was better than carrying the load at the back.

Conclusions

In this chapter, we compared and discussed some of the biomechanical, physiological and motor control parameters of backpack load carriage. We also compared the differences between children and adults. Based on the results from our studies and some other studies, we showed that adults show significant changes in their spatio-temporal parameters when walking with loads as high as 15 per cent of BW. Children do not show changes until 20 per cent of BW load, but these changes are larger than those seen in adults. Children seem as good as adults in attenuating shock transmitted due to ground reaction forces. We strongly recommend that walking speeds should be below or around the optimal walking speed for children to minimize excessive strain on the joints. Lastly, it seems that motor control mechanisms that stabilize posture and spinal curvature are still evolving between the age groups of 11 and 15. It is possible that they are likely to evolve as children progress into adulthood.

References

Bastien, G. J., Schepens, B., Willems, P. A. and Heglund, N. C. (2005a) 'Energetics of load carrying in Nepalese porters', *Science*, 308(5729): 1755.

Bastien, G. J., Willems, P. A., Schepens, B. and Heglund, N. C. (2005b) 'Effect of load and speed on the energetic cost of human walking', *European Journal of Applied Physiology*, 94(1–2): 76–83.

Burdett, R., Skrinar, G. and Simon, S. (1983) 'Comparison of mechanical work and metabolic energy consumption during normal gait', *Journal of Orthopaedic Research*, 1(1): 63–72.

Cappozzo, A. (1981) 'Analysis of the linear displacement of the head and trunk during walking at different speeds', *Journal of Biomechanics*, 14(6): 411–25.

Cappozzo, A., Figura, F., Leo, T. and Marchetti, M. (1978) 'Movements and mechanical energy changes in the upper part of the human body during walking', in E. Assmussen and K. Jorgansen (eds), *Biomechanics*, Baltimore: University Park Press, pp. 272–9.

Cavagna, G. A., Heglund, N. C. and Taylor, C. R. (1977) 'Mechanical work in terrestrial locomotion: two basic mechanisms for minimizing energy expenditure', *American Journal of Physiology*, 233(5), R243–61.

Charteris, J. (1998) 'Comparison of the effects of backpack loading and of walking speed on foot-floor contact patterns', *Ergonomics*, 41(12): 1792–809.

Charteris, J., Scott, P. A. and Nottrodt, J. W. (1989) 'Metabolic and kinematic responses of African women headload carriers under controlled conditions of load and speed', *Ergonomics*, 32(12): 1539–50.

Cotes, J. and Meade, F. (1960) 'The energy expenditure and mechanical energy demand in walking', *Ergonomics*, 3(2): 97–119.

Dingwell, J. and Marin, L. (2006) 'Kinematic variability and local dynamic stability of upper body motions when walking at different speeds', *Journal of Biomechanics*, 39(3): 444–52.

England, S. and Granata, K. (2007) 'The influence of gait speed on local dynamic stability of walking', *Gait and Posture*, 25(2): 172–8.

Epstein, Y., Stroschein, L. A. and Pandolf, K. B. (1987) 'Predicting metabolic cost of running with and without backpack loads', *European Journal of Applied Physiology and Occupational Physiology*, 56(5): 495–500.

Epstein, Y., Rosenblum, J., Burstein, R. and Sawka, M. (1988) 'External load can alter the energy cost of prolonged exercise', *European Journal of Applied Physiology and Occupational Physiology*, 57(2): 243–7.

Goh, J., Thambyah, A. and Bose, K. (1998) 'Effects of varying backpack loads on peak forces in the lumbosacral spine during walking', *Clinical Biomechanics*, 13(1/1): S26–31.

Grimmer, K. and Williams, M. (2000) 'Gender-age environmental associated of adolescent low back pain', *Applied Ergonomics*, 31(4): 343–60.

Harman, E., Han, K., Frykman, P., Johnson, M., Russell, F. and Rusenstein, M. (1992) 'The effects on gait timing, kinetics, and muscle activity of various loads carried on the back', *Medicine and Science in Sports and Exercise*, 24: S129.

Heglund, N. C., Willems, P. A., Penta, M. and Cavagna, G. A. (1995) 'Energy-saving gait mechanics with head-supported loads', *Nature*, 375(6256): 52–4.

Hof, A. L., Gazendam, M. and Sinke, W. E. (2005) 'The condition for dynamic stability', *Journal of Biomechanics*, 38(1): 1–8.

Holewijn, M. (1990) 'Physiological strain due to load carrying', *European Journal of Applied Physiology and Occupational Physiology*, 61(3–4): 237–45.

Holt, K., Wagenaar, R., Lafiandra, M., Kubo, M. and Obusek, J. (2003) 'Increased musculoskeletal stiffness during load carriage at increasing walking speeds maintains constant vertical excursion of the body center of mass', *Journal of Biomechanics*, 36(4): 465–71.

Holt, K., Wagenaar, R., Kubo, M., LaFiandra, M. and Obusek, J. (2005) 'Modulation of force transmission to the head while carrying a backpack load at different walking speeds', *Journal of Biomechanics*, 38(8): 1621–8.

Hong, Y. and Brueggemann, G. (2000) 'Changes in gait patterns in 10-year-old boys with increasing loads when walking on a treadmill', *Gait and Posture*, 11(3): 254–9.

Hong, Y. and Cheung, C. (2003) 'Gait and posture responses to backpack load during level walking in children', *Gait and Posture*, 17(1): 28–33.

Hong, Y., Li, J., Wong, A. and Robinson, P. (2000) 'Effects of load carriage on heart rate, blood pressure and energy expenditure in children', *Ergonomics*, 43(6): 717–27.

Kinoshita, H. (1985) 'Effects of different loads and carrying systems on selected biomechanical parameters describing walking gait', *Ergonomics*, 28(9): 1347–62.

Knapik, J., Harman, E. and Reynolds, K. (1996) 'Load carriage using packs: a review of physiological, biomechanical and medical aspects', *Applied Ergonomics*, 27(3): 207–16.

Knapik, J., Reynolds, K. and Harman, E. (2004) 'Soldier load carriage: historical, physiological, biomechanical, and medical aspects', *Military Medicine*, 169(1): 45–56.

LaFiandra, M., Wagenaar, R., Holt, K. and Obusek, J. (2003) 'How do load carriage and walking speed influence trunk coordination and stride parameters?', *Journal of Biomechanics*, 36(1): 87–95.

Lai, D. (2004) 'Estimating the Hurst effect and its application in monitoring clinical trials', *Computational Statistics and Data Analysis*, 45(3): 549–62.

Legg, S. and Mahanty, A. (1985) 'Comparison of five modes of carrying a load close to the trunk', *Ergonomics*, 28(12): 1653–60.

Legg, S., Ramsey, T. and Knowles, D. (1992) 'The metabolic cost of backpack and shoulder load carriage', *Ergonomics*, 35(9): 1063–8.

Lelas, J., Merriman, G., Riley, P. and Kerrigan, D. (2003) 'Predicting peak kinematic and kinetic parameters from gait speed', *Gait and Posture*, 17(2): 106–12.

Li, J., Hong, Y. and Robinson, P. (2003) 'The effect of load carriage on movement kinematics and respiratory parameters in children during walking', *European Journal of Applied Physiology*, 90(1–2): 35–43.

Liu, B. (2007) 'Backpack load positioning and walking surface slope effects on physiological responses in infantry soldiers', *International Journal of Industrial Ergonomics*, 37(9–10): 754–60.

Lloyd, R. and Cooke, C. (2000) 'The oxygen consumption with unloaded walking and load carriage using two different backpack designs', *European Journal of Applied Physiology*, 81(6): 486–92.

McGraw, B., McClenaghan, B. A., Williams, H., Dickerson, J. and Ward, D. (2000) 'Gait and postural stability in obese and nonobese prepubertal boys', *Archives of Physical Medicine and Rehabilitation*, 81(4): 484–9.

Malhotra, M. and Gupta, J. (1965) 'Carrying of school bags by children', *Ergonomics*, 8(1): 55–60.

Maloiy, G. M. O., Heglund, N. C., Prager, L. M., Cavagna, G. A. and Taylor, C. R. (1986) 'Energetic cost of carrying loads: have African women discovered an economic way?', *Nature*, 319(6055): 668–9.

Martin, P. and Nelson, R. (1986) 'The effect of carried loads on the walking patterns of men and women', *Ergonomics*, 29(10): 1191–202.

Negrini, S. and Negrini, A. (2007) 'Postural effects of symmetrical and asymmetrical loads on the spines of school children', *Scoliosis*, 2: 1–7.

Negrini, S., Carabalona, R. and Sibilla, P. (1999) 'Backpack as a daily load for school children', *Lancet*, 354(9194): 1974.

Ou, Z. (2010) 'The effects of backpack weights and positions on motor control of school children', unpublished master's dissertation, The Hong Kong Polytechnic University.

Pandolf, K., Givoni, B. and Goldman, R. (1977) 'Predicting energy expenditure with loads while standing or walking very slowly', *Journal of Applied Physiology*, 43(4): 577–81.

Pascoe, D., Pascoe, D., Wang, Y., Shin, D. and Kim, C. (1997) 'Influence of carrying book bags on gait cycle and posture of youths', *Ergonomics*, 40(6): 631–41.

Patton, J. F., Kaszuba, J., Mello, R. P. and Reynolds, K. L. (1991) 'Physiological responses to prolonged treadmill walking with external loads', *European Journal of Applied Physiology and Occupational Physiology*, 63(2): 89–93.

Pierrynowski, M., Winter, D. A. and Norman, R. W. (1981) 'Metabolic measures to ascertain the optimal load to be carried by man', *Ergonomics*, 24(5): 393–9.

Pigrrynowsi, M. R., Norman, R. W. and Winter, D. A. (1981) 'Mechanical energy analyses of the human during load carriage on a treadmill', *Ergonomics*, 24(1): 1–14.

Puckree, T., Silal, S. and Lin, J. (2004) 'School bag carriage and pain in school children', *Disability and Rehabilitation*, 26(1): 54–9.

Quesada, P., Mengelkoch, L., Hale, R. and Simon, S. (2000) 'Biomechanical and metabolic effects of varying backpack loading on simulated marching', *Ergonomics*, 43(3): 293–309.

Ratcliffe, R. and Holt, K. (1997) 'Low frequency shock absorption in human walking', *Gait and Posture*, 5(2): 93–100.

Saunders, J., Inman, V. and Eberhart, H. (1953) 'The major determinants in normal and pathological gait', *The Journal of Bone and Joint Surgery*, 35-A(3): 543–58.

Singh, T. and Koh, M. (2009a) 'Effects of backpack load position on spatiotemporal parameters and trunk forward lean', *Gait and Posture*, 29(1): 49–53.

Singh, T. and Koh, M. (2009b) 'Lower limb dynamics change for loaded gait to modulate shock transmission to the head', *Journal of Biomechanics*, 42(6): 736–42.

Smith, B., Ashton, K., Bohl, D., Clark, R., Metheny, J. and Klassen, S. (2006) 'Influence of carrying a backpack on pelvic tilt, rotation, and obliquity in female college students', *Gait and Posture*, 23(3): 263–7.

Sorsdahl, A., Moe-Nilssen, R. and Strand, L. (2008) 'Test-retest reliability of spatial and temporal gait parameters in children with cerebral palsy as measured by an electronic walkway', *Gait and Posture*, 27(1): 43–50.

Stansfield, B., Hillman, S., Hazlewood, M., Lawson, A., Mann, A., Loudon, I. and Robb, J. (2003) 'Normalisation of gait data in children', *Gait and Posture*, 17(1): 81–7.

Stolze, H., Kuhtz-Buschbeck, J. P., Mondwurf, C., Jöhnk, K. and Friege, L. (1998) 'Retest reliability of spatiotemporal gait parameters in children and adults', *Gait and Posture*, 7(2): 125–30.

Stuempfle, K., Drury, D. and Wilson, A. (2004) 'Effect of load position on physiological and perceptual responses during load carriage with an internal frame backpack', *Ergonomics*, 47(7): 784–9.

Wang, Y., Pascoe, D. and Weimar, W. (2001) 'Evaluation of book backpack load during walking', *Ergonomics*, 44(9): 858–69.

Whittfield, J., Legg, S. and Hedderley, D. (2005) 'Schoolbag weight and musculoskeletal symptoms in New Zealand secondary schools', *Applied Ergonomics*, 36(2): 193–8.

Zarrugh, M., Todd, F. and Ralston, H. (1974) 'Optimization of energy expenditure during level walking', *European Journal of Applied Physiology and Occupational Physiology*, 33(4): 293–306.

16

THE EFFECT OF BACKPACK LOAD AND GAIT SPEED ON PLANTAR FORCES DURING TREADMILL WALKING

Yun Wang[1,2] and Kazuhiko Watanabe[2]

[1]TIANJIN UNIVERSITY OF SPORT, TIANJIN
[2]INSTITUTE OF SPORT AND HEALTH SCIENCE, HIGASHI-HIROSHIMA

Introduction

The incidences of osteoporotic hip fracture were increased in both men and women, when data were analysed and compared with that from 30 years ago (Hagino *et al.*, 2005). The crude incidence of osteoporotic hip fracture was 244.8 per 100,000 persons years from 2004 to 2006 in a Japanese population aged 35 years or older. Predominantly due to falls, 30 per cent of individuals after a hip fracture become functionally dependent and require long-term nursing care. To protect against osteoporosis and concomitant fractures, studies of weight-bearing exercise may be of substantial clinical importance. They may be able to provide distributional information related to the vertical ground reaction force and exercise intensity. In particular, force-generating activities have been shown to produce significant effects on attaining optimal bone mass and bone strength (Burr *et al.*, 1983).

Maintaining equilibrium during walking is a challenging task due to a number of factors including the small support area and the high centre of mass location. Several studies show that impact forces associated with walking were responsible for the load distributions of the musculoskeletal system (Fraysse *et al.*, 2009; Wehner *et al.*, 2009). Only currently has dynamic analysis of impact force at the foot-ground interface been possible during walking. Plantar pressure and force measurements provide information about loading to skeletal regions and lower extremities (Chesnin *et al.*, 2000; Han *et al.*, 1999). Evidence suggests that the vertical ground reaction force is dependent on the external factors such as gait speed, carrying weight, shoes and surface involved. Since force-generating activities have positive effects on adaptive skeletal responses, the relationships among gait speed and carrying load with the vertical ground reaction force are important for understanding osteogenic effects on walking (Kai *et al.*, 2003).

Previous studies have evaluated gait adjustments under various load carrying conditions. In a study conducted by Simonsen *et al.* (1995), bone-on-bone forces during unloaded and loaded walking were compared at a self-paced speed. They found that 8.0 body weight (BW) peak compression force generated in the hip joint during loaded walking (20 kg). Kinoshita (1985) and Knapik *et al.* (1996) found that knee flexion after impact was greater when carrying loads in order to absorb increased impact forces. Hsiang and Chang (2002) recorded the vertical ground reaction forces for a number of consecutive steps under three gait speeds and five load carrying positions. They found that some loaded positions and higher speeds reduced reliability of the execution of gait patterns while other loaded positions may actually increase gait stability.

Summing up the present state of our knowledge, loaded walking has the potential to enhance skeletal adaptation. However, it should be noted that experimental evidence for the effectiveness of load carrying and gait speed remains limited. As such, the objective of this study was to assess the effect of backpack load and gait speed on treadmill walking, with a focus on the vertical ground reaction force. We were interested in whether the differences in mechanical adjustments were associated with changes in load and gait speed. The outcome of this study will help us to recommend suitable gait speed and backpack load to provide a greater health benefit.

Methods

Participants

Nine healthy subjects, five males and four females, without any known neurological or motor disorders participated in the experiment. Their mean age, height and mass were 27.4 (± 5.0) years, 172.0 (± 8.1) cm and 69.4 (± 11.8) kg, respectively. Subjects were informed about the experimental procedures and possible risks and benefits of the study, which was approved by the Ethics Committee of the University of Hiroshima. Written informed consent was obtained from the subjects.

Apparatus

The F-scan® Tethered system (Tekscan Inc., USA) was used to collect plantar pressure data with a sampling frequency of 120 Hz. Subjects wore the same kind of walking shoes. The insole was trimmed to their shoe size and the centre of the insole was maintained to coincide with the centre of the foot. The insole was connected via an amplifier attached to the subject's ankle. The plantar loading parameters were then transmitted from F-scan transmission device to a laptop computer. The insole was calibrated for each subject using the subject's own weight before data collection.

Procedures

Subjects were asked to walk on a treadmill (Powerjog, GXC200) for at least 10 minutes for familiarity with experimental environment and ensuring equilibration in the temperature of the insoles. Each participant completed all 12 task conditions. One factor was weight load carried in the backpack (four levels: 0, 10, 20 and 30 per cent of body mass). The second factor was gait speed (three levels: 4, 5 and 6 km.h^{-1}). Under each task condition, subjects walked for approximately 3 minutes. During the last 20 seconds, the vGRF data were collected. The order of task conditions was randomized for each subject.

Data processing

Foot contact and ground reaction forces served to determine gait cycles. Step length was calculated using the equation for gait velocity (m.s^{-1}) = step length (m.step^{-1}) × cadence (step.s^{-1}) and it was normalized with respect to each subject's height. The force signals were normalized as a percentage of body weight (per cent of BW). Coefficient of variation (CV) was used to determine the vertical ground reaction force (vGRF) variability from the consecutive steps. It was calculated as the standard deviation divided by the mean data value, multiplied by 100. The fractions of CV were then transformed into z-scores for statistical analysis using Fisher's z-transformation.

Statistics

All statistical analyses were performed in SPSS 15.0 for Windows XP (SPSS Inc., Chicago, USA). Two-way ANOVA with repeated measures was used to examine effect of the presence of backpack load (four levels: 0, 10, 20 and 30 per cent of body weight) and gait speed (three levels: 4, 5 and 6 km.h^{-1}). When necessary, a one-way ANOVA with repeated measures for each gait speed was performed. If a significant difference was detected, the polynomial test was performed at $p = 0.05$ level of significance to determine if a linear, quadratic or cubic trend existed.

Results

Although we analysed the data separately over gait cycle, there were no significant differences between steps with left and right feet on any of the outcome measures. Therefore, for clarity and brevity, we will report results representing the averaged values of two feet.

Gait performance

Gait cadence averaged across subjects is shown in Figure 16.1. Two-way ANOVA analysis, with the factors backpack load (0, 10, 20 and 30 per cent of body mass) and gait speed (4, 5 and 6 km.h^{-1}) showed no significant speed-by-load interaction ($F(6,48) = 0.58$, $p = 0.0747$) on cadence. There was a main effect of gait speed ($F(2,16) = 108.2$, $p < 0.001$) on cadence, corresponding to cadence increased with gait speed increased. There were significant differences in cadence among each gait speed condition ($p < 0.05$).

For the step length (Figure 16.2), there was no speed-by-load interaction ($F(6,48) = 0.97$, $p = 0.454$). Gait speed showed a main effect ($F(2,16) = 424.0$, $p < 0.001$) on step length. Across backpack loads, step length increased as gait speed increased. There were significant differences in step length under the 4 and 5 km.h^{-1} conditions ($p < 0.05$) and the 5 and 6 km.h^{-1} conditions ($p < 0.05$).

Analysis of plantar forces

The first vGRF peaks (P1) averaged across subjects are shown in Figure 16.3 (top). Overall, we found that P1 increased with the backpack load and gait speed increasing. These observations were confirmed by a two-way ANOVA analysis with factors of backpack load and gait speed. There was no significant speed-by-load interaction for the first vGRF peak ($F(6,48) = 2.0$, $p = 0.091$). Main effects of gait speed ($F(2,16) = 89.5$, $p < 0.001$) and backpack load ($F(3,24) = 35.1$, $p < 0.001$) for P1 were confirmed. Trend analysis showed linear trends of P1 on gait speed ($F(1,8) = 122.5$, $p < 0.001$) and backpack load ($F(1,8) = 54.2$, $p < 0.001$) factors. Across gait speeds, an increase in backpack load resulted in an increased in P1.

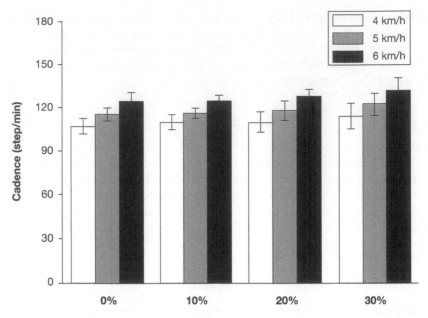

Figure 16.1 Mean and SD of cadence (step.min^{-1}) during gait.

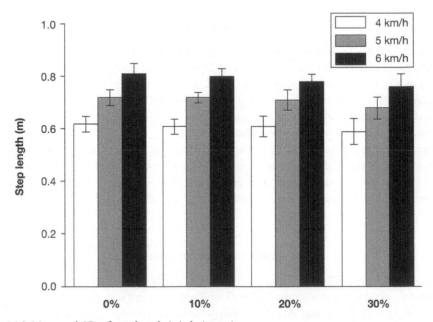

Figure 16.2 Mean and SD of step length (m) during gait.

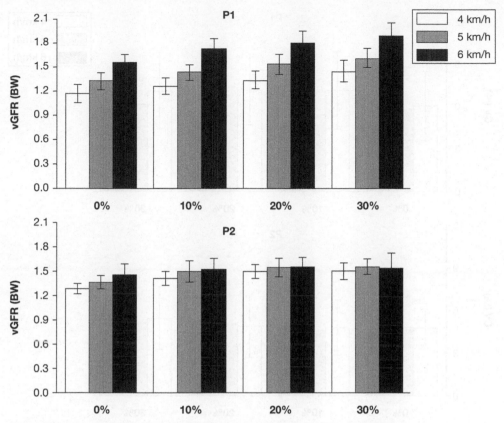

Figure 16.3 Mean and SD of the first (P1) and second (P2) peak of the vGRF (BW).

For the second vGRF peak (P2, Figure 16.3, bottom), there was the main effect of speed-by-load interaction ($F(6,48)$ = 6.7, p < 0.001). The subsequent one-way ANOVA analysis showed a significant backpack load effect for gait speed of 4 km.h^{-1} ($F(3,24)$ = 41.2, p < 0.001) and gait speed of 5 km.h^{-1} ($F(3,24)$ = 27.2, p < 0.001). However, there was no significant load effect for gait speed of 6 km.h^{-1} ($F(3,24)$ = 2.9, p = 0.053). Trend analysis showed a linear trend ($F(1,8)$ = 107.4, p < 0.001) of P2 for gait speed of 4 km.h^{-1}. P2 value increased from 1.28 BW during no load walking to 1.50 BW when backpack load was increased to 30 per cent of body mass. There was also a linear trend ($F(1,8)$ = 95.9, p < 0.001) for gait speed of 5 km.h^{-1}. P2 value increased from 1.36 BW during no load walking to 1.55 BW when backpack load was increased to 30 per cent of body mass.

Figure 16.4 illustrates the coefficient of variation (CV) values of the step to step variation of vGRF from consecutive steps. All were well within the normal variability for experimental data of this type (< 12.5 per cent) (White *et al.*, 1999). The fractions of CV were further transformed into z-scores using Fisher's z-transformation for statistical analysis. Two-way ANOVA with repeated measures, with the factors backpack load (0, 10, 20 and 30 per cent of body mass) and gait speed (4, 5 and 6 km.h^{-1}) were performed. There were no significant effects and no interaction for the z-scores of CV values of P1 and P2.

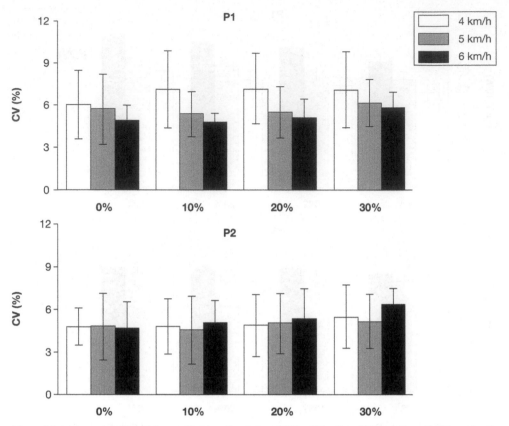

Figure 16.4 Mean and SD of the coefficient of variation (CV) of the first (P1) and second (P2) peak of the vGRF across steps (per cent).

Discussion

This study extends recent work on force-generating activities (Kai *et al.*, 2003; Lloyd *et al.*, 2004), providing a further test that impact force changes with backpack load and gait speed. Our experiment has shown that an increase in gait speed and backpack load led to an increase in the magnitude of the first vGRF peak. Greater magnitudes of the second vGRF peak were only associated with an increase when gait speed was 4 km.h^{-1} and 5 km.h^{-1}. There was no speed-related change in the magnitudes of the second vGRF peak at the speed of 6 km.h^{-1}. These findings are of importance for the purpose of constituting the load-bearing walking programme for protecting against osteopenia and osteoporosis.

Chao *et al.* (1983) provided the largest set of normative data on 148 normal subjects of GRF parameters in adult overground walking. Generally, the magnitude of the two force peaks during level gait was reported between about 1.1 and 1.3 BW (White *et al.*, 1999). Our data are consistent with the previous findings. It would suggest that the analysis of treadmill gait in the present study is functionally equivalent to evaluating with overground gait.

During gait, the foot-ground contact force counteracts the gravitational force of the moving body (Winter, 1995). The vGRF shows a rapid rise at the heel contact to a value (P1) in excess of body weight as full weight bearing takes place. At the pre-swing phase, the plantarflexors are active in generating ankle plantarflexion movement, which causes a second peak (P2) greater than body weight (Winter, 2009). The increases in the magnitude of the vGRF peaks as gait speed and backpack load increased likely reflects an effort by the gait control system to maintain dynamic body stability with respect to the challenging task conditions. In the study by Majumdar *et al.* (2010), a 3D Motion Analysis System was applied to kinematic parameters of gait while carrying different loads (6.5–27.2 per cent of body weight). They found that the ankle was more dorsiflexed, and the knee and hip joints were more flexed during foot strike period for absorbing the increased impact forces. Their findings suggested an adaptive phenomenon to counterbalance load carrying effect.

Evidence shows that vGRF is linearly associated with the strain generated in bone (McKay *et al.*, 2005). Higher strain may contribute to larger osteogenic responses (Wolff *et al.*, 1999; Zanker and Cooke, 2004). A number of studies have shown even moderate impact force may be osteogenic effective (Wallace and Cumming, 2000): a significant increase in bone mineral density has been reported with post-menopausal women walking 1 mile per day (Krall and Dawson-Hughes, 1994). The experiment of Burr *et al.* (1983) found that exercise involving repetitive loading of 1.5 times body weight of the lower limbs could be used to treat or prevent age-related osteoporotic changes in the vertebrae. Under the backpack load condition, the magnitudes of vGRF were above that of unload walking: the magnitudes of two vGRF peaks were both greater than 1.5 times body weight at 6 km.h^{-1}. In combination with the factor of gait speed, it would suggest 20 per cent of body weight load-bearing walking at 5 km.h^{-1} has an optimal influence on osteogenic effects.

The analysis in this study has shown gait length and cadence increased with gait speed and backpack load increasing. This is true with respect to the normal subjects. We have not considered age effect on cadence and gait length. In general, the same expectations would not work with aged people, primarily because cadence increases to the adaptation more than step length. We take it as a major limitation of the study. Since it is an important point to be considered as constituting the load-bearing walking programme, this seems a natural future development of this line of research to explore age effects of different gait speeds and loads on the vGRF.

Conclusions

In summary, the findings on the vGRF parameters indicate that an increase in the first vGRF peak with increased gait speed and heavier backpack could be an adaptive mechanism on the musculoskeletal system in terms of possible higher lower limb impact forces. Results also showed similar CV values of the step to step variation of vGRF indicating adjustment to maintain a dynamic balance for challenging conditions. These findings might be useful in a clinical setting. The vGRF data from this study can provide clinicians with initial values with which to support physical therapists' interventions to maintain and improve bone mass and bone strength. We suggest that backpack load walking may be a complementary approach for protecting against osteopenia and osteoporosis.

References

Burr, D. B., Martin, R. B. and Martin, P. A. (1983) 'Lower extremity loads stimulate bone formation in the ertebral column: implications for osteoporosis', *Spine*, 8(7): 681–6.

Chao, E. Y., Laughman, R. K., Schneider, E. and Stauffer, R. N. (1983) 'Normative data of knee joint motion and ground reaction forces in adult level walking', *Journal of Biomechanics*, 16(3): 219–33.

Chesnin, K. J., Selby-Silverstein, L. and Besser, M. P. (2000) 'Comparison of an in-shoe pressure measure device to a force plate: concurrent validity of center of pressure measurements', *Gait and Posture*, 12(2): 128–33.

Fraysse, F., Dumas, R., Cheze, L. and Wang, X. (2009) 'Comparison of global and joint-to-joint methods for estimating the hip joint load and the muscle forces during walking', *Journal of Biomechanics*, 42(14): 2357–62.

Hagino, H., Katagiri, H., Okano, T., Yamamoto, K. and Teshima, R. (2005) 'Increasing incidence of hip fracture in Tottori Prefecture, Japan: trend from 1986 to 2001', *Osteoporosis International*, 16(12): 1963–8.

Han, T. R., Paik, N. J. and Im, M. S. (1999) 'Quantification of the path of center of pressure (COP) using an F-scan in-shoe transducer', *Gait and Posture*, 10(3): 248–54.

Hsiang, S. M. and Chang, C. (2002) 'The effect of gait speed and load carrying on the reliability of ground reaction forces', *Safety Science*, 40(7–8): 639–57.

Kai, M. C., Anderson, M. and Lau, E. M. (2003) 'Exercise interventions: defusing the world's osteoporosis time bomb', *Bulletin of the World Health Organization*, 81(11): 827–30.

Kinoshita, H. (1985) 'Effects of different loads and carrying systems on selected biomechanical parameters describing walking gait', *Ergonomics*, 28(9): 1347–62.

Knapik, J., Harman, E. and Reynolds, K. (1996) 'Load carriage using packs: a review of physiological, biomechanical and medical aspects', *Applied Ergonomics*, 27(3): 207–16.

Krall, E. A. and Dawson-Hughes, B. (1994) 'Walking is related to bone density and rates of bone loss', *American Journal of Medicine*, 96(1): 20–6.

Lloyd, T., Petit, M. A., Lin, H. M. and Beck, T. J. (2004) 'Lifestyle factors and the development of bone mass and bone strength in young women', *Journal of Pediatrics*, 144(6): 776–82.

McKay, H., Tsang, G., Heinonen, A., MacKelvie, K., Sanderson, D. and Khan, K. M. (2005) 'Ground reaction forces associated with an effective elementary school based jumping intervention', *British Journal of Sports Medicine*, 39(1): 10–14.

Majumdar, D., Pal, M. S. and Majumdar, D. (2010) 'Effects of military load carriage on kinematics of gait', *Ergonomics*, 53(6): 782–91.

Simonsen, E. B., Dyhre-Poulsen, P., Voigt, M., Aagaard, P., Sjøgaard, G. and Bojsen-Møller, F. (1995) 'Bone-on-bone forces during loaded and unloaded walking', *Acta Anatomica*, 152(2): 133–42.

Wallace, B. A. and Cumming, R. G. (2000) 'Systematic review of randomized trials of the effect of exercise on bone mass in pre- and postmenopausal women', *Calcified Tissue International*, 67(1): 10–18.

Wehner, T., Claes, L. and Simon, U. (2009) 'Internal loads in the human tibia during gait', *Clinical Biomechanics*, 24(3): 299–302.

White, R., Agouris, I., Selbie, R. and Kirkpatrick, M. (1999) 'The variability of force platform data in normal and cerebral palsy gait', *Clinical Biomechanics*, 14(3): 185–92.

Winter, D. A. (1995) 'Human balance and posture control during standing and walking', *Gait and Posture*, 3(4): 193–214.

Winter, D. A. (2009) *Biomechanics and Motor Control of Human Movement*, 4th edn, Hoboken, NJ: John Wiley and Sons Inc.

Wolff, I., Croonenborg, J. J., Kemper, C. G., Kostense, P. J. and Twisk, J. W. R. (1999) 'The effect of exercise training programs on bone mass: a meta-analysis of published controlled trials in pre- and post-menopausal women', *Osteoporosis International*, 9(1): 1–12.

Zanker, C. L. and Cooke, C. B. (2004) 'Energy balance, bone turnover, and skeletal health in physically active individuals', *Medicine and Science in Sports and Exercise*, 36(8): 1372–81.

SECTION 5

Measurement in sports and exercise

17

RESISTIVE FORCE SELECTION AND UPPER BODY CONTRACTION DYNAMICS

Relationships with anaerobic cycle ergometry performance

Marie Clare McCormick and Julien S. Baker

UNIVERSITY OF THE WEST OF SCOTLAND, HAMILTON

Introduction

High intensity cycle ergometry is widely used to assess the muscular performance and maximal exercise potential of athletic groups, healthy individuals and special populations (Bogdanis *et al.*, 1995; Stone *et al.*, 2004). Following the initial introduction of the friction braked cycle ergometer test by Cumming (1973), the 30-second Wingate Anaerobic Test was developed in Israel in the 1970s by a team of scientists led by the late Oded Bar-Or (Bar-Or, 1981; McCormick and Baker, 2011). This has since been adapted to assess performance over varying durations. When performing a high intensity cycle ergometer test, the participant initially pedals against no resistance at a fixed speed (Franklin *et al.*, 2006). When resistance is applied, the participant pedals maximally for the specified time period. Some of the variables that are habitually measured include peak power output (PPO), mean power output (MPO) and fatigue indices (Baker *et al.*, 2001a; Dore *et al.*, 2006).

Experimental protocols involving high intensity cycle ergometry commonly use 7.5 per cent of an individual's total body weight as the applied resistive force, and have subsequently attributed the power outputs to the work of the lower limbs. However, evidence would suggest that the assumption that the lower limbs are solely responsible for the power output obtained may be inaccurate, and 7.5 per cent of total body weight may not be the optimal resistance to achieve a true representation of maximal power output.

Resistive force selection

In test protocols using cycle ergometry where a single exercise bout is performed, it is important to set a resistive force that matches the capability of the muscle to contract. In this way, true maximal power output can be measured at, or close to, optimal velocity. Body size, structure and composition differ markedly among individuals, suggesting that a standard ergometer load may not provide optimal resistances for different populations and that the assessment of physique should be considered in any evaluation of high intensity performance. Therefore, optimization procedures should occur prior to testing to ensure more favourable results (McCormick and Baker, 2011).

A number of authors have addressed the possibility of predicting the optimal resistive force from body mass (Aylon *et al.*, 1974; Bar-Or, 1987). Drop loaded, cradle or friction loaded ergometers have permitted rapid applications of load and quantification of the subsequent values for power produced. In the original studies of Aylon *et al.* (1974) using Monark ergometers, the loads were in the order of 75 g.kg^{-1} total body mass. Dotan and Bar-Or (1983) declared that a higher optimal value, namely 87 g.kg^{-1} total body mass, produced greater power outputs. The protocol for friction loaded high intensity cycle ergometry exercise has undergone many modifications and refinements since its introduction in 1974, with researchers indicating that these load ratios may still be too small, especially for athletes involved in sprint- or power-based activities (Nakamura *et al.*, 1985; Winter *et al.*, 1991). Typically, resistive forces used during high intensity cycle ergometry testing have been based on total body mass (TBM) indices. These indices include both active muscle tissue and fat mass. Resistive forces used, which are currently inclusive of the fat component of body composition, may not be representative of the lean tissue mass or muscle mass utilized during maximal cycle ergometer performance.

Fat-free mass (FFM) versus total body mass (TBM)

It would seem appropriate to exclude fat mass from any resistive force protocol that attempts to establish a relationship between power production and the capacity of active muscle. Performance in high intensity experimental procedures has been reported by Van Mil *et al.* (1996) as being highly related to the subjects' lean body mass, or the mass of the muscles that perform the test. To date, during force/velocity relationship assessment, the loads used have been based on total body mass values (TBM) and have ranged from 75 g.kg^{-1} to 130 g.kg^{-1} (Inbar *et al.*, 1996). The resistive forces have also been based on specific guidelines for different populations and sexes (British Association of Sport Science, 1988) or have been derived individually using various optimization procedures. Several investigators are of the opinion that the FFM method of resistive force selection appears to be more representative of active muscle tissue activity (Baker *et al.*, 2000; Inbar *et al.*, 1996; Van Mil *et al.*, 1996).

The direct method of determining the resistive force for individual participants during high intensity cycle ergometry is to provide the subjects with a test protocol that requires them to perform the test repeatedly, each time against a different breaking force, until a maximal value for power is obtained (Dotan and Bar-Or, 1983; Evans and Quinney, 1981). An alternative semi-direct approach has been to assign a braking force that is based on individual subjects' TBM and a performance ratio, normally 75 g.kg^{-1} total body mass (Aylon *et al.*, 1974). The assumption has been that for most healthy individuals, the relationship between total body mass and muscle mass is similar. This is clearly not the case, and the relationship may be compromised further in populations that include the athletic, the undernourished and the obese. This would result in power estimation error during high intensity exercise performance tasks. The differences observed may reflect the inconsistent muscle mass to TBM ratio in individuals. Optimization for FFM appears to provide more accurate and meaningful direct comparisons within and between sport-specific and non-athletic groups. Individuals who weigh the same may have very different body compositions, with differences observed likely to reflect specificity of training status between subjects. The FFM protocol appears to identify more subtle changes in resistive force profiles, which may have resulted from smaller relative load increments during an optimization procedure.

The higher peak power outputs observed for FFM indicate that this method of resistive force selection does not overestimate the capacity of the active muscle mass, and therefore maximizes both resistive force and pedal revolutions. When using the TBM method of resistive force selection, the increases in braking force are greater for any given loading stage; as a result, the increased pedal velocity contribution to power production may be overlooked. The relative strengths of the correlations recorded between power outputs and resistive forces generated for the two protocols (greater for FFM), and the significant differences between loading procedures for TBM and FFM (Baker *et al.*, 2000) suggest that the FFM optimization procedure is related more closely to the active tissue utilized during short term high intensity exercise. When applying the FFM method of resistive force selection in conjunction with a force velocity protocol, the results obtained seem to provide not only a realistic method for determining optimal resistances, but power profiles with greater accuracy and reliability.

Contribution of the upper body musculature to high intensity cycle ergometry

Recent work has demonstrated that in addition to the substantial work of the lower limbs during high intensity cycle ergometry, the upper body may contribute to the power profiles obtained, and therefore we should consider high intensity cycle ergometry as a whole-body exercise (Baker *et al.*, 2001b; Dore *et al.*, 2006; Gregor and Concomi, 2000).

Initial investigations using surface electromyography (sEMG) suggest that during high intensity cycle ergometry with a normal handlebar grip, the amplitude of the sEMG signal of the forearm musculature is similar to, if not greater than, the signal amplitude during a 100 per cent maximum voluntary contraction (MVC) (Figure 17.1). Articulation with the handlebar allows the upper body to isometrically stabilize body position and pull the body downward to help overcome the high resistive loads during cycle ergometry so providing a counterbalancing force for the lower limbs (Baker *et al.*, 2001a, 2001b). Furthermore, research supports the use of a firm handgrip to help maintain body position relative to the ergometer, thus ensuring that the forces generated when forcefully extending the hips and legs are efficiently directed at rotation of the pedals (Baker and Davies, 2009).

Further investigations using sEMG have centred around the activity of the brachioradialis (BR), biceps brachii (BB), triceps brachii (TB) and upper trapezius (UT), all of which were found to be significantly active during high intensity cycle ergometry. The first study was an exploratory investigation that used the amplitude of the sEMG signal to assess any changes in upper body activity during a 30-second Wingate Anaerobic Test, the rationale being that any increase in amplitude would be related to the recruitment of additional motor units (MUs) to compensate for the decrease in the force of contraction and to an increase the MU firing and/or synchronization of MU recruitment (Dimitrova and Dimitrov, 2002). The data revealed that there was no change in signal amplitude over the 30-second test, measured at 5-second intervals, for any of the four muscles investigated. This suggests that the upper body activity remains relatively constant over the 30-second period and is consequently not affected by fatigue, which is likely linked to the submaximal nature of the upper body contractions. The contractions of the upper body also reflect the oscillatory nature of cycling in that the muscles are intermittently active, suggesting that the hyperaemia between contractions is able to provide the muscles involved with sufficient oxygen to maintain aerobic energy metabolism (Vollestad, 1997).

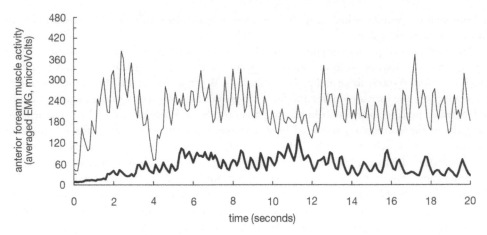

Figure 17.1 The left anterior forearm muscle activity (EMG) is shown for the two test protocols. A schematic diagram of each test protocol is shown. The with-grip protocol consisted of the subject placing their hands upon the handlebars of the cycle ergometer in a traditional gripping fashion (light line). The without-grip protocol (dark line) consisted of the subject placing the posterior aspect of each wrist upon the handlebars so that the open palms faced superiorly. Contact with the handlebar was maintained at the most distal points of the radial and ulnar styloid processes. The figure clearly demonstrates the increase in muscle activity when the with grip protocol is used.

During this exploratory investigation, visual inspection of the raw EMG data obtained during the 30-second maximal cycling test may provide an astute insight into the muscular activity of the upper body activity (Konrad, 2005). The raw EMG signal (Figure 17.2) recorded during the test demonstrates a linkage to the oscillatory nature of cycling, and the bursts of activity are representative of the alternate pushing and pulling motions upon the handlebars (Baker *et al.*, 2001a, 2001b). The raw sEMG signal can also provide some valuable information relating to the working phase of the muscle with respect to the three crank phases as described by So *et al.* (2005) as the downstroke (propulsive), the upstroke (recovery) and the pulling phase where the foot is pushed forward at top dead centre. Observations of participants during the cycle ergometer test revealed that, in general, the bursts of activity observed on the EMG trace (Figure 17.2) in the TB occur during the upstroke of the leg (due to elbow extension), and the bursts of activity in the BR and BB generally occur at the same time during the downstroke of the leg (due to elbow flexion). No clear pattern emerged from the UT data, which may be due to its role as a tonic muscle that is associated with stability during exercise due to the reasonably high percentage of type I fibres (53.7 per cent) (Johnson *et al.*, 1973).

To further scrutinize the contribution of the upper body to high intensity cycle ergometry, muscle fibre recruitment strategies were examined during 8 × 10s (R30) maximal sprints. To determine MU recruitment, the sEMG frequency spectrum is traditionally used, with higher frequencies reflecting the activation of faster MUs (Solomoniv *et al.*, 1990). This is due to fast muscle fibres (MFs) typically having larger fibre diameters and therefore greater muscle fibre conduction velocities (MFCV) than smaller type I fibres (Wakeling *et al.*, 2001). The median frequency (MDF) of the power spectrum is often used as an indication of fatigue. During maximal contractions, the MDF would be expected to decrease due to fatigue of type II fibres and increased recruitment of type I fibres. This is in contrast to the normal 'size principle' recruitment strategies (Henneman, 1957), whereby Renshaw cells provide a mechanism by

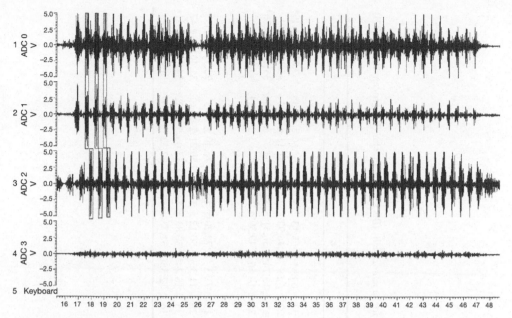

Figure 17.2 sEMG signal of a participant recorded during a 30-second Wingate Anaerobic Test. ADC0 = BR.; ADC1 = BB; ADC2 = TB; ADC3 = UT.

which the size principle recruitment pattern can be reversed. Therefore, if the upper body was fatiguing across the repeated sprints, a decline in MDF would be expected.

The data from the repeated sprint study found no changes in MDF of the power spectrum across the eight sprints and consequently no evidence of upper body fatigue, again confirming the submaximal, intermittent nature of the contractions. This lack of fatigue is reflected in the MDF values for all muscles during cycling, which are generally between 50 and 80 Hz, and is representative of non-fatigued muscles (Table 17.1). The low MDF values during the repeated sprints indicate that primarily slow type I MFs are being recruited, which are unlikely to fatigue when working submaximally for brief 10-second periods.

When the MDF value were normalized (i.e. MDF was calculated as a percentage of a maximal voluntary effort (MVE)), the data suggest that BR, BB and UT, MU recruitment patterns are similar to those during an MVE (Figure 17.3). Interestingly, the MDF of the BR in males during sprints 3–8 was significantly higher than MDF during an MVE ($p < 0.05$). However, in sprints 1 and 2, there were no differences between MDF sprint and MDF MVE, which is when PPO and MPO were found to be significantly higher (Figure 17.4). This suggests that as power drops and legs fatigue, there is increased pulling on handlebars to help overcome the high resistive loads that may reflect the recruitment of a greater number of larger muscle fibres in the forearm musculature and therefore a shift of the MDF to the right of the power spectrum.

On the above evidence, it seems that with the exception of the TB, the large fast fibres of the upper body are unable to be recruited in the seated position on a cycle ergometer, and so during the repeated cycling sprints most of the muscle fibres that are able to be recruited are active. It may be that altering biomechanical aspects on the cycle ergometer will allow the upper body to better recruit larger MUs and therefore contribute more to power profiles generated during high intensity cycle ergometry.

Table 17.1 Values for median frequency of the power spectrum for MVE and during each sprint for brachioradialis (BR), biceps brachii (BB), triceps brachii (TB) and upper trapezius (UT)

	MVC	1	2	3	4	5	6	7	8
MALE									
BR	57.91 ± 11.87	62.60 ± 10.55	63.87 ± 7.98	63.54 ± 7.46*	63.97 ± 8.84*	67.33 ± 6.88*	65.13 ± 9.02*	67.60 ± 8.13*	67.08 ± 11.49*
BB	50.49 ± 14.42	44.57 ± 11.65	45.24 ± 8.00	45.91 ± 7.57	45.55 ± 5.68	46.23 ± 6.59	46.92 ± 7.59	47.11 ± 9.03	45.11 ± 8.39
TB	126.20 ± 37.68	57.89 ± 18.67*	56.10 ± 19.08*	56.55 ± 16.54*	57.16 ± 15.81*	55.61 ± 13.74*	56.51 ± 14.04*	54.57 ± 12.86*	55.22 ± 16.56*
UT	58.96 ± 18.63	45.44 ± 8.81*	45.26 ± 10.16*	47.10 ± 13.93*	47.78 ± 13.77*	51.21 ± 14.66	49.39 ± 15.89	47.03 ± 14.14	49.87 ± 17.07
FEMALE									
BR	65.06 ± 12.06	63.24 ± 6.69	64.83 ± 10.09	65.47 ± 7.46	68.15 ± 7.33	72.15 ± 7.33	72.20 ± 10.96	73.40 ± 8.43	72.57 ± 7.33
BB	49.03 ± 10.74	49.69 ± 9.37	48.38 ± 10.71	50.03 ± 11.32	47.95 ± 12.31	50.28 ± 11.33	50.12 ± 11.06	50.21 ± 13.61	51.40 ± 12.47
TB	131.76 ± 24.50	57.04 ± 18.73*	54.44 ± 18.02*	51.81 ± 18.51*	53.58 ± 14.79*	52.35 ± 15.24*	50.83 ± 14.68*	57.06 ± 20.22*	54.65 ± 13.91*
UT	61.12 ± 22.36	53.21 ± 12.31	51.65 ± 13.80	52.96 ± 13.22	51.13 ± 13.18	50.16 ± 12.35	51.73 ± 13.05	52.32 ± 11.09	51.49 ± 14.93

Values are mean ± SD ($n = 9$).
* Significant differences between MVE and sprint ($p < 0.05$).

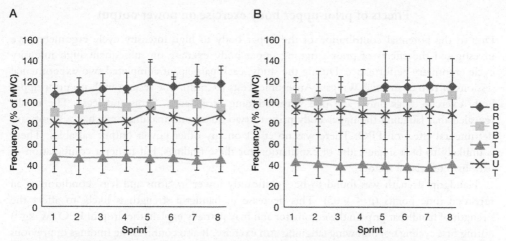

Figure 17.3 Median frequency of the power spectrum (MDF) during sprints calculated as a percentage of MVE MDF for brachioradialis (BR), biceps brachii (BB), triceps brachii (TB) and upper trapezius (UT) (A: male, B: female). Values are mean ± SD ($n = 9$). No significant differences ($p > 0.05$).

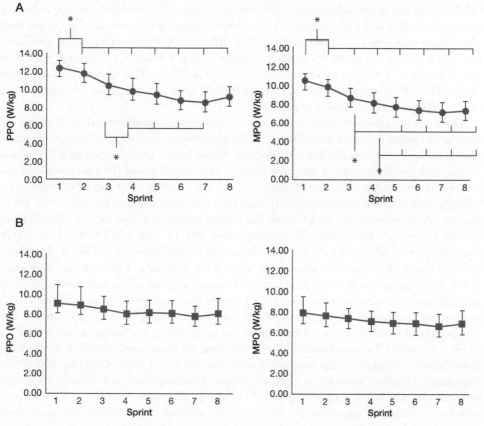

Figure 17.4 Peak power output (PPO, W.kg^{-1}) and mean power output (MPO, W.kg^{-1}) during the repeated sprints (A: male, B: female). Values are mean ± SD ($n = 9$). (* Significant differences ($p < 0.05$).)

Effects of prior upper body exercise on power output

Due to the potential contribution of the upper body to high intensity cycle ergometry, we investigated the effects of prior fatiguing upper body exercise on subsequent high intensity cycle ergometry performance. During the study, each participant completed two experimental sessions of two 30-second Wingate Anaerobic Tests (R 6 m), one session with no prior upper body exercise, 'legs only', and one with fatiguing bicep curls, 'arms and legs'. The results revealed that fatiguing the upper body prior to two 30-second maximal tests had a significant detrimental effect on PPO. There was no effect on any other power output variables. There is unlikely to be a single cause or explanation for these findings, but rather a combination of various interrelated factors.

Handgrip strength was found to be significantly lower in 'arms and legs' condition at all recorded time points ($p < 0.05$). This decrease in handgrip strength is likely to affect the strength of handlebar grip on the ergometer and may partially explain the drop in PPO ($W.kg^{-1}$) during first cycling test following fatiguing arm exercise. It also confirms the findings of previous studies, in that handgrip is key to achieving an optimal PPO and that the forearm muscles are working close to the MVE achievable in the cycle ergometer position for brief intermittent periods, reflecting the oscillating nature of cycling. The handlebar grip is particularly important at the onset of the sprint to help the legs overcome the high resistive loads. During sustained uphill climbs out of the saddle where the resistance cannot be overcome, the upper body is continually pulling and pushing upon the handlebar, suggesting the muscles of the upper body play a more important role in real-world cycling performance. Furthermore, it has been found that when participants adopted a standing position during a maximal cycling test, they were able to produce 12 per cent more power (Davidson *et al.*, 2005). This standing position allows for greater pulling action on the handlebars, which gives subjects more leverage to help overcome high resistance (Baker *et al.*, 2002).

The prior high intensity exercise also causes concurrent metabolic disturbances within the muscles and partial depletion and inhibition of the phosphocreatine and glycolytic energy stores, leading to decline in muscular force production. Blood lactate concentration ($[La^-]$) was used in this study as an estimate of muscular fatigue. The rate of blood $[La^-]$ accumulation and removal can be used as a measure of metabolic efficiency, with trained individuals reported as having a greater lactate transport capacity than their untrained counterparts (Iaia *et al.*, 2011). During intense exercise, the predominate mechanism to move La^- and H^+ out of contracting muscle is through monocarboxylate transporters, MCT1 and MCT4 (Gladden, 2004; Messonnier *et al.*, 2007), with the transport depending on intramuscular and blood pH, density of MCT1 and MCT4 and on blood flow in working muscles and other tissues (Péronnet, 2010). In the present study, blood $[La^-]$ measured post-cycling was similar under both conditions and following the exercise bouts, blood $[La^-]$ measured at 3 m post-exercise did not change at 5 m post-exercise, suggesting a lack of La^- metabolism during the recovery periods. This may be related to the passive recovery used in the experimental conditions, which would not allow for optimal lactate clearance due to pooling of blood, and therefore a decreased redistribution of lactate to the inactive muscles via the blood flow (Gladden, 2004). The importance of lactate clearance is open to debate; however, there is a definite association between elevated blood $[La^-]$ and impaired exercise performance, whether it be a cause or reflection of fatigue (Menzies *et al.*, 2010). Lactate metabolism, following the upper body exercise, may be affected more so, as the upper body is reported to have a higher percentage of type II fibres than the lower body (Sancis-Moysi *et al.*, 2010), which are less efficient in lactate clearance compared to type I oxidative (Gladden, 2000). The high blood $[La^-]$ prior to

Table 17.2 Power output variables during WAnT1 and WAnT2 for both experimental conditions

	WAnT1 PPO (W)	WAnT1 PPO (W.kg^{-1})	WAnT2 PPO (W)	WAnT2 PPO (W.kg^{-1})	WAnT1 MPO (W)	WAnT1 MPO (W.kg^{-1})	WAnT2 MPO (W)	WAnT2 MPO (W.kg^{-1})
Legs only	980.08 ± 158.53	12.71 ± 1.43*	865.47 ± 160.13	11.22 ± 1.63	555.97 ± 80.0	8.51 ± 0.51	589.22 ± 85.21	7.63 ± 0.63
Arms and legs	927.85 ± 167.70	11.91 ± 1.29	820.67 ± 156.60	10.90 ± 1.75	549.30 ± 81.58	8.37 ± 0.65	563.44 ± 69.91	7.50 ± 0.72

All values are means (± SD).
* Significant differences between conditions ($p < 0.05$).

the first Wingate in the 'arms and legs' condition and before the second Wingate in both conditions is likely to contribute to the observed decrease in power outputs (Table 17.2).

It is, however, interesting to note that in the first maximal cycling test, the prior arm exercise seems to have a beneficial effect on sustained power output, as indicated by no differences in MPO between the two conditions. The prior high intensity exercise would have resulted in faster VO_2 kinetics, facilitating an earlier and greater shift to aerobic metabolism in the first sprint in the 'arms and legs' condition. This shift has the potential to improve MPO by reducing the O_2 cost, O_2 deficit and rate of fatigue induction (Ferguson *et al.*, 2007). The effect of the prior upper body exercise is muted in the second 30-second bout due to the exertion during the first cycle ergometer test.

In conclusion, it has been shown that prior fatiguing upper body exercise has a detrimental effect of PPO. This can be related to a number of factors, including the decrease in handgrip strength following the upper body exercise, suggesting the upper body is less able to help overcome the high resistive loads, confirming results of previous investigations, which suggest that the upper body is crucial in achieving an optimum PPO.

Prior upper body exercise also affects PPO due to energy depletion and increase in metabolites. It was also found that MPO was able to be maintained due to the prior intense exercise, resulting in faster VO_2 kinetics and therefore a greater reliance on aerobic metabolism.

Conclusions and future directions

Findings suggest that the present loading methods used for cycle ergometry that are inclusive of TBM significantly underestimate attainable maximal power outputs. FFM is a more exact method of determining resistive force selection to attain more accurate power profiles and make comparison between individuals who weigh the same but have very different body compositions.

Data collected from the upper body musculature, via sEMG, demonstrate that the BR, BB, TB and UT are all active during high intensity cycle ergometry. The upper body does not appear to fatigue, as shown by the lack of changes in the amplitude or frequency of the sEMG signal over the cycling periods. This is likely due to the submaximal and intermittent nature of the contractions reflecting the oscillatory nature of cycling. Results also suggest that during high intensity cycle ergometry, the handlebar grip is key to achieving an optimal peak power output. However, the current design of the cycle ergometer seems to hinder muscle fibre recruitment; therefore, redesign of the bike may allow for a greater upper body contribution during these high intensity tests.

In real-world cycling performance, the upper body is important during sprints and uphill climbs out of the saddle, particularly when the resistance cannot be overcome and there is continual intense pushing and pulling actions upon the handlebars.

References

Aylon, A., Bar-Or, O. and Inbar, O. (1974) 'Relationships among measurements of explosive strength and anaerobic power', in R. C. Nelson and C. A. Morehouse (eds), *International Series on Sports Sciences: Vol. 1. Biomechanics*, Baltimore: University Park Press, pp. 572–7.

Baker, J. S. and Davies, B. (2009) 'Additional considerations and recommendations for the quantification of hand-grip strength in the measurement of leg power during high intensity cycle ergometry', *Research in Sports Medicine*, 17(3): 145–55.

Baker, J. S., Davies, B. and Bailey, D. M. (2000) 'Anaerobic optimisation protocols', *Journal of Human Movement Studies*, 39: 249–64.

Baker, J. S., Davies, B. and Bailey, D. M. (2001a) 'The relationship between total- body mass, fat-free mass, and cycle ergometer power components during 20 s of maximal exercise', *Journal of Science and Medicine in Sport*, 4(1): 1–9.

Baker, J. S., Davies, B., Gal, J., Morgan, R. and Bailey, D. M. (2001b) 'Power output of legs during high intensity cycle ergometry: the influence of hand grip', *Journal of Science and Medicine in Sport*, 4(1): 10–18.

Baker, J. S., Brown, E. and Davies, B. (2002) 'Handgrip contribution to lactate production and leg power during high intensity exercise', *Medicine and Science in Sport and Exercise*, 34(6): 1037–40.

Bar-Or, O. (1981) 'Le test Anaerobie de Wingate. Caracteristiques et applications', *Symbioses*, 13: 157–72.

Bar-Or, O. (1987). 'The Wingate Anaerobic Test. An update on methodology, reliability and validity'. *Sports Medicine*, 4: 381–94.

Bogdanis, G., Nevill, M. and Boobis, L. H. (1995) 'Recovery of power output and muscle metabolites following 30s of maximal sprint cycling in man', *Journal of Physiology*, 482(2): 467–80.

British Association of Sport Science (1988) *Position Statement on the Physiological Assessment of the Elite Competitor*, Leeds: White Line Press.

Cumming, G. R. (1973) 'Correlation of athletic performance and anaerobic power in 12–17 year old children with bone age, calf muscle and total body potassium, heart volume, and two indices of anaerobic power', in O. Bar-Or (ed.), *Pediatric Work Physiology*, Netanya, Israel: The Wingate Institute, pp. 109–35.

Davidson, C. J., Horscroft, R. D., McDaniel, J., Aleksander, T., Hunter, E. L., Grisham, J. D., McNeil, J. M., Gidley, L. D., Carroll, C. and Thompson, F. T. (2005) 'The biomechanics of producing standing and seated maximal cycling power', *Medicine and Science in Sports and Exercise*, 37(5): S393.

Dimitrova, N. A. and Dimitrov, G. V. (2002) 'Amplitude-related characteristics of motor unit and M-wave potentials during fatigue. A simulation study using literature data on intracellular potential changes found in vitro', *Journal of Electromyography and Kinesiology*, 12(5): 339–49.

Dore, E., Baker, J. S., Jammes, A., Graham, M., New, K. and Van Praagh, E. (2006) 'Upper body contribution during leg cycling peak power in teenage boys and girls', *Research in Sports Medicine*, 14(4): 245–57.

Dotan, R. and Bar-Or, O. (1983) 'Load optimisation for the Wingate Anaerobic Test', *European Journal of Applied Physiology*, 51(3): 409–17.

Evans, J. and Quinney, H. (1981) 'Determination of resistance settings for anaerobic power testing', *Canadian Journal of Applied Sport Science*, 6: 53–6.

Ferguson, C., Whipp, B. J., Cathcart, A. J., Rossiter, H. B., Turner, A. P. and Ward, S. A. (2007) 'Effects of prior very-heavy intensity exercise on indices of aerobic function and high-intensity exercise tolerance', *Journal of Applied Physiology*, 103(3): 812–22.

Franklin, K. L., Gordon, R. S., Baker, J. S. and Davies, B. (2006) 'Accurate assessment of work done and power during a Wingate anaerobic test', *Applied Physiology, Nutrition & Metabolism*, 32(2): 225–32.

Gladden, L. B. (2000) 'Muscle as a consumer for lactate', *Medicine and Science in Sports and Exercise*, 32(4): 764–71.

Gladden, L. B. (2004), 'Lactate metabolism: a new paradigm for the third millennium', *Journal of Physiology*, 558(1): 5–30.

Gregor, R. J. and Concomi, F. (2000) 'Anatomy, biochemistry and physiology of road cycling' in R. J. Gregor and F. Concomi (eds), *Road Cycling*, Oxford: Blackwell Science, pp. 1–17.

Henneman, E. (1957) 'Relation between size of neurons and their susceptibility to discharge', *Science*, 126: 1345–7.

Iaia, F. M., Perez-Gomez, J., Thomassen, M., Nordsborg, N. B., Hellsten, Y. and Bangsbo, J. (2011) 'Relationship between performance at different exercise intensities and skeletal muscle characteristics', *Journal of Applied Physiology*, 110(6): 1555–63.

Inbar, O., Bar-Or, O. and Skinner, S. (1996) *The Wingate Anaerobic Test*, Leeds: Human Kinetics.

Johnson, M. A., Polgar, J., Weightman, D. and Appleton, D. (1973) 'Data on the distribution of fibre types in thirty-six human muscles: an autopsy study', *Journal of Neurology and Science*, 18(1): 111–29.

Konrad, P. (2005) *The ABC of EMG: A Practical Introduction to Kinesiological Electromyography*, Scottsdale, AZ: Noraxon Inc.

McCormick, M. C. and Baker, J. S. (2011) 'Considerations in the use of high intensity leg cycle ergometry as a test of muscular performance', *Research in Sports Medicine*, 19(3): 202–16.

Menzies, P., Menzies, C., McIntyre, L., Paterson, P., Wilson, J. and Kemi, O. J. (2010) 'Blood lactate clearance during active recovery after an intense running bout depends on the intensity of the active recovery', *Journal of Sports Science*, 28(9): 975–82.

Messonnier, L., Kristensen, M., Juel, C. and Denis, C. (2007) 'Importance of pH regulation and lactate/H transport capacity for work production during supramaximal exercise', *Journal of Applied Physiology*, 102(5): 1936–44.

Nakamura, Y., Mutoh, Y. and Miyashita, M. (1985) 'Determination of the peak power output during maximal brief pedalling bouts', *Journal of Sport Sciences*, 3(3): 181–7.

Péronnet, F. (2010) 'Lactate as an end-product and fuel', *Deutsche Zeitschrift Fur Sportmedizin*, 61(5): 112–16.

Sancis-Moysi, J., Idoate, F., Olmedillas, H., Guadalupe-Grau, A., Alayon, S., Carreras, A., Dorado, C. and Calbet, J. A. (2010) 'The upper extremity of the professional tennis player: muscle volumes, fibre-type distribution and muscle strength', *Scandinavian Journal of Medicine and Science in Sports*, 20(3): 524–34.

So, R. C. H., Ng, J. K. F. and Ng, G. Y. F. (2005) 'Muscle recruitment pattern in cycling: a review', *Physical Therapy in Sport*, 6: 89–96.

Solomoniv, M., Baten, C., Smit, J., Baratta, R., Hermens, H., D'Ambrosia, R. and Shoji, H. (1990) 'Electromyogram power spectra frequencies associated with motor unit recruitment strategies', *Journal of Applied Physiology*, 68(3): 1177–88.

Stone, M. H., Sands, W. A., Carlock, J., Callan, S., Dickie, D., Daigle, K., Cotton, J., Smith, S. L. and Hartman, M. (2004) 'The importance of isometric maximum strength and peak rate-of-force development in sprint cycling', *Journal of Strength and Conditioning Research*, 18(4): 878–84.

Van Mil, E., Schoeber, N., Calvert, R. and Bar-Or, O. (1996) 'Optimisation of force in the Wingate Test for children with a neuromuscular disease', *Medicine and Science in Sport and Exercise*, 28(9): 1087–92.

Vollestad, N. K. (1997) 'Measurement of human muscle fatigue', *Journal of Neuroscience Methods*, 74(2): 219–27.

Wakeling, J., Pascual, S., Nigg, B. and Tscharner, V. (2001) 'Surface EMG shows distinct populations of muscle activity when measured during sustained sub-maximal exercise', *European Journal of Applied Physiology*, 86(1): 40–7.

Winter, E. M., Brookes, F. B. C. and Hamley, E. J. (1991) 'Maximal exercise performance and lean leg volume in men and women', *Journal of Sport Sciences*, 9(1): 3–13.

18

MEASUREMENT OF POWER IN MECHANICALLY BRAKED CYCLE ERGOMETERS FOR PERFORMANCE EVALUATION

Rae S. Gordon,[1] Kathryn L. Franklin[1] and Julien S. Baker[2]

[1]UNIVERSITY OF GLAMORGAN, PONTYPRIDD
[2]UNIVERSITY OF THE WEST OF SCOTLAND, PAISLEY

Introduction

Since the Industrial Revolution, the measurement of human work has been of great interest. Initially, this interest revolved around determining pay-related performance of miners or navvies digging canals, on the railways and roads. Tate (1870) defines a unit of work as 'the labour requisite to raise one pound through one foot of space', and his texts give examples based around manual labour.

The measure of work done has moved on since then, and it is now common to measure work (or power) as part of ergonomic studies into sports performance and special populations. One of the most common techniques is to determine the work of a subject using a cycle ergometer. A cycle ergometer involves a subject pedalling against some form of measurable resistance. Commonly, the erratic nature of pedalling is smoothed out by introducing a flywheel into the system. The flywheel also provides a suitable means of applying the resistance.

Early cycle ergometers employed spring balances to measure the resistance applied to the flywheel. The system consisted of a flywheel that had a strap around its periphery. The end of each strap was connected to a spring balance. The difference between the two spring balance readings gave the brake force. The work would then be calculated as the brake force multiplied by the circumference of the flywheel multiplied by the number of flywheel revolutions. The system had a number of problems in that it was difficult to set up to get the required brake load, and accurate and constant spring balances were difficult to source. Spring balances are notoriously unreliable for dynamic situations. The motion of the subject causes the pointer on the spring balance to fluctuate, and this makes taking accurate readings difficult.

The first practical cycle ergometer was designed by von Döbeln (1954). The ergometer consisted of straps wound around a flywheel and a pulley with a spring connecting the two ends of the strap. The pulley has an arm to which a mass is attached. The position of the mass can be moved along the arm to alter the brake torque. The pulley is connected to a rack and pinion system, which magnifies the angular displacement to make readings simpler to obtain. The mechanism employed is similar to that used in mechanical weighing systems and is known as a sinus balance. von Döbeln (1954) highlighted the shortcomings of the system in that the work done in overcoming friction was not included. However, he did use an electric cradle dynamometer to estimate the friction losses (using a standard bicycle) to be of the order of 5–10 per cent. von Döbeln (1954) highlighted the effects of the variation in the inertia of the flywheel as it accelerates and decelerates during each revolution of the pedal. He postulated that these losses will be very small and will have little effect on the overall accuracy of the ergometer. In von Döbeln's design, the flywheel has a circumference of 2 m, with a gear ratio of 3:1. This made calculation simple in that for every pedal turn the flywheel periphery travels a distance of 6 m. The work done is then the applied brake force multiplied by 6 multiplied by the number of revolutions of the flywheel:

$$\textit{Work} = \text{Brake Force} \times 6 \times \text{Number of Flywheel Revolutions} \tag{1}$$

The accuracy of the measurement system developed by von Döbeln (1954) was confirmed by MacIntosh et al. (2001). In this study, buckle transducers were placed on the straps of a pendulum-loaded ergometer to measure the tension in the strap on both sides of the flywheel. In a constant load test, the measured resistance in the straps is quoted as 100.5 ± 3.2 per cent of the pendulum setting.

Over the years, a number of different physiological tests have been developed; for those involving a subject to pedal at a constant (or near constant) velocity against a constant load, the pendulum-loaded ergometer is a suitable tool. However, for tests that involve the introduction of or the increasing of load during the test procedure, the use of the pendulum ergometer has severe limitations. One such test is the Wingate Anaerobic Test (WAnT) developed by Inbar et al. (1996). To overcome the limitations of the pendulum ergometer, a basket-loaded ergometer was developed by Monark. In this system, the resistance is provided by means of a weight basket. The subject can pedal against no-load and the basket introduced, or weight can be added or removed from the basket during the test procedure.

The system involves a rope that is wound around a flywheel and attached to a stepped pulley. A basket is hung from the pulley, to which the resistance, in the form of masses, is added. The basket and the rope going to the front of the flywheel is attached to the largest diameter of the pulley, and the rope at the rear of the flywheel is attached to a smaller diameter, as shown in Figure 18.1.

The calculation of work for this ergometer is given as the mass multiplied by the number of revolutions through which the flywheel travels. The derivation of this formula is given in detail by Gordon et al. (2004). The gear ratio of the pedals to flywheel is 52:14 and the circumference of the flywheel is such that for one revolution of the pedals, the flywheel travels through 6 m. The work done is given by:

$$W = \text{Force} \times \text{Distance Travelled} \tag{2}$$

The distance travelled is the number of pedal revolutions multiplied by the circumference of the flywheel (i.e. 6 m). Thus:

$$W = \text{Force} \times 6 \times \text{Number of Pedal Revolutions} \tag{3}$$

The force is assumed to be the resistance placed in the basket, and is therefore the mass multiplied by the acceleration due to gravity (9.81 m.s^{-2}, although in some cases this can be rounded up to 10 m.s^{-2}). The work can now be written as:

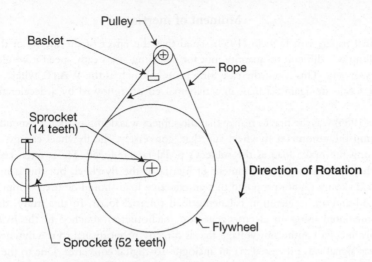

Figure 18.1 Arrangement of mechanically braked ergometer.

$$W = \text{Mass} \times 10 \times 6 \times \text{Number of Pedal Revolutions} \tag{4}$$

As there are 60 seconds in a minute, the number of pedal revolutions per minute and the duration of the test(s) can be substituted into the equation for work. Therefore:

$$W = \text{Mass} \times N \times \text{Time} \tag{5}$$

This is only really useful for tests at which a constant pedal speed is maintained. In cases where the test protocol calls for the subject to accelerate or decelerate, then it is more usual to measure the power output of the subject. As power is the work done per second, then from above it can be deduced that:

$$P = mN \tag{6}$$

where m is the mass and N is the pedal speed (rpm).

The difficulty in calculating the power is determining the speed of the pedals. In a protocol where a subject accelerates, the pedal speed will vary greatly and may change over a small period of time.

When the WAnT was first introduced, the protocol required that the number of pedal revolutions be counted over 5-second intervals to determine the pedal speed. The intervals were measured using a stopwatch. At best, using this measurement system only an average speed will be obtained, and given that in a WAnT a subject can accelerate from a starting cadence of 60 rpm and accelerate to 120–140 rpm in the first 5 seconds, an average speed of 90 rpm results in a large error in calculating the true power.

Over the intervening years, the mechanical analysis of the system for the accurate measurement of power has focused on two main areas. The first area of analysis that has been subjected to close scrutiny concerns correcting the calculation of power to take into account the inertia of the rotating parts of the system. The second is the calibration of the system to determine the losses in the system.

Moment of inertia

In his original paper, von Döbeln (1954) stated that the effect of the inertia of the flywheel while pedalling was difficult to quantify, but for pedalling at a steady speed it would not affect the accuracy greatly. This is not the case for a protocol such as the WAnT, where subjects are required to accelerate against a mass in a maximal effort, followed by a deceleration as they tire.

Lakomy (1986) was the first to realize that the subject was doing work (or expending power) in accelerating the ergometer flywheel and that, conversely, the flywheel energy contributed to overcoming the brake load as the subject's pedal rate reduced. He is often credited with providing the first figure for the moment of inertia of the flywheel, but this is not the case. In his paper, Lakomy (1986) proposed that an effective load should be used comprising of the frictional load and an acceleration balancing load (inertial load). In this study, the flywheel speed was measured using an electric generator (tachometer) attached to the flywheel. The generator produces a continuous voltage that is directly proportional to the flywheel velocity. The electrical signal was processed via an analogue-to-digital converter. Due to the limitations of available computers, the measurements of the velocity were taken as a rate of 20 Hz. To determine the correction factor, Lakomy (1986) measured the deceleration of the flywheel from an equivalent pedal speed of 150 rpm to rest under different brake loads; this is now commonly referred to as a run-down test. The resulting velocity-time plots were linear, showing a constant deceleration. The results from all the tests were plotted as a load-deceleration graph. Lakomy (1986) reasoned the additional load due to the flywheel that the subject overcame when accelerating could be determined by evaluating the load that would produce an equivalent deceleration. This figure was then used to correct the calculation of work or power. As the acceleration is determined by considering the change in velocity over a period of time, Lakomy (1986) examined time steps of 0.2, 0.5 and 1 seconds. This study showed that the maximal power of subjects was underestimated by 36 per cent without the correction for inertia.

Bassett (1989) determined the moment of inertia of the flywheel by calculation. He measured the thickness of the flywheel over a series of concentric rings to determine the volume of the flywheel. Having weighed the flywheel, he used the mass and the volume to determine the density of the material. Having determined the density of the flywheel material, the mass of each ring was calculated. The moment of inertia of the ring was calculated as:

$$I = mr^2 \tag{7}$$

where m is the mass of the ring and r is the average radius of the ring. From this the moment, inertia of the flywheel was determined to be 0.4166 kg.m^{-2}. It should be noted that this figure fails to include the moment of inertia of the drive system components (sprockets, free wheel mechanism, bearings, etc.). The moment of inertia was used to then calculate the total kinetic energy of the flywheel. Bassett (1989) then carried out two deceleration tests: one with an unloaded ergometer, the other with a brake load of 9.8 N. In this study, the flywheel velocity was measured using a magnetic relay switch. This would give the time for one revolution of the flywheel. This gives an average velocity of the flywheel for a single revolution given that the flywheel is accelerating or decelerating. The frequency of readings will vary depending on the speed of rotation using this measuring system. For a pedal speed of 60 rpm, the frequency of readings is 3.7 Hz and at 150 rpm 9.3 Hz. This is considerably less than the frequency of 20 Hz employed by Lakomy (1986). The loaded flywheel had a linear deceleration, as shown by Lakomy (1986). The unloaded flywheel is shown as having a linear deceleration, but only over a small proportion of time (15 seconds). It has been shown (Gordon and Franklin, 2002) that the deceleration of an unloaded ergometer is non-linear, as the braking force is due not only to mechanical friction, but also to windage (air resistance), which is negligible with the loaded ergometer. Gordon and Franklin (2002) also showed that the deceleration of an unloaded ergometer varied depending upon whether the pedals were fixed or free to rotate. From the deceleration test, Bassett (1989) determined the work done by the flywheel in overcoming the brake load during the deceleration. The work was equated to the kinetic energy of the flywheel. This was less than the total kinetic energy of the system, with Bassett attributing the difference to losses due to friction. The power of the subject was corrected as the total power minus the flywheel power based on 5-second intervals. In Lakomy's (1986) study, the WAnT involved a maximal effort after the introduction of a load with the subject initially pedalling at 60 rpm. Bassett (1989) had the subjects pedalling at maximal pedal speed before the introducing the load, and hence only considered the deceleration of the flywheel.

Coleman (1994) measured the moment of inertia of the flywheels of a number of Monark ergometers to investigate the effect on the results of WAnT. In his study, he used a 'run-down' test to determine the moment of inertia of the flywheel; however, this differed from that proposed by Lakomy (1986). The flywheel rim was marked with tape to give equal-sized contrasting segments of black and white that could be distinguished by an opto-sensor connected to a computer. This gives the time taken for the flywheel to travel through 2.88°. An ergometer flywheel was placed at a known height above the ground. A string was attached to a dowel on the rim of the flywheel and then wound around the circumference. A known mass was attached to the end of the string. The mass was released and fell to the ground. The computer recorded the velocity of the flywheel until it came to rest. An energy balance was then used to determine the moment of inertia and the frictional losses. The potential energy of the mass is equated to the rotational kinetic energy and the frictional losses. This is expressed as:

$$mgh = 1/2 \; mv^2 + 1/2 \; I\omega^2 + nf \tag{8}$$

where m is the mass, g is the acceleration due to gravity, v is the linear velocity, I is the mass moment of inertia, ω is the rotational velocity of the flywheel, n is the number of turns of the flywheel before it hits the ground and f is the frictional torque per flywheel turn. The frictional torque is determined by considering the number of turns for the flywheel to come to rest after the weight has struck the ground. At that point, the inertial energy of the flywheel is a maximum and with no other energy in the system it is the friction energy that decelerates the flywheel. This will not give an accurate measure of the frictional losses, as the flywheel has been removed from the ergometer for these tests and hence the friction of the free-wheel mechanism would not be considered. It is interesting to note that the method of determining the moment of inertia of the flywheel employed by Coleman (1994) is that prescribed in the British and European standard, BS EN 957-5 (British Standards Institution, 2009).

Hibi et al. (1996) compared the power measured at the pedals and then at the flywheel with the aim to determine the losses in the system. It was argued that if the power could be measured at the pedals, then the frictional losses and inertial effects would not be an issue. The pedal speed was measured using a magnetic switch and eight magnets (giving the time for the pedal to travel through 45°). The flywheel speed was then calculated using the pedal speed and the gear ratio. The force applied to the pedal was measured using strain gauges attached to the crank. The brake force on the flywheel was measured by modifying the ergometer. The load was applied by means of a mass suspended about a pulley at the front of the ergometer. The brake rope was then wound around the flywheel and then around the pulley above the flywheel where it was attached to a load cell. The brake force was then taken as the difference between the applied mass and the reading from the load cell. There is no explanation as to why this approach was adopted. It would, however, give an accurate measure of the brake force. The moment of inertia of the flywheel was determined using the same technique as described by Coleman (1994), and was found to be comparable with that published by Bassett (1989). The study concluded that there was a significant difference between the powers measured at the pedals compared with the power at the flywheel. The reported percentage difference was between 16.8 and 49.3 per cent. It was found that the percentage difference increased with applied pedal force and acceleration. As the efficiency of a well maintained bicycle is of the order of 98 per cent, it would be assumed that they would have little effect in the overall results.

Coleman and Hale (1998) compared three methods of determining the inertial effects. The three methods were those employed in the previous studies of Lakomy (1986), Bassett (1989) and Coleman (1994). This study found that although the corrected power was significantly higher than the uncorrected value, there was no significant difference in the results between the methods employed to determine the moment of inertia.

Reiser *et al.* (2000) considered not only the inertia of the flywheel, but the inertia of the pedals when determining the power of a subject during a Wingate Anaerobic Test. The moment of inertia was determined using four different methods – spin down, physical pendulum, torsional pendulum and a geometrical estimation. It was reported that the four methods showed good agreement and resulted in a moment of inertia of 0.982 kg.m^2 compared with a value of 0.91 kg.m^2 given by Monark. The moment of inertia of the pedal was taken to be 0.08 kg.m^2 based on an average from the literature. The details of the four methods employed by Reiser *et al.* (2000) are not given, and this gives rise to a number of questions. Were the results of the four tests comparible? In the spin down test, the deceleration of the flywheel, from a given speed to rest, against a given brake load is measured. The deceleration would be aided by factors such as friction and the effects of the free-wheel mechanism. This would not be included in a geometrical estimation. The flywheel is an assembly of parts – which parts were included in the estimation? How were the torsional and pendulum tests conducted? Given that the aim of the paper was to determine the effect of the inertia, there is very little information how this component was actually determined. In this study, the velocity of the flywheel was measured by an optical sensor, which determined the time for the flywheel to travel through 22.5°. The study concluded that there the power was underestimated by 31.7 per cent against uncorrected values and that the inertia of the pedals was evident.

The focus of research into the calculation of the moment of inertia and ultimately the work and power was based around measuring the speed of the pedals or flywheel. It was taken as read that the brake force was equal to the mass (multiplied by gravitational acceleration). However, this was questioned by MacIntosh *et al.* (2001), who attached buckle gauges to the brake ropes to determine the tension. This study discovered that there was tension in both ropes. This has the effect of reducing the brake torque as the forces act against one another. It was found that the power was overestimated by 12 per cent due to this error in determining the brake load. The incorrect assessment of load has two effects on the calculation of the power. The first is that the moment of inertia is reduced. MacIntosh *et al.* (2001) reported a moment of inertia of 0.77 kg.m^2 (compared with a figure of 0.9 kg.m^2 reported by Monark). The second effect of measuring the brake load is in the calculation of the brake power. MacIntosh *et al.* (2001) reported that for a basket mass of 10 kg (98.1 N), 95.5 per cent of this load was transmitted to the front rope and 6.7 per cent to the back rope, giving a resultant brake load of 88.8 per cent. The velocity used in the calculation came from the Monark

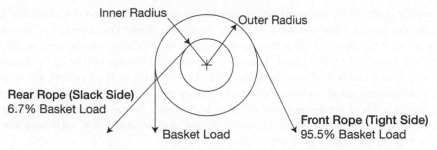

Figure 18.2 Dynamic equilibrium of the basket suspension pulley showing results reported by MacIntosh *et al.* (2001). This shows an anti-clockwise torque of over 100 per cent of brake load, while the clockwise torque is less than 100 per cent. This would result in an anti-clockwise rotation.

ergometer computer. This measures pedal speed using six equally spaced magnetic switches. MacIntosh *et al.* (2001) attributed the incomplete load transmission to the front rope to 'catching' in the mechanism. It is stated that the back rope is never fully unloaded, and this compounded the error. It should be borne in mind that the early ergometers used spring balances on both ends of the brake rope to measure the brake tension. The figures published for the load transmission by MacIntosh *et al.* (2001) were questioned by Gordon *et al.* (2004). The equilibrium of the pulley was considered under the loading conditions outlined and a load imbalance was apparent. The basket load and the front rope are on the same radius of the pulley but act in opposite directions.

Given that there is a load acting on the pulley in the same direction as the applied mass, then the tension in the front rope should actually be greater than 100 per cent of the applied load for equilibrium.

Gordon *et al.* (2004) developed load cells to measure the tension in the rope of a Monark ergometer to determine the braking load. This found a tension in the front rope greater than that of the load applied via the basket and a tension in the rear rope. The results confirmed MacIntosh *et al.* (2001) findings that the brake load could not be taken as the load applied in the basket. Gordon *et al.* (2004) carried out equilibrium checks for the pulley load for both static and dynamic conditions to validate their results. In this study, the velocity of the flywheel was measured using a tachometer, giving a continuous velocity. Gordon *et al.* (2004) provided a theoretical approach to determining the tension in rope of the ergometer. Rope braked dynamometers are often used to measure the power of engines, and the theory is well established. The ratio of tensions is given as (Spotts and Shoup, 1998):

$$\frac{T_1}{T_2} = e^{\mu\theta} \tag{9}$$

where T_1 and T_2 are the tight and slack side tension in the rope, μ is the coefficient of friction between the rope and the flywheel and θ is the angle of lap of the rope on the flywheel circumference. The brake force is the difference in the two tensions T_1 and T_2. As part of the study, experiments were carried out to determine the coefficient of friction. The measured values of tension matched those predicted by the theory very well. As this study was primarily to give a mathematical explanation for the brake forces, it was carried out at constant velocity and hence no inertial effects were considered. It was determined that the power was overestimated by 10.8 per cent. This was of the same order as found by MacIntosh *et al.* (2001).

Franklin *et al.* (2007) measured the tension in the rope to determine the effect this would have on the power calculated for a Wingate Anaerobic Test. The moment of inertia was determined for the flywheel using the run-down method and direct measurement of the brake torque and found to be 0.807 kg.m². This was compared with a value of 0.94 kg.m² determined by assuming the basket load was the brake load. The velocity of the flywheel was measured using a tachometer and all readings taken at a frequency of 50 Hz. The work was then calculated for different levels of acceleration and different brake loads. It was found that the percentage error increased with increasing acceleration. It was also observed that increasing the load increased the error in the calculation of the work done.

As pointed out by Hibi *et al.* (1996), an alternative to measuring the power output at the flywheel and having to determine the inertia load is to measure the power generated by the pedals. A number of studies have taken this approach using instrumented pedal cranks manufactured by Schoberer Rad Messtechnik (SRM). The SRM cranks consist of a series of strain gauges (the number depends on the model), which measure the torque, and a magnet and switch, which measures the pedal velocity. Balmer *et al.* (2004) compared the performance of these cranks in measuring the power output with the conventional (uncorrected) and corrected results. The conventional and unconventional power was determined using a commercial system developed by Cranlea (Birmingham, UK). The Cranlea system consists of an optical sensor that reads black and white segments that are attached to the rim of the flywheel. This study showed that the corrected power was higher than both the uncorrected (23 per cent) and that of the SRM cranks (16 per cent) for the standard 5-second interval. Balmer *et al.* (2004) pointed out that it was difficult to compare the results of different studies employing the WAnT, when it was evident that the different measuring systems provided different results. The results of this study confirm the results of Lakomy (1986), Bassett (1989) and others that the effect of the inertia of the flywheel must be included when determining the power generated by a subject. The fact that the results obtained from the SRM are lower than the corrected values should be a cause for concern. As the SRM is measuring the input power, then it should be greater than the output power due to losses in the system due to friction. This may suggest that the uncorrected values are accurate, as they are less than those obtained using the SRM cranks. This is not the case as shown by MacIntosh *et al.* (2001) and Gordon *et al.* (2004) that the corrected values are based on the incorrect assumption that the basket load is the brake load. One other interesting aspect from the study was the power measured was significantly higher for a 1-second interval compared with a 5-second interval. Franklin *et al.* (2006) carried out a study to compare the power measured using SRM cranks with the power at the flywheel using direct measurement. In this study, the subjects pedalled at a constant rate. This showed that the uncorrected figure for power was greater than both the SRM and direct measure methods. This is not possible, as it would suggest an efficiency of over 100 per cent. When the direct measurement at the flywheel (output power) was compared with SRM results (input power), it was found that they were 12 per cent less. This would suggest that the efficiency of the ergometer was of the order of 88 per cent. This figure was in line with a previous study by Maxwell *et al.* (1998). One of the limitations of the SRM cranks, pointed out by Balmer *et al.* (2004) and Franklin *et al.* (2006), is that although the torque readings are taken at a rate of 100 Hz, the velocity is taken for each pedal revolution. Hence, the SRM calculation for power is based on a constantly changing torque and a slowly changing velocity. The velocity used in the power calculation is identical for each reading of torque between the magnetic switch used for timing being activated.

Balmer *et al.* (2004) showed that the time interval for evaluating power had an effect on the maximum power generated. The power generated over 1 second was greater than that generated over 5 seconds. In the WAnT test, the subject pedals at maximal effort for a period of 30 seconds. The peak power is generated in the first 5–10 seconds and then the subject tires and the power drops. Using a 5-second interval produces an average power output. Reducing the interval to 1 second provides a smaller time over which the power is determined, and hence a higher power due to measuring higher values of acceleration. This gives more detailed information to the researcher. However, setting a fixed time interval will very rarely yield the actual peak power. The calculation of power should be based on the power generated over one pedal revolution or perhaps half a pedal revolution. This will give the maximum torque generated and hence the maximum power. This was considered by Franklin *et al.* (2008). Using a design for experiment technique to consider the measurement and treatment of the parameters that contributed to the calculation of the power, it was found that the time step used for considering the velocity had the greatest influence in the determination of maximal power. The study considered a time step of 0.125 seconds, as this equates to the average time for a single pedal revolution. It was found that this produced significantly higher powers. Santos *et al.* (2010) considered the sampling rate for measurement on the WAnT. Sample rates of 0.2, 0.5, 1, 2 and 5 Hz were considered by extracting the data from experiments where the sample rate was 30 Hz. The study concluded the low sample rates lead to lower values of power output. Sample rates above 2 Hz resulted in similar power output measurements, and this was attributed by Santos *et al.* (2010) to the average input pedal frequency of 2.4 Hz. This argument should be treated with caution because the actual measurements were taken at the flywheel. For a pedal frequency of 2.4 Hz, then taking the gearing into account, the flywheel frequency is 8.9 Hz.

Conclusions

At present, the comparison of data from studies using mechanically braked ergometers and the WAnT in particular is made difficult due to the inconsistencies in the method of carrying out the tests and the manner in which measurements are taken and then used to calculate the power. The results can be both accurate and precise, but only if the measurements are consistent for all studies. Given the improvements in data acquisition systems and the increase in processing power, accuracy and precision can be achieved.

It has been widely accepted that the inertia of the flywheel must be considered in test protocols, such as the WAnT, where there is any acceleration or deceleration. The newer models of ergometer have an option to include the moment of inertia in power calculations. The method used to determine the moment of inertia needs to be decided upon as there are several options. Although some studies have suggested that there is little difference in the results of these methods, it is suggested that those which test the complete system (sprocket, free-wheel mechanism, bearings, etc.) would be the most effective, The fact that carrying out an inertial test on the complete system *in situ* makes the process more straightforward is a bonus. The moment of inertia for each ergometer will vary due to differences in the manufacture of the flywheel and the state of maintenance of the ergometer (rope wear, dirt on flywheel rim, etc.).

The measurement of work or power requires the input of two measureable variables: the flywheel velocity and the brake force. There are two approaches to measuring the velocity; the first being to measure the time taken to travel a certain distance, the second being an instantaneous velocity measured using a tachometer. The major drawbacks of using the time taken to travel through a distance method are: the number of divisions (distance travelled) used in some cases is inadequate to capture the true nature of rapid accelerations, the results are averaged over the period, the measure of velocity lags the actual velocity, and the acceleration is based on two averaged velocities and this introduces further error. The use of a tachometer to give an instantaneous measure of velocity is preferable.

At present, most studies assume the brake load is equal to the load due to the suspended mass. This has been shown not to be the case. There is also the issue that the mass tends to swing about under the exertions of the subject pedalling at maximal rates. This is not helped by the fact that the mass suspension system is attached to the handlebars of the ergometer. Systems measuring the power generated at the pedals measure both torque and velocity, so why not do the same at the flywheel?

The rate at which the measurements are made must be frequent enough to capture the trends in the tension and the velocity. The measurements need to be taken at the same rate and time for all measured quantities.

References

Balmer, J., Bird, S. R., Davison, R. C., Doherty, M. and Smith P. M. (2004) 'Mechanically braked Wingate powers: agreement between SRM, corrected and conventional methods of measurement', *Journal of Sports Sciences*, 22(7): 661–7.

Bassett, D. R. Jr (1989) 'Correcting the Wingate test for changes in kinetic energy of the ergometer flywheel', *International Journal of Sports Medicine*, 10(6): 446–9.

British Standards Institution (2009) BS EN 957–5(3): Stationary training equipment. Stationary exercise bicycles and upper body crank training equipment, additional specific safety requirements and test methods, London: British Standards Institution.

Coleman, S. G. S. (1994) 'The measurement of maximal power output during short-term cycle ergometry', unpublished doctoral dissertation, Loughborough University Institutional Repository.

Coleman, S. G. S. and Hale, T. (1998) 'The effect of different calculation methods of flywheel parameters on the Winagte Anaerobic Test', *Canadian Journal of Applied Physiology*, 23(4): 409–17.

Franklin, K. L., Gordon, R. S., Baker, J. S. and Davies, B. (2006) 'Comparison of methods for determining power generated on a rope braked ergometer during low intensity exercise', *Sports Engineering*, 9(1): 29–38.

Franklin, K. L., Gordon, R. S., Baker, J. S. and Davies, B. (2007) 'Accurate assessment of work done and power during a Wingate anaerobic test', *Applied Physiology, Nutrition and Metabolism*, 32(2): 225–32.

Franklin, K. L., Gordon, R. S., Baker, J. S. and Davies, B. (2008) 'Assessing accuracy of measurements for a Wingate Test using the Taguchi method', *Research in Sports Medicine*, 16(1): 1–14.

Gordon, R. S. and Franklin, K. L. (2002) 'A study into the work done in accelerating a rope-braked flywheel ergometer', *Proceedings of the Fourth International Conference on the Engineering of Sport*, Kyoto: International Sports Engineering Association, pp. 144–8.

Gordon, R. S., Franklin, K. L., Baker, J. S. and Davies, B. (2004) 'Accurate assessment of the brake torque on a rope-braked cycle ergomter', *Sports Engineering*, 7(3): 131–8.

Hibi, N., Fujinaga, H. and Ishii, K. (1996) 'Work and power outputs determined from pedalling and flywheel friction forces during brief maximal exertion on a cycle ergometer', *European Journal of Applied Physiology*, 74(5): 435–42.

Inbar, O., Bar-Or, O. and Skinner, J. S. (1996) *The Wingate Anaerobic Test*, Champaign, IL: Human Kinetics.

Lakomy, H. K. A. (1986) 'Measurement of work and power output using friction-loaded cycle ergometers', *Ergonomics*, 29(4): 509–17.

MacIntosh, B. R., Bryn, S. N., Rishaug, P. and Norris, S. R. (2001) 'Evaluation of the Monark Wingate Ergometer by direct measurement of resistance and velocity', *Canadian Journal of Applied Physiology*, 26(6): 543–58.

Maxwell, B. F., Withers, R. T., Ilsley, A. H., Wakim, M. J., Woods, G. F. and Day, L. (1998) 'Dynamic calibration of mechanically, air and electromagnetically braked cycle ergometers', *European Journal of Applied Physiology*, 78(4): 346–52.

Reiser, F. R. II., Broker, J. P. and Peterson, M. L. (2000) 'Inertial effects on mechanically braked Wingate power calculations', *Medicine and Science in Sport and Exercise*, 32(9): 1660–4.

Santos, E. L., Novaes, J. S., Reis, V. M. and Giannella-Neto, A. (2010) 'Low sampling rates bias outcomes from the Wingate Test', *International Journal of Sports Medicine*, 31(11): 784–9.

Spotts, M. F. and Shoup, T. E. (1998) *Engineering Mechanics: Dynamics*, 7th edn, Hoboken, NJ: John Wiley & Sons.

Tate, T. (1870) *Exercises on Mechanics and Natural Philosophy*, London: Longman, Brown, Green, & Longmans.

von Döbeln, W. (1954) 'A simple bicycle ergometer', *Journal of Applied Physiology*, 7(2): 222–4.

19

METABOLIC TESTING PRINCIPLES FOR OPTIMIZING PERFORMANCE TESTING AND TRAINING GOALS IN SPORT AND EXERCISE

Craig E. Broeder

EXERCISING NUTRITIONALLY, LLC, LISLE

Introduction

Over the last quarter century, many advancements have taken place in the development of metabolic testing systems and procedures. Today's metabolic testing systems are highly automated and instantly provide real-time table and graphical data. Correspondingly, these systems can be programmed to control various ergometers while integrating the devices' respective data into metabolic testing reports (i.e. treadmill speed/grade or cycling watts). Testers can select from a large array of basic or more advanced variable options such as whole-body substrate oxidation rates, ventilatory threshold (VT), respiratory compensation point (RCP), O_2 and CO_2 ventilatory equivalents or oxygen uptake efficiency slopes that help identify key adaptations to training (Balady *et al.*, 2010; Lourenco *et al.*, 2011; Wasserman, 2012). Additionally, most research and clinically based metabolic systems allow the user to develop unique formula-based variables to meet a specific need such as watts per kg of body weight, which is a key indicator of a cyclist's climbing ability.

Many of these systems use interpretation algorithms for analysing raw test data into basic reporting templates to simplify the tester-to-client reporting process. These templates provide information such as current cardiovascular fitness level, ventilatory threshold or functional thresholds (termed aerobic threshold in performance-based systems), respiratory compensation (termed anaerobic threshold in performance-based systems) and a client's corresponding heart rate or watt training zones depending on the ergometer tool used for testing. To gain a competitive edge on the competition, some metabolic cart manufacturers have developed novel uses for metabolic testing parameters, such as plotting whole-body fat oxidation rates based on a person's respiratory exchange ratio (RER) and oxygen uptake responses during an incremental metabolic profiling test from rest to near or maximal exercise effort. Post-testing, the client is provided a training zone report that identifies the estimated ideal fat burn zone according to the testing results. While the use of RER for determining a person's fat-to-carbohydrate utilization crossover point is supported in the literature (Brooks, 1997; Brooks and Mercier,

1994), data regarding the reliability of the testing protocols or the implied benefits on performance improvements before and after a training period are not found in the literature.

Metabolic system start-up costs have dramatically declined over the last decade, especially systems designed for fitness centres. Today, a fitness centre-based metabolic system can be purchased for less than $10,000 versus a research medical-grade system costing between $20,000 and $50,000 depending on the options included. Thus, metabolic measurements are no longer just performed in university and hospital settings. It is not uncommon for personal training facilities, nutritionist offices, health clubs and even bicycle or running stores to offer metabolic testing options. In these facilities, testing is being promoted as an essential part of a person's performance programme development and progress tracking system. However, in many testing locations, individuals involved in running the testing have little to no formal training. Consequently, many of these individuals are unable to actually determine if the test performed was valid or if they are getting reliable results each and every time for their clients. Because many of the systems used in non-medical settings are designed to be fully automated, the tester is left to assume the calibration, data collection, testing results algorithms and final reports are accurate and valid.

This chapter will cover the core principles of metabolic testing, including an overview of current technologies and how to minimize collecting unreliable data. A secondary chapter purpose will be to provide a basic template for developing proper testing procedures related to sports performance settings. This chapter will help the reader understand how to develop a sports performance metabolic testing programme to accurately track and follow an athlete's performance changes over time.

Key aspects for metabolic testing in sports performance

In sports performance, metabolic testing is most often used to determine the athlete's submaximal performance indicators such as VT and RCP along with the athlete's current maximal aerobic fitness level (i.e. $\dot{V}O_2$max) before, during or after a given training periodization (Lucia *et al.*, 2004a; Santalla *et al.*, 2012; Wilmore *et al.*, 2008). Metabolic testing is also used to study the effects that various mechanical or nutritional ergogenic aids have on the metabolic costs of exercise or performance outcomes during an athlete's given event (i.e. aero bars and wheels in cycling, running shoe design differences or the use of various carbohydrate, fat, and protein supplementation feedings, respectively (Burke and Hawley, 2002; Fletcher *et al.*, 2009; Harnish *et al.*, 2007; Krieg *et al.*, 2006; Lucia *et al.*, 2004b; Roltsch *et al.*, 2002)). In all cases, the importance of using a standardized and reliable measurement process is essential for the athlete being tested. Without a standardized process, often times the information provided to the athlete or coach is simply a waste of time and money.

Metabolic Testing Systems. Prior to the development of automated metabolic testing systems, the measurement of a person's metabolic profile required the collection of expired gases for a specific time period using Douglas bags (Haldane and Priestley, 1935) and the micro-Scholander gas analysis technique (Gaudebout and Blayo, 1975; Scholander, 1947). Modified versions of the Douglas bag testing technique are used today primarily as the criterion measurement in validation studies for testing new metabolic systems (Nieman *et al.*, 2005, 2006, 2007). Current metabolic testing set-ups today are either mixing chamber or breath-by-breath (BXB) based (Porszasz *et al.*, 2007).

For mixing chamber-based systems, a subject usually breathes through a mouthpiece or facemask that directs air through a flow-meter interfaced to the mixing chamber (Poole and Maskell, 1975; Wasserman, 2012). Air volume is sampled on a BXB basis from an expired breath. Oxygen and carbon dioxide gas concentrations are measured at various locations within the mixing chamber based on a given manufacturer's design set-up. In most cases, the primary measurement site is the distal end of the mixing chamber. Critical to getting accurate metabolic measurements with a mixing chamber system is assuring that the volume of air measured and gas concentration measurement points are aligned correctly. Mixing chamber systems are prone to error when a person's tidal volume (air per breath) is uneven, making it difficult to align the measured volume with the actual oxygen and carbon dioxide concentrations due to tidal volume noise (Francis *et al.*, 2002). For example, in metabolic systems that automatically identify peak oxygen uptake values, a sudden uneven increase in tidal volume (i.e. a cough), which causes a higher total ventilatory volume than actually was required physiologically at the time the gas concentrations were measured, can artificially elevate a person's peak oxygen uptake above what the person's true oxygen uptake peak value was (Francis *et al.*, 2002). Miniature mixing chamber systems have been developed in an attempt to better align air volume and gas concentration measurements by minimizing gas washout delay errors (Sanjo and Ikeda, 1987).

Beginning in 1973, BXB metabolic systems were used to determine gas exchange and exercise performance (Beaver *et al.*, 1973, 1981; Sue *et al.*, 1980). Today's BXB systems sample a single expired breath 50–125 times per second, breaking down O_2 uptake and CO_2 output into the sum of the sampling frequency per breath used in the system. Similar to mixing chamber systems, BXB systems need to adjust for the delay time for when a gas sample was collected at the mouth for a given breath until that gas sample reaches the O_2 and CO_2 analysers (0.25–1.5 seconds). The exact delay time needed is determined during the pre-testing calibration process (Porszasz *et al.*, 2007).

In research and medical grade metabolic cart systems, although much of the pre-testing calibration process has been automated, the tester can easily review the calibration data at the time of the test along with the systems calibration history. Tracking a system's daily calibration values can help a tester identify potential problems before they lead to inaccurate metabolic data or lead to a system failure. In contrast, fully automated and self-calibrating systems designed for fitness centres do not always provide the tester with detailed calibration information. Thus, it is much more difficult to determine if changes in calibration values that border on acceptable levels are affecting testing results until the automated system denotes a calibration failure. For example, water vapour concentrations highly influence gas analysis measurements. In both BXB and mixing chamber systems, Nafion tubing helps minimize the influences water vapour has on the gas sampling process (Porszasz *et al.*, 2007). However, as the Nafion tubing ages, its ability to properly correct the moisture content as needed for a gas sample declines, leading to inaccurate O_2, CO_2 and RER values, despite initially passing calibration checks. This is especially true when many tests are performed in a row or extended steady-state metabolic testing is being used designed to study substrate utilization at a given percentage of max. Thus, a replacement schedule of expendable items such as Nafion tubing is highly recommended based on the number of tests performed per week and in accordance with the manufacturers' general guidelines.

Today, metabolic testing systems portability ranges from in-lab desktop models to fully portable or wearable systems. As a result, metabolic testing can easily take place in both the laboratory and field settings (i.e. running, rowing, cycling). This allows a testing facility or coach to quantify metabolically the performance needs of a given athlete or to determine if the in-lab measurements are accurately reflected in the real-world setting (i.e. in-lab ventilatory threshold values versus an athlete's actual race pace metabolic responses on the track). Wearable systems can provide valuable information on the metabolic costs of an athlete's body position (upright versus a time trial position in cycling) or the use of various aerodynamic wheel designs (Gnehm *et al.*, 1997; McDaniel *et al.*, 2002).

One concern regarding fitness centre-based metabolic cart systems is the fact that in order to reduce system costs, some systems are designed without a CO_2 analyser. Thus, maximal oxygen uptake criteria such as using RER values ≥ 1.15 cannot be included as an ending test criterion signifying an athlete reached true maximal effort. Despite this limit, previous studies have shown these systems can be both reliable and valid at measuring resting metabolic rate (Nieman *et al.*, 2006; Vandarakis *et al.*, 2013) and maximal oxygen consumption (Nieman *et al.*, 2007) when used by highly skilled and experienced technicians. From a practical perspective, metabolic systems that do not include a CO_2 analyser limit the testing centre's ability to provide additional valuable metabolic information that could help an athlete lose weight or make sure he or she is consuming adequate carbohydrates during endurance events such as marathons, half and full ironman or long-distance bike events. For example, one interesting use of metabolic testing that often occurs in laboratory settings, but has not yet become standard practice in fitness testing centres, is the use of RER values to help identify an athlete's carbohydrate and fat oxidation rates at race pace. Previous research shows that endurance training delays muscle glycogen depletion by enhancing fat oxidation rates at a given relative or absolute workload (i.e. percentage of $\dot{V}O_2$max or watt max, respectively (Holloszy *et al.*, 1998). In metabolic systems that contain O_2 and CO_2 analysers, a metabolic profile test can be performed at various submaximal exercise levels to show the athlete how the training programme has affected the athlete's absolute and relative workloads needed to reach the RER crossover point previously discussed. As an athlete improves his or her aerobic conditioning level, one would observe metabolically that a higher oxygen uptake, running speed or cycling watt output would be needed to reach the 0.85 RER crossover value prior to the performance improvements (Figure 19.1). For example, a study by King *et al.* (2002) in obese women showed a significant increase in both the crossover point and $\dot{V}O_2$max after 8 weeks of interval training that did not occur in a matched group of women for initial fitness and obesity levels performing steady-state endurance exercise. More importantly, before and after the respective training periods, fat oxidation kcals were plotted against various RER values using steady-state exercise at various exercise intensities. The study findings showed that fat oxidation increased in kcals per minute 15 per cent in the interval group only between RER values of 0.80–0.95, indicating the interval training programme dramatically improved fat utilization (Figure 19.2). Most interesting is the fact that both groups exercised in the lab had their oxygen uptake and kcals per minute measured during each training session so that each person oxidized 300 kcals per session, and the interval group's resting period was adjusted so there were differences between the group's overall exercise intensity (50 per cent of $\dot{V}O_2$max). This study highlights how metabolic testing can help a coach or athlete identify specific physiological and metabolic changes resulting from a specific exercise programme (i.e. effects of interval training on performance markers) to optimize an athlete's training needs. In conjunction with these findings, researchers have also shown that metabolic testing incorporating RER values can be used as an excellent predictor of running velocity performance (Bellar and Judge, 2012). Thus, before a fitness testing facility decides on the purchase of a metabolic cart system, they need to clearly identify the primary uses of the system. If the facility wishes to determine a person's resting or exercising substrate whole-body oxidation rates, then the system of choice will need to include both O_2 and CO_2 analysers.

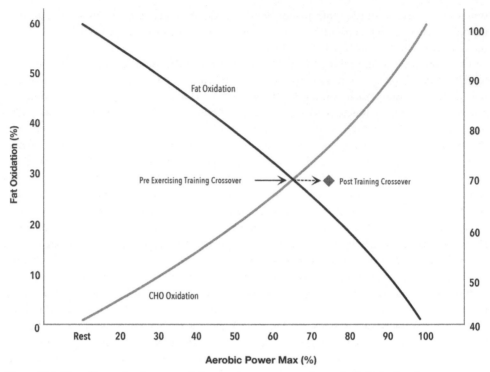

Figure 19.1 The effects of endurance training on the crossover point and whole-body substrate oxidation (adapted from Brooks (1997) and Brooks and Mercier (1994)).

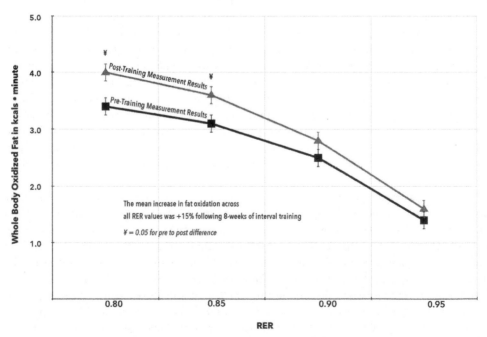

Figure 19.2 The effects of high intensity interval training on whole-body fat oxidation across various exercise intensities and RER values (King *et al.*, 2002).

Developing a sports performance metabolic testing programme

To date, there are no specific standards for the core knowledge, skills and assessment standards a sports performance metabolic testing coordinator should possess. Consequentially, there are no medical or sports performance organizations that have developed specific sports performance metabolic testing accreditations similar to those established by the American College of Sports Medicine (ACSM) for personal trainers, health fitness specialists, clinical exercise specialists or registered clinical exercise physiologists (American College of Sports Medicine, 2011).

The overall goal for all sports performance metabolic assessments should be to provide a consistent, accurate testing process. Key aspects for setting up and developing a quality sports performance metabolic testing programme include personnel, testing equipment quality, proper standardization of testing procedures and protocols, and the development of a scientifically sound data reporting process. Essential to these goals are the use of highly skilled personnel that are well trained in every aspect of metabolic testing. A metabolic test coordinator should have a strong knowledge base about the basic and advanced principles of metabolic testing. That person should understand all aspects of the calibration process and be able to identify when changes in calibration correction values indicate a need to replace gas sensors or drying lines that wear out over time. A testing coordinator should have a very strong understanding of the most commonly used metabolic cart design principles. This knowledge helps the coordinator problem solve when data appears inappropriate for a given testing condition (i.e. an improperly fitted face mask causing ventilation leaks and lower than expected oxygen uptake values for a given workload). Independent of a given manufacturer's interpretation algorithms, the testing coordinator should be able to manually interpret all data for key performance markers such as ventilatory threshold, respiratory compensation and $\dot{V}O_2$max. This knowledge will help assure all testing results are more likely representing an athlete's true performance level. Equally important, the testing coordinator should have a very strong background in the expected physiological and metabolic responses expect during testing based on the athlete's chosen sport or training status. A test coordinator should understand how various test conditions such as sea level versus altitude affect metabolic testing outcomes (Balke *et al.*, 1965; Dill *et al.*, 1980).

No matter how well trained the sports performance testing staff is, the accuracy of an athlete's metabolic results depends on the testing equipment quality used. All testing should take place on ergometers and metabolic systems that are checked and calibrated on a regular basis (Porszasz *et al.*, 2007). For example, many fitness centres use friction braked spin cycles that cannot be calibrated nor provide precise resistances as a subject inadvertently changes the pedalling rate with increasing resistance levels or fatigue setting in. Ideally, electromagnetic cycle ergometers or calibrating ergo trainers should be used to assure accurate power readings independent of a person's pedalling rate (Hellerstein, 1979; Myers *et al.*, 2009; Porszasz *et al.*, 2007). Furthermore, a standard calibration schedule should be maintained similar to those recommended for clinical exercise testing facilities (Myers *et al.*, 2009). Regular calibration checks and maintenance help to prevent poor data collection. Without the use of regularly calibrated and maintained instrumentation, it is very difficult to determine if small changes in metabolic outcomes are the result of calibration errors or actual changes in an athlete's performance outcomes.

In a similar context, it is highly recommended that each metabolic testing lab establish reliability procedures for each of the metabolic protocols performed to help minimize measurement errors (e.g. resting metabolic rate, submaximal and maximal testing protocols). If multiple coordinators oversee testing and data evaluation, each tester should establish his or her own individual test-retest intra-class correlations and standard error (SE) values. At the same time, between coordinator inter-class correlations and SE values should be established on a group of weight-stable athletes to assure that all testing personnel show similar metabolic results. For example, in our lab, we have previously reported intra-class correlations and between trial percentage difference for resting metabolic rate, $\dot{V}O_2$max, treadmill time to exhaustion, and heart rate max at 0.92 (1.2 per cent), 0.99 (3.5 per cent), 0.96 (4.7 per cent) and 0.89 (0.5 per cent), respectively (Broeder *et al.*, 1992). Others have shown similar reliability and between repeat trial differences (Nieman *et al.*, 2007).

A third important aspect critical in the determination of an athlete's performance markers is the development of a consistent and valid testing process. This process must include sport-specific metabolic testing protocols, including the appropriate ergometer for the athlete (e.g. treadmill testing for runners, cycle ergometers for cyclists, or swimming flumes or ergometers for swimmers) along with the correct testing protocol. For example, the maximal oxygen uptake testing protocol used on a beginning cyclist should not be the same one used for a world-class tour cyclist. Previous research shows that inappropriate ergometer use and/or testing protocols does not produce accurate and valid data (McArdle *et al.*, 1973). For example, swimmers tested on a treadmill do not produce the same $\dot{V}O_2$max as they produce in a swimming flume (McArdle *et al.*, 1978; Magel and Faulkner, 1967).The importance of sport specificity in metabolic testing cannot be overemphasized.

Careful attention should also be paid to the exact testing process, including the athlete's pre-testing practices. Important areas to standardized include assuring that an athlete receives 8–12 hours of restful sleep the night prior to testing, asking the athlete to avoid intense strenuous exercise 24 hours prior to testing and making sure the athlete's 48-hour pre-testing dietary intake is representative of the athlete's normal training diet and also assures optimum muscle glycogen storage. This is especially true if the athlete's testing includes measurements of blood lactate and ventilatory threshold measurements. Previous research has shown low muscle glycogen levels affect the accuracy of determining a person's true lactate threshold in relative (percentage of $\dot{V}O_2$max) or in absolute terms (watts of effort) (Hughes *et al.*, 1982).

Regarding the actual testing process, besides applying the appropriate testing protocol for a given athlete, the actual pre-testing calibration process, athlete warm-up and all manual data collection items should be standardized (i.e. RPE, stage changes if not controlled by the metabolic system). These items are important because as an athlete's conditioning level improves, one would expect attenuation in RER, RPE or HR at the same time period or at the same external metabolic demand (i.e. watt resistance level for a given stage). By always following a standard testing pattern, time plots or workload plots provide highly visual data comparisons that an athlete can easily understand and visualize their respective improvements. Also, following the same pre-testing and during testing process every time helps assure the results observed are truly changes that occurred in the athlete.

And finally, there needs to be a clear and consistent set of valid test end points. For example, using common $\dot{V}O_2$max criteria such as RER $\geq$ 1.15, max heart rate $\pm$ 10 bpm of predicted max, with increasing workloads oxygen uptake does not increase $\geq$ 1–2 ml.kg^{-1}, and max lactate levels $>$ 9.0 mmol help to assure true maximal oxygen uptake was measured (American College of Sports Medicine, 2010). These recommendations are especially true when a testing centre will be doing multiple measurements throughout an athlete's race season. In most fitness centres, bike and running shops, true criteria are seldom used because most of the testing performed, although they measure oxygen uptake, often use submaximal testing protocols only. According to the literature, submaximal treadmill and cycle ergometer tested $\dot{V}O_2$max can vary from the actual values by 5 and 20 per cent, respectively (American College of Sports Medicine, 2010). For a competitive athlete, this level of prediction accuracy is not appropriate, especially when these data are the basis of the coach's periodization training zone programme. Thus, it is highly recommended in healthy athletic populations not requiring a physician present for testing, maximal effort testing should be performed (American College of Sports Medicine, 2010).

For example, Table 19.1 shows actual data for one male competitive master triathlete tested (aged 46–48 years old at time of testing) in the same commercial fitness centre for his 2009–11 seasons but by multiple testers. The testing site used a commercially available non-reference gas self-calibrating system following the manufacturer's RER-based standardized submaximal oxygen uptake protocol on both a treadmill and friction-based cycle ergometer. During this protocol, the athlete continued to exercise with increasing workloads until the RER value was ≥ 1.0 on three consecutive 30-second measurements. In 2012, this same athlete volunteered to be tested in an FDA approval study research centre because he did not believe his previous tests were accurately providing him with the training data needed. Prior to testing, he was requested by the research lab coordinator to bring in any past performance testing results and reports available. The data highlighted in Table 19.1 represent this athlete's real client information contained in his automated generated testing reports submitted.

According to the 2012 research centre data results, $\dot{V}O_2$max for this athlete's treadmill test was 56.0 ml.kg^{-1}.min^{-1} (4.535 L.min^{-1}) and for the cycle ergometer test 49.4 ml.kg^{-1}.min^{-1} (4.001 L.min^{-1}). At the time of testing, this athlete's body weight was 80.8 kg with 18.8 per cent body fat. As expected, because this athlete's primary strength was running, his cycle ergometer $\dot{V}O_2$max result was 11.8 per cent lower than his treadmill results. His VT during the treadmill and cycling tests were 68.4 and 58.6 per cent of $\dot{V}O_2$max, respectively.

Looking closely at the fitness centre data, only the initial treadmill testing (1/7/2009) remotely resembled the research lab test results ($\dot{V}O_2$max = 50.0 ml.kg^{-1}.min^{-1} (4.340 L.min^{-1}) when this athlete weighed 86.8 kg. Most alarming is the fact that in 2009, all remaining test results are very inconsistent and underestimated this athlete's true $\dot{V}O_2$max at the time of his testing based on his performance history and the research lab results. The inaccuracy of his testing data are clearly evident by looking closely at his threshold values reported in the printouts that ranged from 82.5 to 92.1 per cent of max. In 2011, while the predicted $\dot{V}O_2$max results are higher, one can see the threshold values are again clearly not consistent or physiological (i.e. 96.9 per cent of max). Consequently, the resulting heart rate training zones are very

Table 19.1 Treadmill performance testing results conducted at the same commercial fitness centre for a male triathlete

Testing date	$\dot{V}O_2$max[¥] (mls.kg^{-1}.min^{-1})	Threshold[¥] (mls.kg^{-1}.min^{-1})	% threshold to max	Lower threshold HR recommendation	Upper threshold HR recommendation
1/7/2009*	50.0	•	•	•	•
12/7/2009 (9 a.m.)*	32.7	28.4	86.9	118 bpm	128 bpm
12/7/2009 (4 p.m.)*	34.3	28.3	82.5	121 bpm	130 bpm
13/7/2009[†]	37.9	34.9	92.1	130 bpm	143 bpm
26/5/2011	44.2	35.4	80.1	134 bpm	142 bpm
16/6/2011	41.3	40.0	96.9	123 bpm	142 bpm

* This data set did not have the any threshold or zone-related data. As a result, a retest was recommended and redone on 12/7/2009. The 13/7/2009 test was a second redo data because the data between the three previous tests did not agree well.
¥ All test results were performed on a treadmill at the same fitness centre facility and metabolic testing system.

Table 19.2 Sample zone training recommendations based on fitness testing centre automated reports versus research lab reports zones

Sport performance centre results heart rate based training zones*			Research lab results heart rate based training zones	
	12/7/2009 and 13/7/2009		4/5/2012	
Active recovery	< 112 bpm	< 117 bpm	Recovery[†]	< 92 bpm (< 68% FTH)
Aerobic development	131–121 bpm	118–130 bpm	Endurance zone[†]	93–113 bpm (69–83% FTH)
Aerobic endurance	122–131 bpm	131–143 bpm	Tempo zone[†]	114–128 bpm (94–94% FTH)
Anaerobic endurance	132–140 bpm	144–153 bpm	Functional threshold zone[†]	128–143 bpm (95–105% FTH)
Speed/power	141–173 bpm	154–172 bpm	$\dot{V}O_2$max zone[†]	143–168[¥] bpm (> 106% FTH)

* Zone names presented as written on the original report. There was no reference for how the heart rate values were determined.
† Functional threshold (FTH) zone names and recommendations were developed according training recommendations by Allen and Coggan (2010). Zone recommendations are based on a percentage of the heart rate observed at the athlete's functional threshold = 135 bpm (i.e. ventilatory threshold during the treadmill test) (Allen and Coggan, 2010; Allen and Cheung, 2012).
¥ 168 bpm was the athlete's actual heart rate at max compared to the estimated heart rate used in the performance centre results from 220 – the athlete's age.

inconsistent within each training year the athlete was tested (Table 19.2). From a practical perspective, this athlete had no clear accurate measurement of his aerobic capacity or his current threshold levels to properly set up a heart rate or watt zone-based training programme. While it is impossible to conclude the core reason(s) for these results, it is clear that the athlete's overall testing results failed to provide accurate, consistent and reliable data.

Summary

In summary, developing a high quality sports performance metabolic testing programme requires careful attention in four main areas, including personnel, equipment used for testing, following standardized testing procedures and the accurate reporting of the testing results. As metabolic sports performance testing continues to gain acceptance in fitness centres around the world, the need for developing sports performance metabolic accreditation standards is needed. Without such standards, more and more clients will not be getting appropriate quality testing and will be simply wasting money on a testing process that is nothing more than a sales gimmick.

References

Allen, H. and Coggan, A. (2010) *Training and Racing with a Power Meter*, 2nd edn, Boulder, CO: Velopress.
Allen, H. and Cheung, S. S. (2012) *Cutting Edge Cycling – Advanced Training for Advanced Cyclist*, Champaign, IL: Human Kinetics.
American College of Sports Medicine (2010) *ACSM's Guidelines for Exercise Testing and Prescription*, 8th edn, Philadelphia, PA: Lippincott Williams & Wilkins.

American College of Sports Medicine (2011) *ACSM Certification*, available at: http://certification.acsm.org/get-certified (accessed 31 August 2012).

Balady, G. J., Arena, R., Sietsema, K., Myers, J., Coke, L., Fletcher, G. F., Forman, D., Franklin, B., Guazzi, M., Gulati, M., Keteyian, S. J., Lavie, C. J., Macko, R., Mancini, D. and Milani, R. V. (2010) 'Clinician's guide to cardiopulmonary exercise testing in adults: a scientific statement from the American Heart Association', *Circulation*, 122(2): 191–225.

Balke, B., Nagle, F. J. and Daniels, J. (1965) 'Altitude and maximum performance in work and sports activity', *Journal of the American Medical Association*, 194(6): 646–9.

Beaver, W. L., Wasserman, K. and Whipp, B. J. (1973) 'On-line computer analysis and breath-by-breath graphical display of exercise function tests', *Journal of Applied Physiology*, 34(1): 128–32.

Beaver, W. L., Lamarra, N. and Wasserman, K. (1981) 'Breath-by-breath measurement of true alveolar gas exchange', *Journal of Applied Physiology*, 51(6): 1662–75.

Bellar, D. and Judge, L. W. (2012) 'Modeling and relationship of respiratory exchange ratio to athletic performance', *Journal of Strength and Conditioning Research*, 26(9): 2484–9.

Broeder, C. E., Burrhus, K. A., Svanevik, L. S. and Wilmore, J. H. (1992) 'The effects of either high-intensity resistance or endurance training on resting metabolic rate', *The American Journal of Clinical Nutrition*, 55(4): 802–10.

Brooks, G. A. (1997) 'Importance of the "crossover" concept in exercise metabolism', *Clinical and Experimental Pharmacology and Physiology*, 24(11): 889–95.

Brooks, G. A. and Mercier, J. (1994) 'The balance of carbohydrate and lipid utilization during exercise: the "crossover" concept', *Journal of Applied Physiology*, 76(6): 2253–61.

Burke, L. M. and Hawley, J. A. (2002) 'Effects of short-term fat adaptation on metabolism and performance of prolonged exercise', *Medicine and Science in Sports and Exercise*, 34(9): 1492–8.

Dill, D. B., Hillyard, S. D. and Miller, J. (1980) 'Vital capacity, exercise performance, and blood gases at altitude as related to age', *Journal of Applied Physiology*, 48(1): 6–9.

Fletcher, J. R., Esau, S. P. and Macintosh, B. R. (2009) 'Economy of running: beyond the measurement of oxygen uptake', *Journal of Applied Physiology*, 107(6): 1918–22.

Francis, D. P., Davies, L. C., Willson, K., Wensel, R., Ponikowski, P., Coats, A. J. and Piepoli, M. (2002) 'Impact of periodic breathing on measurement of oxygen uptake and respiratory exchange ratio during cardiopulmonary exercise testing', *Clinical Science*, 103(6): 543–52.

Gaudebout, C. and Blayo, M. C. (1975) 'Assessment of Scholander micromethod for gas concentrations versus weighing method', *Journal of Applied Physiology*, 38(3): 546–9.

Gnehm, P., Reichenbach, S., Altpeter, E., Widmer, H. and Hoppeler, H. (1997) 'Influence of different racing positions on metabolic cost in elite cyclists', *Medicine and Science in Sports and Exercise*, 29(6): 818–23.

Haldane, J. S. and Priestley, J. G. (1935) *Respiration*, Oxford: Clarendon Press.

Harnish, C., King, D. and Swensen, T. (2007) 'Effect of cycling position on oxygen uptake and preferred cadence in trained cyclists during hill climbing at various power outputs', *European Journal of Applied Physiology*, 99(4): 387–91.

Hellerstein, H. K. (1979) 'Specifications for exercise testing equipment. American heart association subcommittee on rehabilitation target activity group', *Circulation*, 59(4): A849–54.

Holloszy, J. O., Kohrt, W. M. and Hansen, P. A. (1998) 'The regulation of carbohydrate and fat metabolism during and after exercise', *Frontiers in Bioscience: A Journal and Virtual Library*, 15(3): D1011–27.

Hughes, E. F., Turner, S. C. and Brooks, G. A. (1982) 'Effects of glycogen depletion and pedaling speed on "anaerobic threshold"', *Journal of Applied Physiology*, 52(6): 1598–607.

King, J., Broeder, C. E., Browder, K. and Panton, L. (2002) 'The effects of interval training on rmr and body composition in obese women', *Medicine and Science in Sports and Exercise*, 34: S131.

Krieg, A., Meyer, T., Clas, S. and Kindermann, W. (2006) 'Characteristics of inline speedskating – incremental tests and effect of drafting', *International Journal of Sports Medicine*, 27(10): 818–23.

Lourenco, T. F., Martins, L. E., Tessutti, L. S., Brenzikofer, R. and Macedo, D. V. (2011) 'Reproducibility of an incremental treadmill VO_2max test with gas exchange analysis for runners', *Journal of Strength and Conditioning Research*, 25(7): 1994–9.

Lucia, A., Hoyos, J., Perez, M., Santalla, A., Earnest, C. P. and Chicharro, J. L. (2004a) 'Which laboratory variable is related with time trial performance time in the tour de france?', *British Journal of Sports Medicine*, 38(5): 636–40.

Craig E. Broeder

Lucia, A., San Juan, A. F., Montilla, M., CaNete, S., Santalla, A., Earnest, C. P. and Perez, M. (2004b) 'In professional road cyclists, low pedaling cadences are less efficient', *Medicine and Science in Sports and Exercise*, 36(6): 1048–54.

McArdle, W. D., Katch, F. I. and Pechar, G. S. (1973) 'Comparison of continuous and discontinuous treadmill and bicycle tests for max VO_2', *Medicine and Science in Sports and Exercise*, 5(3): 156–60.

McArdle, W. D., Margel, J. R., Delio, D. J., Toner, M. and Chase, J. M. (1978) 'Specificity of run training on VO_2 max and heart rate cganges during running and swimming', *Medicine and Science in Sports and Exercise*, 10(1): 16–20.

McDaniel, J., Durstine, J. L., Hand, G. A. and Martin, J. C. (2002) 'Determinants of metabolic cost during submaximal cycling', *Journal of Applied Physiology*, 93(3): 823–8.

Magel, J. R. and Faulkner, J. A. (1967) 'Maximum oxygen uptakes of college swimmers', *Journal of Applied Physiology*, 22(5): 929–33.

Myers, J., Arena, R., Franklin, B., Pina, I., Kraus, W. E., McInnis, K. and Balady, G. J. (2009) 'Recommendations for clinical exercise laboratories: a scientific statement from the American heart association', *Circulation*, 119(24): 3144–61.

Nieman, D. C., Austin, M. D., Chilcote, S. M. and Benezra, L. (2005) 'Validation of a new handheld device for measuring resting metabolic rate and oxygen consumption in children', *International Journal of Sport Nutrition and Exercise Metabolism*, 15(2): 186–94.

Nieman, D. C., Austin, M. D., Benezra, L., Pearce, S., McInnis, T., Unick, J. and Gross, S. J. (2006) 'Validation of cosmed's fitmate in measuring oxygen consumption and estimating resting metabolic rate', *Research in Sports Medicine*, 14(2): 89–96.

Nieman, D. C., Lasasso, H., Austin, M. D., Pearce, S., McInnis, T. and Unick, J. (2007) 'Validation of cosmed's fitmate in measuring exercise metabolism', *Research in Sports Medicine*, 15(1): 67–75.

Poole, G. W. and Maskell, R. C. (1975) 'Validation of continuous determination of respired gases during steady-state exercise', *Journal of Applied Physiology*, 38(4): 736–8.

Porszasz, J., Stringer, W. and Casaburi, R. (2007) 'Equipment, measurements and quality control in clinical exercise testing', *European Respiratory Monograph*, 40: 108–28.

Roltsch, M. H., Flohr, J. A. and Brevard, P. B. (2002) 'The effect of diet manipulations on aerobic performance', *International Journal of Sport Nutrition and Exercise Metabolism*, 12(4): 480–9.

Sanjo, Y. and Ikeda, K. (1987) 'A small bypass mixing chamber for monitoring metabolic rate and anesthetic uptake: the bymixer', *Journal of Clinical Monitoring*, 3(4): 235–43.

Santalla, A., Earnest, C. P., Marroyo, J. A. and Lucia, A. (2012) 'The Tour de France: an updated physiological review', *International Journal of Sports Physiology and Performance*, 7(3): 200–9.

Scholander, P. F. (1947) 'Analyzer for accurate estimation of respiratory gases in one-half cubic centimeter samples', *The Journal of Biological Chemistry*, 167(1): 235–50.

Sue, D. Y., Hansen, J. E., Blais, M. and Wasserman, K. (1980) 'Measurement and analysis of gas exchange during exercise using a programmable calculator', *Journal of Applied Physiology*, 49(3): 456–61.

Vandarakis, D., Salacinski, A. J. and Broeder, C. E. (2013) 'A comparison of cosmed metabolic systems for the determination of resting metabolic rate', *Research in Sports Medicine*, 21(2): 187–94.

Wasserman, K. (2012) *Principles of Exercise Testing and Interpretation: Including Pathophysiology and Clinical Applications*, Philadelphia, PA: Lippincott Williams & Wilkins.

Wilmore, J. H., Costill, D. L. and Kenney, W. L. (2008) *Physiology of Sport and Exercise*, 4th edn, Champaign, IL: Human Kinetics.

20
POWER METER PRINCIPLES FOR OPTIMIZING TESTING, TRAINING AND PERFORMANCE STRATEGIES IN CYCLING

Craig E. Broeder

EXERCISING NUTRITIONALLY, LLC, LISLE

Introduction

Cycling requires a wide array of physiological, biochemical, mechanical, psychological and strategic needs. For all cyclists, there are four main external forces that either work with or against a cyclist, including gravity, air resistance, friction and rolling resistance (Glaskin, 2012). How these external forces affect a given ride or race are determined by moment-to-moment ride condition factors. These factors include road gradient, wind intensity and direction, the cyclist's current aerodynamic position and the rider's ability to harness neuromuscular power at the time force is needed to alter inertia (Glaskin, 2012). Also, other physiological factors, including muscle glycogen stores at the moment force is needed, thermoregulatory effects on the cardiovascular system, the central governor and psychological factors, play major roles in how well a cyclist can overcome a negative external force (Coyle, 1999; Coyle *et al.*, 1988; Gollnick *et al.*, 1973; Noakes *et al.*, 2001; St Clair Gibson *et al.*, 2001). How these factors impact the actual physiological ride stress is also determined by a rider's anthropometric profile such as current body weight and upper to lower body lean tissue distribution (Martin, 2012), or the cyclist's current condition level (i.e. lactate or functional threshold and maximal aerobic capacity) (Allen and Coggan, 2010; Bentley *et al.*, 2001; Hawley and Noakes, 1992). These factors, along with the effects exerted by other riders (i.e. drafting or breakaway attempts) for a given race event, determines the final imposed physiological and perceived stressors of a given event (Figure 20.1).

Depending on the cyclist's specialty, performance needs vary from just a few seconds of maximal neuromuscular output for a world-class sprinter to the diverse aerobic and anaerobic requirements of a Tour de France rider that must successfully race over flat land, in the high mountains and during near maximal sustained effort time trial stages over several weeks of varying environmental conditions. Whether the cyclist is a world-class sprinter or grand tour rider, the unifying principle is simply: What is the optimum power output needed to be generated and maintained to win the athlete's event? World-class sprint cyclists are capable of generating

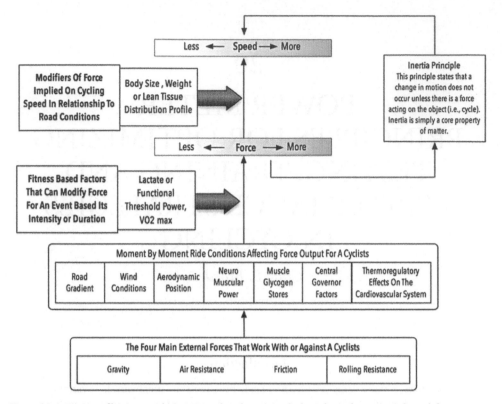

Figure 20.1 Factors affecting a rider's imposed and perceived physiological stresses (adapted from Glaskin, 2012, pp. 12–13; Allen and Coggan, 2010, pp. 40–1; Coyle, 1999).

1,700–2,800 peak watts with steady state per minute power output means of 360–400 W.min^{-1} (Craig and Norton, 2001; Gardner *et al.*, 2005). In contrast, world-class road cyclists generate fewer watts at peak force (1,000–1,250 W) (Fletcher, n.d.). But elite road cyclists are often able to sustain much higher average watts per minute for extended periods of time. For example, it has been reported that top 10 Tour de France riders achieve between 500 and 540 W.min^{-1} or 7–7.7 W.kg^{-1} at $\dot{V}O_2$max using ramp protocols (Lucia *et al.*, 2003; Santalla *et al.*, 2012). Consequently, these athletes typically sustain between 85 and 90 per cent of max aerobic power, which equates to 450–460 W in the final 20–30 minutes of a mountain stage climb (Earnest *et al.*, 2009; Lucia *et al.*, 2003, 2004; Santalla *et al.*, 2012).

As in all sports, cycling success requires that a rider pays careful attention to developing both short- and long-term training strategies that properly focus on the athlete's specific performance needs. Cyclists and other athletes have attempted to accurately quantify training and race performances to gain a competitive edge. With the development of wireless heart rate technology in the late 1970s and early 1980s, coaches had a tool that could help monitor an athlete's training and race responses using real-time physiological quantitative information (Burke, 2002). The Finnish National Cross Country ski team was the first athletic team to incorporate heart rate monitoring into an endurance athlete's training programme (Burke, 1998, 2002). In 1986, Schoberer Rad Messtechnik corporation (SRM) produced the first functional power meter that became commercially available in 1989 and three-time Tour de France winner Greg LeMond was the first professional cyclist to use the SRM power meter system (SRM, n.d.). The development of power meter technologies allowed cyclists for the first time to truly quantify the amount of work produced while training and competing.

Historically, the measurement of heart rate and power are used to assess, quantify and profile the physiological performance characteristics of cyclist in research labs for many years (Coyle, 1999; Coyle *et al.*, 1988). More recently, it has become common to see cyclists at all levels using power-monitoring systems on training rides and in competition. In combination with traditional heart rate monitoring systems, power meters are helping revolutionize how we measure cycling fitness, track performance, improve race results and even prevent overtraining syndrome.

First, this chapter will provide an overview of the power meter system designed for cycling performance monitoring. Second, this chapter will discuss the extent to which power meter training systems can more accurately quantify a cyclist's training load (i.e. watt-based performance measures versus heart responses during a given training condition). Third, this chapter will highlight recently defined watt-based training monitoring terms such as functional threshold, normative power, acute training load scores (ATL), chronic training load scores (CTL), total stress score (TSS) and quadrant analyses that are redefining how we measure, track, quantify and evaluate cycling performance results (Allen and Coggan, 2006, 2010). And finally, this chapter will show how advances in sports performance monitoring software technologies are helping sport scientists and coaches understand and visualize a cyclist's unique individual performance characteristics for developing more efficient training programmes.

Power meter technology history

Since the 1980s, developments in power meter technologies have produced numerous advances. Until recently, power meter hardware development commonly utilized five methods for assessing a cyclist's power output, including: bottom-bracket sensors, crank-based integrated sensors, hub-based integrated systems, chain-stay-mounted sensors and opposing forces methods (Allen and Coggan, 2010; Glaskin, 2012). More recently, two additional power meter systems were developed. Through a partnership between the Look and Polar Corporations, the first pedal-based force sensor system was commercially available (LOOK Cycle USA, n.d.). Pedal-based force sensor systems measure power where it is first applied in cycling, the pedal. As software analysis programmes develop, pedal-based systems will eventually allow for differential analyses between left and right pedal stroke biomechanical patterns as force is being applied throughout the entire 360° pedal stroke.

A second new power system was developed by the Stages Cycling Corporation to be the first super lightweight (20 grams) and inexpensive system directly mounted on the left crank arm using an integrated accelerometer, temperature sensor and strain gauge-based system (Stages Cycling, 2012). To date, the Stages Cycling system is the only power meter set-up that includes a multi-point temperature calibrated set-up. Multi-point temperature point calibration is an important power meter advancement because strain gauge measurement is highly affected by temperature changes. For example, the SRM corporation recommends that if ambient temperature changes more than 20°F (6.7°C), their crank-based system requires a re-zero calibration (SRM, n.d.). One potential measurement issue that needs to be determined with a single crank arm power meter placement is how accurately it measures a cyclist's total power output since the developers assumed that left and right leg contributions to overall power output is similar based on the company's own internal testing (Warner, 2012).

One major disadvantage for several power meter systems (i.e. crank arm and bottom bracket positions) is that most competitive cyclists have multiple bike set-ups and would require that all power meters be installed and calibrated properly on each bike. Besides the additional expenses, cyclists using multiple monitors would need to make sure that each system is properly calibrated and that each power meter system is producing equal results over the same ride conditions. In this context, an advantage of pedal-based power meter systems is the fact the cyclist can easily transfer pedals from one bike to another while avoiding between-system calibration issues (i.e. road versus time trial bike). However, it is important to point out for pedal power systems, especially for left-right-leg pedalling profiling, the between-pedal side calibrations should also be verified between each pedal on the same bike or when switched to a different bike. Table 20.1 and Figure 20.2 highlight key aspects of current power meter systems and their respective placement location.

From a measurement perspective, accuracy measures ≤ 2.5 per cent are considered essential for properly tracking a cyclist's power output (Bertucci *et al.*, 2005; Gardner *et al.*, 2004). The only system listed in Table 20.1 that does not meet this basic measure requirement is the chain stay mounting system (Millet *et al.*, 2003). For all systems, it is important to make sure that the power meter is properly calibrated and zeroed. Most systems are calibrated at the factory. The only system that requires the rider to do a real-time calibration is the opposing forces system by the iBike group. Initially, the calibration process was very complicated for most novices or non-technically savvy riders. With the advent of the iBike Newton and Newton+ models, while still cumbersome to some degree, the calibration process is much more clear and defined. However, one of the underlying assumptions with an opposing force system is a unit's calibration process was performed for the cycling position that a rider will spend a majority of event time. Thus, if a rider calibrates the system for one position but is spending a majority of his or her time in a different aero-position than the original opposing forces, calculation factors will not accurately measure the cyclist's power output. As more and more cyclists use

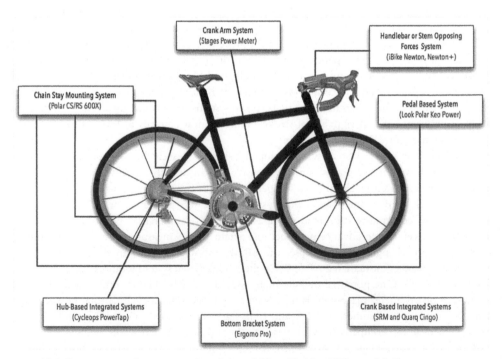

Figure 20.2 Power meter placement options (adapted from Glaskin, 2012, pp. 34–5).

Table 20.1 Power meter options

Location	Power meter manufacturer	Measurement method	Communication method	Reported accuracy	Pedal stroke analysis
Crank-based integrated system	SRM★ Professional	Direct force 4–8 strair gauges	ANT+	± 2.5%	No
	Quarq Cingo	Direct force10 strain gauges across 20 grids	ANT+	± 2.0%	Estimated
Bottom bracket system	Ergomo Pro	Direct force optical sensors	ANT+	± 1.5%	No
Hub-based integrated system	Cycleops PowerTap Comp, Elite+, Pro+, SL+ SLC+	Direct force 3 strain gauges	ANT+	± 1.5%	No
Handlebar or stem-based system	iBike Newton, Newton⁺, IBike Dash	Opposing forces; wind, hills, acceleration, friction	ANT+	± 2–3%	No
Pedal-based system	Look Polar Keo Power	Bilateral pedal direct force 8 strain gauges	ANT+	≤ 2.0%	Yes
Chain stay mounting system	Polar CS/RS 600X	Chain speed and vibration frequency	Polar priority W.I.N.D.	± 5.0%	Estimated
Crank arm-based system	Stages Power Meter	Left crank arm strain gauge. Includes on-board multi-point calibrated thermometer	ANT+, Bluetooth	± 2.0%	No

★ SRM = Schoberer Rad Messtechnik.

power meter values to determine correct pacing strategy during time trials, for a breakaway or climb, inaccurate power measurements have the potential to promote an incorrect pacing strategy (Smith *et al.*, 2001).

Most power meter systems use a standardized area network communication protocol called ANT+. ANT+ is a communication network protocol that is able to collect, transfer and store sensor data used in sports, wellness and home health applications (Dynastream Innovations Inc., 2012). Devices that typically use ANT+ communication protocols include heart rate monitors, speed sensors and small global positioning system (GPS) devices. ANT+ signals transmit over a 2.4 GHz license-free band producing high-quality wireless communication that takes advantage of low-power and low-cost transceivers. Only the Polar Corporation power meter systems do not use ANT+ communication technology. The Polar Corporation uses its own communication technology called a Wireless Integrated Network Device (W.I.N.D.). Unlike ANT+ based systems, which allow various manufacturers to easily transfer data between devices, a W.I.N.D. based system can only use Polar based on-bike monitoring computers, limiting universal data transfer between other manufacturers' devices. Fortunately, to date, most bicycle computer monitors and power meter systems are ANT+ based, thus allowing cyclists to easily transfer data across manufacturers and various analysis platforms. Also, many new monitors and accessories are incorporating both ANT+ and Bluetooth communication technologies, enhancing their overall compatibilities, including smartphone apps.

Most power monitoring systems provide similar variable tracking options. Cyclists, depending on the bike-monitoring computer used to collect data, have a large array of variables and performance-tracking data possibilities. Most on-bike monitoring computers provide current, average and peak data for each measured variable. At the basic level, variables include watts, heart rate, cadence and speed. More advanced monitoring systems also measure per cent grade, altitude, GPS coordinates, environmental temperature, feet climbed, descent feet and net climbing feet. The newest and most advanced monitoring systems provide the cyclist left and right pedal stroke power and torque comparisons, left-to-right pedal balance determinations, race-monitored real-time power output ratios (W/kg^{-1}), normalized power, acute and chronic training load scores, and real-time intensity factor scores relative to the cyclist's current functional threshold. Moreover, these advanced systems now allow cyclists to immediately see total time or per cent time spent at the cyclist's various power and heart rate target training zones. When these data are analysed with performance software analysis programmes (i.e. CyclingPeaks WKO+), cyclists and their coaches have, for the first time, a very comprehensive view into the cyclist's current performance metrics. More importantly, when a cyclist's data are properly tracked and combined with GPS ride profile data, a cyclist and his or her coach can better understand the specific race demands, and where the cyclist needs to focus his or her future training for improving race success.

Traditional versus contemporary performance variables

With the advent of heart rate monitors, athletes could, for the first time, quantify the physiological effects of a given performance in relationship to their current fitness level. Because heart rate responses from rest to maximal effort are linear, it was initially thought that heart rate data provided an accurate insight into an athlete's real-time training load or race intensity performed. As a result, groups such as the American College of Sports Medicine (ACSM) established heart rate-based training intensity guidelines for both health and fitness training (American College of Sports Medicine, 2010).

In general, when heart rate is averaged over a period of time under highly standardized conditions (i.e. 20–60 minutes of continuous exercise), an athlete's average heart rate compared to that athlete's known max heart rate represents a measure of effort. Unfortunately, this information provides little insight into how much actual work was required to produce this summary heart rate value. Although the linear relationship between heart rate and oxygen uptake is valid under standardized conditions in the lab (McArdle *et al.*, 2009; Saltin, 1969; Wilmore *et al.*, 2008), in the real world of athletic performance monitoring, the use of heart rate as a marker of true real-time work output is limited. At best, heart rate is simply an indirect physiological response variable resulting from work performed in combination with the cyclist's ever-changing environmental conditions. Furthermore, a person's acute heart rate responses during exercise are highly influenced by an athlete's pre-exercise rest status, pre-event hydration level, during-event rehydration maintenance ability, environmental temperatures, length of exercise, muscular fatigue status, metabolic efficiency and nutritional factors (e.g. caffeine/ stimulant use, muscle glycogen level) (Benson and Connolly, 2011; Burke, 1998; Wilmore *et al.*, 2008). More importantly, in regards to the real-time workload (current watt demand), heart rate responses are delayed in relationship to a current workload change (i.e. 1–3 minutes).

In cycling, these temporal heart rate delays are especially evident for a ride or racecourse with numerous hills or interval bursts. Figure 20.3 illustrates how a large immediate increase in power output during an uphill climb results in a temporal delay in the cyclist's related heart rate response. At the same time, when power requirements dramatically decline (i.e. during the descent), heart rate still requires time to re-couple with the actual power output being performed. This simple illustration highlights why focusing on developing power-based cycling training programmes is becoming more important for all cyclists. Similar to hill climbing, while

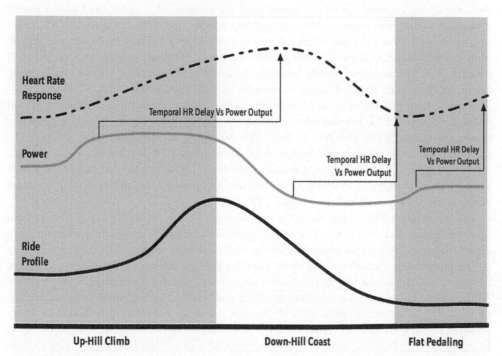

Figure 20.3 Examples of temporal heart rate responses versus immediate changes in power demands (adapted from Friel, 2012, p. 15).

immediate changes in power output can be observed for interval-based workouts, temporal delays in a cyclist's heart rate responses would make it impossible to use heart rate to judge true interval training stress loads. With power-based training programmes, the cyclist can see immediately if he or she is truly working at the target wattage required during a given micro-training segment of the ride. Also, using power monitoring data instead of heart rate during an actual event such as a time trial, the cyclist can more accurately define and ride the proper wattage needed for success independent of how the environmental conditions of race profile, ambient temperature and wind conditions are during the event that might affect heart rate responses (i.e. dehydration during cycling in hot climates).

Allen and Coggan (2006) wrote the first definitive and data-driven scientifically based book detailing key aspects and concepts they believed were needed for a cyclist to successfully use a power meter properly in both training and racing. Based on many years of cycling experience, numerous cycling performance research articles and actual data collected using software they developed specifically for analysing power data, Allen and Coggan introduced the cycling world to a new set of power related training variables that today are used by most athletes and coaches worldwide. In 2010, the second edition of their book *Training and Racing with a Power Meter* continued to refine their concepts (Allen and Coggan, 2010). In 2012, Allen teamed up with Stephen Cheung, PhD, who holds a Canada research chair in environmental ergonomics at Brock University, to further develop these concepts for advanced training concepts and elite cyclists (Allen and Cheung, 2012). Highlighted below are several of the core concepts and variables they introduced to the world of cycling.

Functional threshold power (FTP) is the highest power a cyclist can maintain in a semi-steady state ride for approximately 60 minutes. There are five ways to determine a person's FTP. These include the analysis of a person's power frequency distribution charts over multiple race days, the cyclist's normal sustainable power level for training rides, normalized power during several mass start races lasting 1 hour, normalized power for a 1-hour time trial (TT) event or simulation TT, and the use of critical power plots using TT durations between 3 and 30 minutes. While each of these methods produce similar FTP values, according to specificity of training principles and good testing practices discussed in the previous chapter, FTP testing should be directly determined whenever possible (i.e. 60-minute time trial).

Because time trial racing is very demanding, some sports performance experts recommend doing a 20-minute FTP test and then subtracting 5 per cent from the 20-minute FTP power results (20-minute FTP: 200 W − 5 W = 195 W) (Allen and Coggan, 2010; Friel, 2012). Currently, the most common method used for determining FTP consists of a cyclist doing a 20-minute time trial at the highest sustainable power pace possible after an adequate warm up period (20–30 minutes of cycling). Once the test is completed, 95 per cent of the average power achieved is considered the cyclist's FTP.

Once a person's FTP is determined, watt-training zones can be used to help a cyclist train more efficiently and effectively. The importance of training efficiently and effectively has a differential outcome purpose depending on the cyclist's current training status. For a beginning cyclist, knowing the cyclist's training zones helps that athlete train more effectively while helping the cyclist understand the various training intensity levels of proper sport performance training. At the same time, the sooner a beginning cyclist understands training intensity principles, the more likely the cyclist will train not only smarter, but with a decreased likelihood of injury or overtraining syndrome. In contrast, for the seasoned or elite-level cyclist, in addition to the beginning athlete benefits, using FTP training principles allows the high level cyclist to fine-tune training so that ideal periodization gains are achieved at the appropriate time to maximize race performance. In elite cycling, where races are often won by small margins, ensuring a cyclist trains properly is critical to not only his or her on-field success, but financially, as professional cyclists.

Table 20.2 summarizes how power-based training integrates with heart rate responses, ratings of perceived and continuous or interval training aspects. In the training zone system established by Allen and Coggan (2006, 2010), training zones are based on a cyclist's current FTP results. In addition, this table displays how each training zone would affect various aspects of physiological and biochemical adaptations to exercise training at a given zone (Allen and Coggan, 2010; Coyle *et al.*, 1988).

Normalized power is an expression of a cyclist's power output that can be maintained for a given event if power was perfectly constant (Allen and Coggan, 2010; Allen and Cheung, 2012). Normalized power takes into consideration ride variability due wind, climbs, descents, quick accelerations and long steady grinds in large gears at low RPMs. Simply taking a cyclist's average power output for a given ride does not accurately represent the pacing and environmental variability differences between two rides that may have the same mean power output. Normalized power attempts to take into consideration that many physiological acute responses such as lactate production, glycogen usage, and hormonal responses are curve-linear and have similar temporal responses as heart rate (Allen and Coggan, 2010). The greater the power output variability an event produces, the greater the variability index (VI), which is defined as the normalized power/average power. Thus, a steady-state power workout on an indoor trainer ride would have a VI of 1.00–1.02 compared to a hilly criterium VI of 1.20–1.35 (Allen and Coggan, 2010; Allen and Cheung, 2012).

To further illustrate how important the concept of normalized power is for understanding what true physiological impact a given cycle event might have on a rider, let us compare two distinctly different 1-hour-long workouts with nearly identical average power values. On day one, the athlete completes an upper level FTP workout with several hard 8–10 minute intervals (103–105 per cent of FTP Watts) on a slightly hilly course mixed with recovery in the low to middle end of the rider's endurance zone (69–75 per cent of FTP Watts). After the workout is completed, the cyclist's average watts for the entire interval workout were, say, equal to 268 $W.min^{-1}$. The cyclist's typical rating of perceived exertion (RPE) for such a workout would be 6–9 based on the 10-point Borg scale (Borg, 1982). The next day, the same cyclist completes a steady-state flat course 1-hour ride that also averages 265 $W.min^{-1}$ with an RPE of 4–5. Despite similar mean wattage, physiologically, the interval workout day was much more demanding, yet the average power values do not properly distinguish the difference. However, if we compared the same training ride data using normalized power accounting for the VIs of each ride, we would see a clear distinction between the two ride's perceived intensities because the variability index would be dramatically different. For illustration purposes, let us say that the interval-training day produced a VI similar to what is expected during a slightly hilly criterium course equal to 1.21 (Allen and Coggan, 2010). Despite the two rides having the same mean power averages, factoring in the 1.21 VI would show that the interval ride actually produced a physiological workload equal to a normative power of 324 W (268 W × 1.21 VI), which more closely represents the expected RPE for this cyclist's FTP interval workout. As a result, using normative power instead of overall power averages provides a better insight into the physiological impact that the two rides would have on the cyclist (Figure 20.4).

Intensity factor (IF) data take the concept of normalized power one step further by comparing what acute physiological impact a given workout or race event had on a cyclist. The intensity factor for a given ride, part of a ride or even group of rides is defined by dividing the ratio of a cyclist's normalized ride power by the athlete's current FTP (Allen and Coggan, 2010).

Table 20.2 Watt and heart rate training zones in relationship to potential metabolic and cardiovascular adaptations to training for a specific performance zone

Zone	Active recovery	Endurance	Tempo	Lactate threshold (functional threshold)	$\dot{V}O_2max$	Anaerobic capacity	Neuromuscular
% of Lactate or FTH	< 55	56–75	76–90	91–105	106–120	121–150	N/A
% of FTHR	< 68	69–83	84–94	95–105	> 106	N/A	N/A
RPE	< 2	2–3	4–5	6–7	7–8	> 8	Max
Continuous duration	30–90 min	60–300 min	60–180 min	N/A	N/A	N/A	N/A
Interval duration	N/A	N/A	N/A	8–30 min	3–8 min	30 sec–3 min	< 30 sec
Increased plasma volume		*	**	***	****	*	
Increased muscle mitochondrial enzyme		**	***	****	**	*	
Increased lactate threshold		**	***	****	**	*	
Increased muscle glycogen storage		**	****	***	**	*	
Hypertrophy of slow-twitch fibres		*	**	**	***	*	
Increased muscle capillarization		*	**	**	***	*	
Interconversion of fast-twitch fibres		**	***	***	**	*	
Increased stroke volume/cardiac output		*	**	***	****	*	
Increased $\dot{V}O_2$ max		*	**	***	****	*	
Increased ATP/PC storage						*	**
Increased anaerobic capacity					*	***	*
Fast-twitch muscle hypertrophy						*	**
Increased neuromuscular power						*	***

Source: Adapted from Allen and Coggan (2010: 48–9).

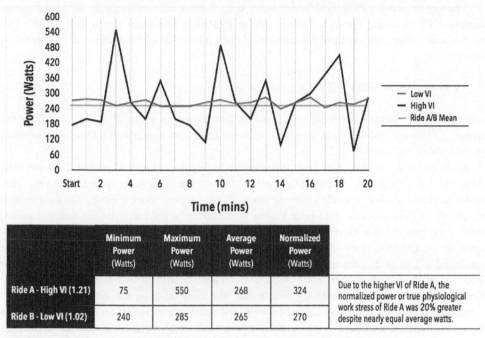

	Minimum Power (Watts)	Maximum Power (Watts)	Average Power (Watts)	Normalized Power (Watts)	
Ride A - High VI (1.21)	75	550	268	324	Due to the higher VI of Ride A, the normalized power or true physiological work stress of Ride A was 20% greater despite nearly equal average watts.
Ride B - Low VI (1.02)	240	285	265	270	

Figure 20.4 How variability index (VI) affects a ride's normative power value.

The larger the ratio produced, the stronger the relative physiological impact of the ride. Using the above VI ride samples for a cyclist with an FTP equal to 275 W, the steady state versus interval ride IF values would be 0.96 and 1.16, respectively. This information is extremely important when considering that cycling is a team event and that teammates will vary in FTP levels. For example, each rider on the team may maintain basically the same pace or even the same normative power for a given training ride. But the physiological impact for any given rider may vary greatly. Similarly, many team-training rides are designed to keep all the riders together. Therefore, some riders needing to maintain a given zone performance wattage to gain physiological improvement may not meet their target wattage goals depending on the drafting effects of where that cyclist is positioned for a majority of the ride. Without actual watt measurements relative the cyclist's FTP, the true physiological effect of the ride would be impossible to establish from heart rate or overall ride speed.

In this context, it is important to consider that cumulative physiological stress on an cyclist is a function of three main aspects of sports performance training; intensity, frequency and duration (American College of Sports Medicine, 2010; Wilmore *et al.*, 2008). Understanding how to balance these factors are the basis of training periodization principles and ensuring an athlete's training programme does not push an athlete from highly trained to either overreaching status or overtraining syndrome (Bompa, 1999). Through the utilization of advanced software programs such as TrainingPeaks WKO+, cyclists and coaches can now carefully monitor a rider's accumulative stress for a given training or race event (i.e. a training stress score). In combination with the basic impulse model, concepts originally developed by Banister used for modelling athletic performance (Banister, 1991), Allen and Coggan (2010) developed a series of similar algorithms to calculate a cyclist's overall training stress balance score (TSB), acute training load (ATL) and chronic training load (CTL).

Training stress score (TSS) is calculated based on a 1-hour time trial ride of the cyclist's most current FTP in watts. For each 1-hour ride at FTP, the ride score equals 100 points. The mathematical formula developed for calculating out a given ride's TSS is shown in the equation below:

$$\text{TSS} = [(s \times W \times IF) \,/\, (FTP \times 3,600] \times 100 \qquad (1)$$

where s = ride duration in seconds, W is normalized power in watts, IF is the ride's intensity factor, FTP is the athlete's most current functional threshold power and 3,600 is the number of seconds in an hour.

Knowing that a cyclist's time trial performance highly correlates ($r = -0.864 \pm 73$ seconds) with the cyclist's power output (Lucia *et al.*, 2004), the TSS score provides a very easy understandable marker of a ride's training stress. For example, riding a mostly flat course with some rolling hill 40K time trial under 1 hour is considered a gold standard for serious cyclists. Such a cycling effort is extremely hard work and requires proper recovery time to perform again at peak performance after an all-out time trial effort. Thus, if a given cycling event produced a TSS of 250 for an age group competitor and world-class professional cyclist, that TSS for both cyclists would still represent the same relative stress. Each cyclist basically experienced the stress of completing two-in-half 40k time trials on the same day.

Acute training load is the exponentially weighted moving average of an athlete's TSS. The ATL is usually set to 7 days, which represents the amount of work an athlete has performed over a 2-week period. In relationship to Bannister's impulse response model (Banister, 1991). ATL represents relative changes in performance ability due to the negative effects of fatigue (the second integral term in the equation).

Chronic training load provides a relative historical marker of the cyclist's training volume in relationship to training intensity calculated by taking a 42-day exponentially weighted moving average of the cyclist's daily TSS representing the athlete's 3-month workload. This value

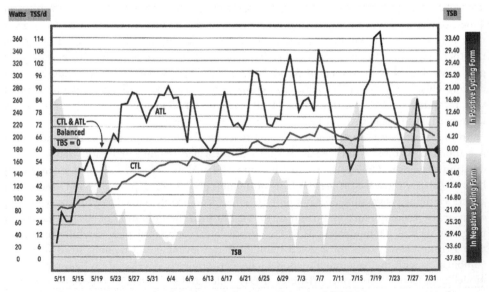

Figure 20.5 How acute training load (ATL) and chronic training load (CTL) interact on a rider's training stress balance (TSB) and current cycling form (adapted from Allen and Coggan, 2010, p. 153).

represents the relative positive effects of training or the first integral term in the Bannister impulse response model equation (Banister, 1991).

Training stress balance (TSB) is the difference between the CTL-ATL scores (Allen and Coggan, 2010; Allen and Cheung, 2012). The TSB score represents how a cyclist's current training compares to the person's historical data. As a result, a cyclist or his or her coach can now easily track the overall acute and chronic effects that a given training or race schedule has on the cyclist's overall training stress. More importantly, this information can be used to carefully design training programmes and race schedules so that the cyclist is in peak form prior to a major event (e.g. Olympic Time Trial or Road Race). These data can also be used during multi-day stage races to determine which riders are maintaining proper form and are the strongest. Additionally, these data provide valuable information regarding which riders are in best form to protect and support the team's leader they are trying to help win the race. The more positive the TSB score, the greater likelihood the cyclist is ready to perform at peak level. Conversely, negative scores imply a need for easier riding or a formal recovery period (i.e. taper). Figure 20.5 highlights how ATL, CTL, and TSB interact to provide a unique view of a cyclist's current training status.

How advanced power analysis software is revolutionizing cycling

Over the past decade, power meter technologies have not only advanced at a rapid pace, but the supporting software tools now assist cyclists and coaches to visualize the data as would be done in a research-like setting. These new software programs are not just providing simple data means and basic data charts. These programs are taking common variables such as heart rate, speed and cadence, along with new variables such as normalized power, ATL, CTL and TSB combined with GPS data, providing cyclists and coaches with extremely insightful views of a given cycling event or series of training sessions. With a simple data download, the click of a few buttons, the data results being produced currently through these advanced software technologies has now reached a level that often exceeds in quality and intricacy the data often presented in many peer review cycling research articles over the last 20 years.

For example, these software programs, in combination with standardized power testing protocols, allow cyclists and coaches to determine what are known as power or fatigue profiles. Power profiling compares a cyclist's watts per kilogram of body weight to known values produced by world-class cyclists at various time intervals (5 seconds, 1 minute, 5 minutes and FTP). Testing requires a warm-up period follow by a series of intervals at various intensity and duration levels. Once the power data are collected, they are analysed for each time segment and plotted accordingly. Figure 20.6 shows the clear distinctions between a category III cyclist and highly trained Ironman triathlete's power profile. These profiles basically tell us the general strengths and weakness of each athlete. Taking these data further, with the use of fatigue profiling, we can use power meter testing to further identify the type of sprinter or endurance cyclist a rider is. Fatigue power profiling protocols helps distinguish if the cyclist is lightening quick with exceptional max power but fatigues quickly or the cyclist, although powerful, can start out at 400 m from the finish line and maintain high power levels with little drop-off. Once a rider or his or her coach knows this type of information, both training and race strategies can be developed to enhance the cyclist's performance for a given race need.

One of the more interesting aspects of advanced power meter analysis software is the fact that the software options can assist a cyclist to more accurately match a specific race's demands with the required training programme for success (i.e. Ironman distance cycle segment). For example, pacing and how a triathlete achieves a given pace during the cycling segment of an

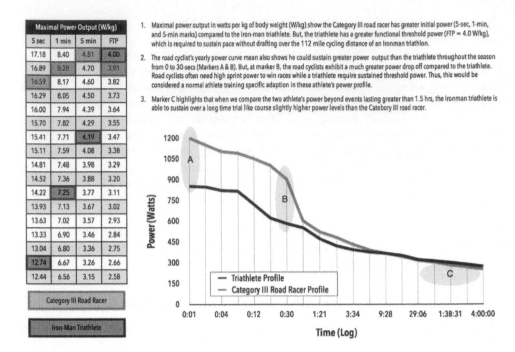

Maximal Power Output (W/kg)			
5 sec	1 min	5 min	FTP
17.18	8.40	4.81	4.00
16.89	8.28	4.70	3.91
16.59	8.17	4.60	3.82
16.29	8.05	4.50	3.73
16.00	7.94	4.39	3.64
15.70	7.82	4.29	3.55
15.41	7.71	4.19	3.47
15.11	7.59	4.08	3.38
14.81	7.48	3.98	3.29
14.52	7.36	3.88	3.20
14.22	7.25	3.77	3.11
13.93	7.13	3.67	3.02
13.63	7.02	3.57	2.93
13.33	6.90	3.46	2.84
13.04	6.80	3.36	2.75
12.74	6.67	3.26	2.66
12.44	6.56	3.15	2.58
Category III Road Racer			
Iron-Man Triathlete			

1. Maximal power output in watts per kg of body weight (W/kg) show the Category III road racer has greater initial power (5-sec, 1-min, and 5-min marks) compared to the Iron-man triathlete. But, the triathlete has a greater functional threshold power (FTP = 4.0 W/kg), which is required to sustain pace without drafting over the 112 mile cycling distance of an Ironman triathlon.

2. The road cyclist's yearly power curve mean also shows he could sustain greater power output than the triathlete throughout the season from 0 to 30-secs (Markers A & B). But, at marker B, the road cyclists exhibit a much greater power drop off compared to the triathlete. Road cyclists often need high sprint power to win races while a triathlete require sustained threshold power. Thus, this would be considered a normal athlete training specific adaption in these athlete's power profile.

3. Marker C highlights that when we compare the two athlete's power beyond events lasting greater than 1.5 hrs, the Ironman triathlete is able to sustain over a long time trial like course slightly higher power levels than the Catebory III road racer.

Figure 20.6 A peak power profile comparison and a yearly best mean maximal power curve (category III road racer versus Ironman triathlete) (adapted from Friel, 2012, pp. 75–6).

Ironman triathlon event is absolutely essential to a successful post-cycle marathon run (Earnest *et al.*, 2009; Foster *et al.*, 1993). This is especially true when the cycling aspect of the triathlon takes place on a hilly course, producing a large variability in power needs on the climbs and descents. According to Friel (2012), the optimum IF value for Ironman distance cycle segment is approximately 70 per cent of that triathlete's FTP value so adequate muscle glycogen and energy stores are available for the marathon. Through the use of power meter data and advanced cycling analysis software, a triathlete can now easily determine the best approach for optimizing pace during the event. This is accomplished by quadrant analysis, which helps the triathlete or coach evaluate the neuromuscular demands of a given cycling training session or race event relative to the triathlete's FTP power and cadence.

Power is determined by both the cadence and force produced at the time of measurement. Through a series of mathematical calculations using these variables, both average effective pedal force in Newtons (AEPF) and the circumferential pedal velocity can be derived (CPV) (Allen and Coggan, 2010). Plotting CPV on the x-axis and AEPF on the y-axis provides valuable information when the resulting graph includes cross-bars representing the triathlete's FTP expressed in AEPF and average cadence expressed in CPV (Figure 20.7). Looking closely at this chart, one can see four distinct quadrants: quadrant 1 – high force/high velocity; quadrant 2 – high force/low velocity; quadrant 3 – low force/low velocity; and, quadrant 4 – low force/high velocity. Additionally, because FTP and lactate threshold generally represent the intensity point in which muscle fibre recruitment patterns begin to include a cyclist's type II muscle fibres (McArdle *et al.*, 2009; Wilmore *et al.*, 2008), data points within a given quadrant help to identify an athlete's neuromuscular activation pattern (i.e. type I versus type II muscle fibres). Consequently, data points falling in quadrants 1 and 2 represent wattage values above FTP indicates, depending how high above the FTP crossbar, the cyclist is working at a rate

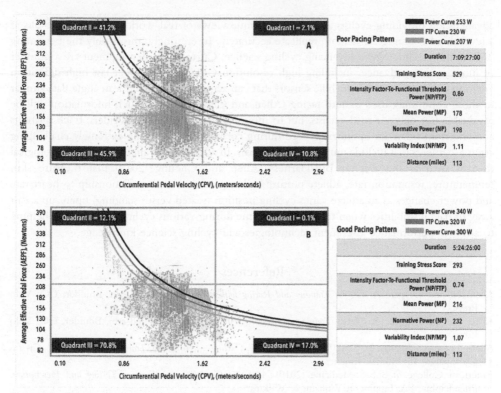

Figure 20.7 The use of quadrant analysis for analysing a triathlete's pacing profile (adapted from Allen and Coggan, 2010, pp. 218–19).

that requires more fast-twitch muscle fibres at that point in time. Conversely, when a cyclist's AEPF to CPV force-velocity plot places a given time point inside quadrants 3 and 4, the athlete is primarily relying on type I muscle fibres unless significant muscle fatigue has set in due to glycogen depletion, which leads to more type II fibre recruitment at lower workloads (Gollnick *et al.*, 1973).

In regards to pacing strategies, quadrant analysis allows a cyclist to visualize how a given pace was actually achieved. In context to our Ironman triathlete example above, the goal for the cycle portion of the race would be to maintain a pace that allowed the athlete to spend a majority of his or her race pace time in quadrants 3 and 4 (Figure 20.7). On the other hand, if pacing was such that the triathlete pushed too large a gear at lower cadence or CPV, this would result in the triathlete spending too much time in quadrant 2. The end result of this type of pacing strategy would lead to unwanted loss of muscle glycogen prior to the start of the marathon race segment diminishing the athlete's run performance. Thus, the use of quadrant analysis allows a triathlete and coach to fine tune effective strategies about pacing, rpm selection, gearing and even optimum crank length to help the rider achieve a target speed with the least detriment to glycogen stores prior to starting the post-ride marathon run.

Summary

Advances in both power meter technologies and analysis software development are revolutionizing and optimizing the training and monitoring of cyclists at all levels. These technological advances are providing cyclists and coaches unique views of real-world cycling data results at a level that lab testing can seldom replicate accurately. Interestingly, this is only the beginning of how new technology is advancing cycling science. Currently in development are a number of more exciting advances including high resolution GPS data and super fast high definition video in combination with on-bike sensors that can acquire braking and lean angle data similar to those commonly used in auto racing (Allen and Cheung, 2012). Such information will be invaluable not only for road cyclists, but to mountain bikers, cycle-cross riders, track sprinters and criterium riders for optimizing speed during corning or negotiating extremely challenging course segments that include jumps and sharp turns. In addition, the application of physiological devices such as the Zephyr Bio-Harness (Allen and Cheung, 2012) that measure skin temperature, respiration rate, athlete posture and acceleration rate in relationship to heart rate and power changes as an athlete varies cycling position (seated versus standing) opens up a vast array of data possibilities when tracked in real time during various cycling events while helping to advance performance assessment technologies and cycling science knowledge.

References

Allen, H. and Coggan, A. (2006) *Training and Racing with a Power Meter*, 1st edn, Boulder, CO: Velo Press.

Allen, H. and Coggan, A. (2010) *Training and Racing with a Power Meter*, 2nd edn, Boulder, CO: Velo Press.

Allen, H. and Cheung, S. S. (2012) *Cutting Edge Cycling – Advanced Training for Advanced Cyclist*, Champaign, IL: Human Kinetics.

American College of Sports Medicine (2010) *ACSM's Guidelines for Exercise Testing and Prescription*, Philadelphia, PA: Lippincott Williams & Wilkins.

Banister, E. W. (1991) 'Modeling elite athlete performance', in J. D. Mcdougall., H. J. Green and H. Wenger (eds), *Physiological Testing of the High Performance Athlete*, 2nd edn, Champaign, IL: Human Kinetics, pp. 403–25.

Benson, R. and Connolly, D. (2011) *Heart Rate Training*, Champaign, IL: Human Kinetics.

Bentley, D. J., McNaughton, L. R., Thompson, D., Vleck, V. E. and Batterham, A. M. (2001) 'Peak power output, the lactate threshold, and time trial performance in cyclists', *Medicine and Science in Sports and Exercise*, 33(12): 2077–81.

Bertucci, W., Duc, S., Villerius, V., Pernin, J. N. and Grappe, F. (2005) 'Validity and reliability of the powertap mobile cycling powermeter when compared with the SRM device', *International Journal of Sports Medicine*, 26(10): 868–73.

Bompa, T. O. (1999) *Periodization: Theory and Methodology of Training*, Champaign, IL: Human Kinetics.

Borg, G. A. (1982) 'Psychophysical bases of perceived exertion', *Medicine and Science in Sports and Exercise*, 14(5): 377–81.

Burke, E. R. (1998) *Precision Heart Rate Training*, Champaign, IL: Human Kinetics.

Burke, E. R. (2002) *Serious Cycling*, 2nd edn, Champaign, IL: Human Kinetics.

Coyle, E. F. (1999) 'Physiological determinants of endurance exercise performance', *Journal of Science and Medicine in Sport*, 2(3): 181–9.

Coyle, E. F., Coggan, A. R., Hopper, M. K. and Walters, T. J. (1988) 'Determinants of endurance in well-trained cyclists', *Journal of Applied Physiology*, 64(6): 2622–30.

Craig, N. P. and Norton, K. I. (2001) 'Characteristics of track cycling', *Sports Medicine*, 31(7): 457–68.

Dynastream Innovations Inc. (2012) *Ant+101: What is Ant+?*, available at: www.thisisant.com/consumer/ant-101/what-is-ant/ (accessed 1 September 2012).

Earnest, C. P., Foster, C., Hoyos, J., Muniesa, C. A., Santalla, A. and Lucia, A. (2009) 'Time trial exertion traits of cycling's grand tours', *International Journal of Sports Medicine*, 30(4): 240–4.

Fletcher, E. (n.d.) *Watt Bike: Training Guide*, available at: http://wattbike.com/uk/guide (accessed 5 August 2012).

Foster, C., Snyder, A. C., Thompson, N. N., Green, M. A., Foley, M. and Schrager, M. (1993) 'Effect of pacing strategy on cycle time trial performance', *Medicine and Science in Sports and Exercise*, 25(3): 383–8.

Friel, J. (2012) *The Power Meter Handbook*, Boulder, CO: Velo Press.

Gardner, A. S., Stephens, S., Martin, D. T., Lawton, E., Lee, H. and Jenkins, D. (2004) 'Accuracy of SRM and power tap power monitoring systems for bicycling', *Medicine and Science in Sports and Exercise*, 36(7): 1252–8.

Gardner, A. S., Martin, D. T., Barras, M., Jenkins, D. G. and Hahn, A. G. (2005) 'Power output demands of elite track sprint cycling', *International Journal of Performance Analysis in Sports*, 5(3): 149–54.

Glaskin, M. (2012) *Cycling Science*, Chicago: The University of Chicago Press.

Gollnick, P. D., Armstrong, R. B., Saubert IV, C. W., Sembrowich, W. L., Shepherd, R. E. and Saltin, B. (1973) 'Glycogen depletion patterns in human skeletal muscle fibers during prolonged work', *Pflugers Arch*, 344(1): 1–12.

Hawley, J. A. and Noakes, T. D. (1992) 'Peak power output predicts maximal oxygen uptake and performance time in trained cyclists', *European Journal of Applied Physiology*, 65(1): 79–83.

LOOK Cycle USA (n.d.) *Keo Power: The Power of Precision*, available at: www.lookcycle.com/en/us/route/pedales/keo-power.html (accessed 5 August 2012).

Lucia, A., Earnest, C. P. and Arribas, C. (2003) 'The Tour de France: a physiological review', *Scandinavian Journal of Medicine and Science in Sports*, 13(5): 275–83.

Lucia, A., Hoyos, J., Perez, M., Santalla, A., Earnest, C. P. and Chicharro, J. L. (2004) 'Which laboratory variable is related with time trial performance time in the Tour de France?', *British Journal of Sports Medicine*, 38(5): 636–40.

McArdle, W. D., Katch, F. L. and Katch, V. L. (2009) *Exercise Physiology: Nutrition, Energy, and Human Performance*, 7th edn, North American Edition, Philadelphia, PA: Lippincott Williams & Wilkins.

Martin, D. T. (2012) 'Winning the Tour de France: a sport science perspective', *Proceedings of the 17th Annual Congress of European College of Sport Science*, Bruges, Belgium.

Millet, G. P., Tronche, C., Fuster, N., Bentley, D. J. and Candau, R. (2003) 'Validity and reliability of the polar s710 mobile cycling powermeter', *International Journal of Sports Medicine*, 24(3): 156–61.

Noakes, T. D., Peltonen, J. E. and Rusko, H. K. (2001) 'Evidence that a central governor regulates exercise performance during acute hypoxia and hyperoxia', *The Journal of Experimental Biology*, 204(18): 3225–34.

Saltin, B. (1969) 'Physiological effects of physical conditioning', *Medicine and Science in Sports and Exercise*, 1: 50–6.

Santalla, A., Earnest, C. P., Marroyo, J. A. and Lucia, A. (2012) 'The Tour de France: an updated physiological review', *International Journal of Sports Physiology and Performance*, 7(3): 200–9.

Smith, M. F., Davison, R. C., Balmer, J. and Bird, S. R. (2001) 'Reliability of mean power recorded during indoor and outdoor self-paced 40 km cycling time-trials', *International Journal of Sports Medicine*, 22(4): 270–4.

SRM (n.d.) *Our Story of Success: Setting the Gold Standard in Sports Power Measurement*, available at: www.srm.de/us/unternehmen/our-story-of-success (accessed 5 August 2012).

St Clair Gibson, A., Lambert, M. L. and Noakes, T. D. (2001) 'Neural control of force output during maximal and submaximal exercise', *Sports Medicine*, 31(9): 637–50.

Stages Cycling (2012) *Technology: Our Power Meter May be Small in Stature, but it Packs a Technological Wallop*, available at: www.stagescycling.com/stagespower-tech-specs (accessed 10 September 2012).

Warner, P. (2012) Phone interview with the Vice president of Stages Cycling and C. E. Broeder (personal communication, 30 October 2012).

Wilmore, J. H., Costill, D. L. and Kenney, W. L. (2008) *Physiology of Sport and Exercise*, 4th edn, Champaign, IL: Human Kinetics.

21

SELECTION OF PARAMETERS USING GROUND REACTION FORCE MEASUREMENT AND 3D MOTION CAPTURE FOR DEVELOPING BIOMECHANICAL FEEDBACK TRAINING IN GOLF

Gongbing Shan,[1,2] *Nils Betzler,*[1,3] *Xiang Zhang*[1,4] *and Daifei Yu*[5]

[1]UNIVERSITY OF LETHBRIDGE, LETHBRIDGE
[2]SHAANXI NORMAL UNIVERSITY, XIAN
[3]UNIVERSITY OF MAGDEBURG, MAGDEBURG
[4]XINZHOU TEACHERS UNIVERSITY, XINZHOU
[5]SHANDONG INSTITUTE OF PHYSICAL EDUCATION AND SPORT, JINAN

Introduction

One of sport medicine goals is to promote people to involve more physical activity in order to develop positive altitude and health lifestyle. Therefore, studies on developing effective human motor skill learning/training will benefit every one of us, as it can help us to develop interests to involve more physical activity during the life span (Chen and Ennis, 2004). Studies, especially the one led by Professor Dr Paffenbarger at Harvard University involving 50,000 alumni who graduated between 1916 and 1950, show that more active involvement in physical activity will achieve healthy ageing by increasing life expectancy and gaining disability-free years during senior time (Nusselder *et al.*, 2008; Paffenbarger *et al.*, 1986). These studies indicate that the two key factors for promoting population health are: (1) to identify types of physical activities that can cover large population (i.e. the popular sports) across all age groups; and (2) to develop effective training methods for the selected sports. Among the top 10 most popular sports played in the world (Chintu, 2012), golf is the only one widely participated by all age groups (Table 21.1). It is well known that the dominant skill in golf is the swing. Therefore, scientific studies on golf swing will benefit both the development of effective training methods and the promotion of population health.

Golf swings are complicated movements that require coordination of all major body segments (Shan *et al.*, 2011). Given the complexity of golf swing, informed training holds the potential

Table 21.1 Comparison among selected top 10 sports (Chintu, 2012) related to the age of participants (shown in per cent)

		#10 Golf (%)		#1 Soccer (%)	#5 Baseball (%)	#6 Basketball (%)
Age breakdown	< 30	5	< 24	77	67	66
	30–39	12	25–34	11	11	14
	40–49	22	35–44	7	12	12
	50–59	24	45–54	4	9	7
	60–69	18				
	> 70	19	> 54	1	1	1

The table indicates that #1 soccer, #5 baseball and #6 basketball have the most youthful profiles while #10 golf is played similarly by all age groups (data are based on the Active Network, Inc, 2007; US Census Department, 2012).

to improve efficiencies, particularly in the acquisition of cognitive and psychomotor skills. Studies on various human motor skills have proven that informed training is resourceful for high-performance activities (Magill, 2001; Raymond *et al.*, 2005; Smith and Loschner, 2002; Visentin *et al.*, 2008). Hence, studies on golf swing should focus on how to develop informed training method.

The dominant component in developing informed training is biofeedback (Schmidt, 1988). Previous studies have shown that when properly understood and applied, biofeedback is an excellent tool for enhancing practice and performance of human motor skills (Egner and Gruzelier, 2003; Jonsdottir *et al.*, 2007; Landers *et al.*, 1994; Markovska-Simoska *et al.*, 2008; Page and Hawkins, 2003; Raymond *et al.*, 2005; Smith and Loschner, 2002). Among numerous types of biofeedback, biomechanical ones (kinematics: joint angles and their coordination; kinetics: force applied and muscle activities) are proven to be valuable by allowing the users to self-adjust problem areas based on the biofeedback provided by devices (Ng *et al.*, 2008; Niemann *et al.*, 1993; Petruzzello *et al.*, 1991; Vernon, 2005). Despite a few successful cases, the application of biomechanical feedback is still rare in practice. After reviewing 666 publications between 1965 and 2007, Tate and Milner (2010) have found that there are only seven studies using real-time biomechanical feedback in rehabilitation. This rarity is caused by the numerous challenges that must be addressed during the development of real-time biomechanical feedback tools. Biomechanical feedback is always specific, requiring different design parameters for different sport skills. Unlike physiological (heart rate, blood pressure, breathing rate, temperature and muscle activities) and neurofeedback (EEG: brain-wave), there is no universal parameter (e.g. heart rate for loading intensity in all sports) that exists for biomechanical feedback. In other words, for developing a biomechanical feedback device, one must first obtain a thorough biomechanical understanding of the selected sport skill in order to select useful parameters for monitoring. Currently, the advance of golf swing study could reach the stage for developing real-time informed training methods/devices for practitioners.

Well-executed golf swings must be both powerful and accurate: the swing must be full speed yet precise enough to ensure a square hit. To help players execute good golf swings, there has been a great deal of golf research in the past decades, investigating various technical aspects of the swing (Betzler *et al.*, 2008; Egret *et al.*, 2003; Hay, 1981; Hume *et al.*, 2005; Neal and Wilson, 1985; Shan *et al.*, 2011; Zhang and Shan, in press). These studies aimed to identify major factors that contribute to better swings by measuring body segment velocities and accelerations, joint angles, ground reaction forces, ball velocities and trajectories, as well as factors related to ball impact and equipment. Such research has successfully yielded insightful instructions on how to execute good golf swings, but none, to the best knowledge of the authors, addresses how to develop an effective informed training based on the results for practitioners.

Studies in the past decades indicate that the synchronized measurement of ground reaction force (GRF) and 3D motion capture holds great potential for developing real-time biofeedback training for golf swing (Betzler *et al.*, 2008; Egret *et al.*, 2003; Hay, 1981; Hume *et al.*, 2005; Neal and Wilson, 1985; Shan *et al.*, 2011; Zhang and Shan, in press), but requires further research before it can become an impactful real-time feedback tool in the real world. Two questions remain to be answered before a practical tool can be developed: (1) the dominant parameters selected for feedback; and (2) the practicality of the measuring devices. So far, there are more than 20 parameters identified in the literature, ranging from kinematics to kinetics (Zhang and Shan, in press). Using multiple sources of information to trainees may impair their practice with overloaded information (Huang *et al.*, 2005). For increasing training efficiency and effectiveness, it is important to choose the dominant information or variables for feedback in order to overcome the information overloading obstacle for practitioners. As for the practicality of the measuring devices, force platforms for GRF collection are sufficiently practical, while the currently marketed 3D motion capture systems are not. Therefore, by applying the synchronized measurement of GRF and 3D motion capture in combination with a 15-segment, full-body biomechanical model (Shan and Westerhoff, 2005), this study tried to: (1) quantify and select the practical/dominant parameters for golf swing training; and (2) determine the minimum number of cameras used during capture in order to simplify the measuring system for developing a user-friendly, real-time biofeedback system for golf swing training.

Method

Subjects and test clubs

Twenty-six experienced, right-handed male golfers were recruited for this study. The subjects averaged 34.6 ± 12.9 years of age, 1.81 ± 0.06 m tall and 91.9 ± 14.0 kg in weight. The subject skill level varied in a remarkable range, from 3 to 29 years of training experience and from 4 to 26 handicaps. Such a test group could supply sufficient evidences related to the quantification of swing skill development and aid to build a foundation for biofeedback training. The Human Subjects Research Committee of the University of Lethbridge scrutinized and approved this protocol as meeting the criteria from the Tri-Council Policy Statement: Ethical Conduct for Research Involving Humans, from the Natural Sciences and Engineering Research Council. All subjects in the study were informed of the testing procedures. They signed an approved consent form and voluntarily participated in the data collection.

For quantification of swing characteristics, a driver and 7 iron were selected to represent a typical clubs used for swing in practice. Each participant used his own driver and 7 iron during the data collection.

Data collection and processing

Two force plates were synchronized with a 3D motion capture system to record the ground reaction forces throughout the swings (Kistler 9826AA, f = 1,050 Hz). A 12-camera VICON motion capture system (VICON Motion Systems, Oxford Metrics Ltd., Oxford, UK) was used to measure full-body movement using 46 reflective markers – 42 on the body, three on golf clubs and one on the ball. The 3D motion capture system tracked the markers at a rate of 250 frames per second. Figure 21.1 shows the synchronized test set-up, a 3D computer recon-struction of a single trial including camera placement, capture volume and a rendered stick figure of a test subject.

The two Kistler force platforms (one under each foot) were used to capture the weight transfer during a golf swing. 2D (anterior-posterior and medial-lateral) weight transfer data were collected to characterize the dynamic balancing/stability of the swing. As mentioned above, the data collection of the ground reaction force was synchronized to the 3D motion capture.

Forty-two body markers (9 mm in diameter) were used for kinematic data collection in order to build a 15-segment full-body biomechanical model for swing quantification (Shan and Bohn, 2003; Shan and Westerhoff, 2005). Markers were placed on subjects as follows: (1) four on the head; (2) trunk markers on the sternal end of the clavicle, xiphoid process of the sternum, C7 and T10 vertebrae, right and left scapula, left and right anterior superior iliac, posterior superior iliac; (3) upper-extremity markers on the right and left acromion, lateral side of upper arm, lateral epicondyle, lateral side of forearm, styloid processes of radius and ulna and distal end of third metacarpal bones; and (4) lower extremities markers on left and right lateral sides of thigh and shank, lateral tibia condyle, lateral malleolus, calcaneal tuberosity, tuberosity of the fifth metatarsal and big toe. Calibration residuals were determined in accordance with VICON's guidelines and yielded positional data accurate within 0.4 mm. Kinematic data collected using this marker set supplied information such as marker position at all times, changes of position, velocities, and accelerations, joint angles and ranges of motion (ROMs), as well as club head speed, ball release angle and speed. The parameters were used to quantify/characterize motor control patterns of golfers with different swing skills.

Before data collection, subjects were allowed to warm up and could perform a sufficient number of swings to get used to the test environment. For testing, they performed three good golf swings (subjective identification of individuals) with a driver and three with a 7 iron. Each subject decided on his own pacing, so that the individual's optimal motor control patterns could be measured. Golf balls were placed on an artificial golf mat (2 × 2 m²) used to mimic

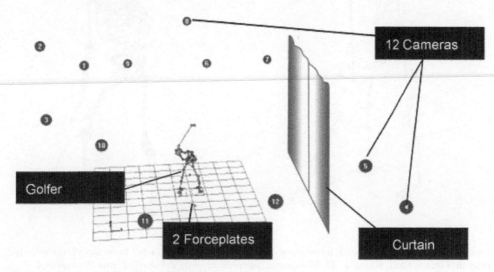

Figure 21.1 Set-up of the test environment.

grass. Subjects stood on the two Kistler force platforms (one platform under each foot) and shot golf balls towards a large vertically hanging curtain (7×7 m², Figure 21.1). The test set-up allowed us to use a relatively large capture volume, which permitted considerable freedom of movement for the subjects, and we placed no restrictions on the subjects. These efforts let the subjects preserve their normal motor control style.

Raw kinematic data were processed using a five-point (1-3-4-3-1 function) smoothing filter and the resultant data were input into the 15-segment biomechanical full-body model in order to determine segment lengths and angles, and subjects' centre of gravity (COG), as well as joint angles and ROMs. Model segments were identified as follows: head, upper trunk, lower trunk, upper arms, lower arms, hands, thighs, shanks and feet. In such biomechanical modelling, inertial characteristics of the body are estimated using anthropometric norms found through statistical studies (Shan and Bohn, 2003). Figure 21.2 shows a still frame of one trial and our 3D computer reconstruction of the full-body, 15-segment model (skeleton) plus golf club and ball.

Data analysis – GRF

A previous study has shown that the centre of ground reaction force (CGRF) measured by force platform and the COG obtained through 3D motion capture and biomechanical modelling are not identical for a golf swing (i.e. they are usually separated with each other) (Shan *et al.*, 2011) (Figure 21.3). Thus, by comparing the dynamic CGRF to the dynamic COG (or timely separation of CGRF and COG), the effects of club on swing control (or how skilful of a subject's swing) can be quantified and revealed. The current study employed this method to identify the influences of swing skill level and anthropometry (i.e. body type heavy – body mass index (BMI) > 25 kg.m⁻² and body type light – BMI < 20 kg.m⁻²) (Vaz de Almeida *et al.*, 1999). There were nine subjects characterized as body type heavy and four as body type light.

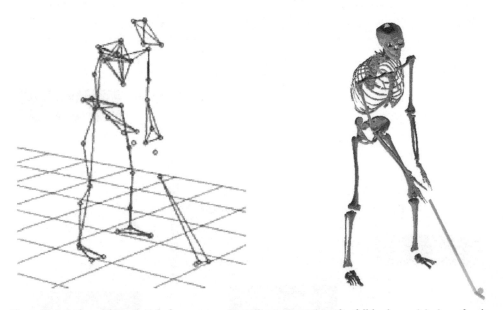

Figure 21.2 Left: a digitized stick figure using 46 markers: 42 markers for full body model, three for the drive and one for ball. Right: a 3D, 17-segment, biomechanical model derived from the captured markers; 15 segments for body, one segment each for golf club and ball.

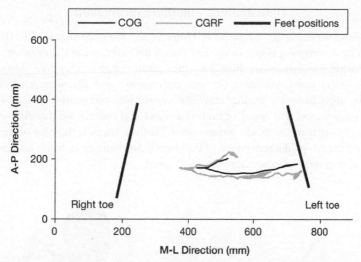

Figure 21.3 The separation of centre of gravity (COG) and centre of ground reaction force (CGRF) during a golf swing. The separation shows an effect of body–club interaction (Shan *et al.*, 2011).

Data analysis – phase definition

Golf literature commonly divides the swing movement into different phases (Ballreich and Schöllhorn, 1992; Maltby, 1995; Trevino, 1992). For analysing the synchronized data in order to identify factors with potential of real-time biofeedback, the current study employed an approach of three events and two phases to examine the swing. The three events are: (1) take-away (begin of a backswing); (2) top of backswing; and (3) ball contact. Between events 1 and 2 is the first phase – backswing – and between events 2 and 3 the second phase – downswing (Figure 21.4).

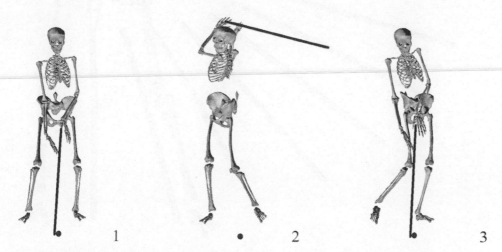

Figure 21.4 Posture characterization of golf swing using 3D 15-segment, full-body model: (1) take-away; (2) top of backswing; and (3) ball contact.

Data analysis – motion capture data

Previous studies (Betzler *et al.*, 2006, 2008; Hume *et al.*, 2005; Shan *et al.*, 2011) have shown that a whip-like downswing is one of the key factors for maximizing the distance of golf shots. Several kinematic parameters are linked to the quality of the whip-like downswing. The parameters are: (1) trunk rotation; (2) arm movement; and (3) wrist extension/flexion, determined by angle between (leading arm) elbow-wrist line and wrist-club line (Figure 21.5). These studies confirmed that speed of both club head and ball release depends on the timely coordination among trunk, arm and wrist control. Further, trunk is the root of the trunk-arm-club chain, and the whip-like movement of the chain should initiate in trunk rotation; therefore, trunk rotation is crucial in increasing club head speed.

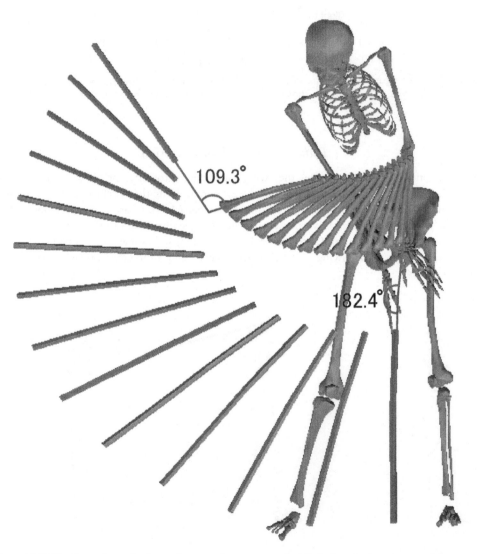

Figure 21.5 The dynamic angle change between lower arm and club during the last quarter of the downswing time.

Among the literature-identified key parameters, trunk rotation could be practically quantified using one camera (an overhead-positioned camera); since the rotation depends on shoulder-hip coordination, a timely difference between these two lines in the transverse (horizontal) plane would characterize the quality of the trunk rotation during a swing. Based on the previous results, the current study focused on the analysis of the timely control of the trunk-arm-club chain (i.e. a degree of a whip-like movement of a chain), as well as the possibility and reliability of quantifying the degree/quality of the whip-like movement in a transverse plan instead of in a 3D space.

Data analysis – numerical quantification

Finally, grouping approach with statistical t-test was applied to both GRF and motion capture data in order to characterize the skill levels among subjects, and correlation analysis was employed to identify the possible influence of the selected parameters on swing quality. The results obtained were used to aid a discussion on the practicality and possibility of developing real-time feedback training for golf swing practice.

Results

The analysis of the synchronized measurement of GRF and 3D motion capture revealed that data exhibit high variations, suggesting the difference of swing quality among the selected subjects was distinguishable. We contrasted the measured data for identifying key parameters that are prone to motor control variations, thus requiring extra attention (or biofeedback) during swing training. Such information could be used to establish a real-time biofeedback practice system in order to increase training efficiency. Our data showed that CGRF, trunk rotation and wrist control confounded with the body and club type had most influence on swing effectiveness or ball release speed.

CGRF and COG excursions

Based on the CGRF excursions in the transverse (horizontal) plane, the swing efficiency of the tested subjects can be grouped into three types: optimal weight transfer, early weight transfer and unstable weight transfer (Figure 21.6). Our data showed that the swing efficiency/control stability was influenced by the body-club interaction. For showing the effect of body-club interaction on the control stability, COG excursion obtained from 3D motion capture and biomechanical modelling has also been added in Figure 21.6. The data indicated that the less skillful subjects experienced more CGRF excursion than more advanced golfers ($p < 0.05$). Correlation analysis showed that the longer the CGRF curve length was, the slower the ball release speed ($|r| = 0.77$). Further, the subjects characterized with unstable weight transfer also demonstrated that the right foot carried more weight than the left one, as well as rear feet were assigned more load than forefeet, while the skilled subjects presented a reversed result ($p < 0.05$).

Additionally, the CGRF and COG results revealed distinguishable differences of club swing between using a driver and 7 iron. It was found that the driver caused more: (1) excursion range; and (2) separation between COG and CGRF than 7 iron in both medial-lateral (M-L) and anterior-posterior (A-P) directions during CGRF and COG excursions ($p < 0.01$, Figure 21.7). Furthermore, the typical weight transfer diagram indicated that both CGRF and COG transferred more in the M-L direction than in the A-P for using both driver and 7 iron clubs

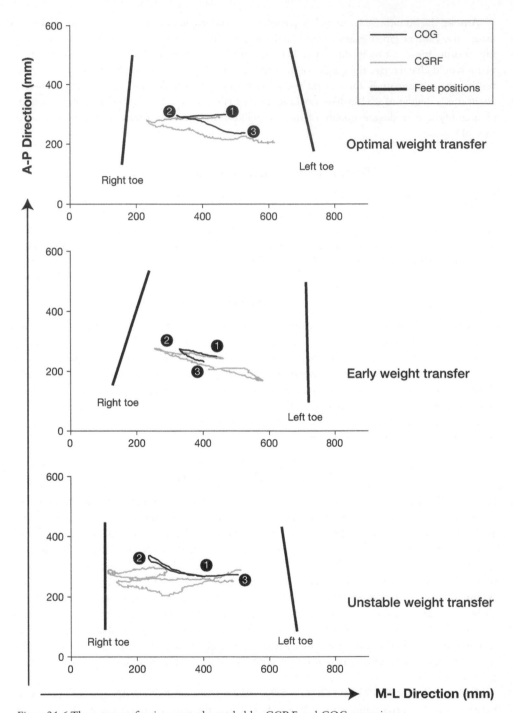

Figure 21.6 Three types of swing control revealed by CGRF and COG excursions.

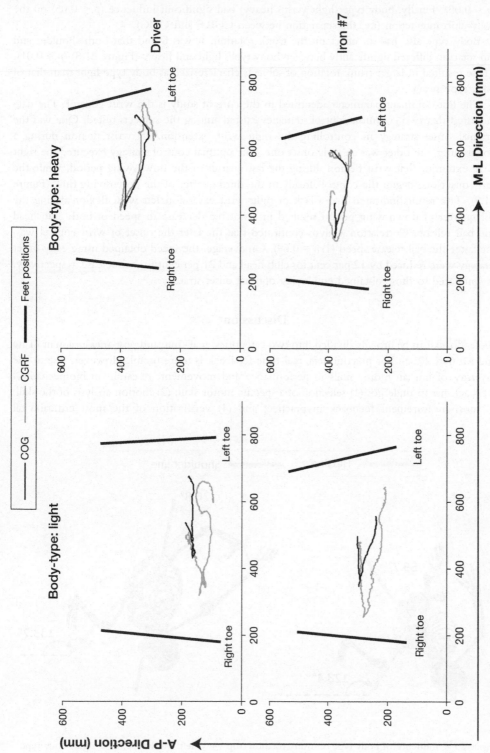

Figure 21.7 Influences of club and body type on weight transfer.

(p < 0.05). Finally, body type (light versus heavy) had significant influence (p < 0.05) on the body-club interaction (i.e. the separation between CGRF and COG).

Body type also had an effect on the trunk rotation. It was found that both shoulder and hip rotation differed significantly between body types light and heavy (Figure 21.8) (p < 0.01). These resulted in larger trunk rotation of subjects characterized as body type light than that of body type heavy.

The last dominant parameter identified in the current study is the wrist control. The data indicated that two common control strategies existed among the subjects tested. One was the optimal onset strategy in controlling the right wrist extension/left wrist flexion during a downswing, the other was an early onset one. The optimal control strategy executed the right wrist extension/left wrist flexion during the last quarter of the downswing period, while the early onset one begun the control already in the third quarter of the downswing time (Figure 21.9). The results indicated that a lack of right wrist extension/left wrist flexion during the last quarter of downswing period resulted in a notable decrease in speed of both club head and ball release. Correlation analysis confirmed that the later the onset of wrist control was, the faster the ball release speed ($|r|$ = 0.69). On average, the speed obtained using early onset strategy were reduced by 12 per cent for club head and 21 per cent for ball release, respectively, as compared to those obtained employing optimal onset strategy.

Discussion

Biofeedback can be broadly divided into two categories: real-time and post-measurement (Tate and Milner, 2010). For practitioners, real-time feedback is more useful. However, due to the diversity of human motor skills in performance and movement, research on biomechanical feedback has to undergo: (1) selection of a specific motor skill; (2) motion analysis of the skill; (3) post-measurement feedback in practice; and (4) verification of the most critical/vital

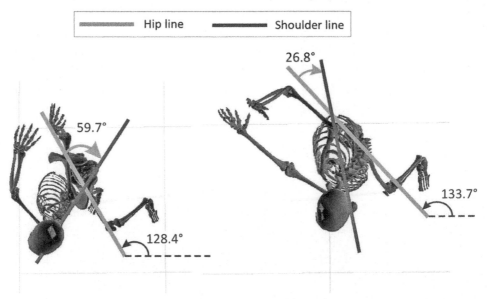

Figure 21.8 Influence of body type on trunk rotation (top view; left: body type light; right: body type heavy).

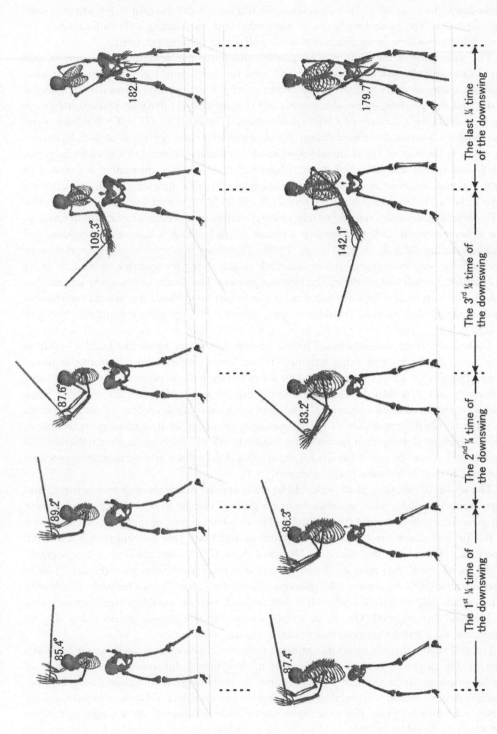

Figure 21.9 Two types of wrist control during the downswing revealed by 3D motion capture (top: optimal onset of wrist control, i.e. right wrist extension/left wrist flexion in the last quarter of the downswing period; bottom: too early onset of wrist control).

parameter(s) for the given motor skill in order to develop a device capable of real-time biofeedback. In other words, post-measurement feedback is the essential step leading to real-time feedback. The current study is a post-measurement one, aiming to lay a foundation for developing a real-time biofeedback system for golf swing training/practice.

The main goal of the study was to quantify and select the dominant parameters of golf swing that could be practically collected and used for developing a real-time biomechanical feedback system in order to improve the efficiency of golf swing training/practice. The results of this and our previous studies (Shan *et al.*, 2011) suggested: (1) dynamic postural stability is the fundament for a delivery of a high-quality swing (Figure 21.6); (2) golf ball release speed mainly depends on the downward swing control of a physics chain (i.e. trunk-arm-club system); (3) trunk is the root of the chain and a whip-like movement/control of the chain increases ball release speed; and (4) a high quality/degree of the whip-like movement is initiated in trunk rotation, followed by arm downswing and finished with a right wrist extension/left wrist flexion shortly before ball contact (Figures 21.8 and 21.9). It is well known that an effective task-oriented biofeedback training system requires orchestrated feedbacks of multiple variables that characterize the task performance without overwhelming a learner's perception and cognitive ability (Magill, 2001; Schmidt, 1988). Therefore, it is vital to select the dominant characteristics of a complicated motor skill such as golf swing for feedback training in order to optimize the skill and accelerate the learning process. The results of this study suggest that real-time biomechanical feedback focusing on the factors listed above (i.e. weight transfer and trunk-arm-club coordination) should have great potential for improving training effects of golf swing.

Technically, three well-established biomechanical devices are needed to build a real-time monitoring system for golf swing training: (1) two force platforms for monitoring dynamic weight transfer; (2) a motion capture system for monitoring the movement of the trunk-arm-club chain; and (3) a radar device for monitoring ball release speed. Practically, there are three challenges that need to be addressed: (1) potential constraints of the selected measuring systems on subjects; (2) the practicality of the measuring systems' set-up in a training environment; and (3) software development for real-time feedback. All evidences so far have indicated that there have been no technical barriers for developing the feedback system; therefore, potential problems remain only in the practical aspects.

The set-up of two force platforms could be easily applied in any training environment. And force platforms usually place no restrictions on golfers' swings; hence, CGRF measurement can preserve a golfer's normal control 'style'. The unsolved aspects of applying force platforms in real-time feedback are to add COG excursion and body type influences to the CGRF monitoring. Based on a study done by Shan and Bohn (2003), one could use a five-segment model (head-trunk, two arms and two legs) and one camera with top view (Figure 21.8) to determine the COG excursion in the transverse (horizontal) plane. Such a real-time monitoring system needs only nine track markers (i.e. one on head, two on shoulders, two on wrists, two on hips and two on feet). Due to its simple set-up, the one camera system places also no restrictions on a golfer's movement within the capture volume.

For golf swing, there is no single optimum movement pattern that can be generalized as a 'best fit' for all golfers because of differences in the physical dimensions of a golfer's body (anthropometry). Anthropometry influences how the body interacts with clubs during a swing, which is directly related to gestural timing. What we perceive of as 'differences in style' among golfers may thus be partly due to anthropometric individualization. As a result, golf swing optimization should be individualized according to anthropometrical variation. Combined with the findings of this study, one could write a programme for integrating COG excursion (obtained through one-camera capture and biomechanical modelling) and the body type/weight influence into CGRF monitoring in order to guide an individualized training for swing optimization. In summary, it is doable and practical to use two force platforms and one overhead camera for a real-time monitoring of CGRF and COG during golf swing training. Proper analysis software should be developed to guide individuals of different body types using different clubs.

Clearly, applying a 3D motion capture system with multiple cameras (like the 3D motion capture system used in this study) for real-time monitoring the movement of the trunk-arm-club chain is not practical at all in a training environment. Simplification of measuring system hardware has to be induced. The ideal solution is that the 3D control characteristics could be represented by using 2D quantification (i.e. using one camera system instead of a multi-camera system). The results of this study indicate that the whip-like movement of the trunk-arm-club chain is initiated in trunk rotation, followed by arm downswing and finished with a right wrist extension/left wrist flexion shortly before the ball contact. Figure 21.8 and our previous discussion (i.e. five-segment model) have indicated that the timely coordination of trunk and arm could be quantified using 2D characteristics in the transverse (horizontal) plane. Similarly, wrist control could also be quantified by the dynamic changes of the golf club length and orientation, as well as left arm orientation in the transverse plane (Figure 21.10). For reaching this, no additional hardware would be required; only adding two reflective markers on the club would be sufficient. The next step is to develop proper analysis software related to the whip-like movement control of the trunk-arm-club chain. Such a programme should also provide optimization feedback for individuals of different body types using different clubs.

Finally, radar gun has been widely used in the training and playing environment for measuring club head and/or ball release speed effectively with minimal set-up, as well as having no intrusion on one's swing during practice (Hellström, 2009; Thompson *et al.*, 2007). Most measuring devices of this kind are extremely portable; as such, they are perfect for taking out on the practice tee.

Summarized above, in the views of the authors, a synchronized measurement using two force platforms, one overhead camera with 11 reflective markers and a mini radar device should be able to supply real-time biomechanical feedback on the swing quality by quantifying: (1) the dynamic weight transfer pattern; (2) the degree of whip-like movement of the trunk-arm-club chain; and (3) the release speed of the golf ball after impact. Up to now, the missing element for developing the real-time feedback system is to write a programme to integrate these three aspects. By linking interpretation of the results to practical realities of the endeavour,

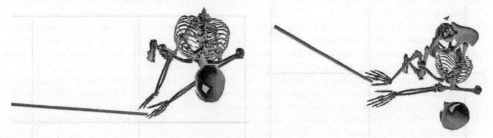

Figure 21.10 The posture comparison of two different subjects at the beginning of the last quarter of the downswing period (top view). The club length in the transverse plane of the left subject is longer than that of right subject, indicating that the left subject employs a strategy of early onset of wrist control. Such a control strategy decreases the ball release speed notably.

it is possible to provide pedagogical meaning that has applications across large cohorts of players, as well as for individuals. Anthropometric differences may be a factor in individual style, but biofeedback training may fundamentally affect the optimization process of individual motor behaviours. Once such a system is available, further studies can be launched to evaluate its efficiency and practical relevance for the swing skill training.

Conclusion

In conclusion, biomechanical feedback holds great potential, but requires much more research before it can become an impactful tool in the real world. This study aimed to establish key foundational work for a development of a real-time biomechanical feedback system for golf swing training. The results of the study have revealed that the effectiveness of a swing could be evaluated by: (1) dynamic weight transfer; (2) degree of whip-like movement of trunk-arm-club chain; and (3) ball release speed. Real-time feedback on these three aspects should hold great potentials for increasing learning/practice efficiency. Technically, synchronization of two force platforms, one overhead camera and a mini radar device is good, and practical enough for delivering a real-time monitoring. So far, the missing element for the real-time feedback has been an evaluation model (i.e. computer program) that integrates the results from all three measurements and visualizes them to learners/practitioners.

Acknowledgement

This work was supported by National Sciences and Engineering Research Council of Canada (NSERC), Sport Science Association of Alberta (SSAA/Canada), Shanxi Scholarship Council of China and Science Research Grant of Province Shanxi/China.

References

Active Network, Inc. (2007) *The Soccer Market – Rewards*, available at: www.activenetworkrewards. com/Assets/AMG+2009/Soccer.pdf (accessed 23 September 2012.

Ballreich, R. and Schöllhorn, W. (1992) 'Golf', in R. Ballreich and A. Kuhlow-Ballreich (eds), *Biomechanik der sportarten*, Stuttgart: Enke Ferdinand, pp. 30–108.

Betzler, N., Hofmann, M., Shan, G. and Witte, K. (2006) 'Biomechanical modelling of a golf swing by means of the multibody-kinetics software ADAMS', *International Journal of Computer Science in Sport*, 5(2): 52–5.

Betzler, N., Monk, S., Wallace, E., Otto, S. and Shan, G. (2008) 'From the double pendulum model to full-body simulation: the evolution of golf swing modelling', *Sport Technology*, 1(4–5): 175–88.

Chen, A. and Ennis, C. (2004) 'Goals, interests, and learning in physical education', *Journal of Educational Research*, 97(6): 329–39.

Chintu, A. P. (2012) *Top 10 Most Popular Sports Played in the World*, available at: http://omgtoptens. com/entertainment/top-10-most-popular-sports-played-in-the-world/ (accessed 11 December 2012).

Egner, T. and Gruzelier, J. H. (2003) 'Ecological validity of neurofeedback: modulation of slow wave EEG enhances musical performance', *Neuroreport*, 14(9): 1221–4.

Egret, C. I., Vincent, O., Weber, J., Dujardin, F. H. and Chollet, D. (2003) 'Analysis of 3D kinematics concerning three different clubs in golf swing', *International Journal of Sports Medicine*, 24(6): 465–9.

Hay, J. G. (1981) *A Bibliography of Biomechanics Literature*, 4th edn, Iowa City, IA: University of Iowa.

Hellström, J. (2009) 'The relation between physical tests, measures, and clubhead speed in elite golfers', *International Journal of Sports Science and Coaching*, 3(1): 85–92.

Huang, H., Wolf, S. L. and He, J. (2005) 'Recent developments in biofeedback for neuromotor rehabilitation', *Journal of NeuroEngineering and Rehabilitation*, 3: 11.

Hume, P. A., Keogh, J. and Reid, D. (2005) 'The role of biomechanics in maximising distance and accuracy of golf shots', *Sports Medicine*, 35(5): 429–49.

Jonsdottir, J., Cattaneo, D., Regola, A., Crippa, A., Recalcati, M., Rabuffetti, M., Ferrarin, M. and Casiraghi, A. (2007). 'Concepts of motor learning applied to a rehabilitation protocol using biofeedback to improve gait in a chronic stroke patient: an A-B system study with multiple gait analyses', *Neurorehabilitation and Neural Repair*, 21(2): 190–4.

Landers, D. M., Han, M., Salazar, W., Petruzzello, S. J., Kubitz, K. A. and Gannon, T. L. (1994) 'Effect of learning on electroencephalographic and electrocardiographic patterns in novice archers', *International Journal of Sports Psychology*, 25(3): 313–30.

Magill, R. A. (2001) *Motor Learning Concepts and Applications*, 6th edn, Boston: McGraw-Hill.

Maltby, R. (1995) *Golf Club Design, Fitting, Alteration and Repair*, Newark, NJ: R. Maltby Enterprises.

Markovska-Simoska, S., Pop-Jordanova, N. and Georgiev, D. (2008) 'Simultaneous EEG and EMG biofeedback for peak performance in musicians', *Prilozi*, 29(1): 239–52.

Neal, R. J. and Wilson, B. D. (1985) '3D kinematics and kinetics of the golf swing', *International Journal of Biomechanics*, 1(3): 221–32.

Ng, G. Y. F., Zhang, A. Q. and Li, C. K. (2008) 'Biofeedback exercise improved the EMG activity ratio of the medial and lateral vasti muscles in subjects with patellofemoral pain syndrome', *Journal of Electromyography and Kinesiology*, 18(1): 128–33.

Niemann, B. K., Pratt, R. R. and Maughan, M. L. (1993) 'Biofeedback training, selected coping strategies, and music relaxation interventions to reduce debilitative musical performance anxiety', *International Journal of Arts Medicine*, 2(2): 7–15.

Nusselder, W. J., Looman, C. W., Franco, O. H., Peeters, A., Slingerland, A. S. and Mackenbach, J. P. (2008) 'The relation between non-occupational physical activity and years lived with and without disability', *Journal of Epidemiology and Community Health*, 62(9): 823–8.

Paffenbarger, R. S., Hyde, R. T., Wing, A. L. and Hsieh, C. C. (1986) 'Physical activity, all-cause mortality, and longevity of college alumni', *The New England Journal of Medicine*, 314(10): 605–13.

Page, P. N. and Hawkins, D. A. (2003) 'A real-time biomechanical feedback system for training rowers', *Sports Engineering*, 6(2): 67–79.

Petruzzello, S. J., Landers, D. M. and Salazar, W. (1991) 'Biofeedback and sport/exercise performance: applications and limitations', *Behavior Therapy*, 22(3): 379–92.

Raymond, J., Sajid, I., Parkinson, L. A. and Gruzelier, J. H. (2005) 'Biofeedback and dance performance: a preliminary investigation', *Applied Psychophysiology and Biofeedback*, 30(1): 64–73.

Schmidt, R. A. (1988) *Motor Control and Learning: A Behavioral Emphasis*, 2nd edn, Champagne, IL: Human Kinetics.

Shan, G. and Bohn, B. (2003) 'Anthropometrical data and coefficients of regression related to gender and race', *Applied Ergonomics*, 34(4): 327–37.

Shan, G. and Westerhoff, P. (2005) 'Full body kinematic characteristics of the maximal instep soccer kick by male soccer players and parameters related to kick quality', *Sports Biomechanics*, 4(1): 59–72.

Shan, G., Zhang, X., Li, X., Hao, W. and Witte, K. (2011) 'Quantification of golfer-club interaction and club-type's affect on dynamic balance during a golf swing', *International Journal of Performance Analysis in Sport*, 11(3): 417–26.

Smith, M. R. and Loschner, C. (2002) 'Biomechanics feedback for rowing', *Journal of Sports Sciences*, 20(10): 783–91.

Tate, J. J. and Milner, C. E. (2010) 'Real-time kinematic, temporospatial, and kinetic biofeedback during gait retraining in patients: a systematic review', *Physical Therapy*, 90(8): 1123–34.

Thompson, C. J., Osness, W. H. and Blackwell, J. (2007) 'Functional training improves club head speed and functional fitness in older golfers', *Journal of Strength and Conditioning Research*, 21(1): 131–7.

Trevino, L. (1992) 'The mechanics of the perfect golf swing', *Popular Mechanics*, 169: 40–3.

US Census Department (2012) *Golf Player Demographic Statistics*, available at: www.statisticbrain.com/golf-player-demographic-statistics/ (accessed 23 September 2012).

Vaz de Almeida, M. D., Graca, P., Afonso, C., D'Amicis, A., Lappalainen, R. and Damkjaer, S. (1999) 'Physical activity levels and body weight in a nationally representative sample in the European Union', *Public Health Nutrition*, 2(1a): 105–13.

Vernon, D. J. (2005) 'Can neurofeedback training enhance performance? An evaluation of the evidence with implications for future research', *Applied Psychophysiology and Biofeedback*, 30(4): 347–64.

Visentin, P., Shan, G. and Wasiak, E. B. (2008) 'Informing music teaching and learning using movement analysis technology', *International Journal of Music Education*, 26(1): 73–87.

Zhang, X. and Shan, G. (in press) 'Where do golf driver swings go wrong? Factors influencing driver swing consistency', *Scandinavian Journal of Medicine and Science in Sports*.

SECTION 6

Influence of playing surface on sports and exercise

22

IN-SHOE PLANTAR LOADS DURING OVERGROUND RUNNING

Lin Wang,[1] *Jing Xian Li*[1,2] *and Youlian Hong*[3]

[1]SHANGHAI UNIVERSITY OF SPORT, SHANGHAI
[2]UNIVERSITY OF OTTAWA, OTTAWA
[3]CHENGDU SPORTS UNIVERSITY, CHENGDU

Introduction

Running is one of the most popular sports activities. Impact force is evaluated to be approximately 2.5 times greater than the runner's body weight in distance running (Cavanagh and Lafortune, 1980). High injury rates have been found in examined runners. The recorded injury rate per 1,000 hours of training is 2.5 hours in long-distance/marathon runners and 5.6–5.8 hours in sprinters and middle-distance runners (Lysholm and Wiklander, 1987).

Plantar loads are widely used to assess injury risks (Queen *et al.*, 2007). Impact forces associated with repetitive loading are responsible for overuse injuries in the lower extremity (Cavanagh and Lafortune, 1980; Hreljac, 2004). A higher plantar pressure underneath the medial side of the foot has been observed in runners with exercise-related lower-extremity pain (Willems *et al.*, 2007) and assumed to be a risk factor associated with sports injury (Tessutti *et al.*, 2010).

Sports surfaces are known to influence the load absorption and absorption mechanism. Many studies have discussed plantar pressures when running and performing specific sports movements on different overground surfaces (Dixon *et al.*, 2000; Ford *et al.*, 2006; Girard *et al.*, 2007; Tessutti *et al.*, 2010; Tillman *et al.*, 2002). A study has found that playing surface affects the plantar load in tennis footwork, and grass courts had higher load in the hallux and lesser toe areas but lower relative load on the midfoot compared with clay surface (Girard *et al.*, 2007). In the cutting movement using soccer boots on natural grass and synthetic turf surfaces, the synthetic turf produced higher maximum pressures on the central forefoot and lesser toes compared with natural grass (Ford *et al.*, 2006). During running on asphalt, concrete, grass and synthetic rubber tracks at a preferred velocity, Tillman *et al.* (2002) have found no significant differences among the surfaces for plantar load; biomechanical compensatory mechanisms of the human body may explain this result. However, the study merely distinguished plantar load of the total foot area, failing to provide comparisons of different areas of the foot during running on varied surfaces. Recently, one study has found higher plantar load in the central rearfoot, lateral rearfoot and lateral forefoot during running on asphalt compared with natural grass at a velocity of 3.3 m.s^{-1} (Tessutti *et al.*, 2010). For natural grass, the researchers likewise observed that contact time and contact area were greater in the central rearfoot (Tessutti *et al.*, 2010).

Common overground surfaces for runners include concrete, asphalt, synthetic rubber sports track and natural turf. Synthetic rubber sports track is the most popular running surface. Concrete and asphalt surfaces are most commonly used for recreational and marathon running (Tessutti *et al.*, 2010). Meanwhile, natural grass surfaces have been used to study plantar loads while running and performing specific sports movements (Ford *et al.*, 2006; Girard *et al.*, 2007; Tessutti *et al.*, 2010).

Identifying impact forces and plantar pressure distribution characteristics during running on different overground surfaces can help reveal risk factors related to sports injury. To date, however, no quantitative information has been made available concerning the comparison of plantar load characteristics during running on concrete, synthetic rubber sports track and natural grass.

Given the contention about running mechanics among different overground surfaces, the aim of the study is to compare plantar loads of running on concrete, natural grass and synthetic rubber surfaces. We hypothesize that plantar loads during running on natural grass are lower compared with running on concrete and synthetic rubber surfaces, and that plantar loads during running on synthetic rubber surfaces are lower compared with running on concrete surfaces. Identifying these differences may be one of the diverse ways to prevent overuse injuries in long-distance running.

Methods

Fifteen amateur male runners (aged 22.0 ± 1.8 years; body mass of 62.8 ± 9.5 kg; body height of 170.4 ± 3.3 cm), all right leg dominant, heel strikers and with a shoe size of 41, participated in the study. All participants were recruited from the long-distance running teams of local universities. Only male participants were recruited to eliminate gender differences in running biomechanics (Ferber *et al.*, 2003). The participants were regular overground surface runners. They had no history of diseases associated with the neuromuscular, vestibular and visual systems; none suffered injuries in the 6 months prior to the study. The participants signed an informed consent. The study was approved by the local Ethics Committee.

Three test surfaces, particularly concrete, synthetic rubber and natural grass, were used in the study. A pair of new running shoes with a European size of 41 (TN600-neutral, ASICS, Japan) was assigned to each participant. The running tests were performed on each surface using the said footwear.

In-shoe loads were measured using a Novel Pedar-X system (Novel, Munich, Germany). Each insole contained 99 force sensors, all of which were calibrated using a standard calibration device (Trublu Calibration, Novel, Munich, Germany). The insole was connected to a Pedar-X box attached to the waist of each participant. Only data from the right foot were collected. The sample frequency was set at 100 Hz.

A synchronized video camera (9800, JVC Inc., Japan) with a sampling frequency of 100 Hz was used to record the feet movement of the participants. At the start of data collection, the Pedar-X insole system generated a flash captured by the video camera as a synchronization signal. The video image was used to identify each right foot stance phase of Pedar-X records used in the data analysis.

Overground running was conducted on a 30 m straight outdoor runway made of concrete, rubber and grass. Running tests on natural grass and rubber surfaces were conducted on a standard natural grass soccer field and standard synthetic rubber running track, respectively. The first 15 m of the runway was the designated acceleration zone, followed by the 5 m (15–20 m) measurement zone, in which the participants ran at a velocity of 3.8 m.s^{-1}. This velocity has been used in previous studies (Dixon *et al.*, 2000; Tillman *et al.*, 2002).

Velocity was timed using an infrared timing system (Brower Timing System, USA). Timers were placed at the start and end points of the measurement zone. Each participant ran for 6 minutes to warm up on a standard running track at his preferred velocity. After warm-up, but prior to data collection, each participant was allowed as many practice trials as necessary to achieve a smooth running pattern, with a controlled velocity of 3.8 m.s^{-1}. A trial was accepted when the running velocity was within 5 per cent of the required 3.8 m.s^{-1} in the 5 m measurement zone.

For each running surface, participants completed five successful trials. In each successful trial, plantar load data of at least one complete right-foot stance were collected. The right-foot stance indicated the phase from heel strike to toe push-off. Five steps on each surface were used in data reduction. Running surfaces were randomly assigned to each participant.

Using the Novel Pedar-X system software, plantar load data of the right-foot stance phase were extracted while the participants ran on each surface. The plantar surface was initially divided into four larger areas: rearfoot (30 per cent of foot length), midfoot (30 per cent of foot length), forefoot (25 per cent of foot length) and toes (15 per cent of foot length). The rearfoot, midfoot, forefoot and toes were subdivided, respectively, into M1 (medial heel, 50 per cent of the rearfoot width), M2 (lateral heel, 50 per cent of the rearfoot width), M3 (medial midfoot, 50 per cent of the midfoot width), M4 (lateral midfoot, 50 per cent of the midfoot width), M5 (medial forefoot, 30 per cent of the forefoot width), M6 (central forefoot, 40 per cent of the forefoot width), M7 (lateral forefoot, 30 per cent of the forefoot width), M8 (great toe, 25 per cent of the toes width) and M9 (lesser toes, 75 per cent of the toes width). The mask determined the plantar pressure of running in our previous study (Hong *et al.*, 2011). Plantar load parameters of the entire foot and the nine selected plantar regions were calculated, including maximum plantar pressure, maximum plantar force, contact area, contact time and relative contact time. The maximum plantar force measurements were normalized to body weight (percentage of BW). The ratio of the contact time of a plantar region in relation to the contact time of the total foot was determined as well. For each subject, plantar load data of five successful stances collected from different trials were used to calculate the mean.

All data are presented as mean and standard deviation (SD) in all subjects. Data were tested for normal distribution using the Kolmogorov-Smirnov's test, and homoscedasticity was verified using Levene's test. Comparison of surfaces was performed using ANOVA for repeated measures analysis on selected plantar loading variables. In each variable, 30 parameters were evaluated; the entire foot and nine plantar regions were assessed for all three running surfaces. Significance was set at alpha < 0.05, and Bonferroni adjustment was used to correct multiple measurements (effective alpha < 0.0017).

Results

The mean and standard deviations of maximum plantar pressure, maximum plantar force, contact area, contact time and relative contact time are presented in Table 22.1.

The maximum plantar pressures were higher when running on concrete than on natural grass at the total foot ($p < 0.0017$, 95 per cent confidence interval for difference (95 per cent CI) = 8.5–91.7 kPa), lateral midfoot ($p < 0.0017$, 95 per cent CI = 8.5–46.3 kPA), central forefoot ($p < 0.0017$, 95 per cent CI = 9.7–49.3 kPa) and lateral forefoot ($p < 0.0017$, 95 per cent CI = 1.8–62.7 kPa). No significant differences were observed in maximum plantar pressure at the total foot and all foot areas between concrete and synthetic rubber, and between synthetic rubber and natural grass. In terms of maximum plantar force, no significant difference in maximum plantar force at toal foot and all foot areas among the three surfaces were observed.

Table 22.1 Comparison of insole loading parameters for running on different surfaces

Variables	Surface	Total	M1	M2	M3	M4	M5	M6	M7	M8	M9
MP	C	451.8	244.2	249.3	130.2	175.3	344.8	366.3	290.2	405.7	228.0
(kPa)		(96.9)	(90.3)	(95.1)	(26.5)	(70.4)	(91.2)	(89.8)	(83.9)	(121.5)	(66.0)
	R	437.1	226.0	232.3	125.3	159.7	338.6	339.3	272.7	365.2	214.2
		(90.8)	(63.9)	(76.6)	(31.9)	(55.1)	(89.6)	(99.9)	(70.1)	(94.8)	(64.7)
	G	401.7	204.9	199.6	122.8	148.0	345.1	336.8	257.9	365.2	212.1
		(83.9)	(47.5)	(44.6)	(29.2)	(52.4)	(93.0)	(84.1)	(70.1)	(119.4)	(55.0)
		★				★		★	★		
MF	C	256.3	59.3	50.3	30.0	43.1	41.7	54.1	37.6	32.9	35.0
(% BW)		(30.5)	(22.5)	(22.0)	(9.0)	(11.6)	(12.2)	(7.3)	(10.6)	(8.3)	(5.0)
	R	256.5	55.1	48.0	28.9	40.4	40.7	51.1	34.7	33.0	35.0
		(39.3)	(16.6)	(18.5)	(8.2)	(10.5)	(12.3)	(9.4)	(10.6)	(8.9)	(5.5)
	G	250.8	49.6	40.0	28.7	40.0	43.7	52.1	34.1	32.1	33.6
		(43.0)	(14.7)	(11.8)	(9.3)	(11.4)	(12.0)	(7.2)	(9.0)	(7.1)	(5.0)
CA	C	182.0	25.7	22.3	24.8	24.5	15.2	18.0	17.8	11.5	22.2
(cm²)		(4.8)	(2.4)	(2.3)	(0.5)	(0.1)	(0.3)	(0.0)	(0.0)	(0.1)	(0.5)
	R	182.6	26.0	22.7	24.7	24.5	15.1	18.0	17.8	11.5	22.1
		(3.8)	(1.6)	(1.4)	(1.3)	(0.0)	(0.5)	(0.0)	(0.0)	(0.0)	(0.8)
	G	182.0	25.7	22.2	24.7	24.5	15.2	18.0	17.8	11.5	22.1
		(4.2)	(1.8)	(1.5)	(0.7)	(0.0)	(0.4)	(0.0)	(0.0)	(0.0)	(0.6)
CT (ms)	C	205.9	81.8	77.1	76.3	112.1	155.5	163.6	152.0	144.5	147.3
		(17.4)	(23.2)	(22.3)	(20.5)	(29.3)	(24.9)	(22.8)	(24.1)	(15.6)	(16.6)
	R	213.5	86.1	83.3	81.9	110.8	161.6	164.7	152.1	152.2	154.1
		(12.1)	(17.6)	(17.8)	(19.7)	(17.4)	(13.5)	(13.8)	(15.1)	(19.2)	(15.8)
	G	214.3	83.4	80.3	79.4	114.1	164.0	179.6	168.5	159.2	159.7
		(19.8)	(18.5)	(19.7)	(19.3)	(23.1)	(37.7)	(37.3)	(39.8)	(19.5)	(18.3)
								★	★	★	★
RCT (%)	C		38.7	36.6	35.3	53.4	75.1	78.8	73.1	70.2	71.7
			(9.0)	(8.7)	(8.4)	(11.1)	(12.2)	(10.2)	(10.0)	(11.6)	(12.9)
	R		40.3	38.5	36.7	51.6	75.7	77.0	71.2	72.8	74.9
			(5.9)	(6.7)	(7.7)	(8.2)	(10.0)	(9.1)	(9.9)	(11.3)	(9.5)
	G		37.9	36.3	37.4	51.9	77.8	81.9	75.2	74.4	74.7
			(6.6)	(5.6)	(8.1)	(7.6)	(10.3)	(9.4)	(10.7)	(14.7)	(14.8)
								★	★		

Values are means (SD).
MP, maximum pressure; MF, maximum force; CA, contact area; CT, contact time; RCT, relative contact time; C, concrete; G, natural grass; R, synthetic rubber.
M1, medial heel; M2, lateral heel; M3, medial midfoot; M4, lateral midfoot; M5, medial forefoot; M6, central forefoot; M7, lateral forefoot; M8, great toe; M9, lesser toes.
★ $p < 0.0017$ natural grass versus concrete.

Among the three surfaces, running on natural grass revealed longer contact time in the medial forefoot ($p < 0.0017$, 95 per cent CI = 4.4–32.6 ms), central forefoot ($p < 0.0017$, 95 per cent CI = 2.2–29.8 ms), great toes ($p < 0.0017$, 95 per cent CI = 4.4–24.9 ms) and lesser toe areas ($p < 0.0017$, 95 per cent CI = 3.3–21.3 ms) than running on concrete. Relative times were longer when running on grass than on concrete at the medial forefoot ($p < 0.0017$, 95 per cent CI = 1.0–7.7 per cent) and central forefoot ($p < 0.0017$, 95 per cent CI = 4.6–5.6 per cent).

Discussion

The results of the current study partially supported our hypotheses. Running on natural grass showed maximum plantar pressures that are lower compared to those recorded when running on concrete. However, the maximum plantar pressures of running on synthetic rubber were not higher than those on natural grass and not lower than those on concrete. The current study found that different plantar loads exist when running on concrete and grass surfaces. This is one of the essential findings of the current study.

Similar maximal forces were found among running on three surfaces at total foot and different plantar areas. Total maximum forces were approximately 2.5 times greater than the runner's body weight. Total maximum force value is similar to the maximum vertical ground reaction force in long-distance running (Cavanagh and Lafortune, 1980). Ferris *et al.* (1998) found that the runners are able to maintain the same ground reaction force during running on different surfaces through adjusting leg stiffness for different surfaces.

Several studies have found that increased surface hardness induces kinematic changes in the lower extremity on the sagittal plane (Dixon *et al.*, 2000; Hardin *et al.*, 2004). Lower-extremity kinematics and stiffness adaptations to different overground running surfaces have been interpreted as a form of active adaptation to maintain similar impact forces (Dixon *et al.*, 2000; Ferris *et al.*, 1998; Hardin *et al.*, 2004). These adaptations include larger ankle and knee flexion (Dixon *et al.*, 2000), and larger knee and hip flexion at heel strike on more rigid surfaces (Ferris *et al.*, 1998).

In the current study, longer contact times and lower maximum plantar pressure were observed at the medial and lateral forefoot while running on natural grass as compared with running on a concrete surface. The results can be explained by the kinematic adaptation of runners to running surfaces of different hardness to maintain similar impact. Compared with running on a concrete surface, lower maximum plantar pressures have been found at the central forefoot region (average of 8.1 per cent lower) as well as at the lateral forefoot region (average of 11.1 per cent lower) while participants ran on natural grass. These results are identical with those reported by Tessutti *et al.* (2010), who found that running on natural grass induces a lower maximum plantar pressure compared with running on concrete in lateral forefoot (average of 10.8 per cent lower). Moreover, in the current study, lower maximum plantar pressure was found while running on natural grass compared with running on concrete in lateral midfoot (average of 15.6 per cent lower). Compared with running on concrete/asphalt surfaces, lower maximum plantar pressures have been reported with natural grass running and certain sport-specific movements (e.g. soccer-specific and tennis-specific movements) (Ford *et al.*, 2006; Girard *et al.*, 2007). However, the lower maximum rearfoot plantar pressures while running on natural grass compared with running on concrete surfaces reported by Tessutti *et al.* (2010) was not found in the current study.

In our work, no significant difference in contact time of right-foot stance has been found between running on concrete and on natural grass surfaces. The results prove the findings of previous studies that different overground running surfaces do not change the duration of the total stance at the same velocity (Ferris *et al.*, 1998; Hardin *et al.*, 2004). Tessutti *et al.* (2010) have reported that running on natural grass induces a longer contact time and larger contact area in the central rearfoot compared with running on a concrete surface. However, in the current study, no significant differences in the contact area in each plantar region have been found between running on concrete and on natural grass. Compared with running on concrete, the longer contact time was determined during running on natural grass in the medial and central forefoot in the current study. The use of different testing shoes (TN600-neutral, Gel, ASICS in our study versus Alpargata-neutral, RAINHA SYSTEM in Tessutti *et al.*'s study), different running velocities (3.8 m.s^{-1} in our study versus 3.3 m.s^{-1} in Tessutti *et al.*'s study), different methods for controlling running speed (infrared timing system in our study versus stopwatch in Tessutti *et al.*'s study) and different plantar region divisions (nine versus six regions) may have resulted in the differences between the contact time and rearfoot plantar pressure presented in our study and Tessutti *et al.*'s research (Tessutti *et al.*, 2010).

In the current study, the contact times and relative contact times in the lateral and medial forefoot during running on natural grass were longer than those during running on concrete. Lower maximum plantar pressures were shown in these areas during running on natural grass. The longer contact time on natural grass running may imply the greater possibility of plantar load absorption during running confirmed by the observed smaller maximum plantar pressure in these areas.

As mentioned above, the runner can adapt kinematic characteristics via adjustment of musculoskeletal system during running on different surfaces to maintain similar impact force (Dixon *et al.*, 2000; Ferris *et al.*, 1998; Hardin *et al.*, 2004). Kinematic adaptation may influence load absorption on different running surfaces. Runners must increase their leg stiffness when running on compliant surfaces (e.g. natural grass) and decrease leg stiffness on hard surfaces (Ferris *et al.*, 1998). Therefore, when runners run on concrete, they run with a more flexed limb posture. These changes may influence the moment arm of ground reaction force, tendons and ligaments (Tillman *et al.*, 2002). Specifically, increased flexion will be accompanied by an increase in muscle forces and joint moments (Tillman *et al.*, 2002).

A previous study has suggested that runners participating in high-impact sports that involve running are at high risk for forefoot injuries, and that higher and repetitive plantar loading may be a risk factor for forefoot injuries (Hockenbury, 1999). In repetitive and long-distance running on concrete surfaces, a higher maximum plantar pressure may lead to an overload of the human locomotor system. With the presence of other risk factors, this may lead to an increased risk of overuse injury in the musculoskeletal system. Thus, running on natural grass is likely to be safer than running on concrete because of lower plantar loads.

Compared with other running surfaces, no significant differences were found in all variables of plantar loads during running on synthetic rubber running track. Tillman *et al.* (2002) used pressure insole to compare plantar loads for running on asphalt, concrete, synthetic rubber and natural grass. The authors found no difference in maximum reaction force and total contact time among different surfaces. The result is consistent with our findings that maximum plantar force and total contact time are similar among concrete, synthetic rubber and natural grass surfaces.

However, the study by Tillman *et al.* (2002) had a few limitations, particularly that the insole used only contained 24 sensors and that it was not divided into different regions. Moreover, maximum plantar pressure was not provided. More recently, Ford *et al.* (2006) measured maximum plantar pressure during cutting on synthetic turf surfaces and on natural grass using the Nover Pedar system. They found that the synthetic turf had significantly higher maximum plantar pressures in the central forefoot (synthetic turf: 646.6 ± 172.6 kPa, grass: 533.3 ± 143.4 kPa) and lesser toes (synthetic turf: 429.3 ± 200.9 kPa, grass: 348.1 ± 119.0 kPa) compared with natural grass. In our study, maximum plantar pressures during running on synthetic rubber and grass were 339.3 and 336.8 kPa in the central forefoot, respectively, and 214.2 and 212.1 kPa in the lesser toes, respectively. Evidently, maximum plantar pressures in running are smaller than those in cutting movements.

Moreover, the difference in maximum plantar pressures between running on synthetic rubber and other surfaces was not detected. This may be explained by several reasons. First, synthetic rubber is a medium-hardness material in the present study and may not induce significant higher maximum plantar pressure than that by the grass and lower maximum plantar pressure than that by the concrete surface. Second, the insole sensor system may not be sensitive enough to distinguish the small difference. The relatively small sample size may be another possible reason to account for no significant difference in plantar pressure. Therefore, compared with running on concrete and natural grass, maximum plantar pressure during running on synthetic rubber is more likely to be centralized on the medium level. Although the difference in maximum plantar pressure is not statistically significant, this difference may have a biomechanical impact. For example, in long-distance running, a slight difference in plantar load may be associated with overuse injury. Therefore, these differences should be interpreted cautiously at present.

Conclusion

The results of the present study indicate that different surfaces affect the plantar loads during running. Running on natural grass induced lower maximum plantar pressure in the lateral midfoot and central and lateral forefoot, and longer contact times in the forefoot than running on a concrete surface. This may be explained by the adjustment in the distal extremity's stiffness. Considering that long-distance running is usually performed on hard surfaces, a more compliant surface can be used to attenuate the impact on the musculoskeletal system and prevent the risk of overuse injuries induced by a more rigid surface. Appropriate preventive strategies (e.g. adapted footwear, alternative running on surfaces with different hardness) should be considered for these spots.

References

Cavanagh, P. R. and Lafortune, M. A. (1980) 'Ground reaction forces in distance running', *Journal of Biomechanics*, 13(5): 397–406.

Dixon, S. J., Collop, A. C. and Batt, M. E. (2000) 'Surface effects on ground reaction forces and lower extremity kinematics in running', *Medicine and Science in Sports and Exercise*, 32(11): 1919–26.

Ferber, R., Davis, I. M. and Williams, D. S. III. (2003) 'Gender differences in lower extremity mechanics during running', *Clinical Biomechanics*, 18(4): 350–7.

Ferris, D. P., Louie, M. and Farley, C. T. (1998) 'Running in the real world: adjusting leg stiffness for different surfaces', *Proceedings Biological Sciences*, 265(1400): 989–94.

Ford, K. R., Manson, N. A., Evans, B. J., Myer, G. D., Gwin, R. C., Heidt, R. S. Jr and Hewett, T. E. (2006) 'Comparison of in-shoe foot loading patterns on natural grass and synthetic turf', *Journal of Science and Medicine in Sport*, 9(6): 433–40.

Girard, O., Eicher, F., Fourchet, F., Micallef, J. P. and Millet, G. P. (2007) 'Effects of the playing surface on plantar pressures and potential injuries in tennis', *British Journal of Sports Medicine*, 41(11): 733–8.

Hardin, E. C., van den Bogert, A. J. and Hamill, J. (2004) 'Kinematic adaptations during running: effects of footwear, surface, and duration', *Medicine and Science in Sports and Exercise*, 36(5): 838–44.

Hockenbury, R. T. (1999) 'Forefoot problems in athletes', *Medicine and Science in Sports and Exercise*, 31(7): S448–58.

Hong ,Y., Wang, L., Li, J. X. and Zhou, J. H. (2011) 'Changes in running mechanics using conventional shoelace versus elastic shoe cover', *Journal of Sports Science*, 29(4): 373–9.

Hreljac, A. (2004) 'Impact and overuse injuries in runners', *Medicine and Science in Sports and Exercise*, 36(5): 845–9.

Lysholm, J. and Wiklander, J. (1987) 'Injuries in runners', *American Journal of Sports Medicine*, 15(2): 168–71.

Queen, R. M., Haynes, B. B., Hardaker, W. M. and Garrett, W. E. Jr (2007) 'Forefoot loading during 3 athletic tasks', *American Journal of Sports Medicine*, 35(4): 630–6.

Tessutti, V., Trombini-Souza, F., Ribeiro, A. P., Nunes, A. L. and Sacco-Ide, C. (2010) 'In-shoe plantar pressure distribution during running on natural grass and asphalt in recreational runners', *Journal of Science and Medicine in Sport*, 13(1): 151–5.

Tillman, M. D., Fiolkowski, P., Bauer, J. A. and Reisinger, K. D. (2002) 'In-shoe plantar measurements during running on different surfaces: changes in temporal and kinetic parameters', *Sports Engineering*, 5(3): 121–8.

Willems, T. M., Witvrouw, E., De Cock, A. and De Clercq, D. (2007) 'Gait-related risk factors for exercise-related lower-leg pain during shod running', *Medicine and Science in Sports and Exercise*, 39(2): 330–9.

23

THE EFFECT OF PLAYING SURFACES ON PERFORMANCE IN TENNIS

Caroline Martin and Jacques Prioux

UNIVERSITY OF RENNES 2, BRUZ

Description of tennis playing surfaces

Competitive tennis players are used to playing multiple tournaments on a variety of court surfaces, more so perhaps than any other sport. In 2011, 210 different court surfaces have been approved by the International Tennis Federation (ITF). The properties of each surface influence the style of the play, the tennis ball rebound and the quality of performance. To facilitate the understanding of these properties, the ITF (2012) classifies court surfaces into categories according to type (acrylic, artificial clay, artificial grass, asphalt, carpet, clay (CL), concrete, grass, other) (see Table 23.1) and court pace rating (CPR): slow ($CPR \leq 29$), medium-slow (CPR 30–34), medium (CPR 35–39), medium-fast (CPR 40–44) and fast ($CPR \geq 45$).

The characteristics of CPR are determined by two main parameters: their coefficient of friction (COF) and their coefficient of restitution (COR):

$$CPR = 100(1 - COF) + 150\,(0.81 - COR_{adj}) \tag{1}$$

where COF is the coefficient of friction and COR_{adj} is the temperature-adjusted coefficient of restitution.

According to the ITF, COF (m.s^{-1}) is the ratio of the horizontal force resisting sliding and the vertical force of the ball normal to the surface:

$$COF = \frac{V_{ix} - V_{fx}}{V_{iy}(1 + COR)} \tag{2}$$

where V_{ix} is the horizontal inbound velocity (m.s^{-1}), V_{fx} is the horizontal outbound velocity (m.s^{-1}), V_{iy} is the vertical inbound velocity (m.s^{-1}) and COR is the coefficient of restitution.

COR (m.s^{-1}) is the ratio of the vertical velocity and after the bounce to that before impact:

$$COF = \frac{V_{fy}}{V_{iy}} \tag{3}$$

Table 23.1 Types and descriptions of playing surfaces

Type	Description
Acrylic	Textured, pigmented, resin-bound coating
Artificial clay	Synthetic surface with the appearance of clay
Artificial grass	Synthetic surface with the appearance of natural grass
Asphalt	Bitumen-bound aggregate
Carpet	Textile or polymeric material supplied in rolls or sheets of finished product
Clay	Unbound mineral aggregate
Concrete	Cement-bound aggregate
Grass	Natural grass grown from seed
Other	e.g. wood, canvas

where V_{fy} is the vertical outbound velocity (m.s^{-1}) and V_{iy} is the vertical inbound velocity (m.s^{-1}).

For a 29 m.s^{-1} groundstroke with a standard type 2 tennis ball on a fast court with pace rating of 60, the ball will reach the other baseline with a speed of about 15.52 m.s^{-1}, or with 53 per cent of its original speed. On a medium-slow court with a pace rating averaging 30, the ball will arrive at the baseline with a speed of 12.96 m.s^{-1}, or 45 per cent of its original speed (Brody, 2003). According to Brody (2003), players should increase their racket head velocity by 25 per cent to maintain the same ball speed at the opposite baseline for medium-slow courts with a pace value of 30 than for fast courts (pace value of 60).

Hard courts (H), CL and grass are the most common surfaces on which professional and leisure tennis are played today (Miller, 2006). In 2006, six tournaments of the Association of Tennis Professionals world tour were played on grass, 30 on H and 25 on CL. During the same year, four tournaments of the Women Tennis Association professional world tour were played on grass, 37 on H and 15 on CL. In the professional circuit, the four Grand Slam tournaments are now played on these different surfaces. Indeed, the US Open moved from the grass courts to the DecoTurf (H) courts in 1978 and the Australian Open moved from the grass surface to the Rebound Ace (H) surface in 1986. Wimbledon remains a grass court tournament and the French Open is still played on the CL of Roland Garros. Consequently, the characteristics of the CL, grass and H surfaces are exposed in the following section.

Grass court

According to Miller (2006) and Brody (2003), the COR of grass court is low (0.77), inducing a lower height of the vertical bounce of the tennis ball than on other surfaces. This reduces the time between the first and the second bounce, which players can also perceive as a 'fast surface' with a CPR value of 46. On grass court, there is a loss of horizontal velocity during the ball rebound since the COF of this surface is low. As a consequence, the player will have less time to get to the ball and prepare its shot than on CL court (Brody, 2003).

Clay court

CL court is considered as a slow surface (CPR = 23), characterized by higher COR (0.86) and COF (> 0.71) than faster surfaces. This results in a high and relative gentle bounce and slows down the ball. On CL, the ball may pick up bits of CL or moisture and become heavier.

Table 23.2 Mean values ($\pm$ SD) of physiological parameters

References	Surface	Sex	Level	HR (bpm)	[La] (mmol L^{-1})	$\dot{V}O_2$ (ml min^{-1} kg^{-1})	% $\dot{V}O_{2max}$
Dansou et al. (2001)	Hard	Male	Club	140.5 $\pm$ 5	3.3 $\pm$ 0.10	32.6 $\pm$ 1.80	56.0 $\pm$ 2.5
Murias et al. (2007)	Clay	Male	National	143 $\pm$ 22	1.65 $\pm$ 0.60	26.33 $\pm$ 3.25	47.6 $\pm$ 6.5
	Hard	Male	National	135 $\pm$ 21	1.16 $\pm$ 0.34	27.48 $\pm$ 2.46	49.5 $\pm$ 4.80
Girard and Millet (2004)	Clay	Male	Club	181.8 $\pm$ 11.9	2.36 $\pm$ 0.47	40.3 $\pm$ 5.70	80.1 $\pm$ 10.80
	Hard	Male	Club	172.8 $\pm$ 17.2	3.08 $\pm$ 1.12	35.9 $\pm$ 7.50	71.6 $\pm$ 15.30
Martin et al. (2011)	Clay	Male	National	154 $\pm$ 12	5.7 $\pm$ 1.80	/	/
	Hard	Female	National	141 $\pm$ 90	3.6 $\pm$ 1.20	/	/
Fernandez et al. (2007)	Hard	Female	International	161 $\pm$ 5.0	2.0 $\pm$ 0.80	/	/
Fernandez et al. (2008)	Clay	Female	International	/	2.2 $\pm$ 0.90	/	/
Fernandez et al. (2009)	Clay	Male	Adv Veterans	143.8 $\pm$ 11.50	/	24.5 $\pm$ 4.10	/
	Clay	Male	Rec Veterans	149.8 $\pm$ 8.40	/	23.3 $\pm$ 3.0	/
Hornery et al. (2007)	Clay	Male	International	152 $\pm$ 15	/	/	/
	Hard	Male	International	146 $\pm$ 19	/	/	/
Smekal et al. (2001)	Clay	Male	National	/	2.07 $\pm$ 0.90	29.1 $\pm$ 5.60	46.4 $\pm$ 7.20

HR : heart rate, [La] : blood lactate concentration, $\dot{V}O_2$: mean oxygen uptake, % $\dot{V}O_2$max : percentage of $\dot{V}O_2$max, RPE : rate of perceived exertion. Adv : advanced, Rec : recreational.

This phenomenon slows down the game more on CL courts because a heavier ball comes off the racket with slightly less speed (Brody, 2003).

Hard court

H courts, such as Rebound Ace in the Australian Open and DecoTurf in the US Open, are usually considered as medium surfaces, with a CPR value between 35 and 39, COF ranging from 0.56 to 0.70 and COR between 0.79 and 0.84.

The physiological demands involved in tennis matches

Tennis is a sport that requires a mixture of complex skills (technical, tactical, psychological) and physical attributes (speed, agility, endurance, strength, balance, flexibility, anticipation, power) (Kovacs, 2007). Match play is defined by intermittent exercise: short bout of high intensity (< 10 seconds) are interrupted by short recovery bouts (10–20 seconds) and periods of longer duration (90–120 seconds). During this time, a player runs about 3 m per stroke (Parsons and Jones, 1998), changes direction four times by point and completes 300–500 explosive efforts during a match (Deutsch et al., 1998). According to Kovacs (2007), 'utilizing the correct energy system during training will improve performance during matches'. As a consequence, it is important to know the involvement of energy systems during tennis matches. As tennis activity is characterized by periods of high-intensity exercise (powerful serves and groundstrokes, rapid changes of direction, explosive nature of the displacements) disrupted by periods of low-intensity exercise of various duration (active recovery between points or sitting periods during changeovers), one may argue to classify it as anaerobic predominant activity requiring high levels of aerobic conditioning to aid in recovery between points and matches (Kovacs, 2006).

Different studies have used portable gas analysers to have an oversight of mean oxygen uptake (VO_2) during tennis matches (see Table 23.2). It has been reported that mean VO_2 levels during matches vary from 23.3 ± 3.0 ml.min^{-1}.kg^{-1} for recreational veterans (Fernandez-Fernandez et al., 2009) to 40.3 ± 5.7 ml.min^{-1}.kg^{-1} for club male players (Girard and Millet, 2004). This corresponds to about 60 per cent of mean VO_2max, with values ranging from 46 to 80 per cent of ,VO_2max (see Table 23.2). During matches, mean VO_2 reached 60 per cent of the mean VO_2max for 80 per cent of the duration of the match. During the points, mean VO_2 varied from 70 to 95 per cent of mean VO_2max and decreased rapidly during the changes of side (Dansou et al., 2001).

Regarding the heart rate (HR), the literature shows that HR is measured as indices to evaluate the intensity and the psychological stress associated during practice (Fernandez-Fernandez et al., 2008). It has been reported that mean HR values during matches vary from 135 to 161 bpm (see Table 23.2), rising to 190–200 bpm during long and intense rallies (Girard and Millet, 2004; Smekal et al., 2001). The mean percentage of maximum heart rate (HRmax) during matches has been reported to approximate 86 per cent and to be not significantly different from the 83 per cent measured during recovery (excluding the rest periods between points and games) (Bergeron et al., 1991). However, care should be taken when looking at the results of mean HR values as they do not accurately represent the intermittent nature of the tennis match (Fernandez-Fernandez et al., 2009; Kovacs, 2007). Indeed, HR values vary continuously during a match due to the continual stop-start movements and intermittent nature of the sport (Bergeron et al., 1991; Dansou et al., 2001) (Figure 23.1). It has been reported that players spent about 13 per cent of match duration at intensities higher than 90 per cent

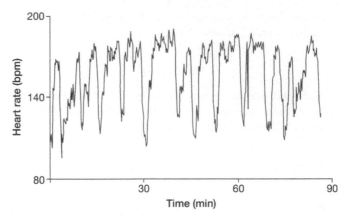

Figure 23.1 Typical evolution of the heart rate of a tennis player during a simulated match, according to Dansou *et al.* (2001).

of HRmax. Moreover, the serving situation influences HR during male and female matches: mean HR values were significantly higher when serving than when receiving (Fernandez-Fernandez *et al.*, 2007; Mendez-Villanueva *et al.*, 2007). This result could be explained by the higher psychological stress and sympathetic activity related to the importance to win the service games (Fernandez-Fernandez *et al.*, 2009).

Finally, in the scientific literature on tennis, the blood lactate concentration ([La]) is measured as indices to evaluate the intensity of tennis match play and to obtain an oversight of the energy production from glycolytic processes (Fernandez-Fernandez *et al.*, 2009). Mean [La] values during matches remain low (from 1.16 to 5.7 mmol.L^{-1}) (see Table 23.2). Indeed, the periods of rest during a match seem sufficient to allow players to reduce the metabolism products (Bergeron *et al.*, 1991; Martin *et al.*, 2011). [La] values can rise to 8 mmol.L^{-1} during long and intense rallies (Martin *et al.*, 2011), suggesting an increased participation of glycolytic processes to energy supply. When [La] exceeds 7–8 mmol.L^{-1}, technical and tactical performance decreases (Ferrauti *et al.*, 2001a, 2001b). So, it is important to prepare players properly to deal with these high-intensity situations and to use optimal resting times. The discrepancies between studies concerning mean [La] values are probably the results of differences in the characteristics of the subjects and the experimental design (number and time of blood taking). However, care should be taken when looking at the results because [La] values only reflect the level of activity during the few minutes before sampling (Martin *et al.*, 2011).

The influence of tennis playing surface on matches' characteristics

As we have seen previously, the court surface influences the tennis ball rebound and the ball speed (Brody, 2003; Miller, 2006) and as a consequence the match's technical characteristics – that is, its effective playing time (EPT), effective resting time (ERT), total match duration (MD), mean rally duration (MRD), resting time between points (RT), number of strokes per rally (SR) and distance ran per point (DRP) (Table 23.3). The EPT, defined as the duration during which the ball is really in play is, on average, significantly longer on CL (20–30 per cent of total match duration) than on faster surfaces such as H courts (10–15 per cent of total match duration) (Table 23.3). O'Donoghue and Ingram (2001) conducted a notational analysis of singles events at all four Grand Slam tournaments between 1997 and 1999 to determine the influence of the surface on tennis matches. Rallies of 6.3 ± 1.8 seconds at the Australian Open

Table 23.3 Mean values (± SD) of match characteristics

References	Surface	Sex	Level	MD (min)	MRD (s)	MRT (s)	EPT (%)	DRP (m)	SR
Murias et al. (2007)	Clay	Male	National	/	8.8 ± 5.3	19.4 ± 8.6	/	11.6 ± 1.5	/
	Hard	Male	National	/	7.2 ± 4.4	20.2 ± 7.7	/	9.3 ± 1.8	/
Girard and Millet (2004)	Clay	Male	Club	/	7.2 ± 1.7	/	/	9.8 ± 2.5	2.5 ± 0.5
	Hard	Male	Club	/	5.9 ± 1.2	/	/	7.7 ± 1.7	1.9 ± 0.4
Martin et al. (2011)	Clay	Male	National	56.9 ± 5.0	8.5 ± 0.2	/	26.2 ± 1.9	/	/
	Hard	Female	National	56.0 ± 10.1	5.9 ± 0.5	/	19.5 ± 2.0	/	/
Fernandez-Fernandez et al. (2007)	Hard	Female	International	/	8.2 ± 5.2	17.7 ± 6.5	21.9 ± 3.8	/	2.8 1.7
Fernandez-Fernandez et al. (2008)	Clay	Female	International	/	7.2 ± 5.2	15.5 ± 7.3	21.6 ± 6.1	/	2.5 ± 1.6
Mendez-Villanueva et al. (2010)	Clay	Male	International	/	7.5 ± 7.3	16.2 ± 5.2	21.5 ± 4.9	/	2.7 ± 2.2
Hornery et al. (2007)	Clay	Male	International	79 ± 13	7.5 ± 3.0	17.2 ± 3.3	/	/	4.5 ± 2.0
	Hard	Male	International	119 ± 36	6.7 ± 2.2	25.1 ± 4.3	/	/	4.7 ± 1.4
O'Donoghue and Ingram (2001)	Clay	Male	International	7.7 ± 1.7	i	19.5 ± 2.1	/	/	/
	Hard	Male	International	5.8 ± 1.9	/	18.3 ± 2.0	/	/	/
	Grass	Male	International	4.3 ± 1.6	/	19.4 ± 1.6	/	/	/
	Clay	Female	International	/	/	18.2 ± 1.6	/	/	/
	Hard	Female	International	/	/	18.1 ± 2.0	/	/	/
	Grass	Female	International	/	/	18.1 ± 1.6	/	/	/

MD: match duration; MRD: mean rally duration; MRT: mean resting time; EPT: effective playing time; DRP: distance ran per point; SR: shots per rally.

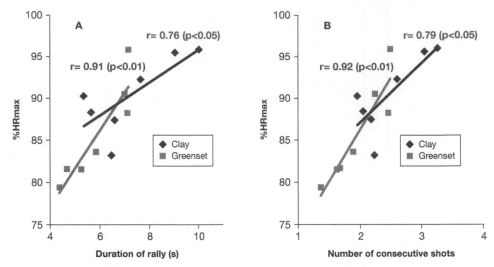

Figure 23.2 Correlations between the percentage of HRmax, duration of rallies and shots played consecutively on clay and hard courts, according to Girard and Millet (2004).

(H), 7.7 ± 1.7 seconds at the French Open (CL), 4.3 ± 1.6 seconds at Wimbledon (grass) and 5.8 ± 1.9 seconds at the US Open (H) were recorded. Rallies were significantly longer at the French Open than at any other tournament and significantly shorter at Wimbledon than at any other tournament. In the same way, it has been shown that SR and DRP are significantly higher on CL than on H. All these results can be explained by the tactical behaviour used by players according to the court surface. For example, a more aggressive and attacking game is associated with a faster surface such as grass. This type of study has been repeated for a more recent period. Indeed, Brown and O'Donoghue (2008) have conducted a notational analysis of singles events at all four Grand Slam tournaments during 2007. They revealed that the difference between rally durations at the French Open (7.3 seconds) and Wimbledon (3.8 seconds) in 1997–9 has decreased in 2007 (7.6 and 5.4 seconds, respectively). Moreover, rallies in men's singles have increased in duration at all four tournaments since 1999. There was a lower percentage of service points (aces, double faults, serve winners and return winners) in men's singles at each tournament in 2007 than reported by O'Donoghue and Ingram (2001). These data reflect two 'evolution points' in elite competitive tennis matches. First, they can be explained by the introduction of new balls by the ITF to reduce the variation between different surfaces. In 2006, the ITF decided to use type 1 balls on the slowest surfaces and type 3 balls on the fastest surfaces. Because the type 3 ball is 6–8 per cent bigger than the standard type 2 ball, it generates greater air resistance, resulting in greater air deceleration before the rebound (Miller, 2006). Second, one may argue that players are fitter and show better technical abilities currently than during the 1990s, allowing them to reach more balls and increase the duration of rallies (Brown and O'Donoghue, 2008).

The influence of tennis playing surface on matches' characteristics and physiological parameters

Studies analysed the effect of court surfaces on the match's technical characteristics in relation to the player's physiological responses during simulated tennis competition (Girard and Millet, 2004; Martin *et al.*, 2011; Murias *et al.*, 2007). They found a relationship between the changes in match characteristics induced by court surface and physiological responses. Court surface influences tennis match characteristics that are probably responsible for the higher mean HR and [La] values measured on CL than on H, suggesting an overall higher physiological demand on that surface (Martin *et al.*, 2011; Murias *et al.*, 2007; Reid *et al.*, 2012). The fact that, on H, the rallies are less long and less intense than on CL could be a factor responsible for higher [La] values on CL. Girard and Millet (2004) found high correlations between the percentage of HRmax, duration of rallies and shots played consecutively on CL and H courts (see Figure 23.2). HR increases when subjects hit more consecutive shots and play longer rallies. In the same way, Fernandez-Fernandez *et al.* (2007) found a significant positive relationship between rally duration, strokes per rally, changes of direction and [La] and HR responses, with stronger correlations when the players were serving on CL. Concerning mean VO_2, Girard and Millet (2004) reported higher mean VO_2 values on CL than on H. According to Murias *et al.* (2007), mean percentage of mean VO_2max was not altered by the playing surface. These results are suggestive of an increased physiological demand on CL. Fernandez-Fernandez *et al.* (2010) have examined how the training surface (CL or carpet) affects the characteristics (ball velocity, running pressure, running volume, physiological responses) of a training session. They reported no significant difference of the court surface on any variables analysed.

The influence of tennis playing surface on fatigue

In tennis, the fatigue may be related to a prolonged or high-intensity physical exertion (Hornery *et al.*, 2007). For these authors, fatigue can be defined as an acute impairment of exercise performance, which ultimately leads to the incapacity to produce maximal force output and/or control motor function. In tennis, fatigue may be resulted in a sequence of long and intense points. To our knowledge, only one study has focused on the effect of the playing surface properties on the development of neuromuscular fatigue in tennis (Fabre *et al.*, 2012). In this study, 10 subjects played randomly two tennis matches on an H court and a CL court for an effective playing duration of 45 minutes, corresponding approximately to a 3-hour game. Before and after each match, the maximal voluntary contraction force of the plantar flexors, the maximal voluntary activation level, the maximal compound muscle action characteristics and the electromyographic activity were determined on the *soleus* and *lateralis gastrocnemius* muscles. Any significant difference between playing surfaces was observed in this study. These results suggest that the ground surface properties influence neither the extent nor the origin of neuromuscular fatigue in tennis.

The influence of tennis playing surfaces on injuries

Most epidemiological studies in tennis players have shown that overuse injuries are very common in all competitive levels (Jayanthi *et al.*, 2005; Pluim *et al.*, 2006). Among these injuries, it has been reported that lower limb problems are nearly equal to or exceed upper limb pains (Pluim *et al.*, 2006). This phenomenon can be explained by the nature of the tennis game that involves quick, intense and repeated start-stop movements, changes in direction, running and sliding side to side (Kovacs, 2006). However, injury rates depend not only of the nature of the sport, but are also caused by a lot of risk factors. Indeed, in sport injury, risk factors are often classified into two main categories: intrinsic athlete-related factors (age, gender, skill level, somatotype, biomechanics, conditioning, maturational stage) and extrinsic environmental factors (weather, rules, equipment, floor surfaces) (Taimela *et al.*, 1990; Van Mechelen *et al.*, 1992). As an extrinsic environmental factor, the court surface has been shown to have

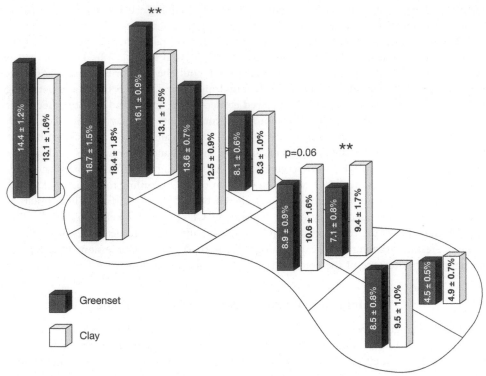

Figure 23.3 Mean and standard deviation relative load (percentage) for each foot region during baseline play on greenset and on clay, according to Girard *et al.* (2007).

an influence on the injury pattern of tennis players (Dragoo and Braun, 2010; Nigg and Yeadon, 1987; Nigg and Segesser, 1988). A study of incomplete matches in Grand Slam professional tennis tournaments from 1978 to 2005 reported the following results: fewer incomplete matches on grass courts (2.0 per cent for men in Wimbledon between 1995 and 2004); higher rates of incomplete matches on Australian Open H courts (1.9 per cent) than on other surfaces (0.6 per cent) in Wimbledon and Roland Garros, 0.8 per cent at the US Open for women; and a higher rate of incomplete matches on US Open H courts for men (4.3 per cent between 1995 and 2004) than on other surfaces (3.1 per cent in Australian Open and 3.6 per cent in Roland Garros) (Cross, 2006). Breznik and Batagelj (2012) clearly confirmed the influence of the surface type, with the proportion of retired matches being higher on H and CL courts compared to grass and carpet surfaces. Moreover, it has been reported that senior players who spent their careers on CL rather than on H surfaces had lower rates of knee problems (Kulund *et al.*, 1979). Bastholt (2000) has examined injury rates in professional male tennis players for three years on CL, H, grass and carpet courts. According to the results, injury treatment during matches was required significantly more often on H than on CL courts. In the same way, Nigg and Denoth (1980) used a retrospective design study over three seasons to question 1,003 tennis players to study the relationship between tennis injuries and court surfaces. They showed that back, knee and ankle joints were the locations the most frequently injured and that athletes playing on surfaces allowed sliding, such as CL courts, were related to significant less pain and injury than athletes playing on surfaces that did not allow sliding (asphalt, synthetic surface). In the literature, possible causes related to court surfaces for such differences have been suggested (Nigg and Segesser, 1988) and will be exposed in the following sections.

Ground reaction forces

Dixon and Stiles (2003) found no significant difference in vertical impact force or peak in-shoe heel pressures across surfaces typically used in tennis when running at a relaxed pace. However, we can suppose that the task in this study ('running at a relaxed pace') was not sufficient to simulate the complex tennis activity and movements that would have revealed impact force differences between court surfaces. Tiegermann (1983) compared the ground reaction forces and the EMG activation of the *soleus* and *peroneus longus* in fast sideways movements on carpet and CL courts. The ground reaction forces and the EMG activity were significantly higher on carpet than on CL. Moreover, Girard *et al.* (2007) compared in shoe-loading patterns during two frequent tennis-specific movements (serve and volley, baseline play) performed on two court surfaces (CL and H) to identify the main loading patterns and locations on the anatomical structures of the foot. Regarding the whole foot, mean force was significantly lower on CL (614 ± 73 N) than on H court (717 ± 133 N) ($p < 0.05$). These results mean that the magnitude of external forces induced by the court surface on the musculoskeletal system is less important. This phenomenon could explain why epidemiological studies reported lower injury rates on CL than on H courts. Furthermore, higher loadings in hallux and lesser toes area were measured on H court than on CL (Girard *et al.*, 2007). Conversely, the CL condition was characterized by higher loadings and relative loadings on medial and lateral midfoot (see Figure 23.3). As a consequence, it was concluded that the type of court surface influences plantar loading at specific foot regions and, as a consequence, differently affects the aetiology of surface-related injuries (Girard *et al.*, 2007).

Cushioning/stiffness

Stiles and Dixon (2006) have evaluated the influence of court surfaces with different cushioning values on the ground reaction forces during tennis running forehand trials. They reported that the surface with the lowest mechanical cushioning induced the lowest vertical force magnitude. However, according to Nigg and Yeadon (1987), the cushioning of a tennis court is less important for load reduction than reduction of frictional forces. Indeed, they showed that the surfaces 'synthetic sand' and 'synthetic turf' have the same stiffness. However, the number of people complaining about pain is higher while playing on 'synthetic turf' than on 'synthetic clay'. This result could be explained by the only difference between these two surfaces. Indeed, the 'synthetic sand' has an additional loose layer of granules on its top that allows tennis players to slide. Consequently, the stiffness of the surface seems less important than the frictional properties for preventing tennis injuries (Nigg and Yeadon, 1987).

Frictional properties

Frictional properties of the tennis shoe-surface interface are a factor that could explain pain/injury frequency and severity (Nigg and Yeadon, 1987). Translational friction determines how much horizontal force will be needed to cause the shoe to slide over the surface. CL courts show a lower coefficient of translation friction than H courts. As a consequence, it has been suggested that playing on CL could produce lower frictional resistance and will decrease the loadings at the joints, which reduce the risk of lower extremity injuries (Girard *et al.*, 2007). Rotational friction determines how much force must be applied as a moment of force to cause the shoe to pivot on the surface. The maximum torque is often measured by researchers comparing various surfaces and shoe combinations to evaluate the rotational friction of the

Table 23.4 Grand Slam match statistics in 2004–5, according to Barnett and Pollard (2007)

	Sex	Roland Garros 2004 (clay)	Australian Open 2005 (Rebound Ace)	US Open 2004 (DecoTurf)	Wimbledon 2004 (grass)
Win per cent on first serve (%)	Men	67.0	70.2	71.6	73.3
	Women	59.2	61.7	56.3	57.9
Serving points won (%)	Men	59.2	62.2	62.1	65.2
	Women	52.5	54.8	56.2	57.9
Aces (%)	Men	4.7	7.2	8.5	8.8
	Women	3.0	3.9	3.8	4.6
Break point conversions (%)	Men	44.5	41.0	41.5	36.4
	Women	51.0	48.7	48.3	44.3
Net approaches (%)	Men	26.4	28.3	30.4	33.4
	Women	17.6	18.1	21.4	21.9

combination. This value corresponds to the maximum torque to produce a shoe rotation on the given surface (Frederick, 1993). It has been reported that surfaces with higher rotational friction demonstrate greater peak torques during pivoting. Conversely, surfaces with lower rotational friction show lower peak torques (Frederick, 1993). For example, executing a guided rotation of 180° on a CL court would result in a peak torque of about 20 Nm (Michel, 1978). Performing the same movement on a grass court and on an asphalt court, the manoeuvre would respectively produce a peak torque of about 25 and 30 Nm (Michel, 1978). High rotational friction on sport surfaces has been shown to cause an increased incidence of knee and ankle injuries (Nigg and Denoth, 1980).

The influence of tennis playing surfaces on strategy

O'Donoghue and Ingram (2001) evaluated the effect of tennis court surfaces on the strategies of elite players in single events at Grand Slam tournaments between 1997 and 1999. According to their results, there were significantly more aces played at Wimbledon than at Roland Garros and significantly more serve winners at Wimbledon than at Roland Garros and at the Australian Open. This result could be explained by the court surface. Indeed, CL courts in Roland Garros induce slower and higher ball bounce, providing the receiver with the opportunity of returning more serves than on faster surfaces such as grass in Wimbledon. Moreover, the players approached the net significantly more at Wimbledon and the US Open than at Roland Garros. Conversely, the proportion of baseline rallies played at Roland Garros (51.9 ± 14.3 per cent of points) was significantly higher than at the Australian Open (46.6 ± 12.5 per cent), Wimbledon (19.7 ± 19.4 per cent) and the US Open (35.4 ± 19.5 per cent). These results suggest that on slow surfaces (such as CL), the tennis players have difficulty in hitting effective approach shots that pressurize their opponent to reduce the risks of successful passing shots or lobs. As a consequence, they prefer to hit baseline strokes. Furthermore, no significant difference was reported between the four tournaments in the percentage of points won at the net and in the percentage of points won when players remained at the baseline by the serving player or the receiving player. In the same way, Barnett and Pollard (2007) analysed various match statistics for men and women during 2004–5 Grand Slams (see Table 23.4). Progressing from left to right in both tables, their results report an increase in the winning percentage on first serve, an increase in the serving points won, an increase in aces and an increase in net approaches. As a consequence, the authors assumed that there was a fundamental ordering of court speeds between Grand Slams: grass, DecoTurf, Rebound Ace, CL.

Acknowledgements

The authors would like to thank Dr Olivier Girard for giving permission to reproduce Figures 23.2 and 23.3.

References

Barnett, T. and Pollard, G. (2007) 'How the tennis court surface affects player performance and injuries', *Medicine and Science in Tennis*, 12(1): 34–7.

Bastholt, P. (2000) 'Professional tennis (ATP Tour) and number of medical treatments in relation to type of surface', *Medicine and Science in Tennis*, 5(2): 9.

Bergeron, M. F., Maresh, C. M., Kraemer, W. J., Abraham, A., Conroy, B. and Gabaree, C. (1991) 'Tennis: a physiological profile during match play', *International Journal of Sports Medicine*, 12(5): 474–9.

Breznik, K. and Batagelj, V. (2012) 'Retired matches among male professional tennis players', *Journal of Sports Science and Medicine*, 11: 270–8.

Brody, H. (2003) 'Bounce of a tennis ball', *Journal of Science and Medicine in Sport*, 6(1): 113–19.

Brown, E. and O'Donoghue, P. (2008) 'Gender and surface effect on elite tennis strategy', *ITF Coach Sport Science Review*, 46(12): 9–12.

Cross, R. (2006) 'Grand Slam injuries 1978–2005', *Medicine and Science in Tennis*, 11(1): 88.

Dansou, P., Oddou, M. F., Delaire, M. and Therminarias, A. (2001) 'Dépense énergétique aérobie au cours d'un match de tennis, du laboratoire au terrain', *Science & Sports*, 16: 16–22.

Deutsch, E., Deutsch, S. L. and Douglas, P. L. (1998) 'Exercise training for competitive tennis', *Clinics in Sports Medicine*, 7(2): 417–27.

Dixon, S. J. and Stiles, V. H. (2003) 'Impact absorption for tennis shoe–surface combinations', *Sports Engineering*, 6(1): 1–10.

Dragoo, J. L. and Braun, H. J. (2010) 'The effect of playing surface on injury rate: a review of the current literature', *Sports Medicine*, 40(11): 981–90.

Fabre, J. B., Martin, V., Gondin, J., Cottin, F. and Grelot, L. (2012) 'Effect of playing surface properties on neuromuscular fatigue in tennis', *Medicine and Science in Sports and Exercise*, 44(11): 2182–9.

Fernandez-Fernandez, J., Mendez-Villanueva, A., Fernandez-Garcia, B. and Terrados, N. (2007) 'Match activity and physiological responses during a junior female single tennis tournament', *British Journal of Sports Medicine*, 41(11): 711–16.

Fernandez-Fernandez, J., Sanz-Rivas, D., Fernandez-Garcia, B. and Mendez-Villanueva, A. (2008) 'Match activity and physiological load during a clay-court tournament in elite female players', *Journal of Sports Sciences*, 26(14): 1589–95.

Fernandez-Fernandez, J., Sanz-Rivas, D. and Mendez-Villanueva, A. (2009) 'A review of the activity profile and physiological demands of tennis match play', *Strength and Conditioning Journal*, 31(4): 15–26.

Fernandez-Fernandez, J., Kinner, V. and Ferrauti, A. (2010) 'The physiological demands of hitting and running in tennis on different surfaces', *Journal of Strength and Conditioning Research*, 24(12): 3255–64.

Ferrauti, A., Bergeron, M. F., Pluim, B. M. and Weber, K. (2001a) 'Physiological responses in tennis and running with similar oxygen uptake', *European Journal of Applied Physiology*, 85(1–2): 27–33.

Ferrauti, A., Pluim, B. M. and Weber, K. (2001b) 'The effect of recovery duration on running speed and stroke quality during intermittent training drills in elite tennis players', *Journal of Sports Sciences*, 19(4): 235–42.

Frederick, E. C. (1993) 'Optimal frictional properties for sport shoes and sport surfaces', in J. Hamill, T. R. Derrick and E. H. Elliott (eds), *Biomechanics in Sports XI*, Amherst, MA: International Society of Biomechanics in Sports, pp.15–22.

Girard, O. and Millet, G. P. (2004) 'Effects of the ground surface on the physiological and technical responses in young tennis players', in T. Reilly, M. Hughes and A. Lees (eds), *Science and Racket Sports III*, London: EFN Spon, pp. 43–8.

Girard, O., Eicher, F., Fourchet, F., Micallef, J. P. and Millet, G. P. (2007) 'Effects of the playing surface on plantar pressures and potential injuries in tennis', *British Journal of Sports Medicine*, 41(11): 733–8.

Hornery, D.J., Farrow, D., Mujika, I. and Young, W. (2007) 'Caffeine, carbohydrate and cooling use during prolonged simulated tennis', *International Journal of Sports Physiology and Performance*, 2(4): 423–438.

International Tennis Federation (2012) *ITF Approved Tennis Balls, Classified Surfaces and Recognised Courts 2012 – a Guide to Products and Test Methods*, 15 February, International Tennis Federation, available at: www.itftennis.com/technical/equipment/courts/courtlist.asp (accessed 16 February 2012).

Jayanthi, N., Sallay, P. I., Hunker, P. and Przybylski, M. (2005) 'Skill-level related injuries in recreational competition tennis players', *Medicine and Science in Tennis*, 10(1): 12–15.

Kovacs, M. S. (2006) 'Applied physiology of tennis performance', *British Journal of Sports Medicine*, 40(5): 381–5.

Kovacs, M. S. (2007) 'Tennis physiology: training the competitive athlete', *Sports Medicine*, 37(3): 189–98.

Kulund, D. N., McCue, F. C., Rockwell, D. A. and Gieck, J. H. (1979) 'Tennis injuries: prevention and treatment. A review', *American Journal of Sports Medicine*, 7(4): 249–53.

Martin, C., Thevenet, D., Zouhal, H., Mornet, Y., Delès, R., Crestel, T., Ben Abderrahman, A. and Prioux, J. (2011) 'Effects of playing surface (hard and clay courts) on heart rate and blood lactate during tennis matches played by high level players', *Journal of Strength and Conditioning Research*, 25(1): 163–70.

Mendez-Villanueva, A., Fernandez-Fernandez, J. and Bishop, D. (2007) 'Exercise-induced homeostasic perturbations provoked by singles tennis match play with reference to development of fatigue', *British Journal of Sports Medicine*, 41(11): 717–22.

Mendez-Villanueva, A., Fernandez-Fernandez, J., Bishop, D. and Fernandez-Garcia, B. (2010) 'Ratings of perceived exertion-lactate association during actual singles tennis match-play', *Journal of Strength and Conditioning Research*, 24(1): 165–70.

Michel, H. (1978). 'Drehbewegungen auf Bodenbelagen (Rotation on surfaces)', unpublished master's dissertation, ETH Zurich.

Miller, S. (2006) 'Modern tennis rackets, ball and surfaces', *British Journal of Sports Medicine*, 40(5): 401–15.

Murias, J. M., Lanatta, D., Arcuri, C. R. and Laino, F. A. (2007) 'Metabolic and functional responses playing tennis on different surfaces', *Journal of Strength and Conditioning Research*, 21(1): 112–17.

Nigg, B. M. and Denoth, J. (1980) *Sportplatzbeläge (Playing surfaces)*, Zurich: Juris Verlag.

Nigg, B. M. and Yeadon, M. R. (1987) 'Biomechanical aspects of playing surfaces', *Journal Sports Sciences*, 5(2): 117–45.

Nigg, B. M. and Segesser, B. (1988). 'The influence of playing surfaces on the load on the locomotor system and on football and tennis injuries', *Sports Medicine*, 5(6): 375–85.

O'Donoghue, P. and Ingram, B. (2001) 'A notational analysis of elite tennis strategy', *Journal of Sports Sciences*, 19(2): 107–15.

Parsons, L. S. and Jones, M. T. (1998) 'Development of speed, agility and quickness for tennis athletes', *Strength and Conditioning*, 20(3): 14–19.

Pluim, B. M., Staal, J. B., Windler, G. E. and Jayanthi, N. (2006) 'Tennis injuries: occurrence, aetiology, and prevention', *British Journal of Sports Medicine*, 40(5): 415–23.

Reid, M., Duffield, R., Minett, G., Sibte, N., Murphy, A. and Baker, J. (2012) 'Physiological, perceptual and technical responses to on court tennis training on hard and clay courts', *Journal of Strength and Conditioning Research*, doi:10.1519/JSC.0b013e31826caedf.

Smekal, G., Von Duvillard, S. P., Rihacek, C., Pokan, R., Hofmann, P., Baron, R., Tschan, H. and Bachl, N. (2001) 'A physiological profile of tennis match play', *Medicine and Science in Sports and Exercise*, 33(6): 999–1005.

Stiles, V. and Dixon, S. (2006) 'The influence of different playing surfaces on the biomechanics of a tennis running forehand foot plant', *Journal of Applied Biomechanics*, 22(1): 14–24.

Taimela, S., Kujala, U. M. and Osterman K. (1990) 'Intrinsic risk factors and athletic injuries', *Sports Medicine*, 9(4): 205–15.

Tiegermann, V. (1983) 'Reaction forces and EMG activity in fast side movements', in B. M. Nigg and B. A. Kerr (eds), *Biomechanical Aspects of Sport Shoes and Playing Surfaces*, Calgary: University Printing, pp. 83–90.

Van Mechelen, W., Hlobil, H. and Kemper, H. C. (1992) 'Incidence, severity, aetiology and prevention of sports injuries. A review of concepts', *Sports Medicine*, 14(5): 82–99.

24

LOADING PATTERNS ON NATURAL GRASS AND SYNTHETIC TURF IN AMERICAN FOOTBALL

Kevin R. Ford[1,2,3]

[1]HIGH POINT UNIVERSITY, HIGH POINT
[2]CINCINNATI CHILDREN'S HOSPITAL MEDICAL CENTER, CINCINNATI
[3]UNIVERSITY OF CINCINNATI, CINCINNATI

Introduction

The popular sport of American football is increasingly played on both natural grass and synthetic turf. For example, in 2005 over one-third (12 out of 31) of the National Football League (NFL) stadiums consisted of artificial surfaces (Ford *et al.*, 2006). Similarly, in the 2009 season, 214 NFL games were played on FieldTurf compared to 366 games played on natural grass (Hershman *et al.*, 2012). The latest synthetic surfaces are developed and marketed to improve performance, provide more natural field and grass characteristics and reduce injuries. They are composed of polyethylene fibres of varying lengths stabilized with ground rubber and/or sand infill, and supported on an engineered foundation. The effects of playing surface on injury risk, athletic performance and movement biomechanics are important to characterize in football from the youth to professional levels.

Injury incidence

Studies have found conflicting results on the injury incidence while playing American football on natural grass and the latest synthetic turf. Hershman *et al.* (2012) recently published the results of 10 years of injury surveillance from the NFL focused on a synthetic turf (specifically FieldTurf) compared to natural grass. During the surveillance period, a total of 20.5 per cent of all team games were played on FieldTurf. Anterior cruciate ligament (ACL) sprains were 67 per cent more likely to occur on FieldTurf compared to a natural grass surface (Hershman *et al.*, 2012). Additionally, eversion ankle sprains were 31 per cent higher on FieldTurf compared to natural grass in professional football players (Hershman *et al.*, 2012).

At the collegiate level, Meyers published a three-year prospective study comparing injury rates on FieldTurf and natural grass (Meyers, 2010). ACL injuries were not specifically described in the collegiate surveillance, so a comparison to the professional level cannot be made. College football players sustained a greater amount of injuries on natural grass compared to FieldTurf (Meyers, 2010). Also of note, fewer severe injuries, defined as 22 days or more of time loss, occurred on FieldTurf (5.8 per cent) compared to natural grass (8 per cent) (Meyers, 2010).

Two hundred and forty high school football games were tracked for injury rates on FieldTurf and natural grass (Meyers and Barnhill, 2004). When the primary type of injury was examined between surfaces in high school football players, a few key differences were evident. For example, a higher rate of ligament tears was found on natural grass (7.2 per cent on natural grass, 3.1 per cent on FieldTurf) (Meyers and Barnhill, 2004). In contrast, greater muscle strains and epidermal injuries were found on FieldTurf (Meyers and Barnhill, 2004). A higher incidence of noncontact/running injuries were found on FieldTurf compared to natural grass (Meyers and Barnhill, 2004).

There is not a consensus from these studies on the effect of synthetic turf on injury incidence in American football. Additional intrinsic and extrinsic variables likely play an important role in the discrepancies found among injury epidemiology studies.

Athletic performance

The physical demands of American football often require high-speed movements with quick decelerations and accelerations. Electronic timing of agility drills or straight ahead sprinting is often performed to evaluate football players at varying levels. Football players have decreased straight-ahead speed on natural grass compared to a rubberized track (Brechue *et al.*, 2005). More specifically, a recent study tested collegiate football players during straight-ahead sprinting and during an agility drill on synthetic turf and natural grass (Gains *et al.*, 2010). There were no differences in time between field surface during the straight-ahead sprint (40-yard dash). However, the agility test (proagility) was performed in less time on synthetic turf compared to natural grass. The authors concluded that the rapid changes of direction necessary in the agility test might have resulted in improved performance on new-generation synthetic turf. In contrast, a slalom course that required moderate changes of direction did not have performance time differences between natural grass and synthetic turf (Ford *et al.*, 2006). The consistency of the latest styles of synthetic turf may enhance the speed of the game (Meyers and Barnhill, 2004). The likely increase in force and momentum with increased speed may, in turn, be a factor to certain types of injuries during football.

Andersson *et al.* (2008) analysed three separate aspects of soccer performance on natural grass compared to synthetic turf. Athlete questionnaires via a visual analogue scale were used to identify subjectively their impression of performing on each surface. Both groups of male soccer players (regularly played on natural grass, regularly played on synthetic turf) reported negative ratings of playing on synthetic turf (Andersson *et al.*, 2008). Females, however, reported a neutral impression regarding synthetic turf (Andersson *et al.*, 2008). Technical performance and movement patterns during matches were also assessed with video analysis and computerized coding. There were no differences in low- and high-intensity running on each surface. The only movement pattern difference found between playing surface was in the lower number of slide tackles on synthetic turf. The majority of soccer skill performances on each surface were not different. However, short passes were performed more often, primarily in the midfield area, on synthetic turf compared to natural grass (Andersson *et al.*, 2008).

Physiological responses are higher during a multistage running test on synthetic turf compared to natural grass (Di Michele *et al.*, 2009). Specifically, higher blood lactate concentration, at specific heart rate levels, was found in 18 young male soccer players. The authors suggest that the mechanical properties of the surfaces likely influenced the physiological responses and may explain higher perceived effort reported previously on synthetic turf (Andersson *et al.*, 2008; Di Michele *et al.*, 2009).

Biomechanical analyses

In-shoe pressure distribution measurement

Flexible and compliant insoles (i.e. pedar system, novel) have been previously used within sport footwear to measure pressure distribution during a variety of movements. The insoles are sized and placed within the footwear to measure the pressure between the foot and the cleat. An advantage of these systems is that they can be used to test differences in footwear on multiple playing surfaces. Typically, regions within the plantar surface of the foot are masked and peak pressure, maximum force or force time integral represented in each of the masked regions (Figure 24.1).

Ford *et al.* (2006) collected in-cleat pressure distribution data during cutting and running on two adjacent football fields (Figure 24.2). Peak pressure was 17.5 per cent higher on the synthetic surface in the central forefoot compared to the natural grass condition. Similarly, the lesser toes region also had increased peak pressure during the cutting steps on synthetic turf compared to natural grass. Interestingly, the total loading (force time integral) was not different between surfaces when considering the entire plantar surface of the foot. However, the

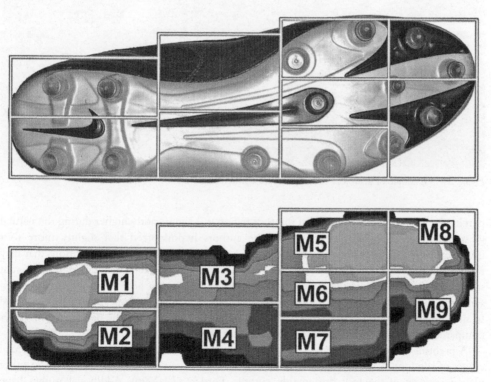

Figure 24.1 Regions of interest at the foot were masked to the size of the Pedar insole. The regions consisted of the following: M1 medial heel, M2 lateral heel, M3 medial midfoot, M4 lateral midfoot, M5 medial forefoot, M6 central forefoot, M7 lateral forefoot, M8 hallux and M9 lesser toes.

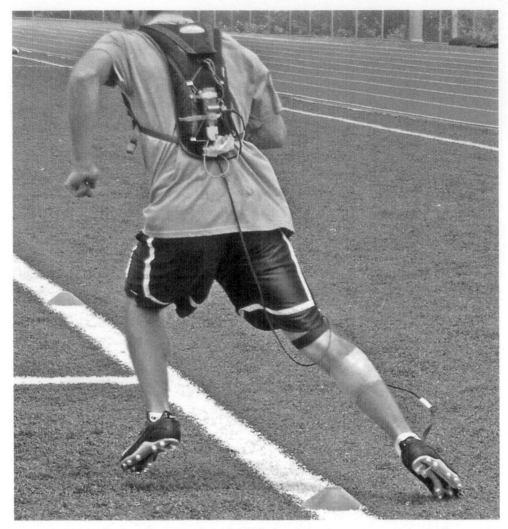

Figure 24.2 Example of a subject cutting on turf with cleated shoe.

percentage of load within the medial forefoot region was significantly higher during the natural grass compared to synthetic turf trials. The authors hypothesized that slightly more foot inversion on synthetic turf may explain the differences in loading between conditions that may result from the cushioning layer in synthetic turf. Orendurff *et al.* (2008) examined two different styles of footwear commonly worn during football. During an acceleration manoeuvre on synthetic turf, the lateral forefoot (fifth metatarsal) experienced elevated peak pressure compared to side-step cuts. Synthetic turf-specific footwear, in general, reduced the peak pressure values compared to a traditional football cleat (Orendurff *et al.*, 2008).

A pivoting or cutting movement requires participants to land and push-off from the medial aspect of the foot. The medial forefoot experiences the largest overall load compared to other plantar surfaces of the foot during side cutting (Ford *et al.*, 2006). Additional studies have demonstrated increases in peak pressure (Eils *et al.*, 2004; Queen *et al.*, 2007; Wong *et al.*, 2007), percentage of load (Eils *et al.*, 2004) and FTI impulses (Queen *et al.*, 2007) on medial aspects of the foot. For example, the hallux is loaded (relative load) only half the magnitude of the medial part of the forefoot (Ford *et al.*, 2006). Increased loading at the plantar surface of the foot may also impact the shoe-surface interface. For example, an increased axial load of 400 per cent can elevate the frictional resistance between 30 and 1,500 per cent (Cawley *et al.*, 2003).

Shoe-surface interface

While insole pressure measurement systems measure the foot-shoe interface, a potentially related and critical variable to injury frequency and severity involves assessment of the shoe-surface interface. High frictional conditions at the shoe-surface interface may contribute to higher injury rates (Nigg and Segesser, 1988). Additionally, the 'cleat-catch' injury may result when long studs are caught or dug into natural grass (Heidt *et al.*, 1996). The surface interface between the grass and cleat may lead to high frictional and rotational forces. Orchard *et al.* (2005) found higher incidence of anterior cruciate ligament injury in Australian football on grass conditions that involved a thick thatched layer (Bermuda) compared to a minimal thatched layer (Rye).

Livesay *et al.* (2006) tested a variety of cleat patterns and surface combinations. The grass-specific cleat on FieldTurf in addition to the turf shoe on Astroturf had the largest peak torque values compared to all other combinations (Livesay *et al.*, 2006). While excessively high peak torque values may increase the risk of injury, a trade-off exists between extremely low and extremely high values for adequate performance and safety.

Rotational stiffness, slope of the torque versus rotation data, has been suggested as a new measure that incorporates the rate at which torque increases (Livesay *et al.*, 2006). Rotational stiffness and peak torque were significantly greater across a variety of footwear on the newer style synthetic surface (FieldTurf and AstroPlay) compared to natural grass (sand-based and native soil) (Villwock *et al.*, 2009). While a variety of shoe-surface combinations are possible, differences in design may not influence lower extremity kinematic and kinetic values. For example, Kaila (2007) found similar knee loading during cutting with bladed versus moulded cleats. Additional studies should be completed to fully assess the full body biomechanical differences among varying levels of shoe-surface combinations.

Summary

The latest synthetic turf surfaces present both subtle and glaring differences in injury risk, athletic performance and movement biomechanics when compared to natural grass. Surface comparisons *in vivo* are challenging due to the variability of the surface, environment, footwear and players. Of concern is the recently identified higher incidence of ACL injury in high-level professional football players on FieldTurf compared to natural grass. Additional research should examine the lower extremity biomechanics of different shoe-surface interface combinations to help delineate high injury risk conditions.

References

Andersson, H., Ekblom, B. and Krustrup, P. (2008) 'Elite football on artificial turf versus natural grass: movement patterns, technical standards, and player impressions', *Journal of Sports Sciences*, 26(2): 113–22.

Brechue, W. F., Mayhew, J. L. and Piper, F. C. (2005) 'Equipment and running surface alter sprint performance of college football players', *Journal of Srength and Conditioning Research*, 19(4): 821–5.

Cawley, P. W., Heidt, R. S., Jr, Scranton, P. E., Jr, Losse, G. M. and Howard, M. E. (2003) 'Physiologic axial load, frictional resistance, and the football shoe-surface interface', *Foot and Ankle International*, 24(7): 551–6.

Di Michele, R., Di Renzo, A. M., Ammazzalorso, S. and Merni, F. (2009) 'Comparison of physiological responses to an incremental running test on treadmill, natural grass, and synthetic turf in young soccer players', *Journal of Srength and Conditioning Research*, 23(3): 939–45.

Eils, E., Streyl, M., Linnenbecker, S., Thorwesten, L., Volker, K. and Rosenbaum, D. (2004) 'Characteristic plantar pressure distribution patterns during soccer-specific movements', *American Journal of Sports Medicine*, 32(1): 140–5.

Ford, K. R., Manson, N. A., Evans, B. J., Myer, G. D., Gwin, R. C., Heidt, R. S., Jr and Hewett, T. E. (2006) 'Comparison of in-shoe foot loading patterns on natural grass and synthetic turf', *Journal of Science and Medicine in Sport*, 9(6): 433–40.

Gains, G. L., Swedenhjelm, A. N., Mayhew, J. L., Bird, H. M. and Houser, J. J. (2010) 'Comparison of speed and agility performance of college football players on field turf and natural grass', *Journal of Strength and Conditioning Research*, 24(10): 2613–17.

Heidt, R. S., Jr, Dormer, S. G., Cawley, P. W., Scranton, P. E., Jr, Losse, G. and Howard, M. (1996) 'Differences in friction and torsional resistance in athletic shoe-turf surface interfaces', *American Journal of Sports Medicine*, 24(6): 834–42.

Hershman, E. B., Anderson, R., Bergfeld, J. A., Bradley, J. P., Coughlin, M. J., Johnson, R. J., Spindler, K. P., Wojtys, E. and Powell, J. W. (2012) 'An analysis of specific lower extremity injury rates on grass and fieldturf playing surfaces in National Football League Games: 2000–2009 seasons', *American Journal of Sports Medicine*, 40(10): 2200–5.

Kaila, R. (2007) 'Influence of modern studded and bladed soccer boots and sidestep cutting on knee loading during match play conditions', *American Journal of Sports Medicine*, 35(9): 28–36.

Livesay, G. A., Reda, D. R. and Nauman, E. A. (2006) 'Peak torque and rotational stiffness developed at the shoe-surface interface: the effect of shoe type and playing surface', *American Journal of Sports Medicine*, 34(3): 415–22.

Meyers, M. C. (2010) 'Incidence, mechanisms, and severity of game-related college football injuries on FieldTurf versus natural grass: a 3-year prospective study', *American Journal of Sports Medicine*, 38(4): 687–97.

Meyers, M. C. and Barnhill, B. S. (2004) 'Incidence, causes, and severity of high school football injuries on FieldTurf versus natural grass: a 5-year prospective study', *American Journal of Sports Medicine*, 32(7): 1626–38.

Nigg, B. M. and Segesser, B. (1988) 'The influence of playing surfaces on the load on the locomotor system and on football and tennis injuries', *Sports Medicine*, 5(6): 375–85.

Orchard, J. W., Chivers, I., Aldous, D., Bennell, K. and Seward, H. (2005) 'Rye grass is associated with fewer non-contact anterior cruciate ligament injuries than bermuda grass', *British Journal of Sports Medicine*, 39(10): 704–9.

Orendurff, M. S., Rohr, E. S., Segal, A. D., Medley, J. W., Green, J. R. and Kadel, N. J. (2008) 'Regional foot pressure during running, cutting, jumping, and landing', *American Journal of Sports Medicine*, 36(3): 566–71.

Queen, R. M., Haynes, B. B., Hardaker, W. M. and Garrett, W. E., Jr (2007) 'Forefoot loading during 3 athletic tasks', *American Journal of Sports Medicine*, 35(4): 630–6.

Villwock, M. R., Meyer, E. G., Powell, J. W., Fouty, A. J. and Haut, R. C. (2009) 'Football playing surface and shoe design affect rotational traction', *American Journal of Sports Medicine*, 37(3): 518–25.

Wong, P. L., Chamari, K., Mao De, W., Wisloff, U. and Hong, Y. (2007) 'Higher plantar pressure on the medial side in four soccer-related movements', *British Journal of Sports Medicine*, 41(2): 93–100.

25

HUMAN MOVEMENT
ON ICE SURFACE

Federico Formenti

UNIVERSITY OF OXFORD, OXFORD

Our walking and running movement patterns require friction between shoes and ground, where we exert downwards and backwards forces ultimately resulting in forward movement. The surface of ice is characterized by low friction in several naturally occurring conditions, for example on frozen lakes or canals; this low friction can limit our walking velocity, increase its energy cost and determine a greater risk of falls and injury. More than 3,000 years ago, humans invented an entirely new form of locomotion to be employed on ice; here, they would stand on skates made of animal bones and push backwards on the ice with a pointy stick in order to move forward, similarly to what one can do on a canoe, rowing with a single-bladed paddle. Ice became a surface where travelling was faster and more economical than other forms of muscle-powered locomotion on ground, especially when skates with metal blades began to be used on Dutch canals in the thirteenth century. The first part of this chapter presents an overview of the physics of ice surface friction, and discusses the most relevant factors that can influence ice skates' dynamic friction coefficient. The second part presents the main stages in the development of human locomotion on ice, describes the associated implications for exercise physiology and shows the extent to which ice skating performance improved through history. This chapter illustrates how technical and material development, together with empirical understanding of muscle biomechanics and energetics, led to one of the fastest forms of human-powered locomotion.

The physics of ice surface, a slippery matter

A few miles from One Ton Depot, Ross Ice Shelf, Antarctica; Saturday, 3 March 1912:

> The (ice) surface, lately a very good hard one, is coated with a layer of woolly crystals [. . .] [that] cause impossible friction to the runners. God help us, we can't keep up this pulling, that is certain.
>
> (Scott, 1913)

The surface of ice is made of a thin layer of molecules that behaves like a liquid, in several natural conditions

Ice as a solid material is truly peculiar: it is a solid, but one of its most distinct characteristics is that even when air is below freezing temperature, its surface is covered with a thin layer of water, the presence of which still puzzles many physicists (Kietzig *et al.*, 2010; Rosenberg, 2005; Watkins *et al.*, 2011). A block of ice floats on water because it is less dense than water. The increase in the volume of water with temperature decreasing below 0°C also explains why a bottle full of water can 'explode' if we forget it in the freezer for too long. The reverse also applies: if we compress ice hard enough, it melts and turns into water. This melting caused by pressure was proposed in the mid nineteenth century as the main mechanism through which a water film would form under ice skates' blades' pressure, which was assumed to be sufficiently high. However, it was later understood that the magnitude of the pressure increase caused by a skater would generally not be sufficient to determine the melting of the ice. In fact, this increase in pressure would result in a small temperature increase, say in the order of 1°C, insufficient to explain the low friction of ice skates at very low temperatures. Moreover, it was observed that the pressure required for melting ice at low temperatures is so great that it would squeeze the water film away from the underside of the skate's blade (Colbeck, 1995). Overall, it is now generally accepted that pressure melting plays a minor role in determining the low friction of skates on ice, other than at temperatures near the melting point.

Whenever motion with friction occurs, some of the kinetic energy is converted to heat. This is why our hands become warmer when we rub them together rapidly; here, some of the heat caused by friction between our hands warms them up, and some heat is lost in the air. Bowden and Hughes (1939) applied this concept to the study of skis sliding on ice and snow. Their experiments took place in an ice cave near the High Altitude Research Station Jungfraujoch in Switzerland, at an altitude of 3,346 m above sea level, where they observed that miniature sliders made of brass were characterized by a considerably greater dynamic coefficient of friction than miniature sliders made of ebonite, and they explained this phenomenon with the materials' thermal conductivity. During the sliding process, brass would take up much of the heat generated by friction, so relatively little heat would be available to melt the ice. Colbeck also supported that heat would decrease the coefficient of friction on ice through experiments where temperature was measured underneath skates (Colbeck, 1995; Colbeck *et al.*, 1997). He observed that blades' temperature increases with velocity, and with thermal insulation of most of the blade; also, he observed that the blade's sliding leaves warm tracks on the surface of ice behind the skates, suggesting that frictional heating may be an important determinant of ice skates' low dynamic coefficient of friction. This finding was replicated in more recent experiments (Baurle *et al.*, 2006).

Neither of the two scenarios presented above, namely pressure melting and frictional heating, can explain why ice is slippery even when we simply stand on it. One of the first experimental observations on the liquid-like nature of the ice surface was presented by Faraday (1859). In simple terms, he observed that although the surface of ice is slippery, two ice blocks would stick if put one on top of the other, as if there were some water that would freeze in between, a phenomenon called regelation. Following these observations made in the mid nineteenth century, studies on the physics of ice surface have not made much progress until the second half of the twentieth century, when the wide multidisciplinary importance of ice as a material became apparent. Several mechanisms have been proposed in order to explain the slippery nature of ice surface. One of the most recent and plausible explanations is that, at a molecular level, the surface of ice vibrates.

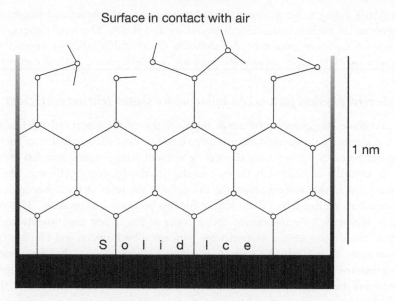

Figure 25.1 The presence of a liquid-like layer on the outermost surface of ice, even at air temperatures below freezing, is possibly one of the main reasons for ice surface slipperiness (adapted from Ikeda-Fukazawa and Kawamura, 2004). This schematic diagram shows a representation of the solid ice layer (bottom), and the liquid-like layer on the outermost surface of ice (top).

In most crystalline materials, each surface molecule has an identical binding energy, while molecules are bound by different forces in the surface of ice (Watkins *et al.*, 2011). In the lower part of Figure 25.1, the solid ice layer is represented by a frame of hexagons with a periodic structure, characterized by several and regular chemical bonds represented by thin lines. In contrast, the liquid-like layer on the surface of ice is represented with relatively fewer and less regular bonds. Due to this weaker physical structure, atoms in the ice surface can move rather freely, similarly to what they do in water. It is thought that the interaction of these moving atoms in the surface of ice with the solid ice immediately underneath generates the superficial lubricating film of water (also known as the liquid-like layer), independently of any frictional heat or pressure generated by ice skates. This can explain why ice is slippery even when we simply stand on it, a situation where we do not generate much frictional heat on the surface of ice and where, as discussed above, the pressure exerted on the ice by our body would not contribute much to the melting of the ice surface. In order to understand the functional significance of the liquid-like layer, a comparison with water slides may help, where the slide itself represents ice, water represents the liquid-like layer on the ice surface and the person sliding represents a skate's blade. In this comparison, with its implicit limitations, it seems clear how friction is greatly reduced by a relatively thin water layer between the person and the slide.

The determinants of the friction coefficient between skates and ice presented above are naturally affected by a variety of factors. Temperature is certainly an important one, as at very low temperatures friction on ice surface can increase dramatically. Captain Scott, quoted in the opening section of this chapter, tragically experienced this increase of skis' and sledges' friction at temperatures below $-30°C$ during the *Terra Nova* expedition at the beginning of the twentieth century, when sadly he and his team did not survive the extremely low temperatures, great resistance to sliding and strong winds. Apart from temperature, other factors such as a skate's sliding velocity, thermal conductivity, area of contact and roughness of the blade determine the friction coefficient between ice and skates. The next paragraph presents an overview of the most important determinants of ice skates' friction coefficient; more extensive reviews on this topic are published elsewhere (Kietzig *et al.*, 2010; Rosenberg, 2005).

Several physical factors can influence ice skates' friction coefficient

Ambient and blades' temperature influence the thickness of the superficial layer of water on ice, which is ultimately the greatest determinant of skates' dynamic coefficient of friction. The layer of water becomes thinner with decreasing ambient temperatures, and this reduction in thickness is normally associated with an increase in the friction coefficient. At ambient temperatures close to the melting point, the thickness of the layer of water becomes relatively excessive, resulting in drag forces that increase friction between ice and skate. This concept is illustrated in Figure 25.2. As mentioned above, some of the earliest experiments investigating the effects of temperature on ice friction were performed by Bowden and Hughes (1939). In their experiments, they used solid carbon dioxide and liquid air to alter temperature, and observed a marked increase in the dynamic coefficient of friction between slider and ice for temperatures decreasing to $-40°C$ and below. Bowden's experimental results showing a relationship between temperature and ice friction were replicated in more recent studies, which considered different materials, sliders' velocities and ice conditions (Albracht *et al.*, 2004; Calabrese *et al.*, 1980; de Koning *et al.*, 1992a; Slotfeldt-Ellingsen and Torgensen, 1983). The minimum coefficient of friction is often recorded at temperatures around $-5°C$ in most of these studies.

Ice surface temperature can also be altered by ice skates' blades' temperature, which in turn is influenced by heat generated through friction. Faster sliding velocities are associated with higher blade temperature, ice surface frictional melting effect and consequently lower dynamic coefficient of friction (Colbeck, 1994; Colbeck *et al.*, 1997; de Koning *et al.*, 1992a). The heat generated by friction can be retained by low thermal conductivity materials, where heat is partly stored in the material itself and contributes to the melting of the ice. This was initially observed by Bowden and Hughes (1939) when they compared the friction coefficient of a copper, 'air-filled' slider with a mercury-filled slider. Air has a much smaller thermal conductivity than mercury, so the air-filled slider appeared to have a smaller coefficient of friction. This finding was replicated in different materials by Itagaki *et al.* (1989). The roughness of skates' blades' material also influences blade temperature and dynamic coefficient of friction (Calabrese *et al.*, 1980; Itagaki *et al.*, 1989). A rough material would determine a great friction, hence a great increase in temperature and great melting effect; however, the roughness of the surface would also be associated with an increased actual contact surface area (for a given apparent contact area), and greater interlocking asperities that would work against the sliding movement. In this respect, a smooth material is preferred for skates' blades because it is characterized by a reduced surface asperity, and ultimately results in a lower coefficient of friction. For a material with a given roughness level, the orientation of polishing marks (e.g. on the blade's lateral or sagittal plane) can also influence the friction coefficient (Itagaki *et al.*, 1989). A large-scale example is the underside of cross-country skis, where the deep groove represents a sagittal plane polishing mark. Clearly, polishing marks that are aligned with the blade's direction of motion are associated with low dynamic coefficient of friction, and may also contribute to the control of the blade during the gliding phase.

The pressure exerted on a surface is a function of a normal force, and the contact area over which the force is applied. As discussed above, pressure does not appear to be a strong determinant of ice skates' friction, so changes in normal force or blades' contact area would not be expected to affect skates' friction coefficient significantly. Studies investigating effects of different normal forces and geometric contact areas on the dynamic coefficient of friction reported contrasting evidence (Albracht *et al.*, 2004; Baurle *et al.*, 2006, 2007; Bowden and Hughes, 1939; Calabrese *et al.*, 1980), where no clear relationship between these variables appeared. It is possible that the variety of experimental conditions (e.g. temperatures, materials, velocities) have determined different outcomes that are difficult to compare. Regardless, possibly through empirical understanding of skates' friction on ice, the geometry of skates' blades has changed through history (Formenti and Minetti, 2007). The apparent contact area of modern ice skates' blades is only about a third of blades used centuries ago. For a given skater's weight, this decrease in the blades' contact area results in a greater pressure exerted on ice, and in a relatively greater pressure-melting effect. However, as mentioned before, a skater is unlikely to generate the amount of pressure required for ice melting. Supporting the minor role of pressure for ice skates' low friction, modern ice skates' blades are relatively long (more than 400 mm). Rather than a small contact area, it seems important for a blade to have a small frontal area in contact with the ice, so that 'frontal' friction is as low as possible (Houdijk *et al.*, 2001), and to distribute the skater's weight over a great length; in other words, modern long blades allow the skate to 'float' on (not sink in) the water layer on the surface of ice. It is possible that the length of modern blades is an optimum in terms of low pressure levels on ice and manoeuvrability. Shorter blades would be associated with greater pressure levels that may still not be sufficient to generate a pressure-melting effect on the ice, but could be sufficient to squeeze part of the water film away from the blade, resulting in greater solid-solid contact and high wear rates; longer blades would be heavier, and could be more difficult to manoeuvre. Recalling the water slide example, a comparison could be drawn with a person sliding in a supine or seated position: when the person slides in a seated position (short blade), the pressure they exert on the water is relatively big, water is squeezed out between the person and the slide, determining solid-solid contact (person-slide) and relatively great friction. In contrast, when the person slides in a supine position (long blade), the smaller pressure exerted on the water allows some water to remain between person and slide, resulting in the presence of a lubricating water layer that reduces friction. This hypothesis needs to be tested with models and experiments.

In conclusion, several physical factors contribute to determining skates' friction on ice. Findings from previous studies have only in part elucidated the physics of ice skates' friction, with results often difficult to compare due to different experimental conditions, including ice properties that change significantly at different temperatures and humidity levels. Nevertheless, it seems generally accepted that an optimum water layer thickness exists where the dynamic coefficient of friction is minimum. The possibility to skate on this optimum water layer thickness depends on a combination of ice skates and ice properties.

Different friction regimes can coexist between skate and ice

Due to the presence of the water layer on the surface of ice, dry friction between an ice skate's blade and ice may be observed only over an extremely limited actual contact area, at least in natural conditions. As discussed in the previous section, the thickness of the water layer varies depending on multiple factors, and is associated with different friction regimes. Figure 25.2 illustrates the three main different friction regimes that characterize ice skates' gliding. Especially at very low temperatures, a very thin liquid-like layer (left, thin grey line) is associated with boundary friction, where the thickness of the liquid-like layer is smaller than the 'height' of ice and blade surface's asperities. This boundary friction regime is similar to that observed when rubbing two solids on each other, but the friction coefficient is lower than in dry friction. In contrast, at ambient temperatures near the melting point or above, an excessively thick liquid-like layer (right, grey icons represent water drops with capillary water bridges between asperities) (Colbeck, 1988) is associated with hydrodynamic friction, a regime similar to that observed between a boat and water. In the hydrodynamic friction regime, the thickness of the liquid-like layer is greater than the 'height' of the surface's asperities. An optimal liquid-like layer thickness, where the dynamic coefficient of friction is minimum, can be observed at intermediate thickness values (middle, thicker grey line). This scenario is often called mixed friction regime, where the thickness of the liquid-like layer is greater than in boundary friction, but still smaller than the 'height' of the surfaces' asperities, so relatively limited capillary water bridges form between surface asperities. Figure 25.2 illustrates these friction regimes together with the relationship between water layer thickness and dynamic coefficient of friction. The drawings at the top of the diagram represent the friction regimes observed between skates' blades and ice for the corresponding liquid-like layer thickness on the horizontal axis beneath. Black and grey arrows represent skates' and ice friction energy respectively (not to scale). Greater friction energy is encountered in boundary (left) and hydrodynamic (right) friction regimes than in the intermediate friction regime; here, the optimum lubricating layer thickness affords the minimum loss of energy caused by friction.

In contrast with this simplified model, a blade most likely shows a variety of friction regimes when we skate. This variety may be influenced by ice surface's irregularity, blade's velocity (even within the gliding phase), blade's orientation, distribution of pressure over the blade,

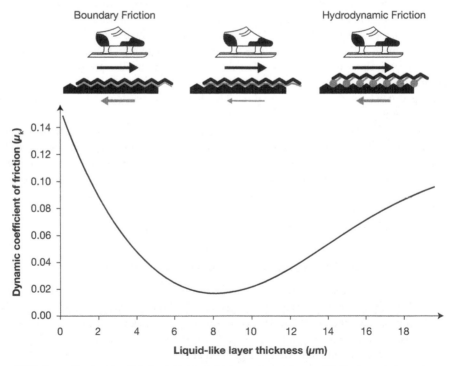

Figure 25.2 An optimal water (lubricating) layer thickness is associated with the lowest dynamic coefficient of friction (adapted from Colbeck, 1988; Kietzig *et al.*, 2010).

blade's and ambient temperature, and several other skater-related factors. The schematic representation above is only a reduced model of a rather complex physics problem: some of the main variables that influence ice friction are fairly well understood (e.g. temperature, velocity), but others (e.g. surface structure) are still an exciting area of exploration.

Human locomotion on ice

Ice was certainly a surface that humans tried to avoid travelling on for millennia, as its slippery nature increases risks of falls and injury, limits walking velocity, and increases walking metabolic energy cost. However, as early as 4,000 years ago, our ancestors realized that this slipperiness could be used to their advantage, and invented an entirely new form of human-powered locomotion: bone skating. The next part of this chapter presents the development of human locomotion on ice through history, and discusses the relevant biomechanical and physiological implications.

Skating on animal bones may have reduced time and energy cost for human-powered transport in Scandinavia more than 3,000 years ago

Most research studies on human locomotion on ice focused on its current relevance for sport and exercise physiology and biomechanics (Allinger and Van den Bogert, 1997; de Groot *et al.*, 1987; de Koning *et al.*, 1992b; Di Prampero *et al.*, 1976; Foster *et al.*, 1999; Houdijk *et al.*, 2000b; Marino, 1977; Rundell *et al.*, 1997; Smith and Roberts, 1990; van Ingen Schenau and Bakker, 1980; van Ingen Schenau *et al.*, 1989). Fewer studies explored the origins and the development of this ingenious form of human-powered locomotion (Blauw, 2001; Brown, 1959; Formenti and Minetti, 2007, 2008; Heathcote *et al.*, 1892; Muhonen, 2005; Munro, 1893).

Humans started skating on ice around the second millennium BC, as suggested by archaeological specimens. The first ice skates were possibly made of animal bones (Jacobi, 1976) on which the skater would stand, and were used together with a pointy stick pushed backwards on the ice surface for propulsion (Olaus, 1555). No clear evidence supports any of the different hypotheses as to why bone skating started. Also, the most ancient archaeological specimens cannot be clearly ordered chronologically, so it is difficult to identify ice skates' birthplace. Archaeological evidence helps to make possible connections between bone skates' qualitative features and tool-making traditions in different European regions thousands of years ago. This approach still leaves a wide spectrum of candidates as for the location of where bone skates might have been used first.

Most of the oldest bone skates were found in areas where water covers more than 5 per cent of the corresponding modern country, namely Finland (with over 60,000 lakes), the Netherlands, Sweden and Norway. Minetti and I hypothesized that the energy-saving principle was a determinant factor in the birth of bone skates (Formenti and Minetti, 2008). We created replicas of ancient bone skates, and measured velocity and metabolic energy cost of bone skating. The average velocity recorded on bone skates was about 1.2m.s^{-1}. In terms of metabolic energy cost, this velocity is similar to the optimal velocity of walking on firm ground, but the metabolic energy cost of skating on bones was $4.6 \text{ J.kg}^{-1}.\text{m}^{-1}$, about two times greater than the cost of walking. We then used the recorded metabolic energy cost values as input for computer simulations of travel in the abovementioned Northern European regions, and in Germany, where relatively many bone skates were found. Assuming a given metabolic power (5.3 W.kg^{-1}) for walking and bone skating, we calculated the energy cost and speed of travelling for a number of simulated journeys (total of 2,400 km over five countries). These journeys were simulated in two conditions: 'walking and skating' and 'walking only'. For the 'walking and skating' simulations, the distance to be travelled was constant (10 km), but the cost and velocity of locomotion varied depending on the presence and dimensions of frozen lakes en route. In contrast, for the 'walking only' simulation, the distance to be travelled varied according to the presence of lakes to be avoided: if lakes were present on the route, we measured the shortest path connecting the starting point to the final destination. We estimated that the greatest reduction in metabolic energy cost of transport would be observed in Finland, where using bone skates allowed saving about half the energy for the average journey considered in the study. The reduction in metabolic energy cost of transport was not as great in the other countries considered. Finally, we estimated that ancient Finnish hunters and fishermen using bone skates for winter travel could have saved almost 10 per cent of the energy needed to survive for a period of 4 months. On the basis of our metabolic energy measurements and computer simulations, we suggested that the use of bone skates in areas characterized by a high density of lakes allowed travelling shorter routes, hence reduced times and metabolic cost of transport. In conclusion, it is fascinating to notice that alongside modern ice skates' models, bone skates were still in use in the eighteenth century 'in Iceland, Gotland and in parts of Hungary and Germany' (Roes, 1963).

Technical and materials' development supported the evolution of human locomotion on ice

Ever since the first bone skates were used, several subsequent modifications led to the current fastest ice skate, called the klapskate. Most of these modifications were based on empirical evidence for ice friction and exercise physiology, as discussed later. Only some of these modifications originated from research studies. The first contribution to understanding the kinematics of ice skating is attributed to Tebbutt (Heathcote *et al.*, 1892). In Amsterdam, he took a series of instantaneous photographs of skaters travelling on three different skates, and consequently adopting different skating techniques. He observed that the fastest skate was the one that allowed for the longest strides and required the smallest lateral deviation from the forward motion, indicating that little of the power generated was wasted laterally. In the 1970s, van Ingen Schenau and colleagues started a most comprehensive and informative series of studies on the biomechanics and physiology of ice skating at the Vrije Univeristeit in Amsterdam. They investigated the effect of air friction on speed skating performance, showing that it accounted for about 70 per cent of energy loss through friction at a speed of 9.2 m.s^{-1} (van Ingen Schenau, 1982). They created the first biomechanical models (van Ingen Schenau and Bakker, 1980) and investigated applied physiology of this form of locomotion, implying peculiar mixed features such as isometric contractions for long periods of time during the gliding phase, as well as fast powerful push-offs (de Groot *et al.*, 1987). The adoption of klapskates at world-level competitions gave a strong impulse for further research trying to explain the reasons for faster velocities on klapskates rather than on traditional skates (de Koning *et al.*, 2000; Houdijk *et al.*, 2000a, 2000b, 2001, 2003; van Ingen Schenau, 1998; van Ingen Schenau *et al.*, 1987). Skating posture does not change during skating on klapskates or traditional skates; consequently, no difference in air frictional losses could be measured. Lower friction between blade and ice was suggested to be a major determinant of faster velocities, because it was thought that the pressure of the tip of the blade in the ice at the end of each push-off could cause a great dissipation of power. Houdijk *et al.* (2000a) showed that this difference in friction determined a relatively small energy dissipation difference (only 0.84 W, compared with a 54 W dissipated by ice friction). Skating velocity increased because of a higher power output, determined by an 11 J increase in work per stroke and a higher stroke frequency (from 1.30 to 1.36 strokes per second). Moving the position of the klapskate hinge along the skate's main axis directly alters the levers' system used by the lower limb muscles. Van Horne and Stefanyshyn (2005) investigated the effects of different klapskate hinge positions, and found an intermediate optimum position in terms of lower limbs' power generation.

One study explored the biomechanics and energetics of skating on more ancient models, and their evolution through history: Minetti and I hypothesized that, similarly to cross-country skiing (Formenti *et al.*, 2005), ice skating developed in order to reduce energy cost and time of travel. We conducted an in-depth historical research, and identified five skates displaying significantly different features from previous models, which could consequently determine a better performance in terms of velocity and energy demand (Formenti and Minetti, 2007). The models used in our experiments are shown at the top of Figure 25.3: from the left, a replica of the bone skates, a replica of the first wooden skates with a metal blade (thirteenth century), skates used in the fifteenth and eighteenth centuries, and a modern conventional ice skate are shown. The main technical steps in the development of ice skates were identified with the use of thinner and longer metal blades, the reduction in skates' dynamic coefficient of friction and weight, the increase in the foot height over the ice, and the use of straps and boots that allowed a better control of the skate (the upper part of Table 25.1 shows further characteristics of the skates included in our study). Being particularly interested in the relative metabolic energy cost associated with the use of different skate models, we carried out our experiments on an ice rink, where ice surface, temperature and other environmental conditions remained unchanged throughout the tests. The metabolic energy cost of modern ice skating was only 25 per cent of that associated with the use of bone skates. Moreover, for the same metabolic power, nowadays skaters can achieve speeds four times higher than their ancestors could. In the range of speeds considered, the cost of travelling on ice was speed independent for each skate model, as for running. This latter finding, combined with the accepted relationship between time of exhaustion and the sustainable fraction of metabolic power, gave the opportunity to estimate the maximum skating speed according to the distance travelled (Figure 25.3). Here, the three lines (black, light grey, dark grey) illustrate the maximum sustainable speed/distance relationships, calculated for constant metabolic cost for each skate model, identified with the approximate time in history when they were in use. The light grey curves are iso-duration speed/distance pairs. The broken line illustrates values for running, and is shown as a means of comparison with the ice-skating speed/distance data. Also reported as a means of comparison are the ice-skating top records (open squares) and records for cross-country skiing (open circles).

Data shown for klapskates in Figure 25.3 were calculated assuming 5 per cent faster speeds, according to Houdijk *et al.* (2000a). The three lines were calculated through equations provided by Wilkie (1980), Saltin (1973) and Davies (1981), and were calculated assuming that the available fraction of the metabolic power used for a given movement pattern (ice skating) is inversely related to the time to exhaustion. From the left, the black, light grey and dark grey lines, respectively, illustrate the maximum sustainable speed calculated for periods of time ranging from 40 seconds to 10 minutes, from 10 minutes to 1 hour, and from 1 to 24 hours. For the calculations, the maximum metabolic power available was set at 21.3 $W.kg^{-1}$. An example might be helpful in order to clarify the information reported in Figure 25.3: the energy cost of skating on bones (1800 BC) is indicated by the thick 345 $J.m^{-1}$ iso-cost line (bottom line in the figure). The intersection between this iso-cost line and the light 10-minute iso-time line shows that in 10 minutes, for an energy cost of 345 $J.m^{-1}$, a person skating on bones could cover a distance of approximately 2.6 km at an average speed of 4.4 $m.s^{-1}$

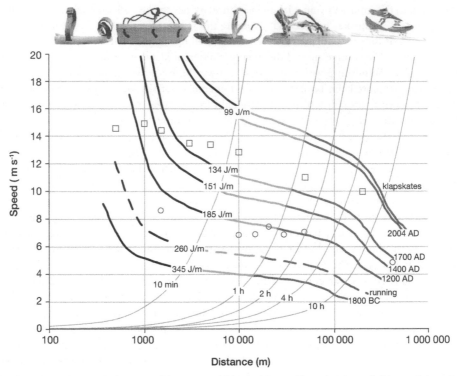

Figure 25.3 Innovative ice skates models improved ice-skating performance through history (adapted from Formenti and Minetti, 2007).

(~ 16 km.h^{-1}) before exhaustion. This is indicated by the intersection of the 345 J.m^{-1} iso-cost and the 10-minute iso-time lines in the figure. In contrast, the energy cost of modern ice skating is only 99 J.m^{-1}, less than one-third of the energy cost associated with skating on bones. On the basis of the equations from Wilkie (1980) and Saltin (1973), it appears that a skater could cover a distance of about 9.2 km in 10 minutes, at an average speed of about 15.3 m.s^{-1} (~ 56 km.h^{-1}) before exhaustion. In the figure, this is indicated by the intersection between the 99 J.m^{-1} iso-cost curve and the 10-minute iso-time line. The 10 km speed skating men's world record at the time of writing is 12 minutes and 41 seconds, achieved at an average speed of about 47 km.h^{-1} (International Skating Union, 2012), not far from the values predicted above. Figure 25.3 can also help to suggest when people could travel faster on ice than on land (moving at their maximum sustainable velocity). On frozen Dutch canals in the thirteenth century, ice skaters could cover a distance of about 26 km.h^{-1}, a much longer distance than the 18 km.h^{-1} that could possibly be travelled by running. This level of performance afforded by ice skates had no equal among other forms of human-powered locomotion until the advent of bicycles centuries later (Minetti *et al.*, 2001).

Ice skates were the first passive tools for human locomotion that took advantage of skeletal muscle biomechanical properties

Contraction of skeletal muscle can generate its maximum power when it shortens at about one-third of its fastest shortening speed. Even when travelling at relatively high speeds, the skating movement pattern requires muscles to shorten slowly, so they can also develop a considerable amount of force; this is the greatest advantage of skating over running. When we run, the velocity of muscle shortening is coupled to the velocity of running: the faster we run, the faster our muscles need to shorten. From a biomechanical perspective, this coupling of muscle shortening velocity and locomotion velocity is the main limiting factor for our fastest running speed. In contrast, when we skate, we can travel faster by taking longer strides, avoiding the need to shorten our muscles very rapidly, hence generating a greater power at each stride. If we compared a runner with a skater travelling at the same speed, the runner would take about six steps for every 'skating step'. For a similar heart rate, say 130 bpm, the skater would travel almost four times as fast as the runner. The stride frequencies and lengths recorded during our study (Formenti and Minetti, 2007) are presented in Table 25.1. Here, ice skate models are identified with the approximate time in history when they were in use. In the upper part of the table, dimensions and weight of each model are reported. Bone skates do not have a blade, so blade measurements reported indicate the dimensions of the underside of the bone skate, the part that is relatively flat on the ice while skating; the mass reported for the bone skates also includes the stick used for propulsion. The dynamic coefficient of friction's average and standard deviation values are reported for each skate model. In the middle part of the table, speed, stride frequency and stride length associated with the use of each skate model are reported for two speeds (i.e. low and high speed). Speed, stride frequency, and stride length average and standard deviation values shown are calculated from data recorded on the three participants who were equipped with inertial sensors. At the bottom of the table, the metabolic cost associated with the use of each skate model is reported; metabolic cost data shown are average and standard deviation values calculated for the speeds considered in the study.

These results suggest that our ancestors empirically understood the abovementioned, important biomechanical properties of skeletal muscle contraction. For example, our participants were asked to skate at a low and at a high speed, defined as sustainable for 8 and 4 hours,

Table 25.1 Relatively longer strides on ice skates allow greater locomotor efficiency: characteristics of five innovative pairs of ice skates developed through history, and associated kinematic parameters recorded at two submaximal speeds

		Ice skate model				
		1800 BC	*1200* AD	*1400* AD	*1700* AD	*2004* AD
Blade length	(mm)	210	230	250	410	460
Blade width	(mm)	14	6	6	1.3	1
Foot height	(mm)	36	59	45	50	62
Mass (pair)	(g)	1,450	1,300	900	950	930
Dynamic μ (10^{-2})		1.03 ± 0.22	1.47 ± 0.11	1.12 ± 0.07	0.84 ± 0.10	0.58 ± 0.04
Low speed	(m.s^{-1})	1.13 ± 0.40	1.80 ± 0.12	2.55 ± 0.16	2.87 ± 0.51	5.09 ± 1.85
Stride frequency	(stride.s^{-1})	0.50 ± 0.01	0.63 ± 0.09	0.54 ± 0.12	0.57 ± 0.15	0.40 ± 0.05
Stride length	(m)	2.68 ± 0.52	2.94 ± 0.44	4.87 ± 0.92	5.17 ± 0.53	13.31 ± 6.09
High speed	(m.s^{-1})	–	2.75 ± 0.73	4.06 ± 0.59	3.96 ± 0.32	6.70 ± 2.39
Stride frequency	(stride.s^{-1})	–	0.90 ± 0.19	0.65 ± 0.20	0.68 ± 0.12	0.45 ± 0.09
Stride length	(m)	–	3.16 ± 1.01	6.44 ± 0.93	5.97 ± 1.71	15.24 ± 5.55
Metabolic cost	(J.kg^{-1}.m^{-1})	4.62 ± 0.91	2.64 ± 0.75	2.01 ± 0.35	1.78 ± 0.28	1.32 ± 0.27

Source: Adapted from Formenti and Minetti (2007).

respectively, simulating the speed that might have been adopted for a journey. It is clear that the 'natural selection' of ice skates favoured models that allowed higher speeds, associated with longer strides and low stride frequencies. Travelling fast on modern skates was associated with a metabolic energy cost that was even lower than that recorded on slow, old skates. Overall, subsequent models of ice skates dramatically improved our locomotion efficiency, allowing faster travel at lower metabolic energy cost.

Modern klapskates require a movement pattern that, in terms of push-off mechanics, is slightly different from that of jumping (or running). When travelling on klapskates, no flexion of the metatarsal joint occurs: the ankle is extended, but the foot rotates as a single element around the hinge between the boot and the blade. In contrast, when we perform a standing jump (or when we run), just before our foot loses contact with the ground, it bends at the metatarsal-phalangeal joint level. The tendons in the arch of the foot, storing some elastic energy during the extension of the metatarsal joint, normally return a substantial portion of energy during these structures' elastic recoil (Hick's windlass effect), possibly playing a role in determining performance. I expect that a block that gives the opportunity to bend the foot at the level of the metatarsal-phalangeal joint in the last stage of the pushing phase would contribute to a small, but perhaps significant, increase in ice-skating performance.

References

Albracht, F., Reichel, S., Winkler, V. and Kern, H. (2004) 'On the influences of friction on ice', *Materialwissenschaft Und Werkstofftechnik*, 35: 620–5.

Allinger, T. L. and Van den Bogert, A. J. (1997) 'Skating technique for the straights, based on the optimization of a simulation model', *Medicine and Science in Sports and Exercise*, 29(2): 279–86.

Baurle, L., Szabo, D., Fauve, M., Rhyner, H. and Spencer, N. D. (2006) 'Sliding friction of polyethylene on ice: tribometer measurements', *Tribology Letters*, 24(1): 77–84.

Baurle, L., Kaempfer, U., Szabo, D. and Spencer, N. D. (2007) 'Sliding friction of polyethylene on snow and ice: contact area and modeling', *Cold Regions Science and Technology*, 47(3): 276–89.

Blauw, W. (2001) *Van glis tot klapschaats*, Franeker: Uitgeverij Van Wijnen.

Bowden, F. P. and Hughes, T. P. (1939) 'The mechanism of sliding on ice and snow', *Proceedings of the Royal Society of London. Series A, Mathematical and Physical Sciences*, 172: 280–98.

Brown, N. (1959) *Ice Skating: A History*, London: Nicholas Kaye.

Calabrese, S. J., Buxton, R. and Marsh, G. (1980) 'Frictional characteristics of materials sliding against ice', *Lubrication Engineering*, 36(5): 283–9.

Colbeck, S. C. (1988) 'Kinetic friction on snow', *Journal of Glaciology*, 34(116): 78–86.

Colbeck, S. C. (1994) 'Bottom temperatures of skating skis on snow', *Medicine and Science in Sports and Exercise*, 26(2): 258–62.

Colbeck, S. C. (1995) 'Pressure melting and ice skating', *American Journal of Physics*, 63(10): 888–90.

Colbeck, S. C., Najarian, L. and Smith, H. B. (1997) 'Sliding temperatures of ice skates', *American Journal of Physics*, 65(6): 488–92.

Davies, C. T. M. (1981) 'Physiology of ultra-long distance running', in P. E. D. Prampero and J. R. Portsman (eds), *Physiological Chemistry of Exercise and Training*, Basel: Karger.

de Groot, G., Hollander, A. P., Sargeant, A. J., van Ingen Schenau, G. J. and de Boer, R. W. (1987) 'Applied physiology of speed skating', *Journal of Sports Sciences*, 5(3): 249–59.

de Koning, J. J., de Groot, G. and van Ingen Schenau, G. J. (1992a) 'Ice friction during speed skating', *Journal of Biomechanics*, 25(6): 565–71.

de Koning, J. J., de Groot, G. and van Ingen Schenau, G. J. (1992b) 'A power equation for the sprint in speed skating', *Journal of Biomechanics*, 25(6): 573–80.

de Koning, J. J., Houdijk, H., de Groot, G. and Bobbert, M. F. (2000) 'From biomechanical theory to application in top sports: the klapskate story', *Journal of Biomechanics*, 33(10): 1225–9.

Di Prampero, P. E., Cortili, G., Mognoni, P. and Saibene, F. (1976) 'Energy cost of speed skating and efficiency of work against air resistance', *Journal of Applied Physiology*, 40(4): 584–91.

Faraday, M. (1859) 'Note on regelation', *Proceedings of the Royal Society of London*, 10: 440–50.

Formenti, F. and Minetti, A. E. (2007) 'Human locomotion on ice: the evolution of ice-skating energetics through history', *Journal of Experimental Biology*, 210(10): 1825–33.

Formenti, F. and Minetti, A. E. (2008) 'The first humans travelling on ice: an energy-saving strategy?', *Biological Journal of the Linnean Society*, 93(1): 1–7.

Formenti, F., Ardigò, L. P. and Minetti, A. E. (2005) 'Human locomotion on snow: determinants of economy and speed of skiing across the ages', *Proceedings of the Royal Society of London, Series B*, 272(1572): 1561–9.

Foster, C., Rundell, K. W., Snyder, A. C., Stray-Gundersen, J., Kemkers, G., Thometz, N., Broker, J. and Knapp, E. (1999) 'Evidence for restricted muscle blood flow during speed skating', *Medicine and Science in Sports and Exercise*, 31(10): 1433–40.

Heathcote, J. M., Tebbutt, C. G. and Maxwell, T. (1892) *Skating*, London: Longmans Green and Co.

Houdijk, H., de Koning, J. J., de Groot, G., Bobbert, M. F. and van Ingen Schenau, G. J. (2000a) 'Push-off mechanics in speed skating with conventional skates and klapskates', *Medicine and Science in Sports and Exercise*, 32(3): 635–41.

Houdijk, H., Heijnsdijk, E. A., de Koning, J. J., de Groot, G. and Bobbert, M. F. (2000b) 'Physiological responses that account for the increased power output in speed skating using klapskates', *European Journal of Applied Physiology*, 83(4–5): 283–8.

Houdijk, H., Wijker, A. J., de Koning, J. J., Bobbert, M. F. and de Groot, G. (2001) 'Ice friction in speed skating: can klapskates reduce ice frictional loss?', *Medicine and Science in Sports and Exercise*, 33(3): 499–504.

Houdijk, H., Bobbert, M. F., de Koning, J. J. and de Groot, G. (2003) 'The effects of klapskate hinge position on push-off performance: a simulation study', *Medicine and Science in Sports and Exercise*, 35(12): 2077–84.

Ikeda-Fukazawa, T. and Kawamura, K. (2004) 'Molecular-dynamics studies of surface of ice Ih', *Journal of Chemical Physics*, 120(3): 1395–401.

International Skating Union (2012) *Speed Skating Records*, available at: www.isu.org (acceesed 10 October 2012).

Itagaki, K., Huber, N. P. and Lemieux, G. (1989) *Dynamic Friction of a Metal Runner on Ice 1. Model Sled Test*, CRREL report 89-14, Hanover: US Army Cold Regions Research and Engineering Laboratory.

Jacobi, H. W. (1976) *RE: De Nederlandse Glissen*, Internal Report, Amsterdam: University of Amsterdam.

Kietzig, A. M., Hatzikiriakos, S. G. and Englezos, P. (2010) 'Physics of ice friction', *Journal of Applied Physics*, 107: 81–101.

Marino, G. W. (1977) 'Kinematics of ice skating at different velocities', *Research Quarterly*, 48(1): 93–7.

Minetti, A. E., Pinkerton, J. and Zamparo, P. (2001) 'From bipedalism to bicyclism: evolution in energetics and biomechanics of historic bicycles', *Proceedings of the Royal Society of London, Series B*, 268(1474): 1351–60.

Muhonen, T. (2005) 'Bone skates', *En Historia*, 1: 42–5.

Munro, R. (1893) 'Notes on ancient bone skates', *Proceedings of the Society of Antiquaries of Scotland*, 28: 185–97.

Olaus, M. (1555) 'Historia de gentibus septentrionalibus', Rome.

Roes, A. (1963) *Bone and Antler Objects from the Frisian Terp-mounds*, Haarlem: Tjeenk Willink, H.D., Zoom, N.V.

Rosenberg, R. (2005) 'Why is ice slippery?', *Physics Today*, 58: 50–5.

Rundell, K. W., Nioka, S. and Chance, B. (1997) 'Hemoglobin/myoglobin desaturation during speed skating', *Medicine and Science in Sports and Exercise*, 29(2): 248–58.

Saltin, B. (1973) 'Oxygen transport by the circulatory system during exercise in man', in J. Keul (ed.), *Limiting Factors of Physical Performance*, Stuttgart: George Thieme, pp. 235–52.

Scott, R. F. (1913) *Captain Scott's Diary*, London: British Library Add. MS 51035, f.39.

Slotfeldt-Ellingsen, D. and Torgensen, L. (1983) 'Water in ice: influence on friction', *Journal of Physics D: Applied Physics*, 16(9): 1715–19.

Smith, D. J. and Roberts, D. (1990) 'Heart rate and blood lactate concentration during on-ice training in speed skating', *Canadian Journal of Sport Sciences*, 15(1): 23–7.

Van Horne, S. and Stefanyshyn, D. J. (2005) 'Potential method of optimizing the klapskate hinge position in speed skating', *Journal of Applied Biomechanics*, 21(3): 211–22.

van Ingen Schenau, G. J. (1982) 'The influence of air friction in speed skating', *Journal of Biomechanics*, 15(6): 449–58.

van Ingen Schenau, G. J. (1998) 'The klapskate: an example of intermuscular coordination', *European Journal of Morphology*, 36(4–5): 269.

van Ingen Schenau, G. J. and Bakker, K. (1980) 'A biomechanical model of speed skating', *Journal of Human Movement Studies*, 6: 1–18.

van Ingen Schenau, G. J., de Groot, G., Scheurs, A. W., Meester, H. and de Koning, J. J. (1987) 'Some technical, physiological and anthropometrical aspects of speed-skating', *International Journal of Sports Medicine*, 8: 371–8.

van Ingen Schenau, G. J., de Boer, R. W. and de Groot, G. (1989) 'Biomechanics of speed skating', in C. L. Vaughan (ed.), *Biomechanics of Sport*, Boca Raton, FL: CRC Press, pp. 122–67.

Watkins, M., Pan, D., Wang, E. G., Michaelides, A., Vandevondele, J. and Slater, B. (2011) 'Large variation of vacancy formation energies in the surface of crystalline ice', *Nature Materials*, 10(10): 794–8.

Wilkie, D. R. (1980) 'Equations describing power input by humans as a function of duration of exercise', in P. Cerretelli and B. J. Whipp (eds), *Exercise Bioenergetics and Gas Exchange*, North Holland: Elsevier, pp. 75–80.

26

SNOW –
THE PERFORMANCE SURFACE
FOR ALPINE SKIING

Lars Karlöf,[1,4] *Matej Supej*[2,3] *and Hans-Christer Holmberg*[4,5]

[1]SWIX SPORT AS, OSLO
[2]UNIVERSITY OF LJUBLJANA, LJUBLJANA
[3]UNIVERSITY OF PRIMORSKA, KOPER
[4]MID SWEDEN UNIVERSITY, ÖSTERSUND
[5]SWEDISH OLYMPIC COMMITTEE, STOCKHOLM

Introduction

Alpine skiing is a popular winter sport. Athletes use their equipment on different courses that are covered with snow. From this perspective, better knowledge of snow conditions and the interaction between the skis and snow is fundamental, because performance and choices between different techniques are directly related to the interaction between the athlete, the ski equipment and the snow.

The snow surface

Snow is a 'hot' material under constant change, meaning that athletes ski on snow at temperatures that are close to its melting point. Changes in the snow's physical properties are influenced by several parameters, such as air and snow temperature, wind, incoming and outgoing radiation, time since last snowfall and how the snow is groomed. At the same time, snow is affected by the number of skiers, their skill level and ski discipline.

Snow in the atmosphere

Snow is solid water that is formed in the atmosphere; the snow crystals studied during precipitation are the result of complex processes before accumulation occurs on the ground. High air humidity (supersaturated air), an air temperature < 0°C and particles that allow condensation (condensation nuclei) are the necessary conditions for snow to form in the atmosphere. The presence of nuclei is necessary for a snowflake embryo to develop at temperatures higher than – 40°C. At lower temperatures, a minute ice particle may form directly from the water molecules in the air.

The further growth and formation of snow crystals is driven by two processes: sublimation and the refreezing/riming of water droplets. Clouds consist of undercooled water droplets, water vapour and small ice particles. These two different processes result in very different snow crystal shapes. Crystals formed by sublimation are well-articulated and well-defined in their shape along the axis of the crystal, whereas the process of refreezing gives more undefined and rounded forms. This means that it is possible to deduce under what atmospheric circumstances the snow has been formed by studying the precipitated snow. Furthermore, the temperature at which a crystal is formed determines the directions in which it grows. The most beautiful and well-known hexagonal star-shaped snow crystals are formed at the coldest temperatures in the plane of the a-axis, more plate-like shapes are formed at higher temperatures, and at temperatures in the range of −6 to −10°C the crystal grows more along its z-axis. Thus, depending on the atmospheric circumstances through which the snow particle descends, three different types of particles may accumulate on the ground: rimed crystals and Graupel (riming), snow crystals (sublimation) and snowflakes (aggregation).

Snow on the ground

As soon as the snow has reached the ground, the crystal continues changing. This process is called metamorphism; the term is borrowed from geology and has the same meaning. The transformation that occurs can primarily take two different paths: equi-temperature or melt temperature metamorphism. The structures of the crystals and grains are under constant change due to the effects of temperature and pressure. Metamorphism changes the snow's properties and, from a thermodynamic point of view, the snow moves towards an equilibrium state in which free energy is at a minimum.

Sintering, the formation of bonds at the snow crystal's point of contact, leads to higher density and structural strength in the snow pack. As the bonding of the snow grains progresses, the permeability, thermal conductivity and electrical properties of the snow also change. One very important result of metamorphism is the change in the snow surface's albedo. With changing reflectivity, more energy may enter the snow pack and further influence the metamorphic process. This external energy interaction is heavily influenced by the surrounding atmosphere.

Equi-temperature metamorphism

Equi-temperature metamorphism (ET) occurs due to thermodynamic instability in well-faceted snow crystals (i.e. with a large surface-to-volume ratio), which provides large surface energy. Thermodynamic equilibrium occurs when the ratio of surface to volume reaches a minimum, and this condition is met when the shape is a sphere. The driving force in ET metamorphism is the vapour pressure difference between the points and crests of the flake. The pressure gradient moves the water molecules from the points towards the crests, thereby rounding off the particle and lowering its surface energy.

Snow crystals with the highest surface-to-volume ratios, such as dendrites, are the most unstable and thus change their form most quickly. When the branches of the dendrites disappear, there is a general decrease in particle size in the snow pack and, after the branches have disappeared, the general size starts to increase. The reason for this is that larger particles grow at the expense of smaller ones, due to more efficient condensation over larger particles. The higher radius of curvature for smaller particles, and therefore higher vapour pressure compared to larger surfaces with lower vapour pressure, drives the process. Or, in other words, sublimation is more efficient from small particles. This type of metamorphism is called equi-temperature metamorphism or destructive metamorphism, as the original forms are destroyed and the density is increased (Colbeck, 1982) and references therein (Figure 26.1).

Snow Metamorphism

Temperature Metamorphism

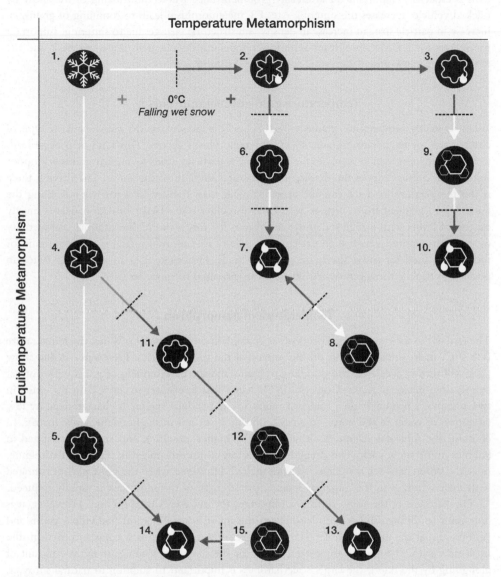

Figure 26.1 A simplified overview of snow metamorphism. The transformation follows two main paths: (1) equi-temperature metamorphism; and (2) temperature metamorphism. The arrows indicate the transition of temperature regime under which the transformation progresses. White is temperatures below 0°C and grey is above.

The breakdown of dendrites initially leads to rounder grains and, eventually, a less stable snow pack. However, during the rounding of the snow grains, contact points between grains also form and grow stronger. Bonding between snow grains occurs through the process of redistributing water molecules from points towards hollows. The redistribution is driven by the same diffusion process as mentioned above, and the rate is determined by the amount of energy available (heat). The rate of metamorphism thus increases with higher temperatures.

Compaction of the snow pack by overburden pressure increases the metamorphosis rate. This is especially important for artificially groomed trails, where the packing of the snow by tracked vehicles increases the sintering rate. ET metamorphism leads to rounding of grains, an increase in particle size, an increase in density and structural change due to sintering. Important parameters for ET metamorphism are a low temperature gradient in the snow pack and the radius of the snow grains' curvature for vapour diffusion.

Temperature gradient metamorphism

When a strong temperature gradient (> 10°C.m^{-1}) is present in the snow pack, a type of constructive or temperature gradient (TG) metamorphism occurs. This kind of process leads to hoar formation, which increases the size of snow particles, leads to angular grains with poor sintering and thus reduces the density and structural strength of the snow. The driving force is the temperature gradient and the accompanying mass transfer of water vapour along the temperature gradient from warmer areas towards colder ones. Hoar formation occurs mostly on top of layers with a higher density; the reason for this is the higher thermal conductivity of the high-density layer. It is an extreme example of metamorphism and is not important for the surface used for snow sports on groomed trails. However, it is an important factor in possible avalanche formation when skiing on ungroomed off-piste areas.

Temperature metamorphism

The rate of the abovementioned processes is dependent on temperature. When the temperature is > 0°C, melt water will form on the surface of the snow particles. Free water in the snow pack will further accelerate the rounding of grains and the development of pores with distinct connections between grains. Colbeck (1973) stated that free water in snow basically exists in two regimes: a pendular and a funicular regime. The pendular regime is characterized by low saturation of water in the pores, so air is found more or less throughout the snow matrix. In contrast, the funicular regime is characterized by higher saturation and any air is trapped in bubbles in the snow pack. The strength of the snow is not influenced in the pendular regime, since the bonds between the grains have not melted. However, when the snow pack is saturated with melt water, as in the funicular regime, the strength of the snowpack is rapidly reduced.

The hardness of the snow surface is important for the skier's total friction. However, it is important to distinguish between hardness at the micro scale (~ 1 mm), individual grains and crystals, and at the macro scale (~ 10 mm), larger snow samples. For waxing and friction, the small micro scale hardness is important, while for the shear and loading strengths (amount of ploughing by the skier), the larger scale hardness is important. In addition to natural snow, as described above, there is also artificial or man-made snow. Artificial snow does not contain snow crystals, but frozen water droplets; these droplets are more rounded and also often smaller in size. Artificial snow is thus more like natural snow in its final stages of metamorphosis.

Gliding on snow

The total friction experienced by the ski in interaction with snow can be divided into the following parameters:

$$\mu = \mu_{plow} + \mu_{dry} + \mu_{wet} + \mu_{cap} + \mu_{dirt} \tag{1}$$

The sum of plowing (μ_{plow}), solid deformation (μ_{dry}), water lubrication (μ_{wet}), capillary attraction (μ_{cap}) and surface contamination (μ_{dirt}) is the total friction (Colbeck, 1992). The size of the parameters varies due to changing snow/ice conditions, slider surface and material, and atmospheric conditions. The time scale of change ranges from microseconds to hours. Air drag is an important friction parameter when skiing at higher velocities, but because it is not determined by the snow's surface it will not be further discussed.

The purpose of ski preparation is to minimize the total friction at the interface between ski and snow. Both the construction of the ski and the material used focus on this. However, the materials used in the ski's construction and in the ski's base are considered to be stable in the temperature range at which skiing is performed. As described above, the snow surface is not stable, so manipulation of the ski base is necessary to optimize the ski's friction properties. The purpose of ski waxes is to aid in this manipulation. Therefore, it is not only the snow's surface that changes over time, but the skiing equipment may also be manipulated to be optimized for the surface that is skied on.

Further preparation of the snow surface is carried out to reduce friction. The friction factor (μ_{plow}) is the only one minimized during snow grooming. Another important reason for grooming the snow surface is for safety reasons in recreational skiing and, in competitive skiing, grooming ensures a homogeneous and fair basis for competition.

Snow surface preparation

The technique used for grooming and preparing the snow's surface is dependent on the type of skiing that will be performed on the surface. Grooming a fresh snow surface changes the surface in two ways: both the density and the particle size are changed by the mechanical treatment. In terms of snow metamorphosis, the transformation is accelerated through rounding the grains, creating smaller grains, and a more inhomogeneous size distribution of the grains. Both the pressure exerted by the grooming machine and the inhomogeneous size distribution accelerate the sintering process and increase the strength of the snow pack. To achieve a long-lasting surface, it is important to let the snow cure before it is used. The ambient meteorological conditions are important to this process, but in general a time frame of about 8 hours is necessary to achieve a homogenous and fair snow surface that will withstand many skiers. The competition rules further dictate the strength and density of the surface of the race course. In alpine skiing, machine grooming is often not enough to achieve the strength and hardness necessary for safe competition; in these cases, the snow's surface can be further strengthened with different techniques such as water injection, artificial snow and chemicals (salts). The aim of adding salts is to induce an endothermic process that will cool and harden the snow pack due to the energy used in the reaction between the salt and snow. The reaction time is short and, when the reaction is finished, the introduced salt will be contra-productive as it lowers the melting temperature of the snow in comparison to snow only. Therefore, the introduction of salt should only be considered close to a competition. In cases where an injection of water and salt is needed, the focus is on making the upper 10–20 cm stronger.

Alpine skiing on a snowy 'playground'

Alpine skiing is a sport that is conducted in an outdoor environment in winter conditions. The skiers use their skis to descend the mountain slopes covered with snow. From this perspective, an understanding of various snow conditions and the interaction between the skis and snow is crucial, and the fundamentals of skiing straight, turning and slowing down are all directly related to this interaction.

Ski-snow friction (the interaction between the skis and the snow) needs to be more broadly defined as regards its basic mechanics. Similar to Coulomb friction, the ski-snow friction represents resistance force that occurs due to the relative motion of solid surface (ski) sliding on the snow. Several investigations have been performed in laboratory conditions and on ski slopes, showing the magnitude of friction and its importance in alpine ski racing (Buhl *et al.*, 2001; Colbeck, 1994; Colbeck and Perovich, 2004; Federolf *et al.*, 2008). In addition, ski-snow friction can be more broadly understood as 'generalised ski-snow friction' (Reid *et al.*, 2009), which occurs when an edged ski is not aligned with the direction of its movement in relation to the snow base. The latter is usually called side-slipping, and besides helping to control velocity, it enables the skiers to turn (change direction) even when skiing on classical (older) skis (i.e. skis with a minimal side cut).

Straight skiing

In order to provide more detailed insight into the interaction between skis and snow, we will begin with straight skiing (Figure 26.2). The force of gravity is a consequence of a skier's mass in the gravitation field. It can be divided into a dynamic and a static component. The first causes the acceleration of the skier and is parallel to the base, and the second is perpendicular to the base and presses the skier to the ground. In accordance with Newton's third law of action–reaction, the normal force is inversely equal to the static component of the gravity force. The stronger the skier acts on the ground, the stronger the ground reacts on the skier. Apart from these forces, drag force and force of friction also oppose the skier's movement. The force of friction is a consequence of the friction between the snow base and the skis and, in accordance with its direction, it is oppositely parallel to the dynamic component of the gravity force.

Friction on hard frozen snow can be compared to the friction of a skater on ice; in such a case, the magnitude of friction would be approximately 2 per cent of the normal force size (Buhl *et al.*, 2001) and the sagging of skis to snow (i.e. how deep the skis sink in the snow)

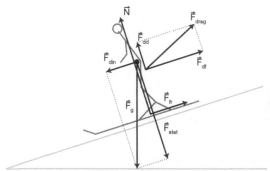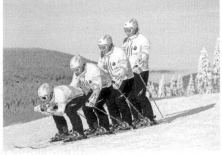

Figure 26.2 Forces of a skier on a slope. $\vec{F}_g$ – gravity force, $\vec{F}_{din}$ – dynamic and $\vec{F}_{stat}$ – static component, $\vec{N}$ – normal, $\vec{F}_{drag}$ – drag force, $\vec{F}_{df}$ – force of frontal drag (drag force), $\vec{F}_{dd}$ – force of dynamic resistance (the lift-induced drag), $\vec{F}_{fr}$ – force of friction and $\vec{F}_{gr}$ – ground reaction force.

is minimal. The force of friction on soft or deep snow depends also on the sagging of the skis to the snow (Federolf, 2005). The force friction is normally greater in deep snow than on hard frozen snow.

Changing direction

Turning with side slipping

When discussing changes in direction, it is necessary to understand why a ski turns on snow. There are two basic principles on groomed slopes that are substantially different to each other from a physical point of view. One is turning the skis with side slipping and the other one is without side slipping (i.e. carving). Different types of models that describe the change in direction when the ski side-slips have been presented previously; the one most commonly referred to for hard snow is from *Snow and Ice Cutting Theories* (Tada and Hirano, 1999, 2002) and when the snow is soft, it is from the *Water Jet Analogy* (Hirano and Tada, 1996). Avoiding the profound mechanical modelling of these theories and analogies, the following can be stated using basic physics. The open ski position (snow plough: see Figure 26.3) is the first one to be discussed; a well-constructed and suitably loaded ski that is set on its edges in the open position turns on its own regardless of whether the ski has a side-cut or not (Kugovnik *et al.*, 2003). The impulse momentum of the ground reaction force acting on the ski causes a change in momentum and consequently the longitudinal and transverse velocities.

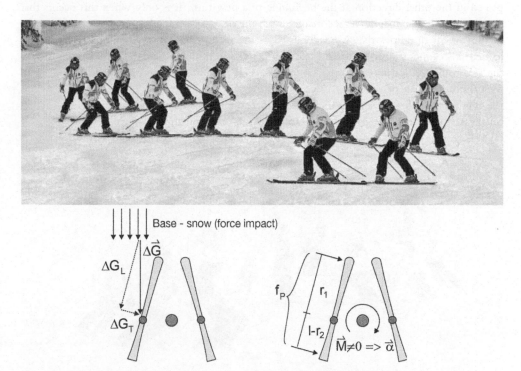

Figure 26.3 Turning using an open ski position (snow plough). The impulse of snow force on a ski changes the momentum $\vec{G}$ in transverse $\vec{G}_T$ and in longitudinal directions $\vec{G}_L$ (left). The torque of specific force in a transverse direction f_p results in torque M and turning the skier round his or her axis (centre of gravity of the body).

The momentum decreases in the longitudinal direction and increases in the transverse direction, or becomes different from zero (Figure 26.3, bottom left). Naturally, a stronger impulse in a transverse direction results in sharper turning and vice versa. If the skier was a 'point-like body', this would cause the skier to turn, but as the skier is a large body in space it has to turn around the longitudinal axis while turning, which is a consequence of various levers and ground reaction forces acting on the tip and tail of the skis and causing torque.

When the torque differs from 0, it results in the angular acceleration and turning of a ski around its axis (Figure 26.3, bottom right). In order to make skiing easier, skis are constructed in such a way that shifting of the centre of gravity forwards and backwards resembles the torque situation; thereby, in the simplest approximation, it is also important that the length from the tip to the centre of the ski is greater than that from the centre of the ski to its tail. This means that the centre of gravity of a balanced skier is shifted backwards because of the position of the ski bindings. In many cases, this difference between the length of the tip and tail helps a skier to turn. Apart from the binding's position, the longitudinal and shear stiffness (Heinrich *et al.*, 2006), as well as the geometry of carving skis (Lind and Sanders, 2010), also contribute to a skier's turning and torques, but these effects are not relevant to this discussion.

Therefore, in the case of snow plough turning, only weight transfer and good balance (weighting of the skis) are necessary (Kugovnik *et al.*, 2003), since the skis complete and begin a new turn simply by transferring weight from one ski to the other. However, this is not the case in parallel skiing (Figure 26.4) where, related to the direction of movement at the end of the turn, both skis are placed slightly transversely in one direction. The skis then need to be placed in the other direction at the beginning of a new turn. It is only when this occurs that the skis turn left and right, in accordance with the physical principles of torque and changes in movement quantities that were discussed in the section on snow ploughing. Because the loaded skis cannot simply be turned from one direction into another, the skier should unload the skis using vertical up-and-down movements. When the skis are unloaded, the skier can turn the upper part of the body in one direction and the lower part of the body, as well as the skis, in the other direction. In addition, the pole plant can help because the force acting on the ski pole from the ground is eccentric to the skier and thus produces torque.

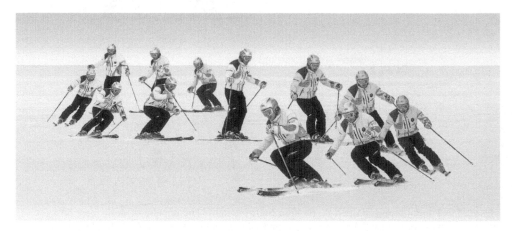

Figure 26.4 Turning with side slipping in a parallel ski position.

Carving

When skiing without side skidding (i.e. carving), there is a different interaction between the skis and the snow compared to turning with side slipping. During carving, the edge of the ski carves the trajectory into the snow and, in an ideal case, each point on the edge travels along the same trajectory (Howe, 1983, 2001). Thus, the skis do not move in a perpendicular (radial) direction to their edge, but in the longitudinal (tangential) direction. The maximal force in the transverse direction to the ski is higher than the radial force in the turn, and therefore the skis do not skid sideways (though skis always skid slightly sideways when they sag into the snow) if the skier is suitably balanced. Skis turn depending on their edge setting or on their inclination to the slope. Using some assumptions, it can be estimated how a ski will turn at a certain inclination, if its geometry is known (Howe, 2001; Kugovnik *et al.*, 2003).

Figure 26.5 demonstrates the radii that can be skied with carving skis. For example, the fun carving skis (declared side cut = 11 m) are limited to turn radii ranging between 3 and 11 m, and the longer skis (declared side cut = 21 m) range between 5 and 21 m. The skis do not allow the remaining radii, although practice slightly deviates from theory, mainly due to minimal side skidding and the skis sagging into the base (Federolf *et al.*, 2010).

Velocity control

Because longitudinal friction between the skis and the snow is minimal, velocity control is crucial to safety in alpine skiing. The problem of controlling velocity appears as soon as the skier can change direction and link several turns, because the skier is descending the inclined slope. An important aspect of skiing is that the skier should remain at a safe velocity for each skiing level; at the beginners' level, the skiers use 'simple' vertical unloading and loading of the skis, which are required for a (quick) change in the position of the skis and for efficient braking. If the skier wishes to push the skis from a less open position (parallel or close to parallel) to a more open position (snow plough or wedge) in order to increase friction, this is usually done by moving downwards. A skier at beginner's level can increase the force of friction

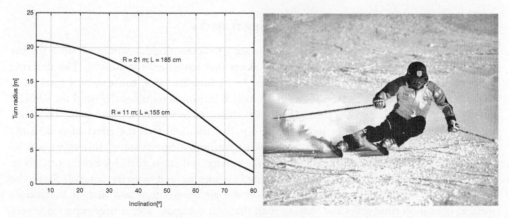

Figure 26.5 The diagram on the left presents the radius of the turn depending on the inclination of the ski to the ground for two different skis: l = 185 cm and R_d = 21 m (top curve); l = 155 cm and R_d = 11 m (bottom curve). The photo on the right shows a skier performing a carved turn in soft snow conditions.

using the position of skis (more or less open) and thus control velocity. Since there are great muscle forces involved in braking, as a consequence of the body's position and increased friction, a skier with a more open ski position finds it easier to brake while skiing diagonally to the slope inclination, or by simply turning uphill, since the dynamic component of the ground reaction force is significantly decreased or even helps braking.

At a higher level of skiing, skiers normally do not use an open ski position in order to slow down or to maintain velocity. Braking with the skis in the open position is not suitable as the 'awkward' position of the skier makes it very tiring for the muscles and joints. Furthermore, it is inefficient at higher velocities and on steeper slopes. A simpler and more efficient way is to place both skis transverse to the direction of movement, which enables the skier to control his or her movement and ski safely at a higher level. In such side gliding, the force of friction increases and, because it acts in the opposite direction to the movement, it directly reduces momentum and thus the velocity.

Besides braking in a snow plough position or by side gliding, which can be combined with turning uphill for the most efficient deceleration, skiers normally control the velocity of almost every turn by ending turns far enough from the fall line, where the dynamic component of the gravity force is less, but where the force of friction and air drag are similar. Maintaining velocity by ending turns far from the fall line can be explained using energy principles. Due to altitude, the skier has potential energy that can be transformed into kinetic energy. Apart from this transformation of potential energy into kinetic energy, the skier constantly dissipates some energy due to the force of friction and air drag. The energy balance can be written as follows: the velocity (kinetic energy) remains constant if energy dissipation equals the change in potential energy. Work of friction and air drag are, simplified, a product of each force and path, which means that a longer path results in higher losses at the same magnitude of friction and air drag, since the force of resistance and the force of friction are inversely parallel to the skiing direction. The above findings are supported by the fact that the path of the skier is longer when making turns far from the fall line at the same altitude difference, which means that it is easier to maintain velocity; this is especially useful on a steep slope. For example, when energy losses are higher compared to the change in potential energy (altitude difference), the skier loses velocity since the kinetic energy decreases, and vice versa.

Concluding remarks

Important factors that influence the playing surface are meteorological conditions since the last snowfall, piste grooming and the number of skiers that have used the surface. The differing properties of snow influence skiing technique. In its simplest form, this can be expressed as the differing frictional coefficient of the snow, which in turn determines the need for velocity control and rate of turning. As described above, there are five different factors that influence the total friction between snow and ski. The one that the skier feels the effect of most is the plowing effect. On a well-groomed track with transformed frozen snow, this effect can be ignored, but as soon as skiers have skied on the surface and snow particles have worn off it, it becomes more important for straight gliding, for turning and velocity control. Since the bulk hardness of the snow surface depends on the air temperature and that of the snow's surface, over short time scales and varying with the solar radiation, a skier may experience very different conditions just from passing from a sunny area to shade. Furthermore, the mechanical hardness of the snow surface changes the way in which a skier edges the ski to perform a directional change or maintain velocity control. In softer snow conditions, it is easier to induce a proper edge because the soft snow helps to balance the ski when edged. When edging on harder snow, the area of contact between ski and snow is much smaller. Hence, a hard snow surface requires a more advanced skiing technique in order to edge the ski correctly and to be able to carve; when edging is not properly performed, a skier will experience side skidding.

The surface used for alpine sports is constantly changing due to external factors that a skier cannot influence. However, in free skiing, a skier can choose to navigate down the ski piste and search for the preferred snow conditions. A competitive racer is limited to the predetermined race course. To be able to ski at ease, following the alternating conditions down the hill at higher speeds, requires long experience and years of training. This makes alpine skiing a demanding and challenging sport.

References

Buhl, D., Fauve, M. and Rhyner, H. (2001) 'The kinetic friction of polyethylen on snow: the influence of the snow temperature and the load', *Cold Regions Science and Technology*, 33: 133–40.

Colbeck, S. C. (1973) *Theory of Metamorphism of Wet Snow*, Research Report 313, Hanover: US Army Cold Regions Research and Engineering Laboratory.

Colbeck, S. C. (1982) 'An overview of seasonal snow metamorphism', *Reviews of Geophysics*, 20(1): 45–61.

Colbeck, S. C. (1992) *A Review of the Processes that Control Snow Friction*, Hanover: US Army Cold Regions Research and Engineering Laboratory.

Colbeck, S. C. (1994) 'A review of the friction of snow skis', *Journal of Sports Sciences*, 12(3): 285–95.

Colbeck, S. C. and Perovich, D. K. (2004) 'Temperature effects of black versus white polyethylene bases for snow skis', *Cold Regions Science and Technology*, 39: 33–8.

Federolf, P. (2005) 'Finite element simulation of a carving snow ski', unpublished doctoral dissertation, Swiss Federal Institute of Technology Zurich.

Federolf, P., Scheiber, P., Rauscher, E., Schwameder, H., Lüthi, A., Rhyner, H. U. and Müller, E. (2008) 'Impact of skier actions on the gliding times in alpine skiing', *Scandinavian Journal of Medicine and Science in Sports*, 18(6): 790–7.

Federolf, P., Roos, M., Lüthi, A. and Dual, J. (2010) 'Finite element simulation of the ski–snow interaction of an alpine ski in a carved turn', *Sports Engineering*, 12(3): 123–33.

Heinrich, D., Mössner, M., Kaps, P., Schretter, H. and Nachbauer, W. (2006) 'Influence of ski bending stiffness on the turning radius of alpine skis at different edging angles and velocities', in E. F. Moritz and S. Haake (eds), *The Engineering of Sport 6, Vol. 2: Developments for Disciplines*, New York: Springer, pp. 207–12.

Hirano, Y. and Tada, N. (1996) 'Numerical simulation of a turning alpine ski during recreational skiing', *Medicine and Science in Sports and Exercise*, 28(9): 1209–13.

Howe, J. (1983) *Skiing Mechanics*, Laporte, CO: Poudre Publishing.

Howe, J. (2001) *The New Skiing Mechanics: Including the Technology of Short Radius Carved Turn Skiing and the Claw Ski*, Waterford, MI: McIntire Publishing.

Kugovnik, O., Supej, M. and Nemec, B. (2003) *Biomehanika alpskega smučanja*, Ljubljana: Fakulteta za šport, Inštitut za šport.

Lind, D. A. and Sanders, S. P. (2010) *The Physics of Skiing: Skiing at the Triple Point*, New York: Springer.

Reid, R., Gilgien, M., Moger, T., Tjørhom, H., Haugen, P., Kipp, R. and Smith, G. (2009) 'Turn characteristics and energy dissipation in slalom', in E. Müller, S. Lindinger and T. Stöggl (eds), *Science and Skiing IV*, Maidenhead: Meyer & Meyer, pp. 419–29.

Tada, N. and Hirano, Y. (1999) 'Simulation of a turning ski using ice cutting data', *Sports Engineering*, 2(1): 55–64.

Tada, N. and Hirano, Y. (2002) 'In search of the mechanics of a turning alpine ski using snow cutting force measurements', *Sports Engineering*, 5(1): 15–22.

SECTION 7

Influence of footwear on sports and exercise

27

EFFECTS OF ELASTIC SHOE COVER ON RUNNING MECHANICS

Youlian Hong,[1] Lin Wang[2] and Jing Xian Li[2,3]

[1]CHENGDU SPORTS UNIVERSITY, CHENGDU
[2]SHANGHAI UNIVERSITY OF SPORT, SHANGHAI
[3]UNIVERSITY OF OTTAWA, OTTAWA

Introduction

Running is one of the most popular leisure sports activities (van Mechelen, 1992). However, when doing this activity, runners usually experience impact force due to the collision of the foot with the ground. Impact force has been evaluated to be approximately 2.5 times the runner's body weight in distance running (Cavanagh and Lafortune, 1980). High injury rates have been found in examined runners. The recorded injury rate per 1,000 hours of training is 2.5 in long-distance/marathon runners and 5.6–5.8 in sprinters and middle-distance runners (Lysholm and Wiklander, 1987). A 12-month follow-up survey participated in by 1,680 runners showed that 48 per cent of them experienced at least one musculoskeletal injury (Walter et al., 1989).

Athletic footwear has been linked to the prevention of injuries and to increased comfort in running (McKenzie et al., 1985; Riddle et al., 2003; Taunton et al., 2003) since it influences running biomechanics. Research in footwear biomechanics has demonstrated that differences in the design of running shoes, including heel height, insole materials and height of the shoe cup, can influence rearfoot motion (Cheung and Ng, 2007; DeWit et al., 1995; Hamill et al., 1992; Kersting and Brüggemann, 2006), plantar pressure loading (Dixon, 2008; Henning and Milani, 1995; Verdejo and Mills, 2004), and shoe comfort (Cheung and Ng, 2007; Chiu and Wang, 2007; Hong et al., 2005; Milani et al., 1997; Mündermann et al., 2001), which have been widely used as indicators of running biomechanics.

Among others, the shoelace has been considered an important part of running shoes and has drawn the attention of many scientists. Frey (2000) suggested that a shoelace provides a more comfortable shoe fit and can distribute stress evenly across the dorsum of the foot. However, no direct evidence has been given to support this suggestion. Among soccer players who showed excessive pronation in running, a study of soccer boots has revealed that a pair of soccer shoes with the pronated lacing technique is superior in rearfoot motion control than a pair of soccer shoes with other lacing conditions (Sandrey et al., 2001). Hagen and Henning (2008, 2009) and Hagen et al. (2010) studied plantar pressure distribution, shock attenuation and rearfoot motion in running shoes with different lacing conditions. In their study, participants

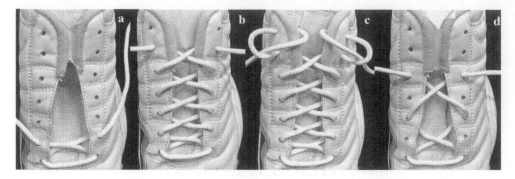

Figure 27.1 Simulated lacing conditions in the study by Hagen and Henning (2009): (a) eyelets 1–2; (b) eyelets 1–6; (c) eyelets 1–7; (d) eyelets 1, 3, 5.

were made to wear the same shoes for a number of times, with different lacing patterns each time: eyelets 1–2; eyelets 1–6; eyelets 1–7; and eyelets 1, 3 and 5 (see Figure 27.1). In the six-eyelet lacing condition, the participants laced the shoes at different tightness according to their own perception of weak, regular and tight conditions. It was found that shoe-lacing conditions have a significant influence on foot-shoe coupling in running. Tighter fitting due to stronger lacing results in the better use of running shoes. Although the number of scientific publications that discuss shoe lacing and running biomechanics are limited, existing published studies have shown that the shoelace has impacts on running biomechanics. Recently, some shoe companies have planned to design a new type of running shoe with an elastic upper envelope, replacing the traditional lacing structure. However, the effects of the new design on running biomechanics in terms of comfort, cushioning and rearfoot motion control during running have not yet been examined. Therefore, this study aims to examine whether there are differences in the perceptions of comfort, cushioning and rearfoot motion control between running shoes that utilize the shoelace system and those that do not. The null hypothesis of the study is that there is no difference in the perceived comfort, plantar pressure and rearfoot movement between conventional laced shoes and elastic-covered shoes.

Methods

Participants

Nineteen male amateur runners (age: 21.4 ± 2.0 years; body weight: 60.7 ± 4.8 kg; body height: 169.0 ± 3.0 cm), who are all heel strikers and have shoe size of 41 (European shoe size), were recruited to participate in the study. Included among the requirements were that they should not have had history of disease in the neuromuscular, vestibular and vision systems, and that they had not experienced any injury in the past 6 months prior to the study. Four subjects were excluded since they either had experienced lower extremity injury in the last 6 months or have a flat foot. The available sample size was therefore 15. Only male participants were recruited for the study to prevent any possible gender differences in running capacity. The participants signed an informed consent. The study was approved by the local institutional review board.

Shoes

The prototype running shoes were provided by a professional shoe manufacturer. The shoes differ only in terms of having shoelaces or elastic shoe cover, as seen in Figure 27.2. Each participant was given two pairs of shoes, one with laces and the other with an elastic shoe cover. This study used the mathematical model on shoe lacing that recommends the X-lacing pattern (conventional crisscross pattern) as the best and strongest way of lacing shoes (Polster, 2002). The participants adjusted the shoelaces according to their preferred tightness.

Experimental protocol

Perceived comfort test

A questionnaire with visual analogue scale (VAS), which has been used in previous studies and has been proven to be reliable (Cheung and Ng, 2007; Clinghan *et al.*, 2008; Mündermann *et al.*, 2001), was used to analyse the perceived comfort rating of running shoes. Nine questions were included in the questionnaire: Q1 (overall comfort), Q2 (heel cushioning), Q3 (forefoot cushioning), Q4 (medial-lateral control), Q5 (arch height), Q6 (heel cup fitting), Q7 (shoe heel width), Q8 (shoe forefoot width) and Q9 (shoe length). The perceived comfort test was conducted on a normal running track. The participants completed a trial involving a 450 m run at a comfortable speed. After the trial, each subject was instructed to answer two sets of questions: one for laced running shoes and the other for elastic-covered running shoes. This study adopted a 150 mm scale, in which the right-hand end was labelled as the 'most comfortable imaginable', while the opposite end was labelled as the 'least comfortable imaginable'.

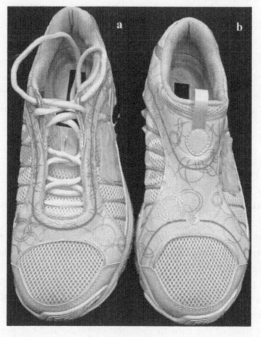

Figure 27.2 Testing shoes in this study: (a) laced running shoes; and (b) elastic-covered running shoes.

Rearfoot movement test

The participants were asked to run on a treadmill at 3.8 m.s^{-1}. A video camera (9800, JVC Inc., Japan) with a sampling frequency of 200 Hz was positioned behind the treadmill to record the rearfoot movement of the runners. Four light reflective spherical markers were attached to the shoe on each participant's dominant leg. This approach has been described in previous studies (Cheung and Ng, 2007; Nigg and Morlock, 1987) and is one of the standard test methods for the comparison of the rearfoot motion control properties of running shoes stipulated by the American Society for Testing and Materials (ASTM, 2006). The first marker was glued over the Achilles tendon, 4 cm above the ankle joint. The second marker was placed at mid-distance on a line defined by the bisector of the knee and the marker on the Achilles tendon. The third marker was placed at the centre heel cap at the insertion of the Achilles tendon. The fourth marker was attached to the centre of the heel cap just above the shoe sole. The angle between the line linking the first and second markers, and the line linking the third and fourth markers, represents the rearfoot inversion or the eversion angle. To correct the differences in marker position between participants, the participants were asked to stand in a standard position. The standard position involves standing with the medial edges of the shoe heels 5 cm apart, with the feet abducted for 7° (ASTM, 2006). The rearfoot angle of each participant was then measured as a reference in determining the same angle measured during the running test. After the reference-neutral position angle was determined, the participants were made to run for 3 minutes in each type of shoe, and the 10 footstrikes in the last 30 seconds were filmed. The video images were then processed using the Ariel Motion Analysis System (APAS, Ariel Dynamics Inc., USA) to determine the rearfoot motion. A positive value against the reference position indicates the inversion of the heel to the shank, which implies a supinated position. Conversely, a negative value indicates eversion, which implies pronation. The dominant leg was determined by kicking a ball. All participants in the study identified their right leg as their dominant leg.

Plantar pressure test

An in-shoe force sensor system (Novel Pedar System, Germany) was used to collect the plantar local loading data during running. Only the plantar pressure of the dominant leg was collected. The sampling frequency was set at 100 Hz. The participants were asked to run on a treadmill at 3.3 m.s^{-1} for 2 minutes. Ten successful trials were subsequently used for data analysis.

Data reduction

The APAS software was used in digitizing and analysing the video images. To evaluate the rearfoot motion, four parameters were analysed: rearfoot touchdown angle (TDR), rearfoot maximal pronation angle (RMP), total rearfoot motion angle (TRM) and peak velocity of the rearfoot angle (PV).

In analysing plantar loading, the insole was divided and masked into nine areas according to the human foot anatomy: M1 (medial heel), M2 (lateral heel), M3 (medial midfoot), M4 (lateral midfoot), M5 (first metatarsal head), M6 (second metatarsal head), M7 (third, fourth and fifth metatarsal heads), M8 (great toe) and M9 (lesser toes), as seen in Figure 27.3. Similar masks have been used in previous studies (Bontrager *et al.*, 1997; Burnfield *et al.*, 2004; Mao *et al.*, 2006). Using the Novel Pedar software, parameters such as peak pressure in each mask, contact area in each mask, support time of the foot in each stance phase and the percentage of the contact time of each mask in relation to the total contact time of the foot were determined.

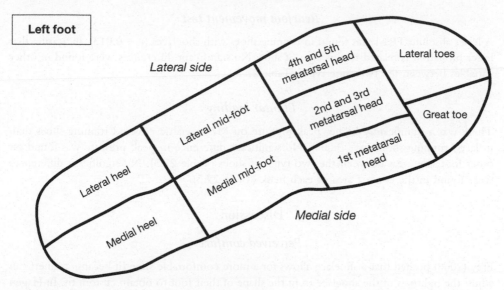

Figure 27.3 Insole masks.

Data analysis

All data were presented as mean and standard deviation. A paired-samples t-test was used to determine whether the performance of the laced running shoes was different from that of the elastic-covered running shoes. The number of independent variables compared between the laced and elastic-covered running shoes was 9 for perceived comfort, 4 for rearfoot motion and 10 for plantar pressure, respectively. Statistical significance was set at $p < 0.05$.

Results

Perceived comfort test

The laced running shoes showed better perceived comfort than the elastic-covered running shoes in Q3 ($p = 0.029$), Q6 ($p = 0.013$), Q7 ($p = 0.036$), Q8 ($p = 0.002$) and Q9 ($p = 0.013$), as seen in Table 27.1.

Table 27.1 Comparison of the perceived comfort scores between laced running shoes and elastic-covered running shoes

		Q1	Q2	Q3	Q4	Q5	Q6	Q7	Q8	Q9
SL	mean	8.79	7.87	8.21	8.47	8.70	9.53	9.36	9.33	9.40
	SD	1.52	2.63	1.79	1.72	1.55	1.35	2.12	1.26	1.47
EC	mean	7.69	7.29	6.73	7.70	7.35	7.99	8.22	6.92	7.63
	SD	1.89	1.77	1.74	1.58	2.36	2.06	1.70	1.60	1.61
				⋆			⋆	⋆	⋆	⋆

SL = laced running shoes; EC = elastic-covered running shoes.
Q1 = overall comfort; Q2 = heel cushioning; Q3 = forefoot cushioning; Q4 = medial-lateral control; Q5 = arch height; Q6 = heel cup fitting; Q7 = shoe heel width; Q8 = shoe forefoot width; Q9 = shoe length.
⋆ $p < 0.05$, significant difference from SL.

Rearfoot movement test

A lesser absolute TRM was found in running shoes with shoelaces ($p = 0.013$), indicating that lesser pronation is related to this type of shoe. No significant differences were found in other variables between the two shoe types (Table 27.2).

Plantar loading

There was a significantly higher peak pressure on M7 in elastic-covered running shoes than in laced running shoes ($p = 0.005$). No significant difference in peak pressure was found on other foot sole areas between the two types of shoes (Table 27.3). No significant differences were found in the contact area of each mask (Table 27.3).

Discussion

Perceived comfort

Frey (2000) posited that a shoelace allows for a more comfortable shoe fit because runners can adjust the tightness of the shoelace to fit the shape of their foot to obtain custom fit. In Hagen and Henning's study (Hagen and Henning, 2009), a questionnaire using a seven-point

Table 27.2 Parameters in the rearfoot motion testing

	TDR (degree)	TRM (degree)	RMP (degree)	MV (degree/s)
SL	6.3 (3.9)	13.5 (2.7)	−6.6 (2.5)	−381.6 (84.8)
EC	5.8 (3.7)	14.2 (3.4)	−7.7 (2.7)★	−359.3 (94.8)

Values are mean (SD).
TDR (rearfoot touchdown angle); RMP (rearfoot maximal pronation angle); TRM (total rearfoot motion angle); PV (peak velocity of the rearfoot angle).
★ $p < 0.05$, SL = laced running shoes; EC = elastic-covered running shoes.

Table 27.3 Parameters in plantar load testing

	Total	M1	M2	M3	M4	M5	M6	M7	M8	M9
Peak pressure (Kpa)										
SL	367.6	214.0	215.1	96.2	124.6	308.9	279.1	204.8	317.3	195.1
	(65.9)	(37.2)	(41.0)	(20.0)	(23.2)	(84.6)	(59.5)	(46.6)	(88.7)	(34.0)
EC	369.9	219.3	219.1	96.8	136.0	302.4	281.9	223.5	316.2	186.2
	(81.2)	(34.1)	(30.0)	(18.2)	(35.6)	(96.7)	(50.9)	(53.4)	(94.9)	(43.7)
p-value	0.847	0.364	0.537	0.884	0.073	0.64	0.669	★0.005	0.918	0.326
Contact area (cm²)										
SL	182.2	26.3	23.5	24.1	24.5	14.9	17.8	17.7	11.4	21.9
	(4.6)	(1.4)	(0.4)	(2.7)	(0.0)	(0.8)	(0.50)	(0.2)	(0.2)	(0.6)
EC	182.9	26.5	23.6	24.2	24.5	15.0	17.7	17.7	11.4	22.2
	(3.0)	(1.1)	(0.3)	(1.5)	(0.0)	(0.8)	(0.6)	(0.3)	(0.1)	(0.2)
p-value	0.394	0.466	0.753	0.818		0.873	0.406	0.483	0.426	0.073

Values are mean (SD).
M1 (medial heel); M2 (lateral heel); M3 (medial midfoot); M4 (lateral midfoot); M5 (first metatarsal head); M6 (second metatarsal head); M7 (third, fourth, and fifth metatarsal head); M8 (great toe); M9 (lesser toes).
★ $p < 0.05$, SL = laced running shoes; EC = elastic-covered running shoes.

perception scale was adopted. In this study, a reliable questionnaire to evaluate running shoe comfort was used. We found that laced running shoes scored higher than their counterparts in terms of shoe length, width and heel cup comfort. Thus, our study supports Frey's assumption that shoelaces may help runners in ensuring that their shoes better fit the shape of their feet (Frey, 2000).

In this study, elastic-covered running shoes had a lower score in comfort evaluation in forefoot cushioning. The pressure distribution of the foot's sole has been found to be associated with comfort (Chen *et al.*, 1995; Milani *et al.*, 1997). A higher plantar pressure would decrease the perceived plantar comfort (Jordan and Bartlett, 1995). In some studies, an in-sole plantar pressure system has been used to investigate the cushioning effects of different running shoes (Clinghan *et al.*, 2008; Dixon, 2008; Wegener *et al.*, 2008). The higher plantar pressure found in M7 in elastic-covered running shoes in this study might have contributed to the lower score in the perceived comfort of forefoot cushioning in this type of shoe. Compared with the shoes with elastic shoe cover, the shoes with shoelaces showed better comfort in length, forefoot and heel width, but not in overall comfort. This might be due to the fact that the two types of shoes showed no difference in terms of the five other comfort ratings. The limited number of participants in this study might be another reason why the shoes with shoelaces showed moderate ($p = 0.074$), but not significant, advantage in the overall comfort rating over the other type of shoe.

Plantar loading

In this study, a higher peak plantar pressure was found in M4 in elastic-covered running shoes. Comparable results were reported by Hagen and Henning (2009). In their study, the participants were made to wear the same shoes, which were laced in different patterns (eyelets 1–2; eyelets 1–6; eyelets 1–7; and eyelets 1, 3 and 5). The lacing pattern using all seven eyelets resulted in the lowest peak pressure, while the weak six-eyelet lacing pattern resulted in the highest peak pressure. The results indicated that the more tightly laced shoes (eyelets 1–7 and tighter eyelets 1–6) were linked to lower pressure on the lateral midfoot. In this study, the higher peak plantar pressure in M7 was found to be higher in the elastic-covered running shoes than in the laced running shoes.

Rearfoot motion

Pronation is a special motion in human walking and running. It is defined as a tri-planar motion of the foot and ankle consisting of eversion in the calcaneal, abduction in the forefoot and dorsiflexion in the ankle (Lafortune *et al.*, 1994; Soutas-Little *et al.*, 1987). Excessive foot pronation in walking or running is believed to be an important risk factor of injuries in the lower extremities (Hintermann and Nigg, 1998). It has been found that a special pronated shoe-lacing technique is effective in controlling the rearfoot motion in soccer players with excessive pronation in normal running (Sandrey *et al.*, 2001). Hagen and Henning (2009) hypothesized that the looser the lacing, the greater would be the maximum pronation; however, their study did not confirm this hypothesis. Hagen and Henning (2009) also explained that the maximum pronation value in the loosest lacing condition (two-eyelet lacing pattern) could not be detected because the fitting between the heel and the heel counter was not maintained. In this study, elastic-covered running shoes showed a larger maximum eversion than laced running shoes. It is therefore suggested that a shoelace structure helps fit the heel and the heel counter, thus contributing to the control of rearfoot motion.

It has been reported that a lesser pronation is associated with a higher plantar pressure on the lateral side and a lower plantar pressure on the medial side of the foot (O'Sullivan *et al.*, 2008; Willems *et al.*, 2006). In this study, the lesser absolute TRM and lower peak plantar pressure in the M7 area (lateral side of the forefoot) were associated with laced running shoes, which supports previous findings.

Overall, footwear has been linked to the prevention of injuries and to the increased comfort in running (McKenzie *et al.*, 1985; Riddle *et al.*, 2003; Taunton *et al.*, 2003). A study conducted by Avramakis *et al.* (2000) has demonstrated that the shoe shaft and shoe sole height can influence lateral movement of foot and ankle complex and the stabilizing effect of the shoe upper in respect to supination. In our current study, the better perceived comfort, lesser absolute TRM and lower peak plantar pressure were associated with laced running shoes. Laced running shoes may help prevent injury in running by controlling the aforementioned factors compared with elastic-covered running shoes.

Conclusion

Shoelaces help runners to have better foot-shoe fit. They also increase the perceived comfort, and decrease the maximum pronation and plantar pressure. Moreover, they may help prevent injury in running by controlling the aforementioned factors. Therefore, shoelaces play a vital role in running. A shoelace system, or any other means that can secure the foot within the footbed and heel counter, must be necessarily integrated in running shoes.

References

American Society for Testing and Materials (2006) *Standard Test Method for Comparison of Rearfoot Motion Control Properties of Running Shoes*, ASTM F1833, West Conshohocken: American Society for Testing and Materials.

Avramakis, E., Stakoff, A. and Stüssi, E. (2000) 'Effect of shoe shaft and shoe sole height on the upper ankle joint in lateral movements in floorball (uni-hockey)', *Sportverletzung Sportschaden*, 14(3): 98–106.

Bontrager, E. L., Boyd, L. A., Heino, J. G., Mulroy, S. J. and Perry, J. (1997) 'Determination of novel pedar masks using Harris mat imprints', *Gait and Posture*, 5(5): 167–8.

Burnfield, J. M., Few, C. D., Mohamed, O. S. and Perry, J. (2004) 'The influence of walking speed and footwear on plantar pressures in older adults', *Clinical Biomechanics*, 19(1): 78–84.

Cavanagh, P. R. and Lafortune, M. A. (1980) 'Ground reaction forces in distance running', *Journal of Biomechanics*, 13(5): 397–406.

Chen, H., Nigg, B. M., Hulliger, M. and de Koning, J. (1995) 'Influence of sensory input on plantar pressure distribution', *Clinical Biomechanics*, 10(5): 271–4.

Cheung, R. T. H. and Ng, G. Y. F. (2007) 'Efficacy of motion control shoes for reducing excessive rearfoot motion in fatigued runners', *Physical Therapy in Sport*, 8(2): 75–81.

Chiu, M. C. and Wang, M. J. (2007) 'Professional footwear evaluation for clinical nurses', *Applied Ergonomics*, 38(2): 133–41.

Clinghan, R., Arnold, G. P., Drew, T. S., Cochrane, L. A. and Abboud, R. J. (2008) 'Do you get value for money when you buy an expensive pair of running shoes?', *British Journal of Sports Medicine*, 42(3): 189–93.

DeWit, B., DeClercq, D. and Lenoir, M. (1995) 'The effect of varying midsole hardness on impact forces and foot motion during foot contact in running', *Journal of Applied Biomechanics*, 11(4): 395–406.

Dixon, S. J. (2008) 'Use of pressure insoles to compare in-shoe loading for modern running shoes', *Ergonomics*, 51(10): 1503–14.

Frey, C. (2000) 'Foot health and shoewear for women', *Clinical Orthopaedics and Related Research*, 372: 32–44.

Hagen, M. and Henning, E. M. (2008) 'The influence of different shoe lacing conditions on plantar pressure distribution, shock attenuation and rearfoot motion in running', *Clinical Biomechanics*, 23(5): 673–4.

Hagen, M. and Henning, E. M. (2009) 'Effect of different shoe-lacing patterns on the biomechanics of running shoes', *Journal of Sports Sciences*, 27(3): 267–75.

Hagen, M., Homme, A., Umlauf, T. and Henning, E. M. (2010) 'Effects of different shoe-lacing patterns on dorsal pressure distribution during running and perceived comfort', *Research in Sports Medicine*, 18(3): 176–87.

Hamill, J., Bates, B. T. and Holt, K. G. (1992) 'Timing of lower extremity joint actions during treadmill running', *Medicine and Science in Sports and Exercise*, 24(7): 807–13.

Henning, E. M. and Milani, T. L. (1995) 'In-shoe pressure distribution for. running in various types of footwear', *Journal of Applied Biomechanics*, 11(3): 299–310.

Hintermann, B. and Nigg, B. M. (1998) 'Pronation in runners. Implications for injuries', *Sports Medicine*, 26(3): 169–76.

Hong, W. H., Lee, Y. H., Chen, H. C., Pei, Y. C. and Wu, C. Y. (2005) 'Influence of heel height and shoe insert on comfort perception and biomechanical performance of young female adults during walking', *Foot and Ankle International*, 26(12): 1042–48.

Jordan, C. and Bartlett, R. (1995) 'Pressure distribution and perceived comfort in casual footwear', *Gait and Posture*, 3(4): 215–16.

Kersting, U. G. and Brüggemann, G. P. (2006) 'Midsole material-related force control during heel-toe running', *Research in Sports Medicine*, 14(1): 1–17.

Lafortune, M. A., Cavanagh, P. R., Sommer, H. J. III and Kalenak, A. (1994) 'Foot inversion–eversion and knee kinematics during walking', *Journal of Orthopaedic Research*, 12(3): 412–20.

Lysholm, J. and Wiklander, J. (1987) 'Injuries in runners', *The American Journal of Sports Medicine*, 15(2): 168–71.

McKenzie, D. C., Clement, D. B. and Taunton, J. E. (1985) 'Running shoes, orthotics, and injuries', *Sports Medicine*, 2(5): 334–47.

Mao, de. W., Li, J. X. and Hong, Y. (2006) 'Plantar pressure distribution during Tai Chi exercise', *Archives of Physical Medicine and Rehabilitation*, 87(6): 814–20.

Milani, T. L., Henning, E. M. and Lafortune, M. A. (1997) 'Perceptual and biomechanical variables for running in identical shoe constructions with varying midsole hardness', *Clinical Biomechanics*, 12(5): 294–300.

Mündermann, A., Stefanyshyn, D. J. and Nigg, B. M. (2001) 'Relationship between footwear comfort of shoe inserts and anthropometric and sensory factors', *Medicine and Science in Sports and Exercise*, 33(11): 1939–45.

Nigg, B. M. and Morlock, M. (1987) 'The influence of lateral heel flare of running shoes on pronation and impact forces', *Medicine and Science in Sports and Exercise*, 19(3): 294–302.

O'Sullivan, K., Kennedy, N., O'Neill, E. and Ni Mhainin, U. (2008) 'The effect of low-dye taping on rearfoot motion and plantar pressure during the stance phase of gait', *BMC Musculoskeletal Disorders*, 9: 111.

Polster, B. (2002) 'Mathematics: what is the best way to lace your shoes?', *Nature*, 420(6915): 476.

Riddle, D. L., Pulisic, M., Pidcoe, P. and Johnson, R. E. (2003) 'Risk factors for plantar fasciitis: a matched case-control study', *The Journal of Bone and Joint Surgery. American Volume*, 85-A(7): 872–7.

Sandrey, M. A., Zebas, C. J. and Bast, J. D. (2001) 'Rear-foot motion in soccer players with excessive pronation under 4 experimental conditions', *Journal of Sport Rehabilitation*, 10(2): 143–54.

Soutas-Little, R. W., Beavis, G. C., Verstraete, M. C. and Markus, T. L. (1987) 'Analysis of foot motion during running using a joint co-ordinate system', *Medicine and Science in Sports and Exercise*, 19(3): 285–93.

Taunton, J. E., Ryan, M. B., Clement, D. B., McKenzie, D. C., Lloyd-Smith, D. R. and Zumbo, B. D. (2003) 'A prospective study of running injuries: the Vancouver Sun Run "In Training" clinics', *British Journal of Sports Medicine*, 37(3): 239–44.

van Mechelen, W. (1992). 'Running injuries: a review of the epidemiological literature', *Sports Medicine*, 14(5): 320–35.

Verdejo, R. and Mills, N. J. (2004) 'Heel-shoe interactions and the durability of EVA foam running-shoe midsoles', *Journal of Biomechanics*, 37(3): 1379–86.

Walter, S. D., Hart, L. E., McIntosh, J. M. and Sutton, J. R. (1989) 'The Ontario cohort study of running-related injuries', *Archives of Internal Medicine*, 149(11): 2561–4.

Wegener, C., Burns, J. and Penkala, S. (2008) 'Effect of neutral-cushioned running shoes on plantar pressure loading and comfort in athletes with cavus feet: a crossover randomized controlled trial', *The American Journal of Sports Medicine*, 36(11): 2139–46.

Willems, T. M., De Clercq, D., Delbaere, K., Vanderstraeten, G., De Cock, A. and Witvrouw, E. (2006) 'A prospective study of gait related risk factors for exercise-related lower leg pain', *Gait and Posture*, 23(1): 91–8.

28

CUSHIONING PERFORMANCE OF RUNNING SHOES WITH EVA AND PU MIDSOLES DURING 500 KM RUNNING

Lin Wang,[1] *Youlian Hong*[2] *and Jing Xian Li*[1,3]

[1]SHANGHAI UNIVERSITY OF SPORT, SHANGHAI
[2]CHENGDU SPORTS UNIVERSITY, CHENGDU
[3]UNIVERSITY OF OTTAWA, OTTAWA

Introduction

During running, repetitive impact loads are applied to running shoes. A running shoe midsole absorbs shock during running and limits the peak impact force from heel strikes. Running shoes may play an important role in preventing injuries by absorbing external shock attributable to ground impact (Cook *et al.*, 1990; Verdejo and Mills, 2004a). Shoe age may be an important factor in running injuries. One prospective study showed that running injury was associated with shoe age (Taunton *et al.*, 2003).

Cook *et al.* (1985) demonstrated that running shoes, tested in continuous machine-simulated mileage, retain approximately 67 per cent of their initial shock-absorbing capacity after 160–240 km and less than 60 per cent after 400–800 km. In the same study, the shoes tested by two volunteer runners retained approximately 70 per cent of their initial shock absorption at 800 km. However, Miles *et al.* (2003) found that four out of six pairs of running shoes, tested in machine-simulated running up to 600 miles, did not demonstrate any significant change in shock absorption with mileage. The different findings may be attributable to different machine-simulated loading conditions. Also, as the properties of midsole materials in these two studies (Cook *et al.*, 1985; Miles *et al.*, 2003) were not reported, so the different results may likewise be attributable to the different materials and structure of the shoes.

A recent study used a standard impact tester to determine the cushioning characteristics of running shoes at different *in vivo* running distances (Wang *et al.*, 2010). The peak force of running shoes with ethylene vinyl acetate (EVA) midsoles was found to increase by approximately 5 per cent after 500 km of running. These results suggest that machine-simulated running studies may overevaluate the cushioning deterioration of running shoes. Running shoes are generally evaluated either through a mechanical impact test or a human subject test. For the mechanical impact test, a known mass is dropped from a preset height to simulate the mass and velocity of the foot at touchdown. For the human subject test, force platforms, in-shoe pressure sensors or tibial accelerometry have been used to evaluate the cushioning properties of running shoes (Hamill, 1999).

To study the durability of running shoe midsoles, the cushioning characteristics of shoes are tested per regular running distance. In measuring the cushioning characteristics of shoes after running, the mechanical impact test on shoes is more suitable than the biomechanical test on runners because the former is simple, consistent, repeatable and can provide equal comparisons across shoes.

Zadpoor *et al.* (2007) demonstrated a mass-spring-damper human model for the computation of the vertical impact force during running. The study showed that numerous factors can affect the heel touchdown impact force, such as variations in the lower-body and upper-body touchdown velocities. Kong *et al.* (2008) investigated the effect of shoe degradation (new and worn shoes) on running kinetics and kinematics measured using a force platform and video motion analysis. The study found that as shoe cushioning capability decreased, runners modified their running patterns to maintain constant external loads. The adaptation strategies of runners in response to shoe degradation were unaffected by the different cushioning technologies employed in shoe design (e.g. air, gel and spring). One study showed that the use of human subject testing, using a force plate and video camera, to determine the change in the cushioning characteristics of running shoes per regular running distance would be very difficult because various factors need to be controlled (Kong *et al.*, 2008).

Two common types of foam materials, EVA and polyurethane (PU), are widely used in shoe midsoles. However, the effect of midsole materials on the cushioning characteristics of running shoes in *in vivo* situations and the mileage dependence of this effect remain unclear. One study suggested that slight modifications in the mechanical characteristics of shoes result in kinematic changes after a long distance of actual running (Kong *et al.*, 2008). The slight changes in cushioning deterioration of running shoes may be associated with running injuries (Taunton *et al.*, 2003).

The purpose of the present study was to examine the durability of running shoes made from midsole materials with different chemical categories and hardness/densities in terms of changes in cushioning and energy return. The intention of the present study was not to investigate why chemical categories affect durability, but to explore whether chemical category and hardness/density affect the durability of running shoes. The current study could provide a better understanding of the mechanical durability of running shoes.

Methods

Running shoes

Three kinds of prototype shoes that differed from one another only in terms of the midsole material used were manufactured by a professional sporting goods company. Each shoe type was made in two sizes (41 and 43, Europe). The three midsole materials were the EVA that is currently used by the company for their running shoe midsoles (hardness Asker C, 54; density, 200 kg.m^{-3}), the currently available PU that has high hardness and density (PU2 (hardness Asker C, 60; density, 380 kg.m^{-3})) that was available for casual footwear midsoles, and the newly developed PU that has low hardness and density (PU1 (hardness Asker C, 55; density, 280 kg.m^{-3})). The hardness of these three materials varied within Asker C 54–60, whereas 55 had been reported as an average value for typical running shoes (DeWit *et al.*, 1995).

Participants

A total of 15 healthy male amateur runners who were heel strikers, had no lower extremity injury in the past half year and matched the sizes of the prototype shoes were recruited from a local club. Each participant wore one type of running shoe for normal training at concrete surfaces and ran approximately 30 km per week. Participants changed to another type of running shoes after completing a 500 km run using one type of shoe. The participants determined running distance using the Polar S3 Stride Sensor W.I.N.D. (Polar Electro, USA). The three types of shoes were randomly assigned to each subject. Finally, only eight participants completed the 500 km run (age 21.2 ± 1.8 years; body mass 62.9 ± 5.5 kg; height 172.4 ± 4.1 cm) because the other seven participants did not have time to complete the run. Participants signed an informed consent form that described the experimental protocol before the experiment started. The present study was approved by the University Research Ethics Committee.

Impact testing

An impact tester (Impact Plus 3.0, Exeter Research, Inc., USA), which conformed to ASTM F1976 (American Society for Testing and Materials, 2006), was used to determine the peak impact force and energy return characteristics of shoes at the heel position (Figure 28.1) before and after each 50 km run. The tester and testing protocol have been described in a previous study (Wang *et al.*, 2010). The energy applied by the impact tester to the shoe heel was 5 J, suggesting that the maximum impact energy of 5 J is used for shoes that are subject to moderate impacts (such as running shoes and multipurpose fitness shoes) during normal use (American

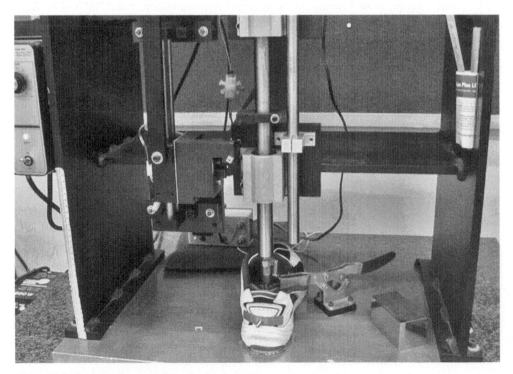

Figure 28.1 Running shoe tested by the impact tester.

Society for Testing and Materials, 2006). As suggested by the equipment manufacturer, the dropping mass and height selected were 8.5 kg and 50 mm, respectively, and the energy return was calculated as the rebound height of impact missile head divided by the drop height of impact missile head (Energy return (per cent) = (rebound height/drop height) × 100 per cent). Peak force is interpreted as a reflection of the shock-absorbing capabilities of the shoe material system, with lower values indicating better shock absorbency.

Statistical analyses

All variables were presented as mean and standard deviations. Two-way ANOVA (midsole type × running distance) with repeated measures was applied on each dependent variable to determine the significant effects of the midsole materials (EVA, PU1 and PU2) and running distance (from 0 to 500 km). A Bonferroni correction method was performed at the location of the variance. Statistical significance was set at the 0.05 level.

Results

Peak force

Peak force showed a significant difference among the shoes at different running distances. EVA and PU1 shoes had lower peak forces than PU2 shoes at all running distances (Figure 28.2), indicating that EVA and PU1 shoes had better cushioning properties than PU2 shoes.

For PU2 shoes, the peak force was lower after 50 km of running, and better cushioning was found from 50 to 450 km. At a distance of 500 km, the peak force again increased. For PU1 shoes, pairwise comparisons showed that the shoes had lower peak forces from 200 to 300 km compared with the peak force at 0 km. For EVA shoes, a significant difference in the impact peak force was only found between 0 and 500 km (Figure 28.2).

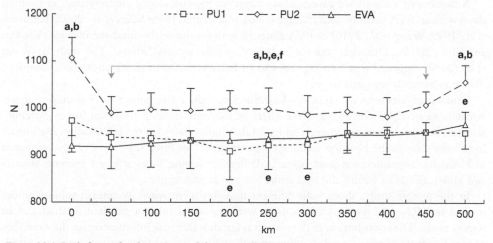

Figure 28.2 Peak forces for three types of shoes at different running distance – (a) significant difference from EVA ($p < 0.05$); (b) significant difference from PU1 ($p < 0.05$); (e) significant difference from 0 km ($p < 0.05$); (f) significant difference from 500 km ($p < 0.05$).

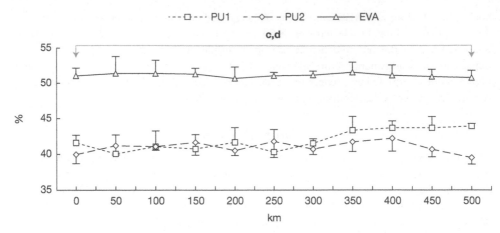

Figure 28.3 Energy returns for three types of shoes at different running distance – (c) significant difference from PU1 ($p < 0.05$); (d) significant difference from PU2 ($p < 0.05$).

Energy return

For shoes with EVA, PU1 and PU2 midsoles, the energy returns fluctuated from 50.8 to 51.7 per cent, 40.1 to 44.0 per cent and 39.6 to 42.3 per cent, respectively. For each type of shoes, no significant differences were observed among running distances. EVA shoes had a higher energy return than PU1 and PU2 shoes at all running distances (Figure 28.3).

Discussion

The results of the present study provided primary information on the changes in the cushioning of running shoes with three midsole materials in actual long-distance running. Different patterns of cushioning characteristics of midsole materials with increasing mileage were observed.

A number of studies have investigated changes in the cushioning characteristics of running shoes with an EVA midsole with mileage (Cook *et al.*, 1985, 1990; Miles *et al.*, 2003; Thomson *et al.*, 1999; Wang *et al.*, 2010) or EVA materials with mechanically simulated mileage (Verdejo and Mills, 2004b). However, the methods used in these studies differed. The study by Wang *et al.* (2010) suggested that running shoes had a less severe loss of shock absorption compared with mechanically repeated tests.

Human subjects tend to adjust the kinematics to reduce the impact force during running. Azevedo *et al.* (2005) investigated the effect of different running shoes on lower extremity kinetics, kinematics and the knees, and found that human subjects tended to adjust the impact force very early in the heel-toe running contact phase. This force regulation can be attributed to kinematic adjustments at heel contacts. Different running shoes affected running kinetics and kinematics at or before the heel strike but not at mid-stance.

In the present study, shoes with different midsoles were worn by human subjects under normal use. The cushioning characteristics were measured using a standard method and an impact tester. The contribution of the current research is that true information on the durability of three midsole materials used in conventional running shoes under normal use were given. As previously mentioned, the material with higher hardness and density (PU2) was associated with higher peak force compared with the other two materials.

Runners are able to adapt to the impact force through kinematic adjustment. Runners typically increase leg stiffness when running on compliant surfaces (e.g. natural grass) and decrease leg stiffness on hard surfaces (Ferris *et al.*, 1998). These changes may affect the moment arm of the ground reaction force (Tillman *et al.*, 2002). Specifically, increased flexion will be accompanied by an increase in muscle forces and joint moments (Tillman *et al.*, 2002). Therefore, the poor cushioning characteristics of casual footwear may result in a higher risk of injury for runners.

Moreover, PU2 was associated with a considerable fluctuation in peak force at 50 and 500 km, showing unstable cushioning properties (Figure 28.2). The present study suggested that materials with high density and hardness, such as PU2, seemed inappropriate for use as midsoles.

A material with low hardness and density, PU1, was newly developed for use as a running shoe midsole. In the present study, similar peak forces were found between running shoes with EVA and PU1 midsoles. Different patterns in peak forces were also found between PU1 and EVA. For PU1, a slow decrease in peak force at the first 300 km of running was observed, and the peak force was then maintained at a stable level through 500 km. For EVA, a slow but homogeneous increase in peak force as running distance increased was observed. PU1 appeared to have better durability than EVA.

In the present study, the parameters for energy return showed patterns that were different from the parameters for cushioning. A number of running shoe companies promoted high energy return running shoes, but only a limited percentage of energy return was found to be used to improve running economy (Shorten, 1993; Thomson *et al.*, 1999). Moreover, energy return sometimes occurs at the wrong time, frequency, location and direction during running, thereby compromising the ultimate effect on performance. As a result, the actual effect that energy return has on performance is probably minimal (Stefanyshyn and Nigg, 2000).

Therefore, although EVA foam midsoles had a higher energy return than other midsoles, the ultimate advantage of these characteristics for running shoes is questionable.

At present, the cushioning performance of shoes in longer distances remains unknown. Therefore, a longer running distance should be considered in further study. A number of studies indicate that the collapse of air cells (Even-Tzur *et al.*, 2006) and the wrinkling of cell faces (Verdejo and Mills, 2004b) affect the shock-absorption capacity of running shoes. An observation of the microstructure of the midsole materials of shoes at different mileages will greatly extend the understanding on the changes in the mechanical properties of midsole materials with running mileage.

Conclusion

The cushioning characteristics of midsole materials changed continuously as running distance increased. Midsole materials with different hardness, densities and chemical patterns showed different patterns of changes in cushioning and energy return. The change in the peak force at a 500 km running distance was approximately 5 per cent. Moreover, PU and EVA, which have a similar hardness and density, showed comparable cushioning properties (peak force) but different energy returns. The two PU materials with different harnesses and densities showed different cushioning properties but comparable energy returns. These findings provided information for chemical engineers and footwear research and development professionals in their endeavour to provide better shoes for consumers.

References

American Society for Testing and Materials (2006) *Test Method for Shock Attenuating Properties of Materials Systems for Athletic Footwear*, ASTM F1614–99(R06), West Conshohocken: American Society for Testing and Materials.

Azevedo, L. B., Schwellnus, M. P., Lambert, M. and Vaughan, C. L. (2005) 'Effect of running shoes on biomechanics and subject variability', *Proceedings of the Seventh Symposium on Footwear Biomechanics*, Cleveland, OH: International Society of Biomechanics, pp.112–13.

Cook, S. D., Kester, M. A. and Brunet, M. E. (1985) 'Shock absorption characteristics of running shoes', *American Journal of Sports Medicine*, 13(4): 248–53.

Cook, S. D., Brinker, M. R. and Poche, M. (1990) 'Running shoes. Their relationship to running injuries', *Sports Medicine*, 10(1): 1–8.

DeWit, B., DeClerq, D. and Lenoir, M. (1995) 'The effect of varying midsole hardness on impact forces and foot motion during foot contact in running', *Journal of Applied Biomechanics*, 11(4): 395–406.

Even-Tzur, N., Weisz, E. Hirsch-Falk, Y. and Gefen, A. (2006) 'Role of EVA viscoelastic properties in the protective performance of a sport shoe: computational studies', *Bio-medical Materials and Engineering*, 16(5): 289–99.

Ferris, D. P., Louie, M. and Farley, C. T. (1998) 'Running in the real world: adjusting leg stiffness for different surfaces', *Proceedings Biological Sciences*, 265(1400): 989–94.

Hamill, J. (1999) 'Evaluation of shock attenuation', *Proceedings of the Fourth Symposium on Footwear Biomechanics*, Canmore: International Society of Biomechanics, pp. 7–8.

Kong, P. W., Candelaria, N. G. and Smith, D. (2008) 'Running in new and worn shoes – a comparison of three types of cushioning footwear', *British Journal of Sports Medicine*, 43(10): 745–9.

Miles, K. A., Smith, J., Riemer, E., Echaefer, M. P., Dahm, D. L. and Kaufman, K. (2003) 'Wear characteristics of common running shoes', *Medicine and Science in Sports and Exercise*, 35(5): S237.

Shorten, M. R. (1993) 'The energetics of running and running shoes', *Journal of Biomechanics*, 26(1): 41–51.

Stefanyshyn, D. J. and Nigg, B. M. (2000) 'Energy aspects associated with sport shoes', *Sportverletz Sportschaden*, 14(3): 82–9.

Taunton, J. E., Ryan, M. B., Clement, D. B., McKenzie, D. C., Lloyd-Smith, D. R. and Zumbo, B. D. (2003) A prospective study of running injuries: the Vancouver Sun Run "In Training" clinics, *British Journal of Sports Medicine*, 37(3): 239–44.

Thomson, R. D., Birkbeck, A. E., Tan, W. T., McCafferty, L. F., Grant, S. and Wilson, J. (1999) 'The modelling and performance of training shoe cushioning systems', *Sports Engineering*, 2(2): 109–20.

Tillman, M. D., Fiolkowski, P., Bauer, J. A. and Reisinger, K. D. (2002) 'In-shoe plantar measurements during running on different surfaces: changes in temporal and kinetic parameters', *Sports Engineering*, 5(3): 121–8.

Verdejo, R. and Mills, N. J. (2004a) 'Heel-shoe interactions and the durability of EVA foam running-shoe midsoles', *Journal of Biomechanics*, 37(9): 1379–86.

Verdejo, R. and Mills, N. J. (2004b) 'Simulating the effects of long distance running on shoe midsole foam', *Polymer Testing*, 23(5): 567–74.

Wang, L., Li, J. X., Hong, Y. and Zhou, J. H. (2010) 'Changes in heel cushioning characteristics of running shoes with running mileage', *Footwear Science*, 2(3): 141–7.

Zadpoor, A. A., Nikooyan, A. A. and Arshi, A. R. (2007) 'A model-based parametric study of impact force during running', *Journal of Biomechanics*, 40(9): 2012–21.

29

THE EFFECT OF ALTERATIONS TO CALCANEAL MOVEMENT DURING RUNNING

Uwe G. Kersting

AALBORG UNIVERSITY, AALBORG

Introduction

The mechanics of foot-shoe-ground interaction has been the focus of running shoe-related research from the early 1980s. It was believed that mechanical factors such as the impact force peak or force rate (Cavanagh and Lafortune, 1980; Nigg, 1986; Stacoff et al., 1988) or the amplitude or velocity of rearfoot eversion during the ground contact phase (Nigg and Morlock, 1987; Stacoff et al., 1988) may be related to or be the cause of injuries. The concept followed on from epidemiological studies that have demonstrated a high proportion of long-distance runners suffering from overuse injuries (Clement et al., 1981; James et al., 1978; Krissoff and Ferris, 1979) in combination with mechanistically based statements on fundamental requirements of a good running shoe (Nigg, 1986). As a logical consequence resulting from these concepts, it was aimed at altering the shoe as the modulating element to potentially change the resulting load on the body system and, with that, the injury rates in runners.

It was shown that midsole hardness alone may not necessarily relate to variations in impact magnitude when assessed during overground running (Krabbe and Baumann, 1995; Nigg and Bahlsen, 1988; Stacoff et al., 1988). It was therefore realized that the physical characteristics of midsole material alone are not uniquely linked to impact magnitude. Numerous studies have been conducted varying the geometry of the midsole, its hardness or a combination of geometrical and material changes (Bates et al., 1982; DeWit et al., 1995; Kersting and Brüggemann, 2006; Nigg and Morlock, 1987; Nigg et al., 1987). From these studies, it may be concluded that it is possible to alter rearfoot movement in a desired direction by changes in midsole construction but how such changes will influence force characteristics is less predictable.

A potential methodological difficulty of relating rearfoot movement and impact force may lie in the fact that virtually all footwear-related experiments used the relative movement of the shoe against the leg as a measure for skeletal movement. Ultimately, only skeletal movement of the calcaneus and the remaining foot will relate to loading of medial muscles, tendons, ligaments or capsular structures. Stacoff et al. (1992), and more recently Stacoff et al. (2001), have provided evidence that foot and shoe movement can differ substantially. The authors reported discrepancies of up to 17° between shoe measurements and calcaneal eversion, which may make it difficult to interpret changes to shoe movement as an indicator of kinematic changes to skeletal movement.

These observations were the motivation for using an in-shoe goniometer to characterize rearfoot movement in foot-shoe-ground contact investigations within our research group. The results presented in this chapter are a synthesis of two studies on rearfoot movement control in running (Kersting and Brüggemann, 2006; Kersting *et al.*, 2006), together with data from a more recent, yet unpublished experiment. The purpose of this chapter was to assess the effects of midsole hardness, external ankle stabilization and rearfoot inserts on calcaneal movement and ground contact mechanics during submaximal, steady-state running.

Method

Experiments discussed in this chapter were carried out with subjects running at submaximal running speeds (i.e. at a steady state). If data were collected on a treadmill, they were given sufficient time to familiarize to the treadmill running situation (minimum 5 minutes). All were experienced and regular runners who took part in occasional running races but they were not training or competing at an elite level. They were all screened for foot strike patterns by being tested running overground crossing a force platform. The inclusion criterion was to show a double-peaked vertical ground reaction force pattern (Cavanagh and Lafortune, 1980). Their feet were also visually inspected and had to be free from any abnormal alignment such as severe planus or cavus foot. They were all equipped with the same rearfoot goniometer, as described in Kersting and Brüggemann (2006), and filmed in the sagittal plane with six retroreflective markers attached to anatomical landmarks (Figure 29.1). As the application of the goniometer with the thermoplast piece is linked to an offset, a static reference measurement was carried out. The subjects were asked to align the medial sides of their feet to a defined rectangular object on the ground between their feet while standing upright with straight knees and hips. This reference was carried out barefoot and repeated with shoes or ankle stabilization to assess static changes in calcaneus alignment.

In one of the experiments, a treadmill with inbuilt force plates (C. Steppat, Cologne, Germany) was used such that vertical ground reaction force parameters could be presented while in the third experiment a standard treadmill was employed (Quinton Inc., Bothell, MA).

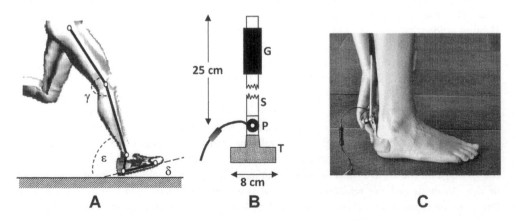

Figure 29.1 Kinematic measurements – (a) sagittal plane kinematics, marker positions and definitions in sagittal plane: γ = knee angle, ε = leg angle, σ = sole angle; (b) schematic of the goniometer: G = guiding sleeve, P = potentiometer, S = lever arm, T = thermoplastic; (c) adjustment to the heel after heating up the thermoplastic.

Running velocities were set to 3.1–4 m.s^{-1} depending on the training level of the runners. Data analysis of accelerometer, force and goniometer data was performed as described in Kersting *et al.* (2006) and Kersting and Brüggemann (2006).

Midsole hardness and calcaneal movement – experiment 1

A commercially available running shoe (Asics Gel 121) was equipped with midsoles of different hardness. In the first shoe type, the rear half of the midsole (53 Shore C) was replaced by an extremely hard material (EH) (approximately 100 Shore C). Models H, M and S comprised a single density midsole of 61 (hard), 53 (medium) and 45 Shore C (soft), respectively, whereas 55 Shore C has been reported as an average value for typical running shoes (DeWit *et al.*, 1995). The fifth shoe used was an extremely soft (ES) shoe, equipped with a block of 35 Shore C in the centre region under the calcaneus. The medial and lateral edges of the midsole under the heel area were made of 53 Shore C material to prevent the construction from bottoming out (Bates *et al.*, 1982). Shoes were tested in a randomized order and data collected from five platform contacts with running speed controlled by timing gates. The instant of first contact of the foot with the ground was identified as touch-down (TD) and the last contact as take-off (TO) with a threshold of 20 N of the vertical ground reaction force (GRF).

Restriction of calcaneal movement – experiment 2

In this experiment, a commercially available (Asics Gel 121) running shoe was used. To restrict rearfoot movement, the ankle joint was either taped medially (tape), they wore an ankle stabilization cast (cast; Air-Stirrup, Aircast, Germany) or both tape and cast simultaneously (tp&ca). The fourth condition was unrestricted running (neutral) while all interventions were applied in a random order. After the familiarization time, the participants were given a short period of rest during which the instrumentation was applied. To provide an optimum adhesion of the tape, the legs of the runners were shaved and wiped with alcohol. For the taped condition, the ankle joint was taped using standard medical tape (4 cm width). On the medial side of the ankle, five to six main strips were attached and horizontal anchors taped across at the proximal end. Distally, the tape was wrapped around the foot and a second anchor was fixed just above the ankle joint level. It was ensured that the taping did not interfere with the fixation of the goniometer (Figure 29.2a). The application of the cast was performed according to manufacturer's instructions. For a combined application of the tape and the brace the cast was worn on top of the tape (Figure 29.2b). In this experiment participants were running on a treadmill at a speed of 4 m.s^{-1} and data were collected and averaged over 12–14 steps.

Wedges and calcaneal movement – experiment 3

In this experiment, three different minimal inserts were used. The inserts were a medial wedge (MW) and a lateral wedge (LW) of approximately 3 mm height (+/−3° inclination) and a neutral control insert (NW), which was 1.5 mm thick but had the same geometry as the wedges covering the heel area up to halfway across the midfoot (Figure 29.3). A standard running shoe was used (Pegasus, Nike Inc.). Muscle activations were recorded using bipolar surface electromyography (EMG) on eight muscles of the right leg (Biovision, Germany). Following standard skin preparation, pairs of electrodes were attached to the *tibialis anterior* (TA), *peroneus longus* (PL), *soleus* (SO), *gastrocnemius medialis* (GM) and *lateralis* (GL), *vastus medialis* (VM), *vastus*

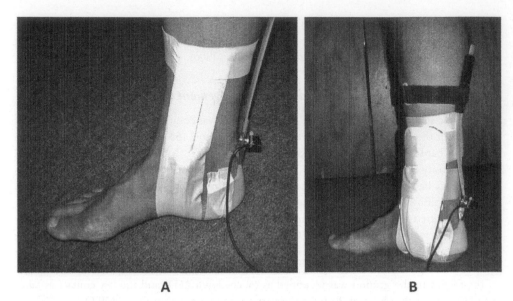

A   **B**

Figure 29.2 Application of taping and bracing. (a) Five to six longitudinal strips of tape were applied on the medial side with the foot in a mildly inverted position. The first three tape strips were fixated by an anchoring horizontal strip (this stage is shown in the picture). A few more strips were applied on top of that, plus another anchor to secure the second layer of tape. It was made sure that no connection between the goniometer and the taping occurred. (b) The cast was applied on top of the tape. Velcro straps were wrapped around the leg under the lever arm of the goniometer. Air was pumped into the cushions of the brace to maintain a good fixation of the joint.

lateralis (VL) and *biceps femoris* (BF) muscles according to SENIAM guidelines (SENIAM, 2006). EMG amplitudes were integrated over the whole stride to express neuromuscular effort according to Moritani *et al.* (1993). Rated perceived exertion (RPE) and shoe comfort (COMF) were assessed using visual analogue scales. Heart rate (HR) was measured throughout the running test to confirm runners were running at a steady state (Polar Heart Rate Monitor). For this experiment, subjects performed three trials in one testing session while running on a treadmill at 3.1–4 m.s^{-1} depending on their training status. Each session consisted of three times running for up to 16 minutes with each of the three inserts at a constant running speed. Data were collected at minute 11 for 12 steps per condition. A repeated measures ANOVA was used to test for significant differences between inserts similar to Kersting *et al.* (2006) with the significance level set to $p < 0.05$.

Results

Results of experiment 1 showed only slight variations in impact force peak measured from the vertical component of the GRF (Kersting and Brüggemann, 2006). There was a significant reduction of rearfoot movement amplitude for the extremely hard shoe (Figure 29.4a), as well as a notable but not significant reduction of rearfoot eversion for the ES shoe. While the eversion amplitude was reduced, the eversion velocity was increased for EH (Figure 29.4b). All other shoe modifications demonstrated similar eversion velocities. Further observations from this paper were that inter-individual variation was considerable with the changes induced by the shoes varying in opposite directions depending on the individual.

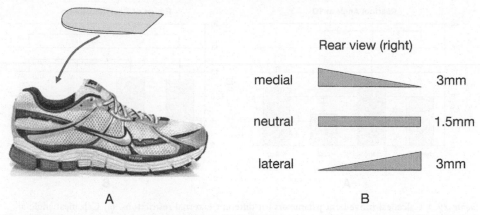

Figure 29.3 Geometry of inserts for experiment 3. (a) The inserts covered the rear half of the midsole and was placed under the standard insole of the shoes. (b) Rear view of inserts. The medial (MW) and lateral (LW) wedges were simple inclined pieces of EVA with a thickness of 3 mm on one side. The neutral (NW) control insert was 1.5 mm thick to produce a similar amount of heel lift inside the shoe.

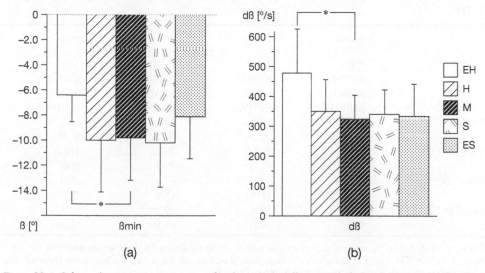

Figure 29.4 Calcaneal movement parameters for shoes with different midsole hardness. (a) Minimum rearfoot angle βmin indicating the maximum eversion. (b) Maximum eversion velocity dβ. Five shoes were compared: EH = extremely hard, H = hard, M = medium, S = soft, ES = extremely soft. * $p < 0.05$.

Results from experiment 2 confirmed that the pattern of skeletal rearfoot kinematics could be systematically altered by providing the described external movement restrictions. In summary, it was shown that the rearfoot angle at touch-down, as well as the minimum angle during contact, could be changed depending on which intervention was applied. With regard to the range of rearfoot movement, there were two interventions each with similar ranges (Figure 29.5). In this experiment, significant changes to the impact magnitude were identified while the sole angle and knee angle at TD also showed some significant alterations (Table 29.1).

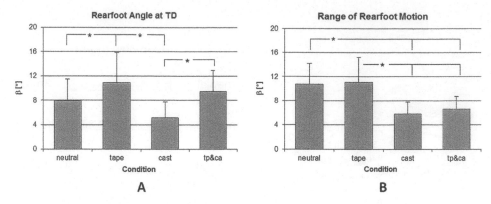

Figure 29.5 Calcaneal movement parameters for different external restrictions. (a) Calcaneal angle at TD. (b) Total range of calcaneal movement from TD to minimum angle (representing maximum eversion, respectively). Neutral, unrestricted running was compared to medially taped, wearing a cast and the combination of tape and cast (tp&ca). ⋆ $p < 0.05$.

Table 29.1 Mean and standard deviations of parameters taken from GRF data and sagittal plane angles at TD

	neutral	*tape*	*cast*	*tp&ca*
StrideF (s⁻¹)	1.461	1.469	1.460	1.457
	(0.039)	(0.043)	(0.050)	(0.053)
tcont (s)	0.2462	0.2401	0.2377[a]	0.2349[b]
	(0.0193)	(0.0192)	(0.0187)	(0.0186)
Fp (BW)	1.62[b]	1.69	1.61[b]	1.67
	(0.20)	(0.23)	(0.20)	(0.15)
Knee_TD (°)	162.7	160.6[c]	162.9	161.6
	(6.0)	(6.1)	(5.0)	(6.6)
Sole_TD (°)	−7.0	−5.6[c]	−7.0	−6.0
	(2.4)	(2.9)	(2.2)	(2.7)
Leg_TD (°)	89.1	89.4	89.9	89.8
	(3.4)	(4.1)	(4.3)	(3.8)

StrideF = stride frequency; tcont = time of ground contact of the right foot; Fp = impact maximum of the GRF; Knee_TD, Sole_TD, Leg_TD = angle of the knee joint, shoe sole and leg at TD; defined in the kinematic data as the respective angle in the last frame prior to ground contact.
Values in brackets are standard deviations, a = significantly different to neutral; b = significantly different to tape and neutral; c = significantly different to neutral and cast.

Results from experiment 3 showed an altered standing position when inserting the wedges into the shoes. The effect is less than the actual geometric change imposed by the insert, with only the difference between the medial support and lateral being significant (Figure 29.6a). For the dynamic measurement of minimum rearfoot angle, a systematic variation was shown with a reduced inversion for the medial insert and increased inversion for the lateral insert compared to the neutral insert (Figure 29.6b). Differences were significant for all conditions. In this study, no ground reaction forces were collected but the tibial accelerometer measurements did not show any significant differences between inserts. For the integral of muscle activity over one stride, there were significant differences for the PL and SO muscles

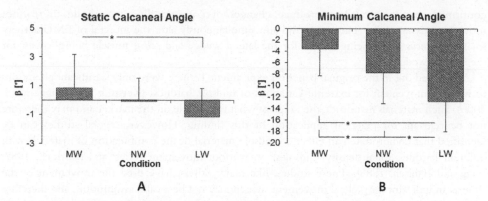

Figure 29.6 Calcaneal movement parameters for different inserts. (a) Static angle inside the shoe in relation to a barefoot standing position. (b) Minimum rearfoot angle indicating maximum eversion for medial wedge (MW), neutral insole (NW) and lateral wedge (LW). * $p < 0.05$.

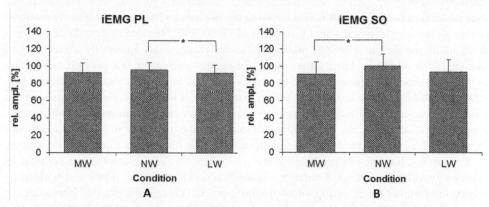

Figure 29.7 Integrated muscular activity (iEMG) of two leg muscles for running in MW, NW and LW condition. (a) *Peroneus longus.* (b) *Soleus.* EMG amplitudes were scaled to the EMG obtained in NW condition. * $p < 0.05$.

only (Figure 29.7), with the PL showing lower activity for the LW condition and SO showing reduced activity for the MW condition when compared to NW.

Discussion

The purpose of this chapter was to assess the effect of foot-shoe-ground contact manipulations on calcaneal movement during steady-state running. Three experiments, which all used an in-shoe goniometer to identify calcaneal movement, were reviewed where the first showed that a manipulation of midsole hardness alone was not linked to systematic changes in rearfoot movement or impact magnitude. The second experiment revealed that systematic restrictions of movement by taping or casting do provoke strictly systematic changes to rearfoot movement, which affects the touch-down angle and the range of movement of calcaneal eversion. This systematic change of rearfoot movement leads to some related changes in impact magnitude and was not coupled to sagittal plane changes to ankle and knee joint kinematics. The third experiment assessed the effect of minimal varus and valgus wedges on rearfoot movement and confirmed that these wedges produce changes of corresponding magnitude in rearfoot movement dynamically. The inserts did also simultaneously alter the integral of EMG activity for the *peroneus longus* being lowest for the lateral wedge and *soleus* muscle being lowest for the medial wedge.

As pointed out in the original paper on experiment 1, there were only significant alterations to rearfoot movement for extreme variations of midsole hardness (Kersting and Brüggemann, 2006). Such materials lie outside the range of what is available on the market and may therefore not be relevant for practical application of this finding. However, several studies can be identified that demonstrated an effect of midsole material or the combination of materials with different hardness (dual density midsoles) on rearfoot movement (Nigg and Morlock, 1987; Nigg and Bahlsen, 1988). These studies, like many others, have used the movement of the shoe as an indicator for skeletal movement, which may not be a valid assumption, and therefore need to be discussed further.

There are several studies that clearly indicate that these two measures may significantly deviate from each other. Stacoff *et al.* (1992) pointed at the difference between shoe- and calcaneus-eversion by cutting holes into the heel counter of a running shoe and comparing shoe movement to markers on the skin covering the calcaneus. Using markers directly mounted to the calcaneus bone, two studies by Stacoff *et al.* (2000, 2001) showed that modified orthotics worn inside the shoem as well as midsole geometry changes only minimally altered skeletal motion of the calcaneus. Their results show that skeletal movement was only changed about 1–3°, while shoe-based measurements deviate 5–20° from bone measurements (Stacoff *et al.*, 2001). On this background, our data confirm that alterations to midsole hardness alone, within a range of currently used material properties, do not affect calcaneal movement substantially. It may be speculated that the effects shown in studies focusing on shoe motion are simply due the shoe shifting around the foot, shoe acceleration during early contact or shoe deformation.

The original purpose of experiment 2 was to confirm Stacoff's concept of greater rearfoot eversion providing an extended distance for deceleration (Stacoff *et al.*, 1988) and with that a reduction of impact forces during initial ground contact. To avoid the possible interactions of altered shoe construction, the approach was inverted and it was aimed at changing rearfoot movement characteristics independently of footwear. It was demonstrated that calcaneal inversion could be affected systematically by taping and/or bracing, but the effects on impact forces were minimal. In fact, there was a statistically higher impact magnitude for the condition that provided the largest inversion at TD, and with that the largest range for potential eversion during contact, and also the largest range of rearfoot motion. This result would contradict the mechanism suggested by Stacoff *et al.* and therefore confirms that skeletal movement does not relate to impact magnitude.

In experiment 3, the methodology was applied to varus and valgus wedges in the heel area of a running shoe, which only had an incline of ± 3°, a comparably subtle amount of wedging compared to previous studies (Milani *et al.*, 1995; van Woensel and Cavanagh, 1992). These wedges lead to a systematically altered static position of the rearfoot, as well as a reduction of minimum rearfoot angle of about the amount of the intervention. This clearly shows that calcaneal movement can be systematically altered by inserts that cover only the heel area. Mündermann *et al.* (2003) investigated the effect of moulded and posted inserts on foot motion and joint loading. The authors used a sports sandal for testing, allowing for measuring calcaneal movement by skin-mounted markers. They could show significant kinematic changes, as in the current study, which may not be detectable when placing markers on the shoe. In our study, there were no changes observed in regard to tibial acceleration, a measure for impact magnitude, and no changes in sagittal plane kinematics were observed.

This study was the only experiment where muscle activity was recorded, and it was shown that two out of the eight muscles investigated showed significant differences between insole conditions. Both the *peroneus longus* and the *soleus* showed reduced activity for LW and MW respectively. This result strongly indicates that muscle activity is 'tuned' in relation to subtle footwear interventions. Nigg and Wakeling (2001) have proposed that muscle activations might be modulated in response to soft tissue vibrations triggered by impact forces during running. This concept may allow for impact forces being kept constant or otherwise regulated by muscle activation (Nigg, 2001; Potthast *et al.*, 2010). In view of the results from experiment 3, a slightly different interpretation is possible: assuming that the cushioning properties of the shoes are not different between MW, NW and LW, a subtle change in calcaneal movement leads to altered muscle activity in muscles that are likely to have a guiding or stabilizing role during foot contact. If the body system is aiming at maintaining a 'preferred path of movement' (Mündermann *et al.*, 2006; Nigg, 2001), a deviation from this preferred direction of movement may lead to an increased muscular effort in muscles controlling the movement path.

From this point of view, as none of the runners in this study showed severe deviations from a 'normal' foot, running in a neutral shoe may be close to the optimal while a slight medial or lateral support may offload certain muscle groups. If that applies, a slight medial or lateral support may be beneficial for certain runners. However, the situation may be very different if runners with cavus or planus feet would be tested. Then, the approach presented here, including the measurement of muscular activity, may be used to identify an optimal shoe or insert for individual runners.

Based on the data presented here, as well as recent suggestions from the literature, it is possible to alter skeletal rearfoot movement and, with that, affect muscle activations. An important observation is that even very subtle changes to inserts or shoe construction may have significant effects on muscle activity, which may relate to the development of overuse injuries. Such a situation could either affect the muscle groups directly by overloading them when training with a suboptimal shoe, or the increased loading of stabilizing muscles could fatigue these during long training sessions and, as a secondary effect, lead to overloading of passive tissues such as ligaments or capsular structures. To investigate this concept further, longitudinal clinical outcome studies paired with detailed biomechanical analyses would be necessary.

The goniometer method used in the three studies has the advantage that it can be used in any running shoe without the requirement of damaging the footwear by cutting holes or removing substantial elements from it. In fact, we did remove the top foam parts of the shoe covering the top of the heel cup around the Achilles tendon and covered the cut part by a smooth tape to omit catching of the thermoplastic by these foam parts. This modification was considered minimal and not affecting the mechanical integrity of the shoes. Another problem with the goniometer is that while the axis of the potentiometer is aligned in parallel to the axis of the subtalar joint, there is a parallax due to an offset between the locations of the two axes. Therefore, the angles measured will not represent the true calcaneal movement. Furthermore, the alignment was done manually, not accounting for individual differences in the three-dimensional alignment of the subtalar joint. Despite these limitations in using the device, it was viewed as an advantage that it can be used reliably as long as its fixation is secured between changing to a new shoe condition.

Another limitation of these experiments was that surface EMG is limited only to muscles that lie directly under the skin, making it impossible to assess the deeper muscles or intrinsic muscles of the foot. Therefore, it may well be that other muscle groups (i.e. the intrinsic foot muscles or *tibialis posterior*) are affected to a much greater extent. However, such changes will remain undetected by the suggested approach. Finally, the goniometer measurements were not compared to shoe measures in this study. Referring to the results of Stacoff *et al.* (2000, 2001), we expect substantial differences between shoe and calcaneal movements, which were considered irrelevant, as the focus of this chapter was on calcaneal movement alone.

Conclusions

In this chapter, it was demonstrated that calcaneal movement in running is not directly affected by changes in midsole hardness as long as variations in material stiffness remain within what is used in commercially available shoes. When calcaneal motion was altered by external stabilization of the ankle, certain conditions showed significant changes to impact forces linked to kinematic alterations in the sagittal plane, but these changes did not match a previously proposed model. It was discussed that runners may use individual strategies to adapt to altered constraints in foot-shoe-ground contact. When applying a minimal medial or lateral wedge, muscular activity of key muscles crossing the ankle joint complex was changed, indicating effects on neuromuscular effort. Such changes may have implications for overuse and injuries in running, which need to be assessed by prospective studies in the future.

References

Bates, B., James, S. L., Osternig, L. R., Sawhill, J. and Hamill, J. (1982) 'Effects of running shoes on ground reaction forces', in A. Morecki and E. Fidelus (eds), *Biomechanics VII-B*, Champaign, IL: Human Kinetics, pp. 226–33.

Cavanagh, P. R. and Lafortune, M. A. (1980) 'Ground reaction forces in distance running', *Journal of Biomechanics*, 13(5): 397–406.

Clement, B. E., Taunton, E., Smart, W. and McNicol, K. L. (1981) 'A survey of overuse running injuries', *Physician and Sports Medicine*, 9(5): 47–58.

DeWit, B., DeClerq, D. and Lenoir, M. (1995) 'The effect of varying midsole hardness on impact forces and foot motion during foot contact in running', *Journal of Applied Biomechanics*, 11(4): 395–406.

James, S. L., Bates, B. T. and Osternig, L. R. (1978) 'Injuries to runners', *The American Journal of Sports Medicine*, 6(2): 40–50.

Kersting, U. G. and Brüggemann, G. P. (2006) 'Midsole material-related force control during heel-toe running', *Research in Sports Medicine*, 14(1): 1–17.

Kersting, U. G., Kriwet, A. and Brueggemann, G. P. (2006) 'The influence of restricted rearfoot motion on impact forces during running', *Research in Sports Medicine*, 14(2): 117–34.

Krabbe, B. and Baumann, W. (1994) 'Mechanical properties of running shoes: measurement and modelling', *Proceedings of Symposium on the Biomechanics of Functional Footwear*, Calgary: University of Calgary, pp. 20–1.

Krissoff, W. B. and Ferris, W. D. (1979) 'Runners injuries', *Physician and Sports Medicine*, 7(12): 55–64.

Milani, T. L., Schnabel, G. and Hennig, E. M. (1995) 'Rearfoot motion and pressure distribution patterns during running in shoes with varus and valgus wedges', *Journal of Applied Biomechanics*, 11(2): 177–87.

Moritani, T., Takaishi, T. and Matsumoto, T. (1993) 'Determination of maximal power output at neuromuscular fatigue threshold', *Journal of Applied Physiology*, 74(4): 1729–34.

Mündermann, A., Nigg, B. M., Humble, R. N. and Stefanyshyn, D. J. (2003) 'Foot orthotics affect lower extremity kinematics and kinetics during running', *Clinical Biomechanics*, 18(3): 254–62.

Mündermann, A., Wakeling, J. M., Nigg, B. M., Humble, R. N. and Stefanyshyn, D. J. (2006) 'Foot orthoses affect frequency components of muscle activity in the lower extremity', *Gait and Posture*, 3: 295–302.

Nigg, B. M. (1986) 'Biomechanical aspects of running', in B. M. Nigg (ed.), *Biomechanics of Running Shoes*, 1st end, Champaign, IL: Human Kinetics, pp. 1–25.

Nigg, B. M. (2001) 'The role of impact forces and foot eversion: a new paradigm', *Clinical Journal of Sport Medicine*, 11(1): 2–9.

Nigg, B. M. and Morlock, M. (1987) 'The influence of lateral heel flare of running shoes on pronation and impact forces', *Medicine and Science in Sports and Exercise*, 19(3): 294–302.

Nigg, B. M. and Bahlsen, H. A. (1988) 'Influence of heel flare and midsole construction on eversion, supination, and impact forces for heel-toe running', *International Journal of Sport Biomechanics*, 4: 205–19.

Nigg, B. M. and Wakeling, J. M. (2001) 'Impact forces and muscle tuning: a new paradigm', *Exercise and Sport Sciences Reviews*, 29(1): 37–41.

Nigg, B. M., Bahlsen, H. A., Luethi, S. M. and Stokes, S. (1987) 'The influence of running velocity and midsole hardness on external impact forces in heel-toe running', *Journal of Biomechanics*, 20(10): 951–9.

Potthast, W., Bruggemann, G. P., Lundberg, A. and Arndt, A. (2010) 'The influences of impact interface, muscle activity, and knee angle on impact forces and tibial and femoral accelerations occurring after external impacts', *Journal of Applied Biomechanics*, 26(1): 1–9.

SENIAM (2006) *Surface Electromyography for the Non-invasive Assessment of Muscles (SENIAM)*, available at: www.seniam.org (accessed 30 December 2012).

Stacoff, A., Denoth, J., Kaelin, X. and Stussi, E. (1988) 'Running injuries and shoe construction: some possible relationships', *International Journal of Sport Biomechanics*, 4: 342–57.

Stacoff, A., Reinschmidt, C. and Stussi, E. (1992) 'The movement of the heel within a running shoe', *Medicine and Science in Sports and Exercise*, 24(6): 695–701.

Stacoff, A., Reinschmidt, C., Nigg, B. M., van Den Bogert, A. J., Lundberg, A., Denoth, J. and Stussi, E. (2000) 'Effects of foot orthoses on skeletal motion during running', *Clinical Biomechanics*, 15(1): 54–64.

Stacoff, A., Reinschmidt, C., Nigg, B. M., van Den Bogert, A. J., Lundberg, A., Denoth, J. and Stussi, E. (2001) 'Effects of shoe sole construction on skeletal motion during running', *Medicine and Science in Sports and Exercise*, 33(2): 311–19.

van Woensel, W. and Cavanagh, P. R. (1992) 'A perturbation study of lower extremity motion during running', *Journal of Sports Biomechanics*, 8(1): 30–47.

30

INFLUENCE OF SOCCER SHOE CONSTRUCTION ON PERFORMANCE AND INJURIES

Ewald M. Hennig and Katharina Althoff

UNIVERSITY DUISBURG-ESSEN, ESSEN

Introduction

The game of soccer is the most watched and played sport on earth, and it still grows in popularity. From a scientific point of view, coaching, game analysis, physiological demands and medical considerations were of primary interest in soccer-related research. In a review, based on 370 scientific papers, Shephard (1999) summarized the research on anthropometric, physiological and medical aspects of male and female soccer players. Surprisingly few research results were published to date on how the type of footwear, ball properties and field surface conditions influence the game. Only recently, the more frequent use of artificial turf triggered a discussion on how this playing surface changes the game and the injury incidence in comparison to the traditional natural grass. Entering the keywords 'running shoes' and 'soccer shoes' into a PubMed (NHL) literature search, approximately eight times more scientific articles are found originating from running shoe studies. This is a surprise, because footwear in soccer has to fulfil many more functions in comparison to the role of running shoes. Running shoe research concentrates primarily on the prevention of overuse injuries with little emphasis on performance. From soccer shoes, players expect primarily a performance enhancement. This footwear has to provide adequate traction for acceleration, stop, and cutting movements on a variety of dry and wet surface conditions. Furthermore, handling of the ball requires special upper material constructions to guarantee a good touch of the ball. Against running, many more injury risk situations are encountered during playing soccer. Therefore, protective shoe features for avoiding skin cuts, preventing ankle turns and knee injuries should be part of modern soccer shoe constructions. In this chapter, we want to summarize and discuss the influence of soccer shoe construction on performance and injury protection.

Shoe requirements: results from soccer game analyses and player questionnaires

The requirements for soccer shoes are best studied by analysing the game and asking players what features of their shoes are most important to them. Game analyses provide information about the situations encountered on the field. Which kicking techniques are used most frequently, how fast are the movement speeds of players and what are the resulting traction needs? A detailed analysis of soccer games thus provides useful insights about the demands for soccer shoes.

Running distance and speed

In recent years, soccer has become faster, more dynamic and the players cover longer distances on the field. Winterbottom (1954) reported running distances of only 3.2 km for the players during a game. Reilly and Thomas (1976) found running distances of 8.7 km and Bangsboe *et al.* (1991) measured average distances of 10.8 km. Using satellite navigation (GPS), our laboratory determined the covered distances and speed profiles of five different player types in professional and non-professional teams (Hennig and Briehle, 2000). It was found that the midfield and wing players showed the longest running distances of approximately 11 km during 90 minutes. The classical defender covered approximately 8 per cent and the playmaker 5 per cent less distance during a game. Overall, the wing players did not only cover the longest distances, but also achieved the highest velocities. Thus, they have the highest physical demands during a game. Between the first and the second half of the game, players covered 4 per cent more distance during the first half. Di Salvo *et al.* (2007) studied 300 professional soccer players in 20 Spanish Premier League and 10 Champions League games during the 2002/03 and 2003/04 seasons. Compared to our GPS evaluation, they reported a similar distance coverage of 11.4 km across all player positions. They also found the lower values for the central defenders, followed by the forward, and the largest covered distances for the central midfield and wing players.

Game analyses from two World Cups

From the men's World Cup 2002 in South Korea/Japan and the women's World Cup 2003 in USA, the last eight games were studied (Althoff *et al.*, 2010). Video recordings were used to analyse the finals, semi-finals and quarter-finals in both world cups. All ball actions were analysed and characterized by two experts and kicking techniques were recorded for all passes and shots. All actions with the ball were recorded: short pass (less than 25 m), long pass (more than 25 m), cross pass, shot on goal, ball control, dribbling with feint, dribbling for speed, dribbling to keep the ball. Activities that did not fit into the above categories (e.g. contact with other body parts) were collected in the category 'others'. The used techniques for the above actions were recorded (inside, instep, full instep, outside kick and head balls). Movements close to the player in possession of the ball were characterized as one-against-one fight (subdivided into air and ground), sliding tackling or jump. From the 16 games in the two World Cups, more than 10,000 short and long passes, almost 8,000 ball control activities, 3,000 cross passes and kicks on goal and more than 5,000 dribblings and tacklings were analysed. Overall, a total of more than 26,000 actions were evaluated. Surprisingly, the men's game had only 8 per cent more overall ball actions as compared to the women s game. Although the men's game appears much more dynamic, this is not apparent in the number of actions. To make the results comparable, the following data are normalized as percentages of the total number of activities in the eight men's and the eight women's games.

Women had approximately 10 per cent more one-against-one fights per game, and the men used 20 per cent more often sliding tacklings. Women also jumped nearly 20 per cent more often than men. This can be explained by the higher number of long passes, which are

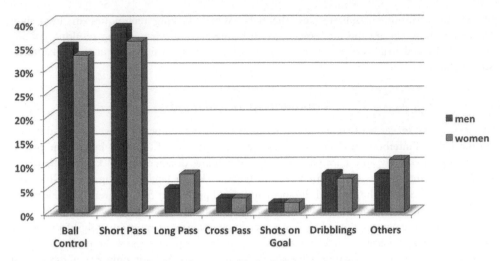

Figure 30.1 Normalized distribution of actions with the ball (percentages).

Table 30.1 Kicking technique percentages of female and male soccer players

	Kicking techniques					
	Inside (%)	Instep (%)	Outside (%)	Full instep (%)	Head (%)	Others (%)
Men	60	9	9	6	8	8
Women	52	14	7	8	10	9

often received by the head. Important for soccer shoe design is the percentile distribution of kicking techniques in a game. As seen in Table 30.1, women showed a higher percentage of head balls, instep and full instep kicks, whereas men kick the ball more often with the inside and outside of the foot.

Muscle strength is probably the most important factor for the different kicking techniques between female and male soccer players. Inside kicks are used for short distances. Because the contact area between ball and foot is largest in inside kicks, best precision is achieved with this technique. Because of a lower muscle mass and strength, women have to use other kicking techniques to achieve the same kicking distances as men. This, however, is accompanied by less kicking precision. A male soccer player can still use good accuracy inside kicks for a midrange pass to his teammate, whereas female players may have to use instep kicks to cover the same distance. For shots on goal, the full instep kick is the preferred technique for the men (60 per cent) and the women (46 per cent). Compared to men, women try to score a goal more often with the instep, inside or head. In general, women try to score from a closer distance to the opponent's goal. Therefore, they try to kick more accurately rather than with more power. The women s soccer game has changed substantially from 2003 until now. It became faster and more powerful. Therefore, it will be interesting to do another analysis for an update of these findings.

Questionnaires

The focus of running shoe research has always been the protection against overuse injuries. Soccer footwear, however, has to fulfil many game-related requirements and is primarily linked to performance. In 1998, a first questionnaire was sent out from our laboratory to 249 male soccer players. From 11 given shoe features, the players selected and ranked their five favourite shoe characteristics. Shoe comfort was ranked as most important, followed by traction and shoe stability. Soccer players also prefer shoes that feel like a glove to provide a good touch of the ball during play. Therefore, shoes are sometimes bought too small to get this close fit between shoe and foot. Surprisingly, protection against injuries received a low ranking. In 2006, the same questionnaire was sent out again and was answered by 73 male players. Figure 30.2 shows a comparison of the questionnaire results from 1998 to 2006 for the top four properties and 'injury protection'.

In both questionnaires, comfort was ranked best by the players. Traction, shoe stability and shoe weight became more important in 2006. These shoe features influence the speed of the player on the field. Because the soccer game became increasingly faster and more dynamic in recent years, the players favour shoe characteristics that improve their performance on the field. The importance of the shoe providing protection against injuries was low in 1998 and became even lower in 2006. Overall, players are much more concerned about performance aspects of the shoe rather than the protection against injuries. Therefore, nowadays lightweight and low-cut shoes with good traction characteristics are most desirable for players. High-tech synthetic materials and carbon fibre outsoles allow the production of comfortable lightweight shoes that offer good traction and shoe stability, and also allow a good touch of the ball.

Recently, Althoff and Hennig (2012) distributed a new questionnaire and extended it by asking the players which parts of their shoes they would like to have modified (stud configuration, outsole, width of the shoe, etc.). This questionnaire was distributed to 105 male and 200 female players. Similar to our previous questionnaires, comfort, traction, stability and touch of the ball were again identified as the four most desirable shoe features for both sexes.

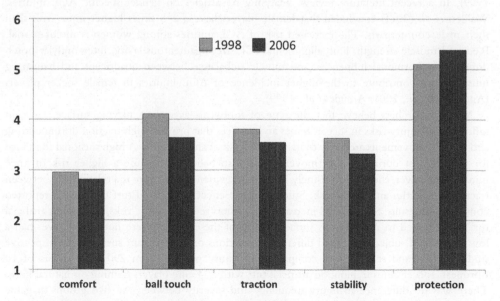

Figure 30.2 Ranking of shoe properties 1998 and 2006 (lower values = better ranking).

For female players, injury protection was more important, although protection had a low priority for both sexes. About 50 per cent of the male and female soccer players are satisfied with the fit of their shoes in the mid- and forefoot region. 35 per cent of the women want a narrower mid- and forefoot region. For those men not satisfied with the shoe fit, half of them prefer narrower- and the other half wider-cut shoes in the mid- and forefoot. Nearly 40 per cent of the female against 25 per cent of the male players prefer a more flexible outsole and 37 per cent against 26 per cent want a softer upper material. Except for 16 per cent, all female players would play with a specific women's soccer shoe. Most of them expect a tighter fit in these shoes. However, women's soccer shoes are often just copies of men's shoes, simply differing in colours. The different foot morphology between men and women has been well documented by Krauss *et al.* (2010). For a better fit and comfort, as well as shoe function, women's soccer shoes should be built on different lasts, taking anatomical features of the female foot into account.

Injury prevention – influence of footwear and turf

Injury rates are higher during games as compared to practices in soccer (Agel *et al.*, 2007; Babwah, 2009). A prospective study on 266 elite players from five European countries found 30.5 soccer injuries for 1,000 playing hours in a match and 5.8 injuries for 1,000 training hours (Walden *et al.*, 2005). From 1988 to 2003, collegiate men's soccer injuries were recorded (NCAA injury surveillance) and analysed in the USA (Agel *et al.*, 2007). The authors reported a four times higher incidence of injuries during games as compared to practices. Almost 70 per cent of all injuries were located in the lower extremities. Ankle sprains were the most common injury, and the knee caused most often severe injuries. A similar NCAA injury surveillance between 1988 and 2003 looked at the injury type and rate for women's soccer (Dick *et al.*, 2007). For them, the lower extremities were affected approximately 70 per cent and ankle sprains were also the most common injury. Data from both NCAA studies show that the frequency of ACL knee injuries was 2.4 times higher for the women (Arendt *et al.*, 1999). In a recent literature review, analysing 33 articles on gender specific ACL injuries, Walden *et al.* (2011) concluded that female players have a 2–3 times higher injury risk than their male counterparts. The increased risk of ACL injuries among women is multifactorial. Reduced muscle strength, limb alignment, ACL size, ligamentous laxity, intercondylar notch dimensions, hormonal influences, and muscle imbalance between quadriceps and hamstring muscles may contribute to the higher incidence of ACL injuries in female soccer players (Anderson *et al.*, 2001; Arendt *et al.*, 1999).

Many researchers believe that the type of footwear, as well as playing surface, have an influence on injury risks in soccer. Shoes and surfaces that provide high traction during cutting and turning movements are likely to increase the risk of ankle sprains. A high torsional resistance for the forefoot during turning movements is also believed to cause a higher risk of knee injuries. However, there is surprisingly little or no evidence that there is a relationship between traction properties and injury risk. Studies on the effect of artificial turf on injuries reported controversial results. Some found increased and others reduced injury risks, playing on artificial turf as compared to natural grass surfaces. Most of these studies were not prospective, had a low number of subjects and used different generations of artificial turf surfaces. A prospective study by Ekstrand *et al.* (2006) compared the injury patterns from 290 elite players of 10 European soccer clubs training on artificial turf with 204 elite players training on natural grass. There was no difference in injury frequency and severity between the two groups in game situations or during practices on the two surface conditions. More recently, Ekstrand *et al.*

(2010) also reported a prospective study with 15 men's and 5 women's soccer teams, playing matches on third-generation artificial turf. A comparison to results from playing on natural grass showed no difference in the overall injury risk for neither the male nor female players in match and practice situations. However, during matches the male players had a reduced risk of quadriceps strains and a higher risk of ankle sprains on artificial turf. Although the overall rate was the same between the two surface conditions, the types of injuries may change.

The soccer shoe industry tries to build footwear that offers good traction for acceleration and cutting movements on the field but low resistance against rotational movements on the forefoot. Using a mechanical testing apparatus to mimic turning movements on the forefoot, Villwock *et al.* (2009) tested 10 different soccer shoe models on Field Turf, AstroPlay and two natural grass surfaces. The authors found higher peak torques and rotational stiffness for both artificial surfaces. Furthermore, the influence of the artificial surface was much larger than the effect of the shoe cleat patterns between the 10 different soccer shoe designs. From these results, it appears surprising that there is little influence of the traction behaviour on the risk of injuries. A possible explanation for this phenomenon is an adaptation behaviour of the player to the traction conditions on the field. In a comparison of playing on artificial turf against natural grass, Andersson *et al.* (2008) examined ball skills and movement patterns of Swedish male and female elite soccer players. The authors reported no differences in total covered distance in a game, speed profiles of the players and number of sprints. However, there were fewer sliding tacklings and more short passes on artificial turf. The players also filled out a perception questionnaire and reported a worse overall impression and poorer ball control for playing on artificial turf. Thus, there is an adaptation of movement patterns to the playing surface. Mueller *et al.* (2010) combined mechanical testing, perception ratings, biomechanical evaluations and performance scores of four soccer shoes with different outsole cleat designs. The experiments were performed on a FIFA third-generation artificial turf. For acceleration, cutting and turning movements, the ground reaction forces showed large differences, especially for the shear force parameters. The shoe with the lowest peak shear force in the cut and turn movements had the worst performance time on a predefined slalom course. The perception ratings from the subjects also identified the soft ground shoe as footwear with the worst performance. Shear ground reaction force parameters and the dynamic coefficient of friction were mentioned by various authors as most important variables, to identify the traction characteristics of soccer shoes (Shorten *et al.*, 2003; Valiant, 1988). Studies from our laboratory (Althoff *et al.*, 2009) confirm these results by analysing the time of greatest likelihood for a slip to occur. The risk of slipping for cutting, rapid turns and sudden stop movements was found to be highest immediately after ground contact and shortly before leaving the ground.

Pressure distribution measurements for better comfort and performance

All questionnaires, analysed by our laboratory during the last 15 years, showed that fit and comfort were always the most important properties that soccer players expect from their shoes. Pressures under the foot are closely related to the perception of comfort (Hennig *et al.*, 1996). Therefore, in-shoe pressure distribution measurements are a good method to identify comfort properties of shoes in soccer-specific movements. The presence of studs and cleats as part of the outsole may cause high local pressures under the foot during running and other activities on the field. Especially on a soft ground surface, long studs are used for good traction. In these soft ground shoes, typically six to eight studs are part of the outsole. Such a stud configuration concentrates the acting forces to a few relatively small areas of the foot, potentially creating high local pressures under the foot. To avoid discomfort by high plantar pressures, manufacturers use pressure distribution measuring insoles during the design process of their products. For peak pressure reduction, conical shaped studs and stiff interface plates between the studs and shoe sole are employed to reduce high pressure peaks under the foot. Anatomically shaped shoe designs are a good way to reduce plantar pressures. Cupping of the heel by a curved rearfoot outsole limits the displacement of the heel fat pad to the side. In a conventional flat outsole construction, the heel fat pad thickness is reduced during loading because it is squashed to the sides. Because the fat pad is a natural shock-absorption and pressure-distributing structure, a cupping of the heel through the shoe will maintain heel pad thickness and thus reduce high pressures. Furthermore, no additional cushioning material is needed in the heel seat design and thus also helps to reduce shoe weight. Anatomical shaping of the outsole may also be used for other areas of the foot (e.g. under the first metatarsal head).

To study the different foot loading patterns during soccer-specific movements, our laboratory measured the plantar pressures for running, cutting movements and kicks on goal. Figure 30.3 shows the peak pressures from 18 male soccer players (averaged across four different shoe constructions).

For the cutting movements, high medial forefoot pressures are present under the first metatarsal head. These medial forefoot loads can lead to overuse injuries. High impact loads on the forefoot are suspected to cause foot problems such as metatarsal stress fractures, metatarsalgia and interdigital neuroma (Hockenbury, 1999). Nihal *et al.* (2009) identified a high incidence of first ray disorders for soccer players. Similar to our study, Eils *et al.* (2004) and Wong *et al.* (2007) measured the plantar pressures in soccer-specific movements, and both research groups concluded that the medial side of the plantar surface may be more prone to injuries in soccer. The knowledge of the pressure distribution under the foot is also interesting from a performance point of view. Cleat placement and design can be modified to provide a better traction on the grass surface. Because the medial forefoot exerts increased forces to the ground during cutting movements, a larger penetration of the cleat or stud under this part of the foot will occur. Thus, the cleats under the medial forefoot are important outsole structures for providing good traction for better performance. The foot of the support leg during kicking (Figure 30.3, right side) shows a completely different loading pattern to the one for cutting movements. The lateral fore- and midfoot areas of the support leg experience the highest mechanical loads. In view of these results, it is not a surprise that Sims *et al.* (2008) found a high incidence of fifth metatarsal stress fractures in soccer players. Again, the knowledge of the high lateral foot loads may help in improving the traction of the stance leg. Better stability of the stance leg through higher traction will improve kicking speed (Sterzing and Hennig, 2008) and may also enhance kicking accuracy.

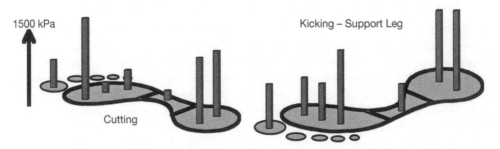

Figure 30.3 Pressure patterns for cutting movements (right foot) and kicking (support leg, left foot).

Traction properties and performance

Traction was ranked as the second most important shoe feature according to our player's surveys on soccer shoe properties. Mechanical devices for the measurement of shoe traction properties are of very limited value in predicting player performance on the field. Whereas mechanical testing devices normally exert a uniform load application, there are no uniform pressures across the whole foot or even parts of the foot. Depending on the movement, time-dependent pressure patterns will be present under the foot. Simulation of time-dependent foot pressure patterns by a mechanical device is almost impossible to achieve . Most important, however, players interact with the shoe and its properties. They will modify their movement patterns, depending on comfort and traction characteristics of the shoes, as well as different turf conditions. No mechanical device is able to mimic this interaction between the footwear and its wearer. A functional traction test (FTC) was introduced in our lab in 1998 and was performed many times until today. This FTC testing is similar to motor performance tests in which subjects are asked to show their best performance for a given task. The principle behind this functional traction test is simple. If subjects do not have the confidence in the traction properties of their shoes, they will run slower on a given parcours. To avoid slipping, they will run more cautiously. An FTC parcours should incorporate sections with multiple acceleration, deceleration, cutting and turning movements. From many FTC studies, carried out at our laboratory, we found significant differences in running times for stud type, stud geometry and stud length on the same parcours at given weather conditions. Sterzing *et al.* (2009b) identified in a series of eight studies between 2002 and 2007 the effects of different footwear and surface conditions on running performance. Removing studs from the outsole resulted in as much as 26 per cent slower running times. Stud type and stud geometry influenced running times on artificial surface by almost 3 per cent and different surface conditions (ice and snow versus dry firm grass) resulted in running time differences of approximately 20 per cent.

Shoe construction and maximum kicking speed

In an early study, we found that soccer shoe construction has an influence on maximum kicking speed during maximum effort full instep kicks (Hennig and Zulbeck, 1999). Although the possible gain in maximum speed is only a few per cent, it may still be the centimetres that the goalkeeper would need to reach the ball with his hands. Ball velocity is dependent on the impulse transfer from the leg to the ball. Top soccer players achieve maximum speeds above 130 km.h^{-1}. Tsaousidis and Zatsiorsky (1996) pointed out that the foot to ball interaction can not be modelled as a pure impact situation. It is also determined by a throwing-like movement, because the foot follows the ball after initial impact for more than 25 cm. The authors concluded that more than 50 per cent of the ball's speed is determined without the contribution of the potential energy from ball deformation. Our laboratory performed a number of experiments to investigate soccer shoe properties on kicking speed (Sterzing and Hennig, 2008). Outsole stiffness and shoe weight did not have an influence. However, better traction for the stance leg improved kicking speed. Amos and Morag (2002) found higher foot velocities during kicking in shoes with a lower mass. However, we did not find increased ball speeds with lower shoe weight in our studies. According to the impulse physics of colliding bodies, the increased mass of the foot with a heavier shoe apparently compensates for the higher foot velocities when kicking in lighter shoes. However, to our surprise, the soccer players achieved the highest ball velocities with their bare feet (Sterzing *et al.*, 2009a). A cinematographic analysis showed that during barefoot kicking the players have a higher degree of foot plantarflexion. This seems to allow a stronger mechanical coupling between the foot and the lower leg. As a consequence, the higher effective impact mass results in a larger impulse and increased kicking speed. Depending on shoe construction, the stiffness of the outsole prevented the foot to go to the same amount of plantarflexion as found for barefoot shooting.

Shoe construction and kicking accuracy

Good precision in passing and kicking belongs to the most important skills in soccer. Comparing different kicking techniques, it is common knowledge that a large contact area between the foot and the ball (e.g. inside kick) leads to good kicking precision. It is also known from tennis that an increase in racket string tension will improve hitting accuracy. This is caused by a larger contact area and a more uniform pressures distribution between the strings and the ball at contact. A similar principle should also apply to the interaction of the shoe with the ball in soccer. But most players are not aware that a shoe can influence their kicking accuracy. In a series of studies on kicking accuracy, we found that different shoe constructions do have an influence on shooting precision. The experiments were conducted using a circular electronic target with a diameter of 120 cm. Thirty electrically conducting wires were fastened in a concentric pattern on a wooden board. During contact with the board, electrostatic charges are transferred from the ball surface to the wires. Each of these wires is connected to its own charge amplifier. The 30 amplifier outputs were sampled at a frequency of 2 kHz with a data acquisition system, and the centre of the charge distribution across the wire arrangement was determined. In our first study, we investigated the effect of five different shoe modifications and barefoot kicking on kicking precision (Hennig *et al.*, 2009). From a distance of 10 m, the subjects had to perform best accuracy kicks to the centre of the electronic target at a height of 115 cm above the ground. During barefoot kicking, socks were worn on the kicking foot to avoid skin pain as a consequence of friction between ball and skin. The mean accuracy from 20 repetitive kicks was determined in each of the six experimental conditions. The repeated measures ANOVA showed differences ($p < 0.01$) between the conditions. Figure 30.4 shows

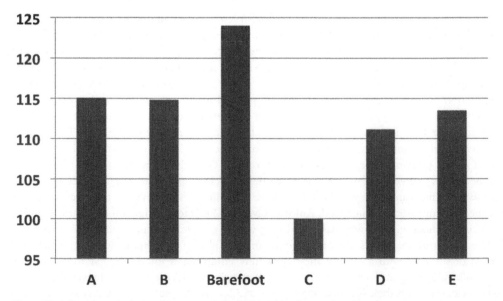

Figure 30.4 Accuracy deviation (in per cent) for kicking barefoot against five shoe constructions.

a per cent deviation of kicking accuracy against the best precision shoe, C. Barefoot kicking was least accurate compared to all footwear conditions ($p < 0.05$). Shoe C showed better precision against each of the four remaining shoe constructions ($p < 0.05$).

Based on these results, we performed a series of subsequent studies to identify the cause of improved precision. The following five hypotheses were tested:

1   higher friction between shoe and the ball will prevent slipping during contact and thus cause better precision;
2   increased spin of the ball will cause a more stable path of flight in the air and increase precision;
3   a higher shoe mass on the kicking leg will create a higher moment of inertia, stabilize the path of the foot, and thus enhance precision;
4   better skin sensation improves the 'touch' of the ball and will enhance accuracy; and
5   a more even pressure distribution across the ball will enhance kicking accuracy.

Based on several studies, no influence of the first three factors was found. We already had found that barefoot kicks resulted in the worst precision performance. Therefore, good skin sensation for perceiving the touch of the ball does not seem to enhance accuracy. We already suspected that uneven pressures across the ball to foot surface, caused by anatomical structures (bony prominences), could be one of the reasons for the lower kicking accuracy. To test whether a more uniform pressure distribution between the shoe and ball surface is the key factor for improving kicking precision, the following study was performed. We mounted a Pedar (Novel Inc.) pressure distribution measuring insole on the upper of the shoes. Using an elastic rubber band, the insole was positioned and fastened to the medial mid- to forefoot of the shoe, where players hit the ball during instep kicks. The pressure distribution patterns between ball and shoe upper were measured for 20 subjects for instep kicks on the target at a frequency of 571 Hz (Hennig *et al.*, 2009). The results confirmed our hypothesis that a more homogenous pressure distribution between shoe and ball improves kicking precision. Further subsequent studies on kicking accuracy always pointed towards the same finding. Avoiding high pressure gradients across the foot during ball contacts is the main factor in achieving better kicking accuracy.

Summary and conclusions

Soccer players prefer shoes that provide comfort, traction, stability and allow touch of the ball. The players are primarily interested in performance rather than injury protection qualities of the shoes. Because the game is played differently, and due to the female foot anatomy, specific women's soccer shoes are needed. Traction properties of the shoes and playing grounds have been linked to the likelihood of injuries. However, conflicting results in the literature do not confirm this hypothesis. Adaptation of the movement behaviour by soccer players to different traction conditions is probably the reason for this finding. Pressure distribution information serves to build comfortable shoes but can also be helpful to identify areas for best stud placement for improved traction performance. Mechanical devices for measuring traction properties of shoes are not suited to predict their grip behaviour on the field. Therefore, we suggest the use of a functional traction test that is based on the confidence that players have in the grip properties of their footwear. Shoe constructions have an influence on maximum ball velocity and the accuracy of kicking. Barefoot shooting leads to the highest ball velocities in maximum effort full instep kicks. However, barefoot shots are less accurate when compared to shod kicking. A more even pressure distribution across the contact area between shoe and ball is the key factor for an improved shooting accuracy.

References

Agel, J., Evans, T. A., Dick, R., Putukian, M. and Marshall, S. W. (2007) 'Descriptive epidemiology of collegiate men's soccer injuries: National Collegiate Athletic Association Injury Surveillance System, 1988–1989 through 2002–2003', *Journal of Athletic Training*, 42(2): 270–7.

Althoff, K. and Hennig, E. M. (2012) 'What female and male soccer players expect from their shoes', *Proceedings of the 3rd World Conference on Science and Soccer*, Ghent, Belgium: Victoris & Gent BC, p. 82.

Althoff, K., Hennig, E. M. and Hömme, A.-K. (2009) 'Analysis of slip events during soccer specific movements', *Footwear Science*, 1(1): S13–14.

Althoff, K., Kroiher, J. and Hennig, E. M. (2010) 'A soccer game analysis of two world cups: playing behavior between elite female and male soccer players', *Footwear Science*, 2(1): 51–6.

Amos, M. and Morag, E. (2002) 'Effect of shoe mass on soccer kicking velocity', *Proceedings of the Fourth World Congress of Biomechanics*, Calgary: Omnipress, pp.150–3.

Anderson, A. F., Dome, D. C., Gautam, S., Awh, M. H. and Rennirt, G. W. (2001) 'Correlation of anthropometric measurements, strength, anterior cruciate ligament size, and intercondylar notch characteristics to sex differences in anterior cruciate ligament tear rates', *The American Journal of Sports Medicine*, 29(1): 58–66.

Andersson, H., Ekblom, B. and Krustrup, P. (2008) 'Elite football on artificial turf versus natural grass: movement patterns, technical standards, and player impressions', *Journal of Sports Sciences*, 26(2): 113–22.

Arendt, E. A., Agel, J. and Dick, R. (1999) 'Anterior cruciate ligament injury patterns among collegiate men and women', *Journal of Athletic Training*, 34(2): 86–92.

Babwah, T. J. (2009) 'Incidence of football injury during international tournaments', *Research in Sports Medicine*, 17(1): 61–9.

Bangsboe, J., Noerregaard, L. and Thorsoe, F. (1991) 'Activity profile of competition soccer', *Canadian Journal of Sport Sciences*, 2(16): 110–16.

Di Salvo, V., Baron, R., Tschan, H., Calderon Montero, F. J., Bachl, N. and Pigozzi, F. (2007) 'Performance characteristics according to playing position in elite soccer', *International Journal of Sports Medicine*, 28(3): 222–7.

Dick, R., Putukian, M., Agel, J., Evans, T. A. and Marshall, S. W. (2007) 'Descriptive epidemiology of collegiate women's soccer injuries: National Collegiate Athletic Association Injury Surveillance System, 1988–1989 through 2002–2003', *Journal of Athletic Training*, 42(2): 278–85.

Eils, E., Streyl, M., Linnenbecker, S., Thorwesten, L., Volker, K. and Rosenbaum, D. (2004) 'Characteristic plantar pressure distribution patterns during soccer-specific movements', *The American Journal of Sports Medicine*, 32(1): 140–5.

Ekstrand, J., Timpka, T. and Hagglund, M. (2006) 'Risk of injury in elite football played on artificial turf versus natural grass: a prospective two-cohort study', *British Journal of Sports Medicine*, 40(12): 975–80.

Ekstrand, J., Hagglund, M. and Fuller, C. W. (2010) 'Comparison of injuries sustained on artificial turf and grass by male and female elite football players', *Scandinavian Journal of Medicine and Science in Sports*, 21(6): 824–32.

Hennig, E. M. and Zulbeck, O. (1999) 'The influence of soccer boot construction on ball velocity and shock to the body', in E. M. Hennig and D. J. Stefanyshin (eds), *Proceedings of Fourth Symposium on Footwear Biomechanics*, Canmore: University of Calgary, pp. 52–3.

Hennig, E. M. and Briehle, R. (2000) 'Game analysis by GPS satellite tracking of soccer players', *Archives of Physiology and Biochemistry*, 108(1/2): 44.

Hennig, E. M., Valiant, G. A. and Liu, Q. (1996) 'Biomechanical variables and the perception of cushioning for running in various types of footwear', *Journal of Applied Biomechanics*, 12(2): 143–50.

Hennig, E. M., Althoff, K. and Hoemme, A.-K. (2009) 'Soccer footwear and ball kicking accuracy', *Footwear Science*, 1(1/1): S85–7.

Hockenbury, R. T. (1999) 'Forefoot problems in athletes', *Medicine and Science in Sports and Exercise*, 31(7): S448–58.

Krauss, I., Valiant, G., Horstmann, T. and Grau, S. (2010) 'Comparison of female foot morphology and last design in athletic footwear – are men's lasts appropriate for women?', *Research in Sports Medicine*, 18(2): 140–56.

Mueller, C., Sterzing, T., Lange, J. and Milani, T. L. (2010) 'Comprehensive evaluation of player-surface interaction on artificial soccer turf', *Sports Biomechanics*, 9(3): 193–205.

Nihal, A., Trepman, E. and Nag, D. (2009) 'First ray disorders in athletes', *Sports Medicine and Arthroscopy Review*, 17(3): 160–6.

Reilly, T. and Thomas, V. (1976) 'A motion analysis of work-rate in different positional roles in professional football match-play', *Journal of Human Movement Studies*, 2: 87–97.

Shephard, R. J. (1999) 'Biology and medicine of soccer: an update', *Journal of Sports Sciences*, 10(17): 757–86.

Shorten, M. R., Hudson, B. and Himmelsbach, J. A. (2003) 'Shoe-surface traction of conventional and infilled synthetic turf football surfaces', in P. Milburn, B. D. Wilson and T. Yanai (eds), *Proceedings of XIX International Congress of Biomechanics*, Dunedin: University of Otago, pp. 6–11.

Sims, E. L., Hardaker, W. M. and Queen, R. M. (2008) 'Gender differences in plantar loading during three soccer-specific tasks', *British Journal of Sports Medicine*, 42(4): 272–7.

Sterzing, T. and Hennig, E. M. (2008) 'The influence of soccer shoes on kicking velocity in full-instep kicks', *Exercise and Sport Sciences Reviews*, 36(2): 91–7.

Sterzing, T., Kroiher, J. and Hennig, E. M. (2009a) 'Kicking velocity: barefoot kicking superior to shod kicking?', in T. Reilly and F. Korkusuz (eds), *Science and Football VI: The Proceedings of the Sixth World Congress on Science and Football*, New York: Routledge, pp. 50–6.

Sterzing, T., Müller, C., Hennig, E. M. and Milani, T. L. (2009b) 'Actual and perceived running performance in soccer shoes: a series of eight studies', *Footwear Science*, 1(1): 5–17.

Tsaousidis, N. and Zatsiorsky, V. (1996) 'Two types of ball-effector interaction and their relative contribution to soccer kicking', *Human Movement Science*, 15(6): 861–76.

Valiant, G. A. (1988) 'Ground reaction forces developed on artificial turf', in T. Reilly, A. Lees, K. Davids and W. J. Murphy (eds), *Science and Football I*, London: E & FN Spon, pp. 406–15.

Villwock, M. R., Meyer, E. G., Powell, J. W., Fouty, A. J. and Haut, R. C. (2009) 'Football playing surface and shoe design affect rotational traction', *The American Journal of Sports Medicine*, 37(3): 518–25.

Walden, M., Hagglund, M. and Ekstrand, J. (2005) 'UEFA Champions League study: a prospective study of injuries in professional football during the 2001–2002 season', *British Journal of Sports Medicine*, 39(8): 542–6.

Walden, M., Hagglund, M., Werner, J. and Ekstrand, J. (2011) 'The epidemiology of anterior cruciate ligament injury in football (soccer): a review of the literature from a gender-related perspective', *Knee Surgery, Sports Traumatology, Arthroscopy*, 19(1): 3–10.

Winterbottom, W. (1954) *Voetballen*, Antwerpen: De Vlijt.

Wong, P. L., Chamari, K., Mao de, W., Wisloff, U. and Hong, Y. (2007) 'Higher plantar pressure on the medial side in four soccer-related movements', *British Journal of Sports Medicine*, 41(2): 93–100.

31

EFFECT OF SHOE HEEL MODIFICATION ON SHOCK ATTENUATION AND JOINT LOADING DURING EXTREME LUNGE MOVEMENT IN ELITE BADMINTON PLAYERS

Ki-Kwang Lee

KOOKMIN UNIVERSITY, SEOUL

Introduction

Lunging is one of the most important and frequent movements in badminton, tennis, squash and fencing. In badminton, lunging is essential and frequently performed, accounting for approximately 15 per cent of all badminton movements in a competitive game (Kuntze *et al.*, 2010). General injuries in badminton have focused mainly on lower extremity (Fahlström *et al.*, 2002a). Jørgensen and Winge (1990) reported that 58 per cent of badminton injuries occurred in lower extremities, while 31 per cent on upper extremities, and 11 per cent on the back. Of these injuries, 74 per cent are injuries that are overused, 23 per cent are various sprains, 1.5 per cent are bone fracture and 1.5 per cent are contusion (Jørgensen and Winge, 1990). The foot experiences a great amount of stress, which may cause fatigue and painful conditions. It has been reported that injuries to the lower extremities account for 58 per cent of all injuries, including pain in the achilles tendon during badminton games (Boesen *et al.*, 2006). Players exhibited ground reaction forces of about 2.5 times body weight (BW) during the impact phase of lunging (Kuntze *et al.*, 2010). This repetitive and high magnitude of loading was suggested to be one mechanical risk factor of injuries and painful symptoms in the lower extremities, especially the patellar tendon or other knee joint problems (Boesen *et al.*, 2006; Fahlström *et al.*, 2002a, 2002b; Peers and Lysens, 2005).

In competitive badminton game situations, players often performed powerful and long-distance lunges, having larger shoe-ground landing angle that may result in greater impact force and joint loading than less extreme lunges. During the heel impact phase of a lunge step, the geometry of a badminton shoe heel may have a great influence to the biomechanical responses such as loading and movement characteristics of the foot and knee joints. However, most badminton shoes in the current market are questioned to be developed based on those characteristics and guarantee to provide shock absorption and stability to the foot. Furthermore, there are not many researchers who studied the relationship between the structure of badminton shoes and the performance and/or injury potential.

Therefore, this study was designed to investigate the effect of different shoe heel radius on shock attenuation, and joint loading during extreme lunge movements in elite badminton players.

Methods

Experimental shoe conditions

Three pairs of test shoes were modified from Li Ning, a badminton shoe model (SAGA, AYAZ005), and they were identical except for the heel shape modifications. The rounded heel (RH) shoe had a 5 mm extension posterior from the heel counter. The square heel (SH) shoe had 90° at the heel. The regular shoe had the commonly used heel shape provided from the shoe manufacturer (Figure 31.1). Developed test shoes were identical in size, last, midsole and outsole materials, except the degree of heel radius. Shoe conditions were tested in randomized order across the participants.

Participants

Eleven male elite badminton players who were in the high rankings at a Korea Collegiate Athletic Association were recruited (age: 21.1 ± 1.2 years; height: 178.5 ± 5.6 cm; weight: 70.6 ± 5.9 kg; career: 9.6 ± 1.1 years) for this study. All of them were on the level of semi-national teams and had served as university team players without ankle or knee injuries in the past 12 months or surgery or fracture of lower extremities in the past 24 months. Only subjects being fitted to US shoe size 8.5, 9 and 9.5 were included in the test. Before participating, all participants read and signed the informed consent.

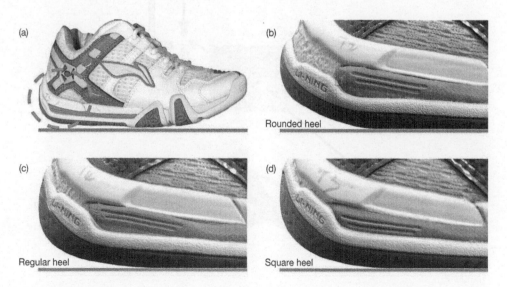

(a)

(b) Rounded heel

(c) Regular heel

(d) Square heel

Figure 31.1 Badminton shoe conditions.

Maximal lunge protocol

Prior to data collection, each participant was asked to perform maximal lunge to measure the individual maximal lunge distance. Participants were instructed to stand at the start positions, where marking was done based on the measured distance for each participant. From the start position, each participant performed maximal lunge and hit the target, and then returned to the starting position (Figure 31.2). If a player completely accomplished all three steps, contact of the force plate, hit the shuttlecock and recovery to the starting position, we considered it a successful lunge task. Each participant performed five successful tasks with each shoe model.

Experimental setup

A 40 × 60 cm force platform (AMTI, Watertown, USA), which was covered by standard badminton court mat, was used for recording ground reaction forces at 2,400 Hz. This force platform was also synchronized with 10 motion-capturing cameras (Oxford Metrics Ltd., Oxford, sampling at 240 Hz) to measure the kinematics data of the lower extremities. Twenty-four markers (diameter 14 mm) were placed on the following anatomical landmarks: three metatarsal markers on medial side of first metatarsal head, upper side of second metatarsal head and lateral side of fifth metatarsal head; three calcaneus markers on posterior upper, posterior lower and lateral aspects of calcaneus, each marker on medial and lateral malleolus, medial and lateral femoral epicondyles, greater trochanters, ASIS, PSIS; and lastly two four-marker rigid clusters on thigh and leg segments. The marker of medial calcaneus, malleolus and medial femoral epicondyle were removed during data acquisition.

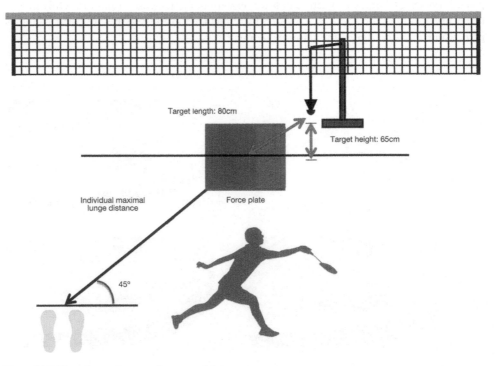

Figure 31.2 Experimental set-up (not to scale).

A spline interpolation was performed for minor missing marker trajectories using three frames of data before and after the missing data. A Butterworth Bidirectional Filter (i.e. a fourth order filter) with cut-off frequency equal to 6 was used to smooth kinematic data. Cut-off frequency at 100 Hz was applied to GRF data, which was normalized with body mass.

During foot contact period, all kinematic and ground reaction force (GRF) variables were analysed with Visual3D software (C-Motion Inc.) for the definition of body segments and calculation of ankle and knee joint kinematics variables. The cut cycle was defined as the period from initial contact of the heel to toe-off, as indicated by the force platform. The instant of foot contact and take-off from the force platform was defined as the time points of the first vertical GRF rise above 10N (foot contact) and reduction to 10N (take-off), respectively.

Data reduction

Kinematic and kinetic data were analysed from initial heel contact to toe-off. Strike phase was defined as the period of time from initial contact to foot flat (Figure 31.3). Contact time, time to shoe flat and peak GRFs slip distance, shoe sole angular kinematics, peak ground reaction forces loading rate, horizontal and vertical force ratio, and knee and ankle joint loads were selected in the present study because this data may provide direct influences on shock attenuation and joint loading by heel shape of badminton footwear.

Statistical analysis

To determine heel curvature effect, contact time, time to shoe flat and peak GRFs, and slip distance, shoe sole angular kinematics, peak ground reaction forces and loading rate, and knee and ankle joint loads were analysed using one-way ANOVAs with repeated measures. A Greenhouse-Geisser adjustment was used if the assumptions of sphericity were violated. Alpha was set at 0.05 for all analysis.

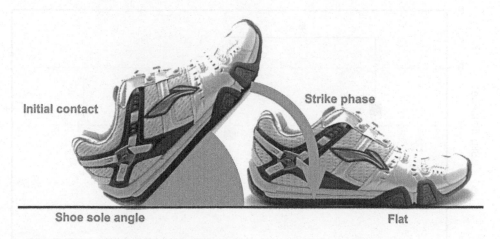

Figure 31.3 Strike phase and shoe sole angle.

Results

Spatio-temporal variables

Contact time and time to shoe flat were not affected by different heel modification (Table 31.1). However, considering the time from initial contact to peak ground reaction forces, the SH shoe demonstrated a shorter time to peak vertical force, compared to RH and regular shoes ($p < 0.05$), whereas heel shape showed no effect on the time to peak horizontal force. In addition, SH shoe demonstrated longer slip distance compared to RH shoe ($p < 0.05$) (see Figure 31.4).

Shoe-ground kinematics

Using one-way ANOVAs with repeated measures, shoe-ground kinematics including shoe sole angle at initial contact, angular velocity and acceleration of this sole angle, and shoe sole angles

Table 31.1 Spatio-temporal parameter

Variables/shoes	SH	Regular	RH	Sig
Contact time (s)	0.67 ± 0.14	0.68 ± 0.13	0.68 ± 0.13	–
Time to shoe flat (ms)	64.2 ± 8.2	65.4 ± 9.0	64.6 ± 6.8	–
Time to peak vertical force (ms)*	10.8 ± 0.7	11.1 ± 1.0	11.20 ± 0.9	SH < regular, RH
Time to peak horizontal force (ms)	63.4 ± 23.5	62.1 ± 17.8	68.1 ± 21.4	–
Slip distance (cm)*	7.28 ± 0.85	6.85 ± 0.95	6.97 ± 0.83	SH > RH

*Statistical significant difference with p < 0.05.

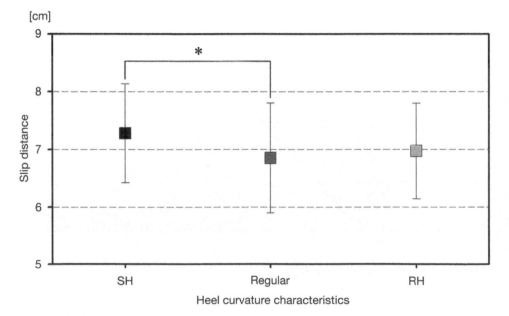

Figure 31.4 Slip distance. * $p < 0.05$.

at peak vertical ground reaction force and loading rate were evaluated (Table 31.2). None of the shoe-ground kinematics showed significant effect of heel modification ($p > 0.05$).

Ground reaction forces

Peak vertical ground force occurred around 20 per cent of strike phase, and peak loading rate appeared just after initial heel contact (Figure 31.5). The SH shoe demonstrated a greater vertical loading rate, and resultant GRF compared to the regular. RH shoes ($p < 0.05$) (see Figures 31.6 and 31.7), moreover, indicated significant higher horizontal and vertical force ratio compared to the rounded heel condition (see Figure 31.8); whereas horizontal ground reaction force and loading rate did not show significant difference by heel modification ($p > 0.05$).

Ankle and knee joint loads

Just after initial heel contact, ankle moment showed dorsiflexion direction, then turned to large amounts of plantar flexion through entire stance phase (Figure 31.9). During early phase of contact, a lager ankle dorsiflexion moment was observed in the regular shoe compared with the RH shoe ($p < 0.001$) (see Table 31.4). Whereas, knee moment started with flexion direction from initial heel contact to shoe sole flat, then turned to extension direction until final phase of contact (Figure 31.10). However, knee flexion moment before shoe sole flat did not show significant difference by heel shape ($p > 0.05$) (see Table 31.4).

Table 31.2 Shoe-ground kinematics

Variables/shoes	SH	Regular	RH	Sig
Sole angle @ contact (deg)	45.64 ± 4.00	45.37 ± 4.20	45.82 ± 5.05	–
Peak foot slap angular vel. (rad/s)	−20.01 ± 1.11	−20.24 ± 1.00	−19.86 ± 1.47	–
Peak foot slap angular acc. (rad/s²)	28.81 ± 12.53	33.90 ± 15.49	31.63 ± 14.14	–
Sole angle @ peak vertical force (deg)	32.47 ± 3.54	31.12 ± 3.68	31.79 ± 4.03	–

Table 31.3 Ground reaction forces

Variables/shoes	SH	Regular	RH	Sig
Peak vertical force (BW)	2.19 ± 0.28	2.22 ± 0.32	2.12 ± 0.32	–
Peak vertical loading rate (BW/s)**	248.53 ± 47.11	232.74 ± 46.21	219.26 ± 49.15	RH < SH, regular
Peak breaking force (BW)	1.47 ± 0.31	1.46 ± 0.23	1.41 ± 0.30	–
Peak breaking loading rate (BW/s)	68.11 ± 11.50	66.31 ± 14.29	69.56 ± 17.92	–
Peak resultant GRF (BW)*	2.36 ± 0.27	2.37 ± 0.33	2.29 ± 0.33	RH < SH, regular
Peak horizontal/vertical force ratio	0.88 ± 0.08	0.88 ± 0.10	0.84 ± 0.07	RH < SH

*Statistical significant difference with $p < 0.05$. ** Statistical significant difference with $p < 0.01$

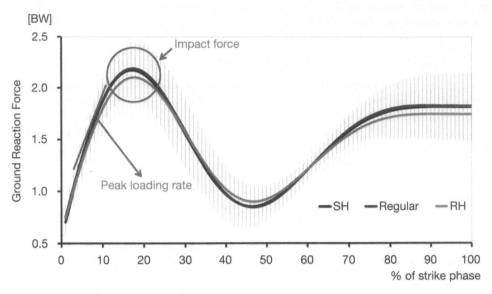

Figure 31.5 Vertical ground reaction force in strike phase.

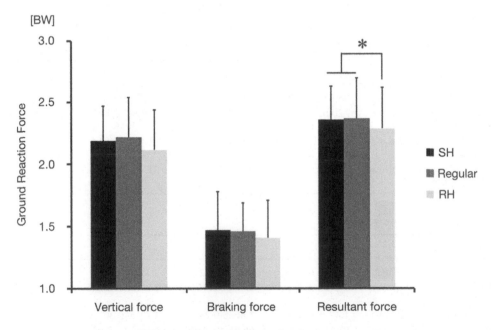

Figure 31.6 Vertical, horizontal and resultant ground reaction force.

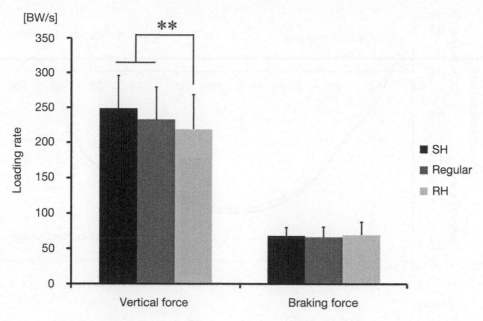

Figure 31.7 Vertical and horizontal loading rate.

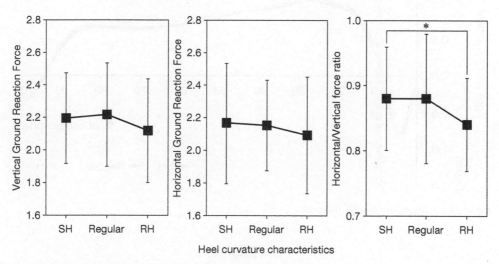

Heel curvature characteristics

Figure 31.8 Vertical GRF, horizontal GRF and H/V force ratio.

Table 31.4 Knee and ankle joints loads

Variables/shoes	SH	Regular	RH	Sig
Knee flexion moment (Nm/kg)	−0.98 ± 0.28	−0.98 ± 0.27	−1.06 ± 0.25	–
Ankle dorsiflexion moment (Nm/kg)	0.14 ± 0.07	0.25 ± 0.06	0.19 ± 0.10	Regular < SH

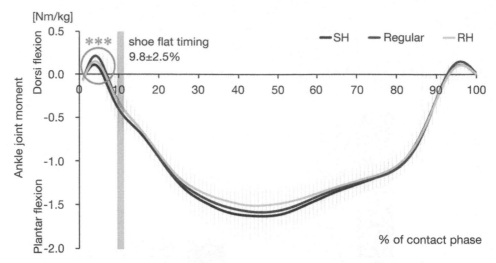

Figure 31.9 Ankle joint sagittal moment.

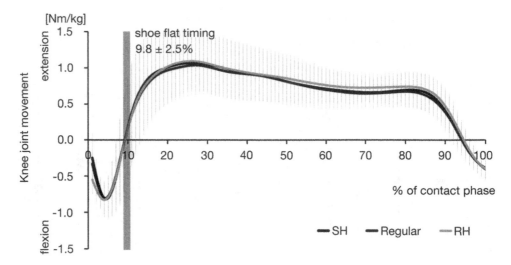

Figure 31.10 Knee joint sagittal moment.

Discussions

The application of heel modification of badminton footwear in this study was to evaluate whether rounded heel shape would reduce impact shock and lower extremity joint loads during maximal lunge movement. The rounded heel shoe was associated with longer time from heel contact to peak vertical ground reaction force that might reduce impact shock. Also, the increased heel curvature showed less slippery phenomenon, which might be associated with better traction during initial contact phase. These results might affect the reduced dorsiflexion moment of ankle joint just after initial heel contact with the rounded heel shoe compared to the square shape shoe. Although it was expected that rounded heel shape induced greater shoe sole angle at heel contact, there was no heel modification effect.

Potential injury mechanism of Achilles tendonitis, which is a major badminton injury, may be the fast forward (Bunn, 1972; Grice, 1996). Contraction of *gastrocnemius* or *triceps surae* during posterior landing may produce excessive load on the Achilles tendon (Jørgensen and Winge, 1999). High stress on the Achilles tendon during fast and powerful foot work in badminton may result in microtrauma in muscle, tendon and ligament (Gowitzke and Milner, 1988). As we expected, the rounded heel shape could lessen both the vertical impact force and the loading rate. The RH shoe reduced the resultant GRF and vertical GRF loading rate by 3.1–3.5 per cent and 6.1–13.3 per cent, respectively. Interestingly, while there was no heel modification effect on braking force and its loading rate, RH shoe reduced the ratio of horizontal and vertical forces, which means there were relatively small amounts of braking force for the foot planting during the early strike phase. However, there was no heel modification effect on knee joint load in the early strike phase.

Although the average distance of extreme lunges in this study was about 2.3 m, and much longer than 1.5 times leg length in the study by Kuntze *et al.* (2010), the value of peak GRFs were similar. This similarity in peak GRF may be due to different skill levels of participants while two groups performed different tasks. Because all athletes in this study were on international competition level, they performed extreme lunges more efficiently than the intermediate level. Also, knee and ankle joint moments identified in this study were generally less than those presented by Kuntze *et al.* (2010). This discrepancy in knee joint moment may be due to a different kinematic data collection system. Overestimation of angular acceleration might due to the lack of number of cameras employed in their study.

In conclusion, the rounded heel shoe demonstrated superior impact attenuation compared to regular and square-type shoes. However, the shoe sole thickness, midsole hardness and material properties should also be taken into account for optimizing cushioning properties. In future study, female and intermediate groups should be included to ascertain if rounded-heel shape is functionally beneficial for badminton.

References

Boesen, M. I., Boesen, A., Koenig, M. J., Bliddal, H. and Torp-Pedersen, S. (2006) 'Ultrasonographic investigation of the Achilles tendon in elite badminton players using color doppler', *American Journal of Sports Medicine*, 34(12): 2013–21.

Bunn, J. W. (1972) *Scientific Principles of Coaching*, 2nd edn, Englewood Cliffs, NJ: Prentice-Hall.

Fahlström, M., Lorentzon, R. and Alfredson, H. (2002a) 'Painful conditions in the Achilles tendon region: a common problem in middle-age competitive badminton players', *Knee Surgery, Sports Traumatology and Arthroscopy*, 10(1): 57–60.

Fahlström, M., Lorentzon, R. and Alfredson, H. (2002b) 'Painful conditions in the Achilles tendon region in elite badminton players', *American Journal of Sports Medicine*, 31(1): 51–4.

Grice, I. (1996) *Badminton: Step to Success*, Champaign, IL: Human Kinetics.

Gowitzke, B. A. and Milner, M. (1988) *Scientific Bases of Human Movement*, Baltimore: Williams & Wilkins.

Jørgensen, U. and Winge, S. (1990) 'Injuries in badminton', *Sports Medicine*, 10(1): 59–64.

Kuntze, G., Mansfield, N. and Sellers, W. (2010) 'A biomechanical analysis of common lunge tasks in badminton', *Journal of Sports Sciences*, 28(2): 183–91.

Peers, K. H. and Lysens, R. J. (2005) 'Patellar tendinopathy in athletes: current diagnostic and therapeutic recommendations', *Sports Medicine*, 35(1): 71–87.

32

THE EFFECTS OF FOOTWEAR ON THE ECONOMY OF MOVEMENT

Edward C. Frederick

EXETER RESEARCH, INC., BRENTWOOD

It is common sense that certain types of footwear are more difficult to move in than other types. For example, we all know from personal experience that heavy and inflexible shoes can be a struggle to walk in and lighter, more flexible shoes seem to ease the burden of walking or running. These obvious differences can express themselves as differences in the energy we require for movement. But there is much more than these obvious results to be revealed in reviewing the effects of footwear on the economy of movement.

The relative energetic demands of movements in various types of footwear has been a topic of study for decades. The preferred bottom-line terminology for discussing this topic is *energetic economy*. This phrase highlights the fact that the effects are expressed and quantified by measuring energy expenditure; and it incorporates the assumed objective of minimizing relative energetic cost.

Although some authors use the term *efficiency* in place of economy, that terminology is misleading and usually wrong. Efficiency implies a complete understanding of the total work done for a given metabolic energy cost. Because neither the total work done nor the total energy expended is completely measured in such cases, it is really not possible to talk about efficiency. Instead, the term *economy* is used as a measure of the relative energetic cost of performing similar activities.

Knowledge of energy expenditure is a critical element in our understanding of the effects that shoes and surface characteristics have on the ergonomics of sports and exercise. Of particular importance is the assessment of the effects of these factors on the energetic economy of locomotion.

The economy of locomotion, a subset of economy of movement, is a measure of the apparent efficiency (Pugh, 1971) of walking or running under specified conditions. For example, if we ask two persons of equal body weight to walk at the same speed while we measure energy expenditure, and one subject requires less energy to perform that task, we may be tempted to say that person is a more 'efficient' walker.

This is an inaccurate and crude way of estimating efficiency because the amount of total work done is not controlled or measured, and this can mislead us about the actual efficiency of the two subjects. The subject who used less energy, for example, may actually have been doing significantly less work as well. This would negate any suspected efficiency gains and, in fact, the less-economical subject who expends more energy might even be more the more efficient of the two people used in this hypothetical example.

By using terms such as *economy*, we escape some of the rigours of true efficiency measurements while we gain some insight into the effects various types of footwear may be having. This may be viewed as a form of intellectual escapism, but there is some bottom-line sense to this approach.

In athletic performance, for example, greater economy of locomotion contributes to excellence. If an athlete requires less energy than others to perform a given defined task, he or she is more likely to be successful. It may not matter whether a particular athlete's enhanced economy of locomotion is due to true improved efficiency or to a disproportionate reduction in the work done – a feat that can be accomplished by moving more economically.

Saunders *et al.* (2004a, 2004b) analysed the potential performance benefits as well as the resolving power of measurements of running economy and concluded that differences of ~ 2.4 per cent or greater are 'real' and 'worthwhile'.

Measuring the economy of locomotion

Open-circuit oxygen uptake measurement is the method of choice for evaluating the energy requirements of locomotion at submaximal steady-state workloads. Even though this is the best method we currently have for measuring energy expenditure, it is still rather limited in its ability to resolve very small treatment effects such as those that might be produced by slight differences in the biomechanical properties of various shoes and surfaces. The resolving power of the measurement, as it is used here, refers to the ability to find statistically significant differences between treatment groups. Resolution is expressed as a percentage difference between means. Lower percentages of resolution are better because they reflect an ability to detect smaller differences between means.

Depending on the number of subjects used, the number of replicate measurements made and the variability resulting from biological and technical sources, the resolving power of oxygen uptake measurements may range from less than 1 per cent to more than 10 per cent. Many physiologists regard a 1 per cent resolving power for the measurement of oxygen uptake as unattainable. They mistakenly assume that the maximal resolving power cannot be less than the reproducibility of the measurement, which is generally regarded as being in the range of 3–5 per cent.

Day-to-day variability in oxygen uptake has been shown to produce a coefficient of variability of 3–5 per cent (Armstrong and Costill, 1983; Saunders *et al.*, 2004b). Within day variability in our experience is less and falls within a range of 1–3 per cent depending on the state of fitness of the experimental subjects and, to a lesser extent, on their familiarity with treadmill walking or running. These wide values for the reproducibility of the measurement add to the difficulty of finding statistically significant differences between various treatment effects because they increase the variability term of whatever statistic is used. They do not, however, represent a built-in limit on our ability to find significant differences (Frederick, 1983).

Even with reasonably small sample sizes, it is possible to find significant differences between means of less than 1 per cent, if a low coefficient of variation (CV) of the mean difference is present. Even with a high CV of 5 per cent, it is possible to detect differences of 2 per cent with a sample size of less than 20 subjects. Indeed, it is possible to find significant differences even when the reproducibility of the measurement is higher than the difference that has been recorded. Reproducibility clearly has no direct effect on finding differences between treatment effects.

Even though we can show that the CV of VO_2 measurements does not represent a built-in limit on the resolving power of the method, others may question the physiological significance of differences that fall within the range of day-to-day variability of the measurement.

If we carefully interpret the meaning of a statistical difference between means, however, it is clear that *significant differences* are outside the variability we are measuring. When included in the day-to-day variations, they would not show up as significantly different. If a difference between means is labelled as physiologically trivial, it is because it is considered small in magnitude and not because it is small in relation to the CV of the measurement. Given the 1–2 per cent resolving power of comparative oxygen uptake experiments, it is possible to find out a great deal about the effects that various shoe and surface characteristics have on the economy of locomotion. The following sections review the literature on this subject.

Shoe studies: weight effects

The earliest studies of the effects of shoe type on the economy of locomotion were done during the later stages of World War II. The work of Russell and Belding (1946) was commissioned by the US Army Quartermaster Corps to ascertain the effects of shoe weight on the energy cost of walking. Because of the large within-step changes in the potential energy and the rotational and translational kinetic energies of the foot, it was expected that the relative cost of carrying weight on the feet would be much greater than carrying the same weight on the torso. Results were presented for barefoot walking and for walking in a range of shoe types that were selected presumably because of the wide differences in weight they represented (1.4 to 3.4 kg per pair).

Russell and Belding (1946) found a great deal of variation between shoes in the economy of locomotion. As expected, the heavier models required significantly more energy expenditure, although the authors speculated that only a portion of those differences were due to the weight effects. They were also able to show that at faster walking speeds and on grades the relative cost of carrying weight on the feet went up. This increase in relative cost was also evident when the costs of wearing heavier and heavier shoes were compared. Part of this variation in relative cost with speed, grade and weight might be explained by variations in step frequency and in the vertical excursion of the body's centre of gravity that the authors observed.

In a side experiment, Russell and Belding (1946) compared the effect of adding weights to a pair of standard issue combat boots to carrying the same weight in a pouch at the waist. Their results showed that carrying the weight on the feet was about four times more costly than carrying it at the waist, nearer the centre of gravity of the body. Interestingly, Martin (1985) found that this ratio is approximately seven times for running.

Russell and Belding later discovered that carrying added weight on the feet was less costly than wearing boots of similar additional weight, supporting the observation that only part of the variation in the cost of wearing different boots could be explained by weight alone. This is a theme that repeats itself often in studies of the energetic effects of footwear.

Table 32.1 displays some of the results of the Russell and Belding experiments as well as other studies on the effects of wearing shoes of differing weights on the economy of locomotion. The results of all studies have been recalculated to a common value for the *oxygen cost of transport* in litres of O_2 per kilogram of weight added to both feet per kilometre walked or run. This normalizes all results in a way that eliminates the effect of differences in speed.

Soule and Goldman (1969) and Ralston (1981) performed their experiments by adding weights to the foot rather than comparing the cost of walking in shoes of different weight. Considering the increase in relative cost of carrying progressively heavier weights observed by

Table 32.1 Oxygen cost of transport for carrying added weight on the feet. O$_2$ cost is expressed as litres of O$_2$ per kg of added weight carried per km travelled. Subject body mass is 68 kg for all calculations.

Condition	O$_2$ cost (l O$_2$/ kg/km)	Source
Walking @ 5.6 km/hr in 2.1 kg/pr boots	0.421**	Russell and Belding (1946)
Walking @ 5.6 km/hr, 0.91 kg wt added/both feet	0.241**	Russell and Belding (1946)
Walking @ 4.3 km/hr, 4 kg wt added/both feet	0.785**	Ralston (1981)
Walking @ 4.0 km/hr, 12 kg wt added/both feet	0.634	Soule and Goldman (1969)
Walking @ 5.6 km/hr, 12 kg wt added/both feet	1.004	Soule and Goldman (1969)
Running @ 15 km/hr*, 0.350 kg wt added/both feet	1.185**	Catlin and Dressendorfer (1979)
Running @ 16.1 km/hr, 0.450 kg wt added/both feet	0.616	Frederick *et al.* (1984)
Running @ 12.06 km/hr, 0.600 kg wt added/both shoes	0.755	Frantz *et al.* (2012)
Running @ 12.06 km/hr, 0.900 kg wt added/both barefeet	0.594	Frantz *et al.* (2012)
Running @ 13 km/hr, 0.700 kg wt/pr shoes	0.538	Divert *et al.* (2008)

* Average speed estimated from the range of speeds mentioned for all subjects. ** Value for litres O$_2$ calculated from kilocalorie data by dividing by 4.9.

Russell and Belding (1946), it is not surprising that both Soule and Goldman and Ralston found greater costs of transport than were reported in the earlier study. Ralston added 4 kg to the feet and Soule and Goldman added 12 kg – an amount of weight that would be expected to produce dramatic and energetically costly adjustments in kinematics.

The first two running studies shown in Table 32.1 differ in that the results reported by Catlin and Dressendorfer (1979) were for two different models that differed in weight, whereas the Frederick *et al.* (1984) employed identical shoes to which weights were added. The discrepancy in the oxygen cost of transport between these two studies may be due to the fact that the shoes used by Catlin and Dressendorfer were different enough in design features such as the amount of cushioning they provided to cause effects on the economy of locomotion beyond weight effects alone (Frederick, 1983; Frederick *et al.*, 1983). These and other non-weight effects are discussed in the following section.

Catlin and Dressendorfer (1979) were the first to show that adding weight to the feet while running brings with it a penalty of a roughly 1 per cent increased energy expenditure per 100 g added to each foot. In their study, their subjects ran at moderate speed wearing 870 g and 520 g shoes. The 350 g of weights added to each shoe required 3.3 per cent more metabolic energy at the moderate pace their subjects were running. That is approximately 1 per cent per 100 g added weight per foot.

Frederick *et al.* (1984) found that adding a mass of 100 g per shoe increased aerobic cost of running by 1.2 per cent at 3.83 m.s^{-1} (7 minutes per mile) and 0.8 per cent at 4.88 m.sec^{-1} (5 minutes and 30 seconds per mile). This 1 per cent estimate has been found in other more recent studies (Divert *et al.*, 2008; Frantz *et al.*, 2012), and it is generally considered a good rule of thumb for the energetic costs of carrying added weight on the feet.

Shoe studies: non-weight effects

Numerous studies have shown that various non-weight-related aspects of shoe design can have significant effects on the kinetics and kinematics of locomotion (Frederick, 1984; Nigg, 1986).

With such biomechanical effects in evidence, it is not surprising that significant differences in the economy of locomotion caused by various shoe properties have been reported.

Mathews and Wooten (1963) compared the economy of locomotion of 10 female subjects walking barefoot and in three different shoe styles. There was no difference between the mean oxygen uptakes reported for the barefoot, loafer and saddle style shoes. However, walking either on the level or on a 6 per cent grade in high heels was significantly more costly than all of the other conditions. The difference between walking on the level in the high heels and in the saddle shoes and loafers was 11 per cent and 10 per cent, respectively. High heel walking on the level was 15 per cent greater than barefoot walking.

Although Mathews and Wooten (1963) did not make any kinematic measurements, it seems likely that the greater cost of walking in the 3-inch high heels may be due to greater instability and to the added muscle tension required for walking on the balls of the feet. Such extreme instability may be energetically costly but the results are mixed in studies of the energetic effect of orthotics, supports designed to control rearfoot movement and stabilize the foot on the economy of locomotion.

Hennacy (1973) measured VO_2 on subjects walking with and without orthotics. He used subjects who had 'foot problems' and a normal control group. The subjects with foot problems showed twice as much variation in VO_2, and three of these subjects showed a lower VO_2 when walking with orthotics. Although Hennacy states that these three subjects showed a 'definite improvement' with the orthotics, he did not test for statistical significance and judging from the large variation in his results, it is unlikely that he would have found significance had he tested for it. Given this lack of statistical treatment of the data, it is fair to conclude that no change in VO_2 occurred as a result of wearing orthotics.

Tests of runners wearing orthotics have shown either no difference or an increase in VO_2 while wearing the devices. Clement et al. (1982) found no effect of wearing orthotics on VO_2 in a group of 10 subjects running at three speeds on the treadmill. Hayes et al. (1983), however, showed that wearing either semi-rigid (RO) or flexible orthotics (FO) caused a significant increase in VO_2 while running on the treadmill at two common speeds (230 and 268 m.min^{-1}). Hayes et al. found VO_2 values significantly greater than no orthotics for both the RO and FO conditions while running at the slower speed. At 268 m.min^{-1} only the RO condition was significantly different. No significant differences were found between the two orthotic conditions. Most of the increase in VO_2 found by Hayes et al. (1983) with orthotics may be explained by the difference in weight of the devices.

Little information is presented in the Clement et al. (1982) abstract so it is difficult to speculate on why they did not also find a significant increase in VO_2 with orthotics. The fact they did not use common speeds but relative speeds, however, would increase variability and might have made it more difficult for them to find significance.

These results do not support the notion often heard in sports medicine circles that orthotics improve 'biomechanical efficiency'; in fact, wearing them appears to bring with it a reduction in the economy of locomotion.

This should not be construed as a recommendation for not wearing the devices. They may perform important clinical biomechanical functions that outweigh any negative energetic effects. But it must be said that improving the control of rearfoot movement in shoes does not appear to have any positive effects on the economy of locomotion.

Other features of shoe design, however, appear to have an effect. Nigg et al. (2003) showed systematic variations in economy attributable to midsole material characteristics. Roy and Stefanyshyn (2006) showed that within a defined range of stiffnesses, stiffer, less flexible soles seemed to induce improved running economy by about 1 per cent in most subjects.

Hamill *et al.* (1988) did not find significant differences in oxygen uptake while comparing racing flats versus a training shoe that had a more stable structure and was heavier. Rubin *et al.* (2009) studied running economy while wearing a motion control versus a cushion shoe using a crossover blind design. They found no difference in running economy between the two shoe conditions. This study is limited to a comparison of the two particular models used in the study. However, the results suggest that choosing footwear to potentially reduce certain overuse injuries does not necessarily have energetic consequences for the runner.

Shorten (2000) has offered the opinion that it is better not to give too much emphasis to lightweight in selecting running shoes. In his view, any energetic savings due to reduced weight may be offset by costly kinematic adaptations in compensation for losses in cushioning.

Anderson (1996) has opined that the 'spring rate' of certain shoes may compliment that of the body and enhance economy by contributing to the exploitation of stored elastic energy. It seems likely that tuning the compliance of running shoes to bring their spring properties more in phase with that of the running leg may explain some of the unusual results found for studies of shoes.

Frederick *et al.* (1980, 1986) reported a 2.8 per cent difference in the energetic cost of running in two-different shoe models. The test shoes used in their study were similar in upper construction but the sole units differed in their physical properties. The shoe with the lower measured energy cost was a softer, air-soled type shoe, and the other shoe was a more conventional (at the time) sole with a firmer, less compliant midsole. The softer shoe was actually heavier by an average of 33 g per pair, despite the fact that the subjects used less energy running in them. The authors have offered no explanation for this other than the speculation that it might be a result of the softer shoe being more complaint and perhaps more closely tuned to the subjects' compliance.

It seems likely that spring effects can have an effect on economy, at least when the spring characteristics of the shoes are capable of significant energy storage and return. Mercer *et al.* (2003) measured similar economies of running when comparing conventional shoes with special spring shoes. The spring shoes were built like ski boots with large leaf springs forming the sole. The spring shoes weighed, on average, 1.727 kg per boot, considerably more than the conventional shoes. Despite the mass and bulk of the spring shoes, running economy was similar for the subjects running in both shoes. This study and the previously cited air sole study (Frederick *et al.*, 1980, 1986) seem to underline the potential role that tuning and energy storage and return may play in strategies to enhance the economy of running by modifying footwear.

More recently, other researchers have suggested that not wearing shoes at all might also lead to improved economy. The results of these investigations are less promising.

Cost of cushioning and barefoot

Frederick *et al.* (1983) observed that there were no significant differences in the oxygen cost of running in six different shod conditions including barefoot and five different types of shoes with a range of cushioning characteristics. If the shod VO_2 data were adjusted downward to account for the known incremental increase in VO_2 due to added mass of the shoes (1 per cent per 100 g per foot), the authors predicted there would have been a significant and relatively greater energetic cost for running barefoot compared with shod running. One would expect that the weight savings alone of barefoot running should have made it more economical. This was not the case, and other studies in the intervening years have shown a similar lacking in the barefoot condition to realize an energetic benefit from the reduced weight.

Frederick *et al.* (1983) hypothesized that this difference between barefoot and shod and the trends in the shod data could be explained by a phenomenon called *the cost of cushioning*. They presented kinematic data showing a significant correlation ($r = 0.802$; $p < 0.05$) between the mean O_2 uptake and knee flexion velocity data in the various shoes for their subjects. These findings support the notion that a portion of the variability in VO_2 response between the shoe conditions may have been due to adjustments in the cushioning provided by controlled knee flexion.

Since then, other studies have indicated that the biomechanical adjustments that runners make when running barefoot on hard surfaces seem to consistently require increased energy relative expenditure.

There have been several other studies that have looked at the energetic demands of running barefoot versus in shoes (shod) (Burkett *et al.*, 1985; Divert *et al.*, 2008; Flaherty, 1994; Frederick *et al.*, 1983; Hanson *et al.*, 2011; Pugh, 1970; Squadrone and Gallozzi, 2009). The majority of these studies have not found a statistically significant difference in the energy cost of barefoot versus shod running. This is quite surprising because of the obvious decrease in mass carried on the foot in the barefoot condition. One would expect a reduction in VO_2 of something on the order of ~ 3 per cent based on the mass differences alone. However, most have found no difference. Two studies found a significant difference (Divert *et al.*, 2008; Flaherty, 1994).

Flaherty (1994) found that running in shoes with a mass of 356 g per foot showed increases in VO_2 of 4.6 per cent on average compared with barefoot running. More recently, Divert *et al.* (2008) compared VO_2 between barefoot running and running in 150 g and 350 g shoes. Only the heavier, 350 g shoes elicited a greater VO_2 (3.4 per cent) than barefoot. Divert *et al.* also found that when masses were equivalent, barefoot and shod running showed equivalent values of oxygen uptake. However, 9 of the 12 participants in the Divert *et al.* (2008) study preferred a midfoot strike pattern when barefoot and all were rearfoot strikers when shod.

It seems likely that these barefoot versus shod comparisons are all confounded by the fact that running in shoes is biomechanically distinct from barefoot running. In many cases, even something as fundamental as foot strike can change between barefoot and shod running. These biomechanical differences can have energetic consequences that undermine the validity of the experiment. In other words, runners who switch from shod to barefoot are doing more than just taking off their shoes (i.e. they may be dramatically altering their kinetics and kinematics. It has often been suggested that these adjustments are responses to the hardness of the surface, be it the treadmill surface or the 'overground' surface of a lab floor.

Frantz *et al.* (2012) overcame some of these limitations. They compared barefoot versus shod running while controlling for barefoot running experience, foot-strike pattern and footwear. Their 12 subjects ran on the treadmill at 3.35 m.s^{-1} with a midfoot strike pattern (all were midfoot strikers), both barefoot and in lightweight cushioned shoes (~ 150 g per shoe). In additional trials to tease out mass effects, the researchers attached small lead strips to each foot/shoe (~ 150, ~ 300, or ~ 450 g).

They found that adding mass to the feet elicited the predicted approximately 1 per cent increases in O_2 uptake per 100 g per foot of added weight, whether running barefoot or shod. However, there were no significant differences in VO_2 when just comparing running barefoot versus running in lightweight cushioned shoes. When they added mass to the barefoot condition to equal the weight of the shoes, running in shoes was more economical by 3 to 4 per cent. This seems to support the notion that there is a non–mass-related added cost of running barefoot.

Hanson *et al.* (2011) is often cited as proof that shod running brings with it increased VO_2, compared with barefoot running. But Hanson *et al.* (2011), like most other studies that have looked looking at this question, did not find statistically significant differences in VO_2 during treadmill running, even when wearing relatively heavy shoes (353 g per foot) compared to barefoot.

They did report a 5.7 per cent increased VO_2 when running shod overground versus barefoot overground in the same paper (Hanson *et al.*, 2011). However, as Kram and Frantz (2012) pointed out in a published commentary on this study, the method used by Hanson *et al.* to monitor and control running speed may not have been calibrated properly and may have introduced a bias that would have lowered the relative oxygen uptake during barefoot compared with shod running overground. This leads this reviewer to question the validity of Hanson's overground data, especially given the fact their treadmill data seemed to agree with the preponderance of published studies on this topic, and the technology used to measure speed overground has not been satisfactorily validated by published reports.

In Divert *et al.* (2008), 12 subjects ran at 3.61 m.sec^{-1} (7 minutes and 26 seconds per mile) while barefoot, in diving socks (simulating a nearly barefoot condition) unloaded, loaded with 150 and 350 g, and in 150 and 350 g shoes for comparison. VO_2 increased the same amount with masses added to socks as when running in shoes with the same masses. The authors concluded that higher metabolic cost was only due to the extra mass induced by the shoe itself and not due to other mechanical properties of the shoe.

Taken en masse, these studies contradict the suggestion by proponents of barefoot running (e.g. Richards and Hollowell, 2011; Sandler and Lee, 2010) that running barefoot is more 'efficient'. It seems more reasonable to conclude after so many studies that have examined barefoot versus shod that, clearly, barefoot is in fact not more economical than shod running.

Conclusions

Several general conclusions about the economy of movement and footwear are in order given the information reviewed in this chapter:

1   The power to resolve a difference as small as 1 per cent is theoretically possible using conventional oxygen uptake measurements.
2   Significant differences as small as 2.4 per cent can be real and meaningful when considering performance.
3   Carrying weight on the feet is relatively more costly than carrying the same weight nearer to the body's centre of mass.
4   The relative cost of carrying weight on the feet during walking and running increases with increasing speed, grade and with the magnitude of the weight carried.
5   Other non-weight-related characteristics of shoes that may influence economy are: the relative shock attenuation properties of the shoes worn, and their compliance, flexibility and use of orthotics.
6   Under most circumstances, running barefoot is not more economical than running in shoes.

References

Anderson, T. (1996) 'Biomechanics and running economy', *Sports Medicine*, 22(2): 76–89.
Armstrong, L. E. and Costill, D. L. (1983) 'Day-to-day variations in respiratory exchange data during cycling and running', *Medicine and Science in Sports and Exercise*, 15(2): 141–2.
Burkett, L. N., Kohrt, W. M. and Buchbinder, R. (1985) 'Effects of shoes and foot orthotics on VO2 and selected frontal plane knee kinematics', *Medicine and Science in Sports and Exercise*, 17(1): 158–63.

Catlin, M. E. and Dressendorfer, R. H. (1979) 'Effect of shoe weight on the energy cost of running', *Medicine and Science in Sports*, 11: 80.

Clement, D. B., Taunton, J. E., Wiley, J. P., Smart, G. W. and McNicol, K. L. (1982) 'Investigation of metabolic efficiency in runners with and without corrective orthotic devices', *International Journal of Sports Medicine*, 2: 14–15.

Divert, C., Mornieux, G., Freychat, P., Baly, L., Mayer, F. and Belli, A. (2008) 'Barefoot-shod running differences: shoe or mass effect', *International Journal of Sports Medicine*, 29 (6): 512–18.

Flaherty, R. F. (1994) 'Running economy and kinematic differences among running with the foot shod, with the foot bare, and with the bare foot equated for weight', unpublished master's dissertation, Springfield College.

Frantz, J. R., Wierzbinski, C. M. and Kram, R. (2012) 'Metabolic cost of running barefoot versus shod: is lighter better?', *Medicine and Science in Sports and Exercise*, 44(8): 1519–25.

Frederick, E. C. (1983) 'Measuring the effects of shoes and surfaces on the economy of locomotion', in B. M. Nigg and B. A. Kerr (eds), *Biomechanical Aspects of Sport Shoes and Playing Surfaces*, Calgary: The University of Calgary, pp. 93–106.

Frederick, E. C. (1984) 'Physiological and ergonomics factors in running shoe design', *Applied Ergonomics*, 15(4): 281–7.

Frederick, E. C., Howley, E. T. and Powers, S. K. (1980) 'Lower oxygen cost while running in air cushion type shoe', *Medicine and Science in Sports and Exercise*, 12(2): 81–2.

Frederick, E. C., Clarke, T. E., Larsen, J. L. and Cooper, L. B. (1983) 'The effects of shoe cushioning on the oxygen demands of running', in B. M. Nigg and B. A. Kerr (eds), *Biomechanical Aspects of Sport Shoes and Playing Surfaces*, Calgary: The University of Calgary, pp. 107–14.

Frederick, E. C., Daniels , J .T. and Hayes, J. W. (1984) 'The effect of shoe weight on the aerobic demands of running', in N. Bachl, L. Prokop and R. Suckert (eds), *Current Topics in Sports Medicine, Proceedings of the World Congress of Sports Medicine*, Vienna: Urban & Schwarzenberg, pp. 616–25.

Frederick, E. C., Howley, E. T. and Powers, S. K. (1986) 'Lower oxygen cost while running in soft-soled shoes', *Research Quarterly*, 57: 174–7.

Hamill, J., Freedson, P. S., Boda, W. and Reichsman, F. (1988) 'Effects of shoe type on cardiorespiratory responses and rearfoot motion during treadmill running', *Medicine and Science in Sports and Exercise*, 20(5): 515–21.

Hanson, N. J., Berg, K., Deka, P., Meendering, J. R. and Ryan, C. (2011) 'Oxygen cost of running barefoot vs. running shod', *International Journal of Sports Medicine*, 32(6): 401–6.

Hayes, J., Smith, L. and Santopietro, F. (1983) 'The effects of orthotics on the aerobic demands of running', *Medicine and Science in Sports and Exercise*, 15: 169.

Hennacy, R. H. (1973) 'Metabolic efficiency of orthotic appliances measured by oxygen consumption', *Journal of the American Podiatry Association*, 63(10): 481–90.

Kram, R. and Frantz, J. R. (2012) 'Is barefoot running more economical?', *International Journal of Sports Medicine*, 33(3): 249.

Martin, P. E. (1985) 'Mechanical and physiological responses to lower extremityloading during running', *Medicine and Science in Sports and Exercise*, 17(4): 427–33.

Mathews, O. K. and Wooten, E. P. (1963) 'Analysis of oxygen consumption of women while walking in different styles of shoes', *Archives of Physical Medicine and Rehabilitation*, 44: 569–71.

Mercer, J. A., Branks, D. A., Wasserman, S. K. and Ross, C. M. (2003) 'Physiological cost of running while wearing spring-boots', *Journal of Strength and Conditioning Research*, 17(2): 314–18.

Nigg, B. M. (1986) *Biomechanics of Running Shoes*, Champaign, IL: Human Kinetics.

Nigg, B. M., Stefanyshyn, D., Cole, G., Stergiou, P. and Miller, J. (2003) 'The effect of material characteristics of shoe soles on muscle activation and energy aspects during running', *Journal of Biomechanics*, 36(4): 569–75.

Pugh, L. G. (1970) 'Oxygen intake in track and treadmill running with observations on the effect of air resistance', *The Journal of Physiology*, 207(3): 823–35.

Pugh, L. G. (1971) 'The influence of wind resistance in running and walking, and the mechanical efficiency of work against gravity', *The Journal of Physiology*, 213(2): 255–76.

Ralston, H. J. (1981) 'Energy expenditure', in V. T. Inman, H. J. Ralston and F. Todd (eds), *Human Walking*, Baltimore: Williams & Wilkins, pp. 62–77.

Richards, C. and Hollowell, T. (2011) *The Complete Idiot's Guide to Barefoot Running*, New York: Alpha Books.

Roy, J. P. and Stefanyshyn, D. J. (2006) 'Shoe midsole longitudinal bending stiffness and running economy, joint energy, and EMG', *Medicine and Science in Sports and Exercise*, 38(3): 562–9.

Rubin, D. A., Butler, R. J., Beckman, B. and Hackney, A. C. (2009) 'Footwear and running cardio-respiratory responses', *International Journal of Sports Medicine*, 30(5): 379–82.

Russell, H. D. and Belding, H. S. (1946) *Metabolic Cost of Wearing Various Types of Footwear*, National Academy of Sciences Committee on Quartermaster Problems Report, Cambridge, MA: Harvard Fatigue Laboratory.

Sandler, M. and Lee, J. (2010) *Barefoot Running*, Boulder, CO: RunBare.

Saunders, P. U., Pyne, D. B., Telford, R. D. and Hawley, J. A. (2004a) 'Reliability and variability of running economy in elite distance runners', *Medicine and Science in Sports and Exercise*, 36(11): 1972–6.

Saunders, P. U., Pyne, D. B., Telford, R. D. and Hawley, J. A. (2004b) 'Factors affecting running economy in trained distance runners', *Sports Medicine*, 34(7): 465–85.

Shorten, M. R. (2000) 'Running shoe design: protection and performance', in T. Pedoed (ed.), *Marathon Medicine*, London: Royal Society of Medicine, pp. 159–69.

Soule, R. G. and Goldman, R. F. (1969) 'Energy cost of loads carried on the head, hands or feet', *Journal of Applied Physiology*, 27(5): 687–90.

Squadrone, R. and Gallozzi, C. (2009) 'Biomechanical and physiological comparison of barefoot and two shod conditions in experienced barefoot runners', *Journal of Sports Medicine and Physical Fitness*, 49(1): 6–13.

SECTION 8

Influence of implements and protective devices in sports and exercise

33

HEAD INJURIES, MEASUREMENT CRITERIA AND HELMET DESIGN

Andrew Post,[1] *T. Blaine Hoshizaki*[1] *and Sue Brien*[1,2]

[1]UNIVERSITY OF OTTAWA, OTTAWA
[2]CENTRE DE SANTÉ ET DE SERVICES SOCIAUX DE GATINEAU, GATINEAU

Introduction

Combatants wearing rudimentary head protection have been depicted in drawings for thousands of years (Hoshizaki and Brien, 2004). While sometimes dramatic in appearance, the effectiveness of these helmets is not well documented; however, they likely provided some protection against impacts from falling to the ground and strikes to the head. In the early twentieth century, motorized travel became more common followed by increases in accidental head injuries. During the same period, recreational sports were becoming popular, also resulting in a higher incidence of head injuries. This increase in head injuries prompted an increase in research designed to measure the effectiveness of helmets. Helmets have been used for decades to reduce the severity and incidence of brain injury during both sporting and non-sporting events. They have been used for military purposes to prevent injury from bullets and shrapnel and in sport to prevent traumatic brain injuries, which often led to death or permanent disability (Hoshizaki and Brien, 2004). Originally, American football players used cloth followed by leather helmets to protect their heads, with subsequent injuries often severe. Over time, as manufacturing capabilities and standards of performance for helmets became more sophisticated, traumatic brain injuries became rare in sport. However, while the incidence of traumatic brain injury in sports such as football, hockey and lacrosse has been reduced through the use of helmets, the incidence of concussion remains high (Casson *et al.*, 2010; Wennberg and Tator, 2003). This is, in part, a result of the method in which helmets are evaluated and subsequently designed (Post *et al.*, 2012, 2013). Currently, helmet performance and certification primarily employs linear acceleration to predict the risk of head injury (Canadian Standard Association (CSA), 2009; National Operating Committee on Standards for Athletic Equipment (NOCSAE), 1998; Snell Memorial Foundation (SNELL), 1995). Linear acceleration is more closely associated with the risk of traumatic brain injury (Gurdjian *et al.*, 1966; Thomas *et al.*, 1966). Research has confirmed that while linear acceleration is effective for the evaluation of helmet performance for the reduction of traumatic brain injuries, it may not be suitable for evaluation of helmets with respect to managing the risk of concussive injury (Gennarelli *et al.*, 1971, 1972; Holbourn, 1943; Hoshizaki *et al.*, 2012; Kendall *et al.*, 2012; Post *et al.*, 2012, 2013). Sport activities with increased risk for traumatic head injuries such as cycling, motorsport and competitive alpine skiing do benefit from what are generally termed crash helmets designed to manage high energy impacts and protect against traumatic brain injuries. These helmets are designed and certified using peak linear acceleration as a measure of performance (Hoshizaki and Brien, 2004).

The following chapter will describe the types of head injuries reported in sport, how head injuries occur and a description of how current head protection systems work to prevent them. Specific helmet designs and their influence on the metrics used to quantify brain injuries will be discussed, as well as the limitations of these systems.

Types of head injuries

All impacts to the head result in both linear and rotational acceleration, which is the root cause of brain injuries from impacts (Viano *et al.*, 1989). Brain injuries can be subdivided into focal or diffuse brain injuries. Focal injuries include fractures of the skull, and hematomas either within the brain tissue or external to the brain but within the skull. All of these injuries, intracerebral, subdural and epidural hematomas are diagnosed using CT and/ or MRI. Subdural and epidural hematoma are commonly the result of severe translations, which cause the brain to lag behind the skull motion and create stresses on the blood vessels of the brain (Viano *et al.*, 1989). Intracerebral hematomas are localized blood volumes found throughout the cerebrum. They typically occur deeper in the brain between tissues with different densities and inertial properties. Contusions occur when head motions cause the brain to rub against the bony protuberances within the skull, causing injury (Gurdjian and Gurdjian, 1976). Contusions can also result in areas of high intracranial pressure from impact. Diffuse injuries are normally associated with high rotational accelerations and, by definition, are diffuse effect matter deep within the brain. These injuries are generally diagnosed using an MRI (Jones *et al.*, 1999). Diffuse axonal injury is the most severe type of diffuse brain injury and commonly results in severe disability and death. Mild traumatic brain injury (mTBI), also known as concussion, is a type of diffuse brain injury (Ommaya and Gennarelli, 1974).

Skull fracture

Skull fracture results from when bone is deformed past its fracture limit (Gurdjian and Webster, 1947). This causes the bone to separate and possibly damage the brain tissue beneath. Descriptions of how skull fractures occur go as far back as the 1800s, where much of the data referred to impacts to the front of the skull relating to car crash injuries (Yoganandan and Pintar, 2004). Skull deformation causes stretching and compressing of the bone, resulting in a fracture (Gurdjian *et al.*, 1947; Yoganandan and Pintar, 2004). The area of the fracture is largely dependent on the geometry of the impacting object. In addition, the varying thickness of bone in the human skull makes it more difficult to fracture in some areas in comparison to others. Typical testing methods for determining skull fracture thresholds involved impacts to human cadavers with proposed tolerance levels between 3,000 and 4,000 N and between 200 and 300 g (Got *et al.*, 1978; Hodgson, 1967; Schneider and Nahum, 1972; Stalnaker *et al.*, 1977; Yoganandan *et al.*, 1995). This data was referenced by many helmet standards associations when developing pass/fail criteria for sports helmets (275–300 g), and has resulted in skull fracture becoming a rare event for contact sports.

Hematomas

Hematomas are collections of blood in the brain tissue resulting from damaged blood vessels. A number of mechanism are proposed that result in this injury, including areas of high and low pressure in the brain, and motion of the brain causing it to bump against bony outcroppings on the interior of the skull. There are two types of contusion, the coup and the contrecoup (Gurdjian *et al.*, 1968). The coup contusion occurs below the impact site and the contrecoup is typically located opposite to the initial impact (Gurdjian *et al.*, 1968). The contusion can be associated with a wide variety of symptoms depending on the location of the brain damage. For example, cortical contusion patients normally remain conscious but brain stem contusion can cause symptoms ranging from unconsciousness to coma depending on severity. Typically, brain contusions resolve, but can require medical interventions.

Cerebral hematomas

Hematomas occur when there is damage to the brain vasculature, resulting in regions of high intracranial pressure from the accumulating blood (Kleiven, 2003). The presence of a large amount of blood can compress the brain tissue and cause severe damage and death. Intracranial hematomas are classed as epidural, subdural, subarachnoid and intracerebral. The mechanism of cranial hematomas is related to the motions of the skull and brain relative to each other. Research using animal models has demonstrated that these types of injuries typically occur with high rates of application of linear or rotational acceleration (Gennarelli, *et al.*, 1983). Subdural and epidural hematomas are thought to occur from similar brain motions, which cause damage to the vasculature tethering the brain to the skull. When this vasculature is damaged, an increase of blood within the cranial cavity causes damaging pressure on brain tissue (Adams *et al.*, 1983; Bradshaw *et al.*, 2001; Kleiven, 2003).

Epidural hematoma

Epidural hematoma is bleeding that is related to local skull fractures and injury to blood vessels occurring between the skull and the dura of the brain. The dura is a double membrane with an inelastic periosteal layer attached to the inner surface of the skull and a meningeal layer forming the external covering of the brain (Marieb, 1998). The source of this bleeding can be from either veins or arteries. The buildup of blood within the cranial cavity creates a dangerous increase in pressure and damage to the dural layer. This is a severe injury, with death occurring in 15–20 per cent of cases (Marieb, 1998).

Acute subdural hematoma

A subdural hematoma is the collection of blood between the brain and the dura. It is usually a result of tears to the bridging veins, which tether the brain to the skull and empty into the venous sinuses. The tearing of these veins is a result of relative brain skull motions caused from motions of the skull from an impact. The location of subdural hematoma can vary, but appear primarily in the frontotemporoparietal regions.

Intracerebral hematoma

Intracerebral hematomas are localized contusions found throughout the cerebrum. These types of hematomas are attributed to motions of the head, which causes deep shearing of brain tissues (Ommaya *et al.*, 2002).

Diffuse brain injury

Mild traumatic brain injury (mTBI)

On the continuum of diffuse brain injury, the mTBI, commonly referred to as concussion, is arguably the mildest form. Concussion is defined as a post-traumatic brain dysfunction In fact, as a result of the specificity of the symptoms of concussion, it has been postulated that it is not really a diffuse injury, but rather an injury to specific regions of brain tissue that are associated with these symptoms. Concussive injuries are characterized by symptoms such as headache, amnesia, dizziness, depression, loss of coordination and unconsciousness (Carroll et al., 2004; Levin et al., 2012). Early research using animal models reported that it is difficult to create a concussion using linear motion (Gennarelli et al., 1971). When using rotational motion, however, this injury becomes prevalent. As a result, this type of injury is thought to occur primarily through rotational acceleration of the brain and has been found to be commonplace in contact sports (Casson et al., 2010; Wennberg and Tator, 2003). As helmets are primarily designed to reduce linear acceleration to the brain tissue, they are not intended to reduce the rotational component of an impact, which is associated with concussion (Post et al., 2012). Rotational acceleration in combination with linear acceleration create diffuse stresses and strains to brain tissue, resulting in transient local deformations leading to symptoms of concussion (Holbourn, 1943). The neural damage appears to be temporary in nature, but can result in long-term debilitating symptoms (McKee et al., 2010). Recently, there has been some evidence that although there appears to be little mechanical damage, there are physiological responses to concussion that can cause long-term degeneration of brain tissue (McKee et al., 2010).

Diffuse axonal injury (DAI)

Diffuse axonal injury is an injury affecting the white matter axons in the brain stem, cerebellum and cerebral hemispheres. This damage is thought to be caused primarily through rotations that contribute to a shearing and stretching effect on the axons of white matter, causing interruption of brain function (Bradshaw et al., 2001). The fact that this injury is influenced by rotations makes it similar to the mechanism of concussion; however, the level of rotation to induce DAI is much larger. This injury is thought to be present in 50 per cent of all head injury cases, and is responsible for 35 per cent of deaths in head injury patients (Meaney et al., 1994). Of all brain injuries, DAI has been found to have the highest rate of mortality (Maas et al., 2008). The symptoms of DAI can vary from short losses of consciousness to deep coma and death (Duncan et al., 2011).

Summary

Brain injuries are a complex and difficult area of research. The brain itself is a complicated structure with many levels of complexity, which is yet to be fully understood, especially on a physiological level. It is also difficult to quantify TBI and mTBI progression post-impact. However, due to the complex nature of brain injury, there is much more research required. What is not in doubt, however, is that the mechanism of these injuries, essentially the way in which they occur, is due to the motions of the head from an impact. These motions are typically measured in linear (translational) and rotational accelerations.

Criterion variables for predicting risk of head injuries

For helmets to be effective at preventing injuries, they must be evaluated using variables associated with the brain injuries they are intended to predict. In the previous section, the primary mechanism of brain injury in sport involves impacts to the head. These impacts cause the head to accelerate, resulting in damaging deformation to the brain tissue. As a result, helmets are evaluated using measurement variables based upon the movement of the head linked to the various mechanisms of injury (Post and Hoshizaki, in press). The following section examines existing and proposed measurement variables used to predict injury and evaluate the performance of helmets.

Linear acceleration

Linear acceleration is the rate of change of velocity over time, measured in m.s^{-2}; however, in terms of brain injury and helmet performance, it is typically measured in units of gravity (g, 1 g = 9.81 m.s^{-2}). Linear acceleration measures the translational movement of the head from an impact. This metric is the most commonly used dependent variable when evaluating the performance of helmets; the pass/fail threshold is generally set around 275–300 g (CSA, 2009; NOCSAE, 1998). This threshold approximates the level of peak linear acceleration associated with a skull fracture (Yoganandan *et al.*, 1995). Peak linear acceleration was also used because it correlated with the presence of pressure waves within the skull, which were thought to create traumatic brain injury (Thomas *et al.*, 1966, 1967).

Gadd severity index (GSI)

The Gadd severity index (GSI) was developed to take into consideration the shape of the linear acceleration time history, effectively adding time duration of linear acceleration from the event to the evaluation of helmet performance (Gadd, 1966). The Gadd severity index was developed from animal and cadaver impact data, which was simplified into what is known as the Wayne State Tolerance Curve (developed at Wayne State University, Detroit, USA). This curve essentially demonstrated that high linear accelerations could be endured for short durations, and lower intensity linear accelerations for longer durations. From this data, the following calculation was derived for the GSI:

$$GSI = \int_{t_0}^{t} a^{2.5} dt \tag{1}$$

where *a* is the linear acceleration, 2.5 is a weighting factor based on the Wayne State Tolerance Curve, and *t* is time. Using this measure was viewed as an improvement over peak linear acceleration, as it incorporated duration into the risk of incurring a brain injury. A threshold value of 1,000 was used for brain injury based on data collected by Wayne State, the FAA and NASA. The Gadd severity index is typically used in American football, baseball and lacrosse helmets. The primary standards association using this measure is the National Operating Committee on Standards in Athletic Equipment (NOCSAE, 1998).

Head Impact Criterion (HIC)

Versace (1971) made some subtle improvements to the GSI by primarily using data from the automotive industry to create the Head Impact Criterion (HIC). Both the GSI and HIC incorporate time duration in predicting injury; however, the HIC selects specific time ranges:

$$HIC = \left(t - t_0\right)\left[\frac{1}{t - t_0} \int_{t_0}^{t} a\left(t\right) dt\right]^{2.5} \tag{2}$$

where a is the linear acceleration, t is time and 2.5 is a weighting factor based on the Wayne State Tolerance Curve. The HIC sets an injury threshold at 1,000, with varying time limits, with recommended time intervals of 36 ms for automotive head impact testing and 15 ms (ISO) for helmet testing.

Using integrations that incorporate time duration into injury prediction and helmet evaluation has a number of limitations. The largest limitation involves the fact that GSI and HIC rely on linear acceleration alone and do not include rotational acceleration, which effectively ignores an important measure of brain injury. Attempts to establish a correlation of these values to injury scales, such as the Glasgow Coma Scale or Abbreviated Injury Score, has met with little success.

Rotational acceleration

Rotational (or angular) acceleration is the rate of change of rotational (angular) velocity over time, typically measured in rad.s^{-2}. This dependent variable is not currently being used in most helmet standards. However, new and revised standards are considering changes to include this metric. The need to use rotational acceleration to evaluate helmets was established by researchers as far back as 1943 (Holbourn, 1943). In fact, it has been demonstrated that it is easier to create concussive and diffuse axonal type injuries than other types of TBI using a pure rotation. Holbourn (1943) demonstrated how important rotational motion is in identifying the risk of head injury from an impact. To date, helmets are only designed to manage peak linear acceleration, and in so doing primarily prevent injuries that are associated with these types of motion (Hoshizaki and Brien, 2004). As any impact can be quantified kinematically with linear and rotational acceleration, it would be useful to include both linear and rotational acceleration when evaluating the capacity of helmets to prevent head injuries. Thresholds of injury for mTBI using linear and rotational acceleration are presented in Table 33.1.

Time histories of dynamic response

Peak linear acceleration, GSI and HIC all ignore the importance of rotational acceleration in predicting brain injury, especially in the case of concussion. Using a peak resultant variable to describe all the motion of the head may over- or under-predict the risk of injury.

Previously discussed risk of injury metrics and standards used to measure helmet performance are all based on a single number to represent the entirety of the dynamic response resulting from an impact (Hoshizaki and Brien, 2004). Peak linear and rotational acceleration, GSI and HIC all use resultant values in their calculations (Gadd, 1966; Versace, 1971). The resultant is a summation of the x, y and z axes of motion into one curve meant to represent the magnitude of the impact over time. Using a complete time history of the linear and rotational acceleration would allow for the interpretation of the impact event over time and measure how the impact management materials function over all phases of the impact event. Using individual components allows for separate analysis of how the helmet performs along each axes, allowing for complex design characteristics to be harnessed to reduce linear motion or rotation in directions that have been identified as more susceptible to produce certain types of brain injury, such as concussion (Post *et al.*, 2011, 2013). While there are many advantages to this analysis, such as providing precise information as to how the helmet performs in three dimensions, and

Table 33.1 Linear and rotational acceleration thresholds for brain injury

Lesion type	Threshold	Measurement method	Reference
mTBI	82 g for 50% chance	Laboratory reconstruction	Zhang *et al.* (2004)
mTBI	81 g	Instrumented helmets	Duma *et al.* (2005)
mTBI	103 g	Instrumented helmets	Brolinson *et al.* (2006)
mTBI	82–146 g	Instrumented helmets	Schnebel *et al.* (2007)
mTBI	103 g	Dynamic modelling	Fréchède and McIntosh (2009)
mTBI	90 g	Primate impacts	Gurdjian *et al.* (1964)
Subdural hematoma	130 g	Laboratory reconstruction	Willinger and Baumgartner (2003)
mTBI	5,900 rad.s^{-2} for 50% chance	Laboratory reconstruction	Zhang *et al.* (2004)
mTBI	3,000–4,000 rad.s^{-2}	Laboratory reconstruction	Willinger and Baumgartner (2003)
mTBI	8,020 rad.s^{-2}	Dynamic modelling	Fréchède and McIntosh (2009)
No lesion	2,700 rad.s^{-2}	Human volunteers	Ewing (1975)
No lesion	16,000 rad.s^{-2}	Human boxers	Pincemaille *et al.* (1989)
Subdural hematoma	4,500 rad.s^{-2}	Cadaver impacts	Lowenhielm (1974)
mTBI	1,800 rad.s^{-2}	Primate impacts	Ommaya *et al.* (1967)
DAI	16,000 rad.s^{-2}	Primate, physical and numerical model impacts	Ommaya *et al.* (1967)

how to control rotation, which can lead to concussion, there are also drawbacks. For the purpose of helmet standards, it would be difficult to establish pass/fail criteria based on time histories. Also, the equipment necessary for this type of analysis (hybrid III dummy systems and the accelerometers) are relatively expensive.

Brain deformation metrics

Describing tolerance to injuries based on the kinematics of the impact ignores how the resulting motions affect the deformation of brain tissue, which is the root cause of the injury (King *et al.*, 2003). The use of brain deformation measures such as stress and strain are a relatively new measurement variable used to evaluate the performance of helmets and other protective equipment (Forero Rueda *et al.*, 2011; Post *et al.*, 2011, 2013). This method requires that the acceleration time histories of an impact in x, y and z axes be collected and then used as input for a three-dimensional finite element model (computational model) of the human brain. This simulates the motion resulting from the impact and how those motions influence the deformation of tissue in regions of the brain. This is viewed by many researchers as an improvement in predicting brain injury because it allows for the interpretation of how linear and rotational accelerations interact with the different brain geometries and tissue characteristics (King *et al.*, 2003; Kleiven, 2007). Currently, there are few commonly used partially validated brain finite element models in use. These validations are conducted using cadaveric impacts and are meant as close approximations, but not perfect representations, of how live tissues would respond to an impact (Hardy *et al.*, 2001; Nahum *et al.*, 1977; Trosseille *et al.*, 1992). However, using finite element models of the human brain is considered by many researchers as the missing link between impact kinematics and injury (Hoshizaki *et al.*, 2012; King *et al.*, 2003; Wright *et al.*, 2012). The most commonly used brain deformation metrics used when simulating impacts using a finite element model of the human brain is maximum principal strain and von Mises stress. Maximum principal strain is a measure of the stretching of a region of brain tissue in one direction. The use of this variable is primarily to allow a comparison with anatomical research, which typically measures failure of brain tissue in terms of strains. Von Mises stress represents a three-dimensional deformation of brain tissue (in this case), which is summed into one value and then compared to failure thresholds. This parameter is commonly used in engineering to estimate failure of three-dimensional structures. Using brain deformation to predict tolerance levels for brain injury and helmet performance is currently viewed as one of the best ways forward for reduction of injury and improve helmet design. While precise geometry can be simulated, the finite element models are not perfect in their representations of brain matter. These parameters are taken from anatomical testing, which in itself has limitations that are exacerbated in the modelling process. As a result, the deformation measured can be specific to the model used and may not be suitable for generalization across all models. Thresholds for concussive injury taken from the literature are presented in Table 33.2.

Types of materials and structures used in sport helmets

Sport helmets are typically comprised of a shell and an inner energy absorbing liner. The types of shell materials can vary according to the sport, but typically the shell materials used include polycarbonate, polyethylene, polycarbonate microshells or various composite materials. The energy absorbing liners used in sport include foams such as vinyl nitrile (VN), expanded polypropylene (EPP) and expanded polystyrene (EPS), as well as a number of engineered structures.

Shell materials

The primary purpose of the helmet shell is to distribute the impact force across the energy-absorbing liner, as well as in some cases to prevent penetration of foreign objects. To accomplish this, some helmets such as the American football helmet use a very stiff shell material to distribute the forces, while in other sports the shell is a softer material and includes shell geometry to manage the impact forces (as in ice hockey). American football uses a polycarbonate shell, which is a very durable material but can fracture under extremely high energy impacts. Ice hockey helmets use a polyethylene shell, which is lighter than polycarbonate shells but has less

Table 33.2 Brain deformation thresholds for mTBI

mTBI threshold value (50% chance)	Dependent variable	Location	Reference
0.21	Max. principal strain	Corpus callosum	Kleiven (2007)
0.26	Max. principal strain	Grey matter	Kleiven (2007)
0.19	Max. principal strain	Grey matter	Zhang *et al.* (2004)
48.5 s^{-1}	Strain rate	Grey matter	Kleiven (2007)
8.4 kPa	Von Mises	Corpus callosum	Kleiven (2007)
7.8 kPa	Von Mises	Brain stem	Zhang *et al.* (2004)
18 kPa	Von Mises	N/A	Willinger and Baumgartner (2003)
65.8 kPa	Intracranial pressure	Grey matter	Kleiven (2007)
90.0 kPa	Intracranial pressure	Grey matter	Zhang *et al.* (2004)

stiffness. To compensate for the lack of stiffness, the hockey helmet employs shell geometries at certain impact sites. Finally, there are some helmets that use a composite material as the shell. An example of this would be in some motorcross helmets. The benefit of this type of shell is that the stiffness qualities can be fine-tuned for the impacts expected within the sport and be more efficient at distributing the load than using polycarbonate. The drawbacks include being more expensive to manufacture, and the failure (delamination) of the shell may not be obvious after an impact, which could lead to an athlete playing with a compromised shell. Polycarbonate microshells are commonly used in bicycle helmets and serve little purpose other than creating a surface upon which to apply graphics and colours.

Impact-absorbing liner materials

There are many liner materials that can be used to absorb the energy from an impact. In sport, the most common energy-absorbing liner materials include: vinyl nitrile (VN), expanded polypropylene (EPP), expanded polystyrene (EPS) and engineered structures (Hoshizaki, 2000). These materials will vary in thickness and density depending on the application and sport in which they are used. Generally, the thicker the liner is, the greater the protection. Having a thick liner does have its drawbacks as it increases the weight and size of helmet. Increasing helmet size can increase the rotational moment upon impact; therefore, it is generally accepted that a smaller helmet is more ideal so long as it effectively manages the impact energy.

Vinyl nitrile

Vinyl nitrile is a resilient foam used for multi-impact conditions. This type of foam can be impacted and then return to its original shape. As a result, it tends to perform similarly across many impacts. This type of foam is commonly used in multi-impact sports such as American football and ice hockey. While VN foams are excellent for lower energy multi-impact scenarios, they tend to not perform well at higher impact energies (Hoshizaki, 2000).

Expanded polystyrene

Expanded polystyrene is an energy-absorbing liner typically used in crash helmets such as bicycle, motocross, alpine and motorcycle (Hoshizaki, 2000). This means that this material is used for a single impact and does not perform well under multiple impacts. In its construction, the polystyrene beads are put into a mould and then the beads are glued together using steam. The beads then form to the shape of the mould, creating the thickness required for the helmet. When impacted, the liner is compressed and the beads break apart, releasing energy (Hoshizaki, 2000). As a result, the impact force transmitted to the head is reduced. This type of liner material is intended for high energy impacts and is used in sports where the helmet would only need to protect against a single high energy impact.

Expanded polypropylene

Expanded polypropylene has a similar manufacturing process as EPS. It is created from beads expanded in a mould designed to fit as the helmet liner. The difference between EPS and EPP is that under impact the EPS is essentially destroyed to manage the energy whereas the EPP is not (Hoshizaki, 2000). The EPP beads have enough compliance and elasticity to deform and then return to their original shape under an impact load. Over time, this material does degrade and become less efficient at managing energy, but is far more resilient than EPS foams. This type of foam is commonly used as an alternative to VN foam in ice hockey helmets, where it is perceived as better at managing higher energy multiple impacts (Hoshizaki, 2000).

Engineered structures

Foams such as VN, EPP and EPS function to reduce the impact force felt by the head by function of their respective thickness and density (Hoshizaki and Post, 2009). This means that, all things being equal, the thicker the liner, the better protection offered; also, denser materials manage higher impact energies. Engineered structures are characterized as a structure where its energy-absorbing characteristics under impact are not solely defined by its thickness (height) or density. Typically engineered structures are composed of a rigid wall of an elastic material, which deforms under impact and often resumes its normal shape post-impact. In order to optimize an engineered structure in a sport helmet, designers manipulate variables including: the shape of the structure – they can be circular, triangular etc.; the material; the stiffness of the material; the thickness of the walls of the material; and the shape of the walls. This creates an environment where the characteristics of the structure combine to match an intended energy attenuation response for a specific sporting helmet. This type of impact-absorbing technology is a recent concept, with few helmets using structures to manage the impacts. Examples of helmets that employ structures to manage energy include the Xenith X1 series, Schutt DNA American football helmets, the Cascade M11 ice hockey helmet and the Cascade lacrosse helmet.

Types of sport helmets

There are a large number of styles and models of sport helmets on the market; however, for the most part they fit into one of two categories. The first can be described as multiple impact helmets and include such helmets as American football helmets, ice hockey helmets, lacrosse helmets and baseball helmets, and the second are described as single impact or crash helmets and include cycling helmets, alpine helmets and motorsport helmets (Hoshizaki, 2000). As described earlier, the objective of multiple impact helmets is to design helmets that can receive an impact and return to their original condition to manage subsequent impacts. The materials used in these types of helmets are elastic and include vinyl nitrile and expanded polypropylene, as well as a variety of other foams (Hoshizaki, 2000). Crash helmets primarily employ impact materials made from polystyrene that crush under the forces of an impact. Once the helmet has received an impact, it is compromised and can no longer effectively manage additional impact energies. The helmet must be discarded and replaced with an undamaged helmet (Hoshizaki, 2000).

Discussion

Sport helmets are designed and tested to provide protection from the head injuries that present the greatest risk to the participant. Originally, football players were concerned about traumatic brain injuries, and this is reflected in the certification requirements used as well as the design of the football helmet. As a result, traumatic brain injuries in football are a rare event, while more recently concussive injuries have become a serious issue. The nature of the game demands that helmets are able to withstand numerous blows and still provide protection; therefore, a multiple impact test standard is used to certify football helmets. Similar demands are required for ice hockey, which also employs a multiple impact standard and resulting helmet design. In activities such as cycling, the only time an impact to the head is expected is during an accident. This is a rare event and the protection the helmet provides involves managing higher energies of a single impact. Thus, a single test impact standard is employed to certify these types of helmets. These helmets are primarily designed to protect against traumatic brain injuries and less so for the prevention of concussions. In activities where the participants are vulnerable to both high energy impacts and multiple lower energy impacts such as recreational alpine skiing, defining the requirements for both certification and design is more challenging. Ultimately, the realistic adoption of helmets that are not too large yet provide adequate protection needs to be sought. Clearly, preventing catastrophic head injuries as described in this chapter is a priority; however, in sports such as football, hockey and lacrosse, where concussive injuries are common, helmets need to provide protection for these injuries as well. Historically, materials such as vinyl nitrile and expanded polystyrene have served the helmet industry well; however, engineered structures are providing opportunities for engineering more effective head protection. As more sophisticated testing protocols are developed for evaluating helmet performance, more effective helmets will be developed.

References

Adams, J. H., Graham, D. I. and Gennarelli, T. A. (1983) 'Head injury in man and experimental animals: neuropathology', *Acta Neurochirurgica*, 32: S15–30.

Bradshaw, D. R., Ivarsson, J., Morfey, C. L. and Viano, D. C. (2001) 'Simulation of acute subdural hematoma and diffuse axonal injury in coronal head impact', *Journal of Biomechanics*, 34(1): 85–94.

Brolinson, P. G., Manoogian, S., McNeely, D., Goforth, M., Greenwald, R. and Duma, S. (2006) 'Analysis of linear head accelerations from collegiate football impacts', *Current Sports Medicine Reports*, 5(1): 23–8.

Canadian Standard Association (2009) *Ice Hockey Helmets*, CAN/CSA Z262.1–09, Mississauga: Canadian Standard Association.

Carroll, L. J., Cassidy, J. D., Peloso, P. M., Borg, J., von Holst, H., Paniak, C. and Pépin, M. (2004) 'Prognosis for mild traumatic brain injury: results of the WHO collaborating centre task force on mild traumatic brain injury', *Journal of Rehabilitation Medicine*, 43: S84–105.

Casson, I. R., Viano, D. C., Powell, J. W. and Pellman E. J. (2010) 'Twelve years of National Football League concussion data', *Sports Health: A Multidisciplinary Approach*, 2(6): 471–83.

Duma, S. M., Manoogian, S. J., Bussone, W. R., Brolinson, P. G., Goforth, M. W., Donnenwerth, J. J., Greenwald, R. M, Chu, J. J. and Crisco, J. J. (2005) 'Analysis of real-time head accelerations in collegiate football players', *Clinical Journal of Sport Medicine*, 15(1): 3–8.

Duncan, C. C., Summers, A. C., Perla, E. J., Coburn, K. L. and Mirsky, A. F. (2011) 'Evaluation of traumatic brain injury: brain potentials in diagnosis, function, and prognosis', *International Journal of Psychophysiology*, 82(1): 24–40.

Ewing, C. L. (1975) *Injury Criteria and Human Tolerance for the Neck*, Charlottesville, VA: Aircraft Crashworthiness, University Press of Virginia.

Forero Rueda, M. A., Cui, L. and Gilchrist, M. D. (2011) 'Finite element modelling of equestrian helmet impacts exposes the need to address rotational kinematics in future helmet designs', *Computer Methods in Biomechanics and Biomedical Engineering*, 14(12): 1021–31.

Fréchède, B. and McIntosh, A. S. (2009) 'Numerical reconstructions of real-life concussive football impacts', *Medicine and Science in Sports and Exercise*, 41(2): 390–8.

Gadd, C. W. (1966) *Use of a Weighted Impulse Criterion for Estimating Injury Hazard*, SAE technical paper No. 660793, Warrendale, PA : SAE International.

Gennarelli, T. A., Thibault, L. E. and Ommaya, A. (1971) 'Comparison of translational and rotational accelerations in experimental cerebral concussion', *Proceedings of the 15th Stapp Car Crash Conference*, Coronado, CA: SEA International.

Gennarelli, T. A., Thibault, L. E. and Ommaya, A. (1972) *Pathophysiological Responses to Rotational and Translational Accelerations of the Head*, SAE technical paper No. 720970, Warrendale, PA: SAE International.

Gennarelli, T. A., Thibault, L. E., Adams, J. H., Graham, D. I., Thompson, C. J. and Marcincin, R. P. (1983) 'Diffuse axonal injury and traumatic coma in the primate', *Annals of Neurology*, 12(6): 564–74.

Got, C., Patel, A., Fayon, A., Tarriere, C. and Walfisch, G. (1978) 'Results of experimental head impacts on cadavers: the various data obtained and their relations to some measured physical parameters', *Proceedings of the 22nd Stapp Car Crash Conference*, Ann Arbor, MI: SEA International.

Gurdjian, E. S. and Webster, J. E. (1947) 'The mechanism and management of injuries to the head', *Journal of the American Medical Association*, 134(13): 1072–7.

Gurdjian, E. S. and Gurdjian, E. S. (1976) 'Cerebral contusions: re-evaluation of the mechanism of their development', *The Journal of Trauma*, 16(1): 35–51.

Gurdjian, E. S., Lissner, H. R. and Webster, J. E. (1947) 'The mechanism of production of linear skull fracture further studies on deformation of the skull by the stresscoat technique', *Surgery, Gynecology and Obstetrics*, 85(2): 195–210.

Gurdjian, E. S., Lissner, H. R., Hodgson, V. R. and Patrick, L. M. (1964) 'Mechanisms of head injury', *Clinical Neurosurgery*, 12: 112–28.

Gurdjian, E. S., Roberts, V. L. and Thomas, L. M. (1966) 'Tolerance curves of acceleration and intracranial pressure and protective index in experimental head injury', *Journal of Trauma*, 6(5): 600–4.

Gurdjian, E. S., Hodgson, V. R., Thomas, L. M. and Patrick, L. M. (1968) 'Significance of relative movements of scalp, skull, and intracranial contents during impact injury to the head', *Journal of Neurosurgery*, 29(1): 70–2.

Hardy, W. N., Foster, C. D., Mason, M. J., Yang, K. H., King, A. I. and Tashman, S. (2001) 'Investigation of head injury mechanisms using neutral density technology and high-speed biplanar x-ray', *Stapp Car Crash Journal*, 45: 337–68.

Hodgson, V. R. (1967) 'Tolerance of the facial bones to impact', *American Journal of Anatomy*, 120(1): 113–22.

Holbourn, A. H. S. (1943) 'Mechanics of head injuries', *Lancet*, 2: 438–41.

Hoshizaki, T. B. (2000) 'Engineering head protection', in R. C. Cantu (ed.), *Neurologic Athletic Head and Spine Injuries*, New York: Saunders Co, pp. 41–50.

Hoshizaki, T. B. and Brien, S. E. (2004) 'The science and design of head protection in sport', *Journal of Neurosurgery*, 55(4): 856–966.

Hoshizaki, T. B. and Post, A. (2009) 'Impact attenuation characteristics of engineered structures used in protective helmets', *Journal of ASTM International*, 6(4): 1–7.

Hoshizaki, T. B., Walsh, E. S., Post, A., Rousseau, P., Kendall, M., Karton, C., Oeur, A., Foreman, S. and Gilchrist, M. D. (2012) 'The application of brain tissue deformation values in assessing the safety performance of ice hockey helmets', *Journal of Sport Engineering and Technology*, 226: 226–36.

Jones, D. K., Simmons, A., Williams, S. C. and Horsfield, M. A. (1999) 'Non-invasive assessment of axonal fiber connectivity in the human brain via diffusion tensor MRI', *Magnetic Resonance in Medicine*, 42(1): 37–41.

Kendall, M., Post, A., Rousseau, P., Oeur, A., Gilchrist, M. D. and Hoshizaki, T. B. (2012) 'A comparison of dynamic impact response and brain deformation metrics of head impact reconstructions representing three mechanisms of head injury in ice hockey', *Proceedings of the 2012 IRCOBI Conference on the Biomechanics of Impacts*, Dublin: International Research Council on the Biomechanics of Injury, IRC-12–53.

King, A. I., Yang, K. H., Zhang, L., Hardy, W. and Viano, D. C. (2003) 'Is head injury caused by linear or angular acceleration?', *Proceedings of the 2003 IRCOBI Conference on the Biomechanics of Impacts*, Lisbon: International Research Council on the Biomechanics of Injury, pp. 1–12.

Kleiven, S. (2003) 'Influence of impact direction to the human head in prediction of subdural hematoma', *Journal of Neurotrauma*, 20(4): 365–79.

Kleiven S. (2007) 'Predictors for traumatic brain injuries evaluated through accident reconstruction', *Stapp Car Crash Journal*, 51: 81–114.

Levin, H., Li, X., McCauley, S. R., Hanten, D., Wilde, E. A. and Swank, P. R. (2012) 'Neuro-psychological outcome of mTBI: a principal component analysis approach', *Journal of Neurotrauma*, doi:10.1089/neu.2012.2627.

Lowenhielm, P. (1974) 'Dynamic properties of the parasagittal bridging veins', *Journal of Legal Medicine*, 74(1): 55–62.

Maas, A. I., Stocchetti, N. and Bullock, R. (2008) 'Moderate and severe traumatic brain injury in adults', *The Lancet Neurology*, 7(8): 728–41.

McKee, A. C., Gavett, B. E., Stern, R. A., Nowinski, C. J., Cantu, R. C., Kowall, N. W., Perl, D. P., Hedley-White, T., Price, B., Sullivan, C., Morin, P., Lee, H., Kubilus, C. A., Daneshvar, D. H., Wulff, M. and Budson, A. E. (2010) 'TDPE-43 proteinopathy and motor neuron disease in chronic traumatic encephalopathy', *Journal of Neuropathology and Experimental Neurology*, 69(9): 918–29.

Marieb, E. N. (1998) *Human Anatomy and Physiology*, 4th edn, San Francisco: Benjamin/Cummings Science Publishing.

Meaney, D., Thibault, L. and Gennarelli, T. (1994) 'Rotational brain injury tolerance criteria as a function of vehicle crash parameters', *Proceedings of the IRCOBI Conference on the Biomechanics of Impacts*, Lyon: International Research Council on the Biomechanics of Injury, pp. 51–62.

Nahum, A. M., Smith, R. and Ward, C. C. (1977) *Intracranial Pressure Dynamics During Head Impact*, SAE technical paper No. 770922, Warrendale, PA : SAE International.

National Operating Committee on Standards for Athletic Equipment (1998) *Standard Performance Specification for Newly Manufactured Football Helmets*, NOCSAE DOC (ND) 002-98m05. Overland Park, KS: National Operating Committee on Standards in Athletic Equipment.

Ommaya, A. K. and Gennarelli, T. A. (1974) 'Cerebral concussion and traumatic unconsciousness: correlation of experimental and clinical observations on blunt head injuries', *Brain*, 97(4): 633–54.

Ommaya, A. K., Yarnell, P., Hirsch, A. E. and Harris, E. H. (1967) *Scaling of Experimental Data on Cerebral Concussion in Sub-human Primates to Concussion Thresholds for Man*, SAE technical paper No. 670906, Warrendale, PA: SAE International.

Ommaya, A. K., Goldsmith, W. and Thibault, L. (2002) 'Biomechanics and neuropathology of adult and paediatric head injury', *British Journal of Neurosurgery*, 16(3): 220–42.

Pincemaille, Y., Trosseille, X., Mack, P., Tarriere, C., Breton, F. and Renault, B. (1989) *Some New Data Related to Human Tolerance Obtained from Volunteer Boxers*, SAE technical paper No. 892435, Warrendale, PA: SAE International.

Post, A. and Hoshizaki, T. B. (in press) 'Mechanical properties describing brain impact injuries: a review', *Trauma*.

Post, A., Oeur, A., Hoshizaki, T. B. and Gilchrist, M. D. (2011) 'Examination of the relationship of peak linear and angular acceleration to brain deformation metrics in hockey helmet impacts', *Computer Methods in Biomechanics and Biomedical Engineering*, doi: 10.1080/10255842.2011.627559.

Post, A., Oeur, A., Hoshizaki, T. B. and Gilchrist, M. D. (2012) 'The influence of centric and non-centric impacts to American football helmets on the correlation between commonly used metrics in brain injury research', *Proceedings of the IRCOBI Conference*, Dublin: International Research Council on the Biomechanics of Injury, IRC-12–52.

Post, A., Oeur, A., Hoshizaki, T. B. and Gilchrist, M. D. (2013) 'An examination of American football helmets using brain deformation metrics associated with concussion', *Materials and Design*, 45: 653–62.

Schnebel, B., Gwin, J. T., Anderson, S. and Gatlin, R. (2007) 'In vivo study of head impacts in football: a comparison of National Collegiate Athletic Association Division I versus high school impacts', *Journal of Neurosurgery*, 60(3): 490–5.

Schneider, D. and Nahum, A. (1972) 'Impact studies of facial bones and skull', *Proceedings of the 16th Stapp Car Crash Conference*, Detroit: SAE International, pp. 186–203.

Snell Memorial Foundation (1995) *Standard for Protective Equipment (1998 Revision): For Use in Bicycling*, North Highlands: Snell Memorial Foundation.

Stalnaker, R., Melvin, J., Nuscholtz, G., Alem, N. and Benson, J. (1977) 'Head impact response', *Proceedings of the 21st Stapp Car Crash Conference*, New Orleans, LA: SAE International, pp. 305–35.

Thomas, L. M., Roberts, V. L. and Gurdjian, E. S. (1966) 'Experimental intracranial pressure gradients in the human skull', *Journal of Neurology, Neurosurgery and Psychiatry*, 29(5): 404–11.

Thomas, L. M., Roberts, V. L. and Gurdjian, E. S. (1967) 'Impact-induced pressure gradients along three orthogonal axes in the human skull', *Journal of Neurosurgery*, 26(3): 316–21.

Trosseille, X., Tarriére, C., Lavaste, F., Guillon, F. and Domont, A. (1992) *Development of a F.E.M. of the Human Head According to a Specific Test Protocol*, SAE technical paper No. 922527, Warrendale, PA: SAE International.

Versace, J. (1971) *A Review of the Severity Index*, SAE technical paper No. 710881, Warrendale, PA: SAE International.

Viano, D. C., King, A. I., Melvin, J. W. and Weber, K. (1989) 'Injury biomechanics research: an essential element in the prevention of trauma', *Journal of Biomechanics*, 22(5): 403–17.

Wennberg, R. A. and Tator, C. H. (2003) 'National Hockey League reported concussions, 1986–87 to 2001–02', *Canadian Journal of Neurological Sciences*, 30(3): 206–9.

Willinger, R. and Baumgartner, D. (2003) 'Numerical and physical modelling of the human head under impact – towards new injury criteria', *International Journal of Vehicle Design*, 32: 94–115.

Wright, R., Ramesh, K. T., Post, A. and Hoshizaki, T. B. (2012) 'A computational approach to estimate axonal damage under inertial loading of the head', *Journal of Neurotrauma*, doi:10.1089/neu.2012.2418.

Yoganandan, N. and Pintar, F. A. (2004) 'Biomechanics of temporo-parietal skull fracture', *Clinical Biomechanics*, 19(3): 225–39.

Yoganandan, N., Pintar, F. A., Sances, A., Walsh, P. R., Ewing, C. L., Thomas, D. J. and Snyder, R. G. (1995) 'Biomechanics of skull fracture', *Journal of Neurotrauma*, 12(4): 659–68.

Zhang, L., Yang, K. H. and King, A. I. (2004) 'A proposed injury threshold for mild traumatic brain injury', *Journal of Biomechanical Engineering*, 126(2): 226–36.

34

THE EFFECTS OF FUNCTIONAL KNEE BRACING ON INJURY PREVENTION AND SPORT PERFORMANCE

Sergej M. Ostojic,[1] Marko Stojanovic[2] and Boris Vukomanovic[3]

[1]METROPOLITAN UNIVERSITY, BELGRADE
[2]UNIVERSITY OF NOVI SAD, NOVI SAD
[3]INSTITUTE FOR ORTHOPAEDIC DISEASE BANJICA, BELGRADE

Introduction

High prevalence and large economic impact of knee injuries related to athletic activities led to the development of different protocols for injury prevention, management and/or rehabilitation in the past decades, with the use of various knee braces among the most popular. Braces have been used to reduce knee injuries in top-level sport since the beginning (Wirth and DeLee, 1990), with their popularity exploding from the early 1980s, when a multitude of manufacturers started to promote several brace models for use in American football and other contact and non-contact sports. Yet, debate over their true efficacy was ongoing in medical circles because injuries did continue to occur despite the use of braces (Najibi and Albright, 2005). Today, with the advance of biomechanical techniques, functional approach and epidemiological investigations into the effectiveness of bracing, the use of functional knee braces in athletes with joint instability is seriously questioned. This chapter provides a review of the applicability of functional knee braces in reinjury prevention and for athletic performance. Besides clinical significance of knee injuries, the design of functional braces will be discussed, as well as the effects of knee bracing for injury prevention in athletes with insufficient knee ligaments, and its effectiveness on physiological parameters of sport performance in anterior cruciate-deficient knees.

Sport-related knee injuries: epidemiology and clinical significance

Sport-related knee injuries (SRKI) results from an acute trauma or repetitive strain associated with athletic activities, which can be caused by accidents, impact, sudden or awkward movements, and gradual wear and tear of the knee joint (Jonasson *et al.*, 2011; Mayor, 2010). Since the knee joint is vulnerable and used extensively in many sport activities, it is prone to injuries. It seems that SRKI compromise 71 per cent of all sport injuries in some sports (e.g. football, skiing, gymnastics, racket sports) (Zarins and Adams, 1988), with approximately one-fourth of all problems treated by orthopedic surgeons (Lubowitz and Appleby, 2011). Furthermore, female athletes are five times more likely to suffer from severe SRKI injuries (Hutchinson and Ireland, 1995). SRKI often impairs both primary and secondary factors of knee dynamic stability, such as major ligaments, capsular components and the muscles acting over the joint. In particular, anterior cruciate ligament (ACL) injuries are widespread in athletic and physically active populations, and can result in a significant functional disability of the knee (Cheatham and Johnson, 2010). Majewski *et al.* (2006) have documented 19,530 sport injuries over a 10-year period of time, with 7,769 injuries (39.8 per cent) related to the knee joint, with almost 50 per cent of the patients between the ages of 20–29 at the time of injury. The most frequently reported knee injury was ACL lesion (20.3 per cent), while other types of SRKI were observed less frequently (> 10 per cent). The activities leading to most SRKI were soccer (35 per cent) and skiing (26 per cent), with ACL injury associated with handball, tennis and volleyball, and causing the most time lost from competition (Alentorn-Geli *et al.*, 2009). These figures have influenced a strong research focus in the past decades to determine the etiology and risk factors for ACL injury. The most common ACL injury mechanism includes a deceleration task with high knee internal extension torque (with or without perturbation) combined with dynamic valgus rotation with the body weight shifted over the injured leg and the plantar surface of the foot fixed flat on the playing surface (Griffin *et al.*, 2000). Therefore, precluding significant valgus stress to the knee and restricting anterior-posterior displacement through different protective strategies and/or devices seems to be the crucial step to decrease ACL injury or reinjury in athletes (Ostojic *et al.*, 2007; Yu and Garrett, 2007).

SRKI can be devastating to an athlete, as this type of injury is often accompanied with long disability time and high economic cost as compared to other common athletic injuries. King *et al.* (2009) reported cost of $8,750,147 for knee injuries requiring medical treatment (19 per cent of total cost for sport injuries, with 225 per 1,000 entitlement claims) during an 8-year Accident Compensation Corporation trial in New Zealand rugby league players, with the high cost of knee injuries a cause for concern, as it reflects the severity of the injuries. High economic cost of SRKI management is particularly observable for ACL injuries, with total treatment price per injury up to $19,000 (Lubowitz and Appleby, 2011). Furthermore, acute SRKI was the first cause of absence in competition greater than 1 week due to injury (Cumps *et al.*, 2007; Jarret *et al.*, 1998). Rupture of the ACL, as one of the most clinically challenging SRKI, is a potentially career-threatening injury in elite athletes, with average absence from the field between 6 and 9 months (Lee *et al.*, 2008; Shah *et al.*, 2010). Since the ACL serves as the primary knee stabilizer, preventing forward displacement of the tibia on the femur, ACL injuries more commonly cause knee instability than do injuries to other knee ligaments (Sarraf *et al.*, 2011). Furthermore, ACL-insufficient knee increases the risk of cartilage damage, additional knee lesions and the development of early osteoarthritis, multiplying the overall cost of injury (Myklebust and Bahr, 2005). Different treatment protocols, both conservative and surgical, have been developed to regain knee stability after ACL injury through strengthening the surrounding muscles, flexibility exercise, proprioceptive training, ligament reconstruction and/or use of knee braces, with the incidence of non-contact reinjury being reduced from 20 to 80 per cent in athletes engaged in retraining programmes (Albright *et al.*, 1994; Myer *et al.*, 2011; Sitler *et al.*, 1990; Stojanovic and Ostojic, 2011). Although 87 per cent of the orthopedic surgeons prescribe functional knee braces after ACL rupture (Decoster and Vailis, 2003), the clinical significance of knee bracing after ACL injury for returning to a pre-injury level of function, and decreasing the risk of reinjury, is still subject to debate.

Functional knee braces: terminology and design

A knee brace is a supportive implement worn by athletes and non-athletes to protect and/or support the knee joint, either after a medial collateral ligament, ACL or other knee injury, or to prevent one. Knee braces fit into several categories: prophylactic braces, functional braces, rehabilitative braces and unloader braces (Paluska and McKeag, 2000; Rishiraj *et al.*, 2009). Functional knee braces (FKBs) gained popularity among elite athletes from the 1970s after a seminal study on the effectiveness of the first FKB (Anderson Knee Stabler, Omni Scientific Inc., Laffayette, IL, USA) in 52 patients following reconstruction of knee anteromedial instability (Nicholas, 1973). Authors reported enhanced stability for injured knees after combined use of knee braces along with a properly directed and strictly executed exercise programme. In general, FKBs are designed to reduce knee instability following injury to the ACL, decrease additional injuries during athletic activities and, following reconstructive surgery, reduce strain in an ACL graft (Rishiraj *et al.*, 2009). FKBs are usually promoted to provide stability for unstable knees in sporting activities that require rapid directional changes (e.g. jumping, twisting, pivoting or cutting activities). They are intended to limit tibial rotation and anteroposterior translation, attenuate knee discomfort and pain, and enhance performance and confidence during sporting events (Chew *et al.*, 2007). Despite much research having been conducted in the area of FKB application, the efficacy of these devices remains in question.

Knee braces are typically made from a combination of metal, plastic, elastic material and foam, and constructed using straps, pads and hinges, with FKB prescription design matching the severity of knee injury as suggested by suppliers. For mild to moderate ligament injuries, the most common style is made of stretchy neoprene material and has metal hinges on either side of the knee. For more severe injuries, a knee brace that uses a rigid frame with hinges may be necessary (Paluska and McKeag, 2000). FKBs are available in custom-made or pre-sized models, with both categories using either a 'hinge-post-shell' or 'hinge-post-straps' design (Paulos *et al.*, 1987). Braces further differ in their thigh and calf enclosures. Shell-shaped models use a moulded shell of plastic and foam, while straps models use a system of straps around thigh and calf (Ott and Clancy, 1993; Paluska and McKeag, 2000). France *et al.* (1990) suggested that shell-designed braces provide improved tibial-displacement control, greater rigidity, enhanced durability and better soft tissue contact as compared to straps models. Custom FKBs require several measurements of the affected leg to be taken (e.g. knee joint angle, thigh and calf circumference, thigh and calf contour, knee width and varus/valgus) to produce a brace that is specific to the patient. Pre-sized or off-the-shelf FKBs are usually sized by thigh circumference measurements taken 6 inches above mid-patella and selecting the corresponding brace size. Pre-sized FKBs are advertised as the least expensive and are easily applicable in a multitude of sizes, while custom-made braces are recommended for patients with abnormal limb contours and top-level athletes for enhanced patient comfort. Yet, several studies questioned differences in protection of injured or reconstructed ACL between pre-sized and custom-made FKBs. Beynnon *et al.* (1992) found no apparent advantages of the more expensive custom-made braces compared with the off-the-shelf designs in the strain-shielding effect on the ACL with an internal torque of 5 Nm applied to the tibia. Similar results were reported by Wojtys and Huston (2001), where a custom-fit ACL functional brace did not reduce anterior laxity or improve standing long jump, muscle strength, endurance or muscle response times significantly more than the off-the-shelf ACL brace. Both braces improved anterior stability over knee taping when the knee muscles were contracted under the low forces used in this study. Furthermore, after 1 hour of exercise, brace migration was significantly greater for the custom brace (18.6 mm) than for the off-the-shelf brace (4.5 mm). There appears to be no advantage to the more expensive custom-fit knee brace over the off-the-shelf brace. It seems that the longest length of FKB the athlete can comfortably wear (Paluska and McKeag, 2000), along with the correct hinge placement relative to the femoral condyles (Beynnon *et al.*, 1992), should be chosen for optimal brace effectiveness. Yet, regardless of which type of knee brace chosen, it should not interfere with normal knee function or increase the risk of injury to any other part of the lower body or to other players.

Functional knee bracing for reinjury prevention

Knee injury prevention should be of great concern when it is considered that statistics on return to sport post-injury, with conservative management and/or ACL reconstruction, illustrate a decreased level of participation, earlier forced retirement and/or continued knee joint discomfort (Rishiraj *et al.*, 2009). Furthermore, it seems that athletes with previous ACL injury are more susceptible to ACL rupture than athletes without previous ACL injury (Sarraf *et al.*, 2011). The elevated risk of recurrent ACL injury has fuelled intensive research regarding the effectiveness of prevention programmes aimed at extrinsic and intrinsic ACL injury risk factors. Although there is evidence that a neuromuscular prevention programme decreases potential biomechanical risk factors for ACL injury and reduce ACL injury/reinjury incidence in athletes (Alentorn-Geli *et al.*, 2009; Griffin *et al.*, 2000; Mandelbaum *et al.*, 2005), the role of FKBs in the prevention of further injury to previously injured knees is not clear, with few trials reporting reinjury rates in braced athletes as an outcome. Theory for the use of knee bracing in ACL injury prevention was mainly due to the 1970s FKB efficacy studies involving cadaveric and surrogate models that showed restricted tibial rotation and anterioposterior translation in braced knees (for a review, see Najibi and Albright, 2005). Since ACL tears usually occurred during non-contact deceleration situation that produces a valgus twisting injury (e.g. when the athlete lands on the leg and quickly pivots in the opposite direction), with knee hyperextension and marked internal rotation of tibia on femur, authors speculated that knee bracing could stabilize the knee during training and competition, and prevent ligamentous injuries to the knee joint. A few recent epidemiological studies in skiers affirm functional knee bracing for athletes with ACL reconstruction who wish to return to sport (Kocher *et al.*, 2003; Sterett *et al.*, 2006). Sterett *et al.* (2006) examined the effect of functional bracing on subsequent knee injury in 820 skiers with ACL reconstruction. Sixty-one subsequent knee injuries were identified, 51 (8.9 injuries/100 knees/ski season) in the non-braced group and 10 (4.0 injuries/100 knees/ski season) in the braced group. Non-braced skiers were 2.74 times more likely to suffer subsequent injury than braced skiers. Logistic regression modelling identified non-bracing as a significant independent multivariate risk factor for subsequent knee injury in the high-demand skiers with ACL reconstruction. On the other hand, several prospective studies in the past 15 years have shown that post-injury functional bracing does not appear to change the clinical outcomes and/or reinjury rates after ACL reconstruction (Kartus *et al.*, 1997; Möller *et al.*, 2001; Risberg *et al.*, 1999). McDevitt *et al.* (2004) recruited 100 volunteers from the three US service academies with surgically treated acute ACL tears in a prospective, randomized, multicentre clinical trial. The braced group was instructed to wear an off-the-shelf functional knee brace for all cutting, pivoting or jumping activities for the first year after surgery, with 95 subjects available with a minimum 2-year follow-up. There were no statistically significant differences between groups in reinjury rates, knee stability, functional testing with the single-legged hop test, International Knee Documentation Committee scores, Lysholm scores, knee range of motion or isokinetic strength testing. Authors concluded that the brace does not contribute to a more stable knee during rehabilitation or the 2-year follow-up. Evidence-based commentary from Mallory *et al.* (2003) clearly pointed to insignificant protection against injury during recovery in braced subjects after surgical ACL reconstruction; neither improved stability nor hastened rehabilitation, either immediately or for up to 2 years. With more recent clinical and functional sophisticated studies, it has been shown that functional bracing may be effective in controlling anteroposterior translation in ACL-deficient knees under low loading conditions, but it may not be effective under high loading conditions that occur during athletic activities (Wright *et al.*, 2008). Contrary to the current brace prescription patterns, the use of the FKB to lower the risk of ACL reinjury is not supported in the literature (except possibly in skiing) (Pezzullo and Fadale, 2010).

Sport performance and functional braces

Although functional knee braces are largely promoted in athletic environments, their effectiveness on sport performance are controversial (Kramer *et al.*, 1997), with only few studies evaluating exercise performance changes in braced subjects with previous ACL injury (Table 34.1).

A seminal study by Wilson *et al.* (1998) assessed the effects of a functional knee brace for ACL insufficiency on physiological and perceptual parameters during treadmill running in 13 subjects with previous ACL injury. Bracing had no effect when exercising at below lactate threshold, but did significantly alter the metabolic profile developed during the performance of the above lactate threshold tests. FKB resulted in elevated blood lactates, oxygen uptake, ventilation, and ventilatory equivalent. Rates of perceived exertion for leg and knee were significantly elevated during running above lactate threshold when the brace was worn. Similar results were found by Wu *et al.* (2001), who assessed speed of running and turning, speed of running and jumping, and accuracy of landing after the jump in 31 subjects with unilateral ACL reconstruction under three bracing conditions: (1) functional knee brace; (2) mechanical placebo brace; or (3) no brace, in cross-sectional comparative clinical trial. Subjects performed similarly in conditions 1 and 2 in all the tests, but the speeds of running and turning were significantly slower in conditions 1 and 2 than condition 3. Results of the run and jump tests were not different among all conditions. On the other hand, Birmingham *et al.* (2001) reported that FKB appears to improve proprioceptive performance during tasks characterized by relatively limited somatosensory input (single-limb standing balance tests), but not during more challenging tasks. A small magnitude of the improvements noted in the present study, coupled with FKB apparent lack of carry-over to more difficult and functionally relevant tasks (such as sport performance), questions the clinical benefit of the effects of bracing. In conclusion, most performance studies indicated compromised performance in braced subjects, with these dynamic outcomes needing to be noted when such a brace is used on this group of subjects.

It seems that, when applied, knee braces compress the soft tissues of the thigh and leg, and external compression may abnormally elevate intramuscular pressure beneath the straps of the knee brace (for up to 20 per cent) (Alerntone-Geli *et al.*, 2009). This will lead to decreased local muscle blood flow and muscular oxygenation, and will induce premature muscle fatigue (Styf, 1999). FKB could also alter muscle recruitment patterns (Wilson *et al.*, 1998), slow voluntary reaction time (Smith *et al.*, 2003) and compromise neuromuscular control (Osternig and Robertson, 1993), which leads to reduced exercise performance. Although braces may give some degree of support to athletes with unstable knees following surgery for knee joint instability, FKBs do not improve performance and may even inhibit exercise capacity. The use of such a brace could actually slow down running and turning, irrespective of the mechanical constraints of the brace. Athletes and coaches should be aware of the serious adverse effects of

Table 34.1 Summary of sport performance studies using functional knee braces

Reference	Subjects	Exercise protocol	Results
Wilson et al. (1998)	Thirteen subjects with insufficient ACL (> 5 years postinjury).	Incremental test to exhaustion and two constant load 20-min tests, one at an intensity bLT, and the other at an intensity aLT with and without the FKB.	Bracing had no effect on peak variables except for higher RPE at the legs at the velocities associated with a [HLa] of 4.0 mM and at peak. Bracing had no effect when exercising at bLT but did significantly alter the metabolic profile developed during the performance of the aLT tests. FKB resulted in elevated [HLa] (23%), VO2 (4%), VE (12%), VCO2 [corrected] (7%), and VE/VO2 (7%). Heart rate and slow component VO2 did not differ between the brace and no brace aLT tests. RPE-legs and RPE-knee were significantly elevated during aLT when the brace was worn.
Wu et al. (2001)	Thirty-one subjects with unilateral ACL reconstruction (> 5 months postinjury).	Running and turning 10 times on a 22-meter figure-8 runway; running and jumping on a semicircular path. Patients were assigned to: (1) functional brace, (2) mechanical placebo brace, or (3) no brace.	Subjects performed similarly in conditions 1 and 2 in all the tests, but the speeds of running and turning were significantly slower in conditions 1 and 2 than condition 3 ($p < 0.008$).
Birmingham et al. (2001)	Thirty individuals after ACL reconstruction.	Series of single-limb standing balance tests completed on a force platform with and without the FKB.	Brace provided improvement in proprioception and postural control ($p < 0.02$), with the brace providing improvement during the test completed on the stable platform with eyes open (mean reduction in centre of pressure path length = 4.2 ± 8.4 cm, $p = 0.02$) but not during the other more challenging test situations.
Ramsey et al. (2001)	Four subjects with ACL rupture.	Maximal horizontal jump with and without the FKB.	Bracing ACL deficient knee resulted in minor kinematic changes in tibiofemoral joint motion. No consistent reductions in anterior tibial translations were observed as a function of the knee brace tested.

Birmingham et al. (2002)	Twenty-seven individuals after ACL reconstruction.	Peak isokinetic concentric knee flexion and extension performed at 90°/s with and without the FKB.	Knee flexion strength decreased significantly with the brace (mean brace effect = −7.3%, $p < 0.05$). The brace effect during knee flexion was significantly related to peak torque observed without the brace ($r = -0.50$, $p < 0.01$).
Smith et al. (2003)	Ten active individuals with ACL-deficient knees (> 18 months postinjury).	Three single-leg hop manoeuvres on ACL-deficient knee with and without the FKB.	Brace use significantly delayed the average onset of vastus lateralis activation before landing (123 ± 47ms versus 109 ± 30 ms, $p < 0.001$). Brace use did not consistently result in more favourable muscle firing patterns during the single-leg hop manoeuvre.
Lu et al. (2006)	Thirty ACL-injured subjects.	Walking at a self-selected pace with and without the FKB.	Bracing significantly increased the peak abductor moments in ACL-deficient knees and reduced the bilateral kinetic asymmetry in the coronal plane ($p < 0.01$). FKB increased peak moments and impulses of the abductors and extensors for the ACL-reconstructed group ($p < 0.01$).
Théoret and Lamontagne (2006)	Eleven ACL-deficient participants.	Running on a treadmill with three-dimensional kinematic and electromyographical data collected from 10 consecutive gait cycles under braced and unbraced conditions.	Bracing significantly reduced total ROM in the frontal and transverse planes ($p < 0.05$) while running. Muscle activity at heel-strike showed a consistent trend to increase for the hamstrings and decrease for the quadriceps under the braced condition when compared to the unbraced.

FKB – functional knee braces; ACL – anterior cruciate ligament; RPE – ratings of perceived exertion; [HLa] – blood lactate concentration; bLT – below lactate threshold, aLT – above lactate threshold; VO_2 – oxygen uptake; VE – ventilation; VCO_2 – rate of elimination of carbon dioxide; VE/VO_2 – ventilatory equivalent for oxygen; ROM – range of motion.

knee bracing. Nonetheless, athletes who use FKBs report subjective improvements that exceed objective measurement of knee stability and performance enhancement, but patients must be guarded against a false sense of security (Möller *et al.*, 2001; Swirtun *et al.*, 2005).

Conclusion

Functional knee braces are devices promoted to provide support for the unstable knee in ligament injury, such as a rupture of anterior cruciate ligament or post-ACL reconstruction. Although beneficial in controlling anteroposterior translation in ACL-deficient knees under low loading conditions, functional bracing, either pre-sized or custom-made, may be ineffective in knee protection during sport activities; neither changed ACL reinjury rates in athletes with ACL insufficiency. Furthermore, the application of FKBs in athletes with ACL lesion demonstrated compromised exercise performance, with decrement in most functional outcomes in braced knee. Contrary to the current brace prescription practice, non-critical and routine use of FKBs in the anterior cruciate ligament-deficient, injured or reconstructed knee lacks scientific support and should be discouraged.

References

Albright, J. P., Powell, J. W., Smith, W., Martindale, A., Crowley, E., Monroe, J., Miller, R., Connolly, J., Hill, B. A., Miller, D., Helwig, D. and Marshall, J. (1994) 'Medial collateral ligament knee sprains in college football. Brace wear preferences and injury risk', *American Journal of Sports Medicine*, 22(1): 2–11.

Alentorn-Geli, E., Myer, G. D., Silvers, H. J., Samitier, G., Romero, D., Lázaro-Haro, C. and Cugat, R. (2009) 'Prevention of non-contact anterior cruciate ligament injuries in soccer players. Part 2: a review of prevention programs aimed to modify risk factors and to reduce injury rates', *Knee Surgery, Sports Traumatology, Arthroscopy*, 17(8): 859–79.

Beynnon, B. D., Pope, M. H., Wertheimer, C. M., Johnson, R. J., Fleming, B. C., Nichols, C. E. and Howe, J. G. (1992) 'The effect of functional knee-braces on strain on the anterior cruciate ligament in vivo', *Journal of Bone and Joint Surgery. American Volume*, 74(9): 1298–312.

Birmingham, T. B., Kramer, J. F., Kirkley, A., Inglis, J. T., Spaulding, S. J. and Vandervoort, A. A. (2001) 'Knee bracing after ACL reconstruction: effects on postural control and proprioception', *Medicine and Science in Sports and Exercise*, 33(8): 1253–8.

Birmingham, T. B., Kramer, J. F. and Kirkley, A. (2002) 'Effect of a functional knee brace on knee flexion and extension strength after anterior cruciate ligament reconstruction', *Archives of Physical Medicine and Rehabilitation*, 83(10): 1472–5.

Cheatham, S. A. and Johnson, D. L. (2010) 'Current concepts in ACL injuries', *Physician and Sportsmedicine*, 38(3): 61–8.

Chew, K. T. L., Lew, H. L., Date, E. and Fredericson, M. (2007) 'Current evidence and clinical applications of therapeutic knee braces', *American Journal of Physical Medicine and Rehabilitation*, 86(8): 678–86.

Cumps, E., Verhagen, E. and Meeusen, R. (2007) 'Prospective epidemiological study of basketball injuries during one competitive season: ankle sprains and overuse knee injuries', *Journal of Sports Science and Medicine*, 6(2): 204–11.

Decoster, L. C. and Vailas, J. C. (2003) 'Functional anterior cruciate ligament bracing: a survey of current brace prescription patterns', *Orthopedics*, 26(7): 701–6.

France, E. P., Cawley, P. W. and Paulos, L. E. (1990) 'Choosing functional knee braces', *Clinics in Sports Medicine*, 9(4): 743–50.

Griffin, L. Y., Agel, J., Albohm, M. J., Arendt, E. A., Dick, R. W., Garrett, W. E., Garrick, J. G., Hewett, T. E., Huston, L., Ireland, M. L., Johnson, R. J., Kibler, W. B., Lephart, S., Lewis, J. L., Lindenfeld, T. N., Mandelbaum, B. R., Marchak, P., Teitz, C. C. and Wojtys, E. M. (2000) 'Noncontact anterior cruciate ligament injuries: risk factors and prevention strategies', *Journal of the American Academy of Orthopaedic Surgeons*, 8(3): 141–50.

Hutchinson, M. R. and Ireland, M. L. (1995) 'Knee injuries in female athletes', *Sports Medicine*, 19(4): 288–302.

Jarret, G. J., Orwin, J. F. and Dick, R. W. (1998) 'Injuries in collegiate wrestling', *American Journal of Sports Medicine*, 26(5): 674–80.

Jonasson, P., Halldin, K., Karlsson, J., Thoreson, O., Hvannberg, J., Swärd, L. and Baranto, A. (2011) 'Prevalence of joint-related pain in the extremities and spine in five groups of top athletes', *Knee Surgery, Sports Traumatology, Arthroscopy*, 19(9): 1540–6.

Kartus, J., Stener, S., Köhler, K., Sernert, N., Eriksson, B. I. and Karlsson, J. (1997) 'Is bracing after anterior cruciate ligament reconstruction necessary? A 2-year follow-up of 78 consecutive patients rehabilitated with or without a brace', *Knee Surgery, Sports Traumatology, Arthroscopy*, 5(3): 157–61.

King, D. A., Hume, P. A., Milburn, P. and Gianotti, S. (2009) 'Rugby league injuries in New Zealand: a review of 8 years of Accident Compensation Corporation injury entitlement claims and costs', *British Journal of Sports Medicine*, 43(8): 595–602.

Kocher, M. S., Sterett, W. I., Briggs, K. K., Zurakowski, D. and Steadman, J. R. (2003) 'Effect of functional bracing on subsequent knee injury in ACL-deficient professional skiers', *Journal of Knee Surgery*, 16(2): 87–92.

Kramer, J. F., Dubowitz, T., Fowler, P., Schachter, C. and Birmingham, T. (1997) 'Functional knee braces and dynamic performance: a review', *Clinical Journal of Sport Medicine*, 7(1): 32–9.

Lee, D. Y., Karim, S. A. and Chang, H. C. (2008) 'Return to sports after anterior cruciate ligament reconstruction – a review of patients with minimum 5-year follow-up', *Annals of the Academy of Medicine Singapore*, 37(4): 273–8.

Lu, T. W., Lin, H. C. and Hsu, H. C. (2006) 'Influence of functional bracing on the kinetics of anterior cruciate ligament-injured knees during level walking', *Clinical Biomechanics*, 21(5): 517–24.

Lubowitz, J. H. and Appleby, D. (2011) 'Cost-effectiveness analysis of the most common orthopaedic surgery procedures: knee arthroscopy and knee anterior cruciate ligament reconstruction', *Arthroscopy*, 27(10): 1317–22.

McDevitt, E. R., Taylor, D. C., Miller, M. D., Gerber, J. P., Ziemke, G., Hinkin, D., Uhorchak, J. M., Arciero, R. A. and Pierre, P. S. (2004) 'Functional bracing after anterior cruciate ligament reconstruction: a prospective, randomized, multicenter study', *American Journal of Sports Medicine*, 32(8): 1887–92.

Majewski, M., Susanne, H. and Klaus, S. (2006) 'Epidemiology of athletic knee injuries: a 10-year study', *Knee*, 13(3): 184–8.

Mallory, N., Kelsberg, G, Ketchell, D. and Lord, J. L. (2003) 'Clinical inquires. Does a knee brace decrease recurrent ACL injuries?', *Journal of Family Practice*, 52(10): 803–4.

Mandelbaum, B. R., Silvers, H. J., Watanabe, D. S., Knarr, J. F., Thomas, S. D., Griffin, L. Y., Kirkendall, D. T. and Garrett, W. Jr (2005) 'Effectiveness of a neuromuscular and proprioceptive training program in preventing anterior cruciate ligament injuries in female athletes: 2-year follow-up', *American Journal of Sports Medicine*, 33(7): 1003–10.

Mayor, R. B. (2010) 'Knee injuries in athletes', *Connecticut Medicine*, 74(8): 473–5.

Möller, E., Forssblad, M., Hansson, L., Wange, P. and Weidenhielm, L. (2001) 'Bracing versus nonbracing in rehabilitation after anterior cruciate ligament reconstruction: a randomized prospective study with 2-year follow-up', *Knee Surgery, Sports Traumatology, Arthroscopy*, 9(2): 102–8.

Myer, G. D., Brent, J. L., Ford, K. R. and Hewett, T. E. (2011) 'Real-time assessment and neuromuscular training feedback techniques to prevent ACL injury in female athletes', *Strength and Conditioning Journal*, 33(3): 21–35.

Myklebust, G. and Bahr, R. (2005) 'Return to play guidelines after anterior cruciate ligament surgery', *British Journal of Sports Medicine*, 39(3): 127–31.

Najibi, S. and Albright, J. P. (2005) 'The use of knee braces, part 1: prophylactic knee braces in contact sports', *American Journal of Sports Medicine*, 33(4): 602–11.

Nicholas, J. A. (1973) 'The five-one reconstruction of anteromedial instability of the knee: indications, technique, and the results in fifty-two patients', *Journal of Bone and Joint Surgery. American Volume*, 55(5): 899–922.

Osternig, L. R. and Robertson, R. N. (1993) 'Effects of prophylactic knee bracing on lower extremity joint position and muscle activation during running', *American Journal of Sports Medicine*, 21(5): 733–7.

Ostojic, S. M., Arsic, M., Prodanovic, S., Vukovic, J. and Zlatanovic, M. (2007) 'Glucosamine administration in athletes: effects on recovery of acute knee injury', *Research in Sports Medicine*, 15(2): 113–24.

Ott, J. W. and Clancy, W. G. Jr (1993) 'Functional knee braces', *Orthopedics*, 16(2): 171–5.

Paluska, S. A. and McKeag, D. B. (2000) 'Knee braces: current evidence and clinical recommendations for their use', *American Family Physician*, 61(2): 411–18.

Paulos. L. E., France, E. P., Rosenberg, T. D., Jayraman, H., Abbott, P. J. and Jaen, J. (1987) 'The biomechanics of lateral knee bracing. Part I: response of the valgus restraints to loading', *American Journal of Sports Medicine*, 15(5): 419–29.

Pezzullo, D. J. and Fadale, P. (2010) 'Current controversies in rehabilitation after anterior cruciate ligament reconstruction', *Sports Medicine and Arthroscopy Review*, 18(1): 43–7.

Ramsey, D. K., Lamontagne, M., Wretenberg, P. F., Valentin, A., Engström, B. and Németh, G. (2001) 'Assessment of functional knee bracing: an in vivo three-dimensional kinematic analysis of the anterior cruciate deficient knee', *Clinical Biomechanics*, 16(1): 61–70.

Risberg, M. A., Holm, I., Steen, H., Eriksson, J. and Ekeland, A. (1999) 'The effect of knee bracing after anterior cruciate ligament reconstruction. A prospective, randomized study with two years' follow-up', *American Journal of Sports Medicine*, 27(1): 76–83.

Rishiraj, N., Taunton, J. E., Lloyd-Smith, R., Woollard, R., Regan, W. and Clement, D. B. (2009) 'The potential role of prophylactic/functional knee bracing in preventing knee ligament injury', *Sports Medicine*, 39(11): 937–60.

Sarraf, K. M., Sadri, A., Thevendran, G. and Vedi, V. (2011) 'Approaching the ruptured anterior cruciate ligament', *Emergency Medicine Journal*, 28(8): 644–9.

Shah, V. M., Andrews, J. R., Fleisig, G. S., McMichael, C. S. and Lemak, L. J. (2010) 'Return to play after anterior cruciate ligament reconstruction in National Football League athletes', *American Journal of Sports Medicine*, 38(11): 2233–9.

Sitler, M., Ryan, J., Hopkinson, W., Wheeler, J., Santomier, J., Kolb, R. and Polley, D. (1990) 'The efficacy of a prophylactic knee brace to reduce knee injuries in football. A prospective, randomized study at West Point', *American Journal of Sports Medicine*, 18(3): 310–15.

Smith, J., Malanga, G. A., Yu, B. and An, K. N. (2003) 'Effects of functional knee bracing on muscle-firing patterns about the chronic anterior cruciate ligament-deficient knee', *Archives of Physical Medicine and Rehabilitation*, 84(11): 1680–6.

Sterett, W. I., Briggs, K. K., Farley, T. and Steadman, J. R. (2006) 'Effect of functional bracing on knee injury in skiers with anterior cruciate ligament reconstruction: a prospective cohort study', *American Journal of Sports Medicine*, 34(10): 1581–5.

Stojanovic, M. D. and Ostojic, S. M. (2011) 'Stretching and injury prevention in football: current perspectives', *Research in Sports Medicine*, 19(2): 73–91.

Styf, J. (1999) 'The effects of functional knee bracing on muscle function and performance', *Sports Medicine*, 28(2): 77–81.

Swirtun, L. R., Jansson, A. and Renström, P. (2005) 'The effects of a functional knee brace during early treatment of patients with a nonoperated acute anterior cruciate ligament tear: a prospective randomized study', *Clinical Journal of Sport Medicine*, 15(5): 299–304.

Théoret, D. and Lamontagne, M. (2006) 'Study on three-dimensional kinematics and electromyography of ACL deficient knee participants wearing a functional knee brace during running', *Knee Surgery, Sports Traumatology, Arthroscopy*, 14(6): 555–63.

Wilson, L. Q., Weltman, J. Y., Martin, D. E. and Weltman, A. (1998) 'Effects of a functional knee brace for ACL insufficiency during treadmill running', *Medicine and Science in Sports and Exercise*, 30(5): 655–64.

Wirth, M. A. and DeLee, J. C. (1990) 'The history and classification of knee braces', *Clinics in Sports Medicine*, 9(4): 731–41.

Wojtys, E. M. and Huston, L. J. (2001) 'Custom-fit versus off-the-shelf ACL functional braces', *American Journal of Knee Surgery*, 14(3): 157–62.

Wright, R. W., Preston, E., Fleming, B. C., Amendola, A., Andrish, J. T., Bergfeld, J. A., Dunn, W. R., Kaeding, C., Kuhn, J. E., Marx, R. G., McCarty, E. C., Parker, R. C., Spindler, K. P., Wolcott, M., Wolf, B. R. and Williams, G. N. (2008) 'A systematic review of anterior cruciate ligament reconstruction rehabilitation: part I: continuous passive motion, early weight bearing, postoperative bracing, and home-based rehabilitation', *Journal of Knee Surgery*, 21(3): 217–24.

Wu, G. K., Ng, G. Y. and Mak, A. F. (2001) 'Effects of knee bracing on the functional performance of patients with anterior cruciate ligament reconstruction', *Archives of Physical Medicine and Rehabilitation*, 82(2): 282–5.

Yu, B. and Garrett, W. E. (2007) 'Mechanisms of non-contact ACL injuries', *British Journal of Sports Medicine*, 41(1): S47–51.

Zarins, B. and Adams, M. (1988) 'Knee injuries in sports', *New England Journal of Medicine*, 318(15): 950–61.

35

INTERACTION OF TENNIS RACKET DESIGN AND BIOMECHANICAL FACTORS

Duane Knudson,[1] *Tom Allen*[2] *and Simon Choppin*[2]

[1]TEXAS STATE UNIVERSITY
[2]SHEFFIELD HALLAM UNIVERSITY

Introduction

Improvements in tennis racket design, testing and manufacturing have had a major impact on the sport. To ensure that these advances do not damage the nature of the game, the International Tennis Federation (ITF) tests equipment and establishes rules for limiting the properties and performance of tennis equipment. These tests are designed and monitored by the ITF Technical Department.

Ergonomics, sports engineering and biomechanics are all fields that have contributed to our understanding of the player/racket system and how to improve performance. Confirming these improvements with evidence has been difficult given the system's complexity. To rectify these validation issues, racket developers have started supplementing traditional design and testing techniques with on-court measurements of ball and racket movements to gain a greater understanding of the interaction of these two systems. Several reviews of the research on tennis racket equipment have been published (Brody, 1987, 2002; Brody *et al.*, 2002; Cross and Lindsey, 2005; Elliott, 1989; Knudson, 2008; Miller, 2006). Unfortunately, there are virtually no prospective studies that have compared common racket equipment with new designs to validate theoretical or experimental research in the laboratory. Comparative testing will inevitability be done by equipment developers, although the results are unlikely to make their way into the public domain.

This chapter integrates the latest and previous research on how racket properties and engineering affect tennis play:

- First, major changes in tennis racket design and construction that have been influential in the sport are briefly summarized.
- Next, we summarize the techniques used by engineers, researchers and developers when systematically evaluating the performance of rackets.
- Third, we summarize the biomechanical characteristics of tennis strokes.
- Fourth, the racket variables that most strongly interact with player biomechanics are reviewed.

423

- Fifth, the research on tennis racket variables hypothesized to be related to overuse injuries in tennis are examined.
- Finally, we discuss future directions for tennis racket design.

Throughout this chapter, the unifying themes are the complexity of the player/racket system in tennis and the interaction of the mechanical factors of the racket/string/ball with the bio-mechanical factors of the player. This interaction needs to be considered for racket innovations to be effective in improving performance or reducing the risk of overuse injury. We will demonstrate that it is insufficient to develop rackets using traditional mechanical engineering techniques without considering the interaction with the player. Integrating mechanics, biology and sport is particularly important in avoiding negative, unintended consequences commonly seen in the implementation of new technologies (Tenner, 1996). In tennis, for example, lighter, more powerful composite rackets have been hypothesized to contribute to increased incidence of new kinds of injuries and decreased spectator interest in the increasing fast play in professional tennis.

Influential changes in racket design

Modern tennis barely resembles its origins of 'jeu de paume' and 'real' tennis (Clerici, 1976), or even the lawn tennis of 100 years ago. Early rackets were made of laminated ash or beech wood with a roughly oval head and a functional hitting area of 450 cm^2 (Figure 35.1a). The shorter (0.68 m), heavier (0.4 kg) and smaller racket faces compared to modern rackets meant that strokes were usually longer and driven by the whole body compared to current stroke technique. The faster play and new stroke techniques in modern play are a result of a series

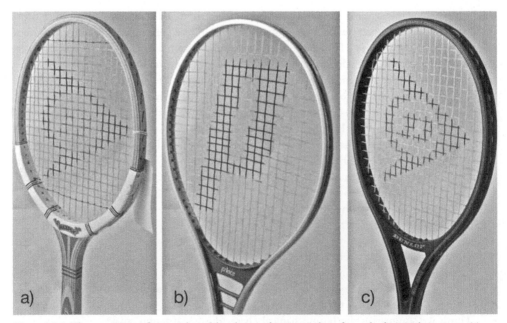

Figure 35.1 The transition of materials and head size of tennis rackets from the late 20th century: (a) standard head wood racket – 1981 Dunlop Maxply; (b) Prince Classic, oversize head aluminum – 1977 Prince; and (c) midsize graphite – 1980 Dunlop Max 200G.

of changes in the racket frame's dimensions and materials (for an extensive review of racket changes, see Haake *et al.*, 2007). Measurements of racket properties and simulations have been used to predict that a player could serve 18 per cent faster with modern equipment compared to what was available in the 1870s (Haake *et al.*, 2007).

Major changes in racket performance occurred in the 1960s and 1970s. At first, rackets constructed of steel and aluminum allowed engineers to experiment with geometries that were not possible with the mechanical constraints of wood (ITF Technical Department, 2012). The larger head size racket (Figure 35.1b) patented by Howard Head increased the hitting area, speed of ball rebound and shot accuracy in impacts offset from the longitudinal axis (off-axis) compared to traditional rackets (Head, 1976). The patent revolutionized the design of tennis rackets, and it is possible that some of the boom in the popularity of the sport in that era was the increased shot success and ease of gameplay for beginners using these lighter, midsize (Figure 35.1c) and oversive head rackets. The longer 'widebody' rackets, with super-oversize heads (as pioneered by Howard Head) led to rackets with substantially faster ball rebounds and resulted in the ITF establishing limits on the dimensions of tennis rackets (ITF Technical Department, 2012; Miller, 2006). Racket length is currently restricted to 73.7 cm and the maximum permissible width is 31.75 cm (ITF Technical Department, 2012).

In the 1980s, racket manufacturers began experimenting with a wide variety of materials with greater strength-to-weight ratio in comparison to wood and metal: graphite, fibreglass, Kevlar and boron. The use of these materials in racket frames (as a composite) has increased overall stiffness and decreased mass. Modern high-end rackets are manufactured by hand from composite lay-ups, and materials can be precisely placed for desired stiffness and mass distribution. The frame's stiffness can be manipulated by changing the amount of composite material, the direction of the composite's fibres (for stiffness in specific directions) or the frame profile (adjusting the second moment of area).

The focus of research and development has shifted from producing the 'lightest' or 'stiffest' racket, to producing equipment that is best for the player. Rackets with piezoelectric fibres have been developed to store and reuse impact energy to dampen frame vibrations (Kotze *et al.*, 2003). While these rackets only utilize energy generated by the ball impact, the ITF moved in 2002 to outlaw rackets with external energy sources.

The aims of racket developers are often to further understand the effect of design parameters on both performance and injury prevention, through the use of simulation, laboratory-based testing and on–court player testing. Rackets are currently marketed to players with stroke styles described as compact, moderate and full-swing. However, these rackets are also marketed with claims of unique design features that minimize the risk of injury. Ironically, many of these features have not been tested by experiments or validated by prospective research. Often there is a trade-off; the potentially positive effects of minimizing injury risk adversely affect the racket performance. The following section will explore the techniques used to characterize the performance of tennis rackets.

Racket performance characterization

The assessment of racket performance is essential in order to explore, appraise and compare design choices. The engineering techniques utilized to measure racket performance have become increasingly advanced over recent years, but they have always involved experimental or mathematical methodologies (or a combination of both).

Performance characteristics of particular relevance are: (1) the coefficient of restitution (COR) of the racket/ball system (which dictates the rebound speed of the ball); (2) the contact time of the ball during impact; (3) post-impact ball spin/angle; and (4) post-impact frame vibration (both frequency and amplitude). Racket manufacturers are often concerned with characterizing less tangible metrics such as feel (Davies *et al.*, 2003), control and power. The engineer will often express these metrics as functions of COR, spin, angle and vibration (for an example, see the work in golf by Roberts *et al.*, 2001a, 2001b).

Early experimental methods often involved projecting a ball normal to the face of a freely suspended racket and measuring the rebound speed with light gates or a high-speed camera. Recently, the desire for more complex and realistic impact conditions has led to the development of more sophisticated experimental methodologies. The International Tennis Federation currently uses a fully automated Racket Power Machine to characterize racket performance (ITF Technical Department, 2012). This machine drops a tennis ball into the path of a semi-clamped racket, which is rotating at a high (but variable) angular velocity. The impact position is controlled by carefully controlling the timing of ball release. To investigate the string bed in isolation, the racket frame is often fixed; this method has been used to investigate oblique spinning impacts (Goodwill and Haake, 2004; Haake *et al.*, 2012). Stereo calibration high-speed camera techniques (Choppin *et al.*, 2005) allow analysis of off-axis and oblique impacts on non-fixed rackets, as ball trajectories can be measured in three dimensions. Recent experimental research has investigated oblique spinning impacts on a freely suspended racket (Allen *et al.*, 2009) and the effect of simulated grip on off-axis impacts (Choppin *et al.*, 2011).

Sophisticated methodologies have also been applied to on-court testing in order to assess the effect of changes in the playing environment and record player movements. Accurate and representative impact conditions has been vital in designing appropriate laboratory-based experiments. Choppin *et al.* (2011) measured ball and racket movements (as summarized in Figure 35.2) using the stereo calibration technique, and Sheets *et al.* (2011) used a marker-less motion capture method called 'visual hulling' to measure player and racket movements. As motion capture systems become more portable and automated, it is likely that racket developers will place more emphasis on evaluating design parameters in simulated or match play. Manufacturers are likely to place more emphasis on developing rackets using a combination of computer-aided engineering techniques and laboratory-based testing, while using player perception and stroke analysis to evaluate on-court performance.

As a cheaper and often quicker way of assessing racket performance, mathematical models of varying complexity have been used. In the simplest case, one-dimensional rigid body models can be used to predict the effect of changing mass and impact location on the longitudinal axis (Brody, 1997; Cross, 1999; Liu, 1983) (Figure 35.3a). Introducing separate segments into the model allows the effect of stiffness to be studied (Cross, 2000; Goodwill and Haake, 2003) (Figure 35.3b). Recent work in this area has introduced another dimension to enable off-axis impacts to be simulated. Glynn *et al.* (2011) presented a model for simulating off-axis non-spinning oblique impacts on a flexible racket. The racket consisted of two coupled rigid segments, while the string bed was modelled as 9 point masses and 24 springs.

The cutting edge of computational impact modelling is currently finite element analysis. Finite element models (Figure 35.3c) can be applied to racket development, as they allow the effect of specific design parameters, such as materials and geometry, to be predicted. Allen *et al.* (2009) developed a finite element model of a tennis ball impacting with a racket, which was later used to predict the effect of string bed friction (Allen *et al.*, 2010a) and racket frame parameters (Allen *et al.*, 2011) on ball rebound velocity, angle and spin. Trajectory simulations, combined with racket impact models (or the results of experiments) allow the effect of changes in ball rebound to be predicted and illustrated in the court frame of reference, as done by

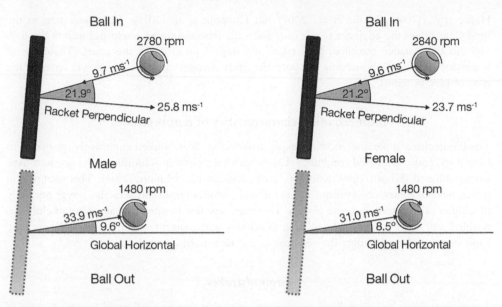

Figure 35.2 A diagrammatic summary of the mean player groundstroke conditions measured at the 2006 Wimbeldon qualifying tournament (Choppin *et al.*, 2011). 106 strokes were analysed from 16 players (10 male and 6 female).

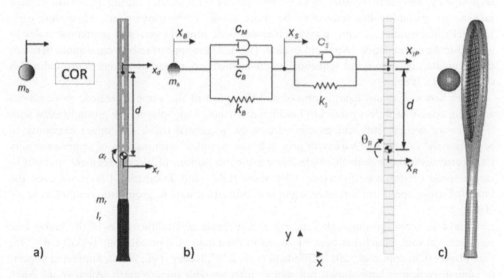

Figure 35.3 (a) Early rigid body models of the racket had few degrees of freedom, and were mostly used to approximate post-impact ball velocities (modified from Goodwill and Haake, 2001); (b) the addition of flexible beam elements and spring-damper ball and spring models allowed racket vibration and ball/string properties to be taken into account; and (c) three-dimensional finite element models simulate complex ball and string deformations throughout impact (Allen *et al.*, 2010b).

Haake *et al.* (2000), Haake *et al.* (2007) and Choppin *et al.* (2010). This extra step in the modelling allows the engineer to not only assess the rebound speed, angle and spin of the ball, but also the distance travelled, time taken and impact location on the court. These are all important criteria when assessing the potential effect changes in racket design will have on the state of play in tennis.

Biomechanical characteristics of tennis strokes

The biomechanical parameters of all tennis strokes have been studied extensively, primarily in laboratory/court-simulated conditions. Extensive reviews of tennis biomechanics research have been published (Elliott, 1989; Knudson, 2006; Knudson and Elliott, 2004). This section will review several robust observations across the main strokes (groundstrokes and serve) primarily in samples of advanced and elite players. There are very few biomechanical studies of children, disabled and older players. This section concludes with current research that explores how hand forces at the grip affect the response of the racket/string system.

Groundstrokes

Tennis groundstrokes are ballistic striking activities that can be performed using a variety of coordination strategies through numerous combinations of multiple body segments and multiple degrees of freedom at the joints between the segments. When implements are heavy, coordination tends to involve simultaneous segment motions. More sequential segment motion is observed as the implement gets lighter and the swing gets faster. As noted in a previous section, early twentieth century rackets were heavier with smaller hitting areas than current rackets, so groundstrokes tended to be more whole-body movements. However, early biomechanical studies of elite players observed both simultaneous and sequential styles of groundstroke coordination (Ariel and Braden, 1979). There appears to be a continuum between simultaneous/single-unit and sequential/multi-segment coordination in tennis groundstrokes (Elliott *et al.*, 1989).

As rackets and strings have improved and the speed of the game increased, more players are using open stance (feet parallel to baseline) forehands. Many players use groundstrokes with less forward weight shift and greater reliance on sequential trunk and upper extremity to accelerate the racket. The variety of grip style and complex combinations of upper extremity joint rotations make it difficult to identify stable contributions of specific segment motions to racket speed or stroke performance. Grip styles (Elliot and Takahashi, 1997) and even the intended stroke speed can influence segment coordination used in groundstrokes (Seeley *et al.*, 2011).

Almost all tennis groundstrokes use fast racket speeds and subtle angles of the racket face to create ball spin, which has been measured in the range of approximately 0–350 rad.s^{-1} for elite players (Choppin *et al.*, 2011; Goodwill *et al.*, 2007; Kelley *et al.*, 2008). Simulated impacts in laboratory studies have shown ball spin to increase with impact speed (Allen *et al.*, 2009; Goodwill and Haake, 2004) and angle (relative to string bed normal) (Goodwill *et al.*, 2006; Haake *et al.*, 2012). Finite element simulations have shown ball spin to be dependent on impact location (Allen *et al.*, 2011), although elite players aim to strike the ball at the node of the fundamental mode of vibration (approximate string bed centre) (Choppin *et al.*, 2011).

Ranges of racket trajectories in space and racket angles relative to the ball have been reported for most strokes (see Choppin *et al.*, 2011; Knudson, 2006; Sheets *et al.*, 2011). The study of these important interactions has been complicated by the short duration of impact (about

5 ms) and data smoothing problems related to impact (Knudson and Bahamonde, 2001; Reid *et al.*, 2012). Skilled tennis players positively accelerate the racket up to impact, reaching peak racket speed just before deceleration created by impact and follow-through.

Serves

Tennis rules require the player to serve from a stationary position, the ball to be tossed and hit before it bounces. There is considerable biomechanical consistency in serving because of the great advantage a player has if they have developed a high-speed overhead service. In general, it is advantageous for the player to develop a high point of racket-ball impact with high racket-head speeds, but with a variety of racket trajectories to vary ball speed, spin and placement in the service box. See Knudson (2006) for a complete review of the biomechanics of the tennis serve.

Players generally use two patterns of stance and a sequential coordination of the lower body, trunk and upper extremity to create high racket speed at impact (Knudson, 2006). Advanced players use a continental or backhand grip to maximize the ability to use forearm and wrist rotations to create ball speed and spin. Higher spin rates have been reported for serves in comparison to groundstrokes (Goodwill *et al.*, 2007; Kelley *et al.*, 2008). Serves are commonly called flat, slice and twist according to the primary racket trajectory through impact. Flat serves are a misnomer. While these serves maximize ball speed, the path of the racket and angle of the racket face create topspin and sidespin (Elliott, 1983; Sakurai *et al.*, 2012). Slice serves emphasize sidespin, while twist serves emphasize topspin with some sidespin (Knudson, 2006; Sheets *et al.*, 2011). While many recreational players feel they hit the ball with an initial downwand trajectory in the serve, this tends not to be the case; only advanced players with high-speed and spin serves can hit the ball on a slightly downward (< 10°) trajectory (Knudson, 2006).

Grip forces

Ball impact on the racket string bed typically lasts from 3 to 5 ms (Brody *et al.*, 2002; Groppel *et al.*, 1987; Kawazoe, 2002). The importance of grip forces applied over this short interval have been a long-standing controversy. From the very origins of the sport, tennis players and instructors advocated that the use of a firm grip at impact would increase the speed of ball rebound. A firm grip at the moment of impact was believed to impart greater force to the ball and, consequently, create greater ball speed and spin. Interestingly, the problem of the effect of grip forces at or during impact on stroke performance variables has been difficult to resolve.

Early studies predominantly focused on the effect of handle constraints for impacts on the longitudinal axis of the racket. Measurements of ball rebound speed showed no differences between unrestrained rackets and rackets rigidly clamped at the handle (Baker and Putnam, 1979; Watanabe *et al.*, 1979). Both modelling and experimental studies have confirmed that handheld tennis rackets behave at impact as unrestrained bodies (Brody, 1987; Casolo and Ruggieri, 1991; Hatze, 1992; Kawazoe, 1997; Knudson, 1997; Vallatta *et al.*, 1993), so studies using rigidly clamped rackets do not represent the mechanics of impact in actual tennis play.

The length and stiffness of a typical tennis racket frame is such that the impulse from impact takes around 8 ms to travel along its length and back again (Brody *et al.*, 2002; Cross, 1998, 1999; Knudson and White, 1989). As such, the ball has left the string bed before the grip at the handle could assert its influence. Rackets would have to be shorter and unusually stiff for forces at the grip to influence ball rebound speed for a standard impact (Missavage *et al.*, 1984). High-speed imaging shows that the ball has rebounded from the strings in groundstrokes before the backward recoil of the frame is completed into the player's hand. Figure 35.4 shows sequence images from high-speed video of the racket recoil and bending in a 35 m.s⁻¹ impact. Notice the frame deformation beyond the impact phase so no frame elastic energy can be returned to the ball.

Off-axis impacts create a torque about the longitudinal axis of the racket. The majority of previous research comparing freely suspended with handheld rackets reported no difference in ball rebound characteristics, which indicates that increasing grip forces cannot normally influence a tennis stroke (Knudson, 1997). Recent laboratory testing of simulated arm off-axis impacts has shown that resistive torques (0, 8, 15 Nm) on the handle simulating different grip levels do not significantly affect ball speed (Choppin *et al.*, 2010). However, moving from a loose grip to some grip torque influenced the rebound angle of the ball by 0.5 to 1.0°. This small change in ball rebound angle can result in a difference of 1–2 m in shot depth for a standard baseline forehand. These results need to be confirmed because even very small changes in ball rebound angles have meaningful performance effects.

Forces on the hand measured during tennis strokes have reported moderate (not maximal voluntary effort) grip forces up to impact, followed by highly variable forces after impact (Hennig, 2007; Knudson, 1991b; Knudson and White, 1989; Plagenhoef, 1982; Savage and Subic, 2006). The hand forces at impact are moderately correlated (r^2 = 25–36 per cent) with post-impact peak forces and vibrations (Knudson, 1991a; Savage and Subic, 2006), but are not related to ball rebound speed (Hennig, 2007; Knudson, 1989). The variability of handheld racket performance and the ethical problems of exposing humans to injury risk are also strong arguments for laboratory-based testing using simulated grips and theoretical testing. Racket manufacturers will likely always use highly skilled human player testers because their perceptions are very important in predicting sales. However, evaluation of performance parameters should be systematically evaluated using robots as surrogates for biomechanical testing as well as theoretical modelling (Kawazoe, 2002).

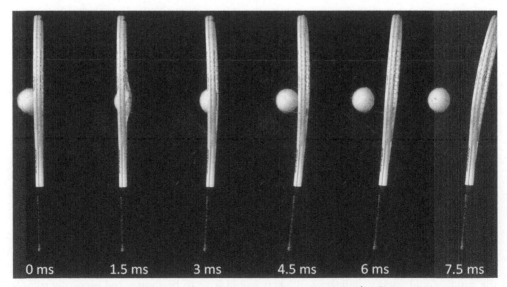

Figure 35.4 High-speed (3,300 Hz) video of the impact phase of a 35 m.s⁻¹ collision of a ball with a free-standing racket. Ball and frame response during the 5 ms impact phase are similar to handheld conditions during a groundstroke.

Several researchers have proposed robotic arms for human surrogate testing of tennis rackets (Choppin *et al.*, 2010; Furusho *et al.*, 2001; Hatze, 1992). Some theoretical models avoid complications of uncertain grip effects by assuming hand mass (about 0.6 per cent of athlete mass) is part of the racket (Kawazoe *et al.*, 2010a, 2010b; Li *et al.*, 2009). Recently, Kentel *et al.* (2011) developed a 3D torque-driven model of the upper extremity in tennis backhands. Use of this model confirmed a lack of an effect of grip forces on speed of ball rebound at all impact locations, but a firm grip (50 times typical elite player grip) was able to increase rebound accuracy for balls impacting below the centre of the racket (King *et al.*, 2012).

Biomechanical research indicates that grip forces during tennis play are not as influential on impact dynamics as most players believe. Grip forces do not affect ball rebound speed, but it is unclear if typical grip forces can influence the accuracy and spin of the shot. Inconsistency of player perception of impact force and sensitivity to the 'feel' and 'comfort' of impacts does not mean that racket design cannot take into account player perception. Engineers and manufacturers must accommodate psychometric and biomechanical factors in racket design (Sol, 1994).

Interaction of racket characteristics with player biomechanics

The following section will explore the interactions between important racket design parameters and the biomechanics of tennis strokes. The challenge for engineers striving to improve racket performance is the complex way in which a change in the racket's parameters (dimensions, inertia and stiffness) interacts with the swing of the player, as well as the impact with the ball. Readers are also referred to articles that have summarized the likely changes in performance, match play statistics and opinions that are a result of changes in tennis racket design (e.g. Arthur, 1992; Coe, 2000; Haake *et al.*, 2000, 2007; McClusky, 2003; Sheridan, 2006).

Racket dimensions

Several changes in racket dimensions (length, width and head size) over the years have allowed the retrospective comparison of the performance effects of these design changes. In general, the increase in head size (Blanksby *et al.*, 1979; Gruetter and Davis, 1985) and racket length (Pellett and Lox, 1997) have created significant improvement on the tennis skills test scores of tennis students. Coaches and players, however, are more concerned with ball speed, spin and accuracy, which they believe to be related to match–play success.

Larger head rackets create significantly higher ball rebound speed and less frame vibration than traditional rackets (Elliott *et al.*, 1980). The initial US patent on an oversize tennis racket was based on a larger 'sweet spot' and higher coefficients of restitution compared to other rackets of the time (Head, 1976). The common notion of the sweet spot is a mix of three mechanical points on the racket face (Brody, 1981; Cross, 1998): the area of maximum rebound coefficient of restitution, the point of minimum vibration (node) and the point of no frame reaction (centre of percussion).

Stiffness

Frame stiffness can be increased by utilizing stiffer materials or changing the geometry of the frame, and it has increased dramatically over time (Haake *et al.*, 2007). Greater racket stiffness can increase ball rebound speed (Cross, 2000; Kern and Zimmerman, 1993) and accuracy (Bower and Sinclair, 1999), although Allen *et al.* (2011) demonstrated stiffness to have only a minor effect on ball rebound velocity for impacts close to the centre of the string bed. The effect of stiffness is likely to be greater for serves (Allen *et al.*, 2009; Goodwill and Haake, 2003), as the ball is struck towards the tip. Stiffness interacts with string tension (Baker and Wilson, 1978; Elliott, 1982), so the player will likely need to adjust stringing when moving to a stiffer frame. The United States Racquet Stringers Association (USRSA) collects racket and string characteristics in an extensive database and provides a model for USRSA members to help players customize their rackets.

Inertial properties

The inertial properties of tennis rackets are important because of their effect on shot performance and their interaction with player stroke mechanics. Modern rackets are lighter and have a lower moment of inertia about the grip (I_s) than the wooden rackets of the mid twentieth century (Haake *et al.*, 2007). The polar moment of inertia (I_p) is the resistance to angular acceleration of the frame about its longitudinal axis and is approximately 20 times smaller than I_s. Polar moments of inertia have remained relatively constant as decreases in racket mass since the 1970s have coincided with increases in head width (Haake *et al.*, 2007).

For constant impact conditions, an increase in the mass or I_s of the racket will increase the impulse applied to a ball. Cross and Nathan (2009) tested 133 rackets and showed ball rebound speed to increase with I_s for normal impacts 0.16 m from the tip. Cross (2010) used an analytical model to show that ball rebound speed increases with I_p for off-axis impacts. Allen *et al.* (2011) used a finite element model to predict that ball rebound velocity and spin increases with racket mass and as the balance point moved towards the tip (effectively increasing I_s). The results presented in these studies appear to contradict the trend of decreasing I_s values over time (Haake *et al.*, 2007). There is a discrepancy between racket performance parameters measured through simulation and laboratory-based testing and player performance and preference on court.

The loss of racket mass in modern frames does not result in a reduction of momentum at impact because players tend to swing the lighter rackets faster. Mitchell *et al.* (2000) reported that skilled players could swing low moment of inertia rackets faster when serving than higher inertia rackets. Cross and Bower (2006) reported a study of the biomechanics of swinging weighted rods and found that the speed of an overarm swing decreases with increasing swingweight. They also noted that given the mass of a tennis ball and typical impact position on the racket face, that racket masses between 0.31 and 0.51 kg were near optimal for momentum transfer to the ball. Most current tennis rackets have masses below 0.3 kg, so rackets may be near the lower biomechanical limit for tennis racket mass. Given these data, one could hypothesize that tennis players currently using very light rackets might experience benefits in performance and lower risks of overuse injury by adding some mass to their rackets. Research concerning racket parameters and overuse injuries will be discussed in the next section.

A lower-mass racket is easier to move and accuracy might, theoretically, improve given less muscular effort required in the stroke. A tennis player, however, is also likely to swing the lower mass racket faster, decreasing accuracy (speed-accuracy trade-off). This is another example of the interaction of racket mechanical characteristics and player biomechanics. Gagen *et al.* (2005) reported that based on speed and accuracy of children's (4–10 years old) strokes using different rackets, there was a 'best' racket for each child. The optimal racket was due to a unique combination of racket size and inertial properties.

Advanced players often customize rackets by adding lead tape to specific frame locations to adjust balance and swing weight (Brody *et al.*, 2002). This is logical given the lower mass of modern frames and the high level of strength of modern athletes. Advanced players are fairly sensitive to changes in I_S of tennis rackets and can detect differences down to 2.5 per cent (Brody, 2000). Cross (2001) reported that the tip of the racket is the most effective location when adding mass in order to increase the speed of ball rebound. There is, however, a compromise between optimum mass distribution for a groundstroke and serve, due to differences in impact location and stroke mechanics.

The performance of a tennis racket is not only a function of its physical properties, but also the manner in which it interacts with the players that wield it. While there is some research on the general effect of several racket design variables (size, inertial properties, stiffness), their combined effect on the several performance variables is difficult to optimize. The interaction between tennis racket design and player biomechanics is a promising area of future research. The next section will focus on the hypothesized connection between racket design and risk of common overuse injuries such as tennis elbow.

Racket design to reduce risk of injury

The majority of tennis players will experience elbow pain sometime in their lifetime (Kamien, 1990; Maffulli *et al.*, 2003). The most common overuse injury is 'tennis elbow', the common term for inflammation and, sometimes, degradation of the common wrist flexor (medial) and extensor (lateral) muscle-tendon attachments. Tennis rackets are often marketed to prevent or alleviate the pain from tennis elbow. However, relatively little is known about the effect of tennis racket parameters on the risk of developing, or recovery from, tennis elbow. This section summarizes the research and logic on tennis racket designs purported to decrease the risk or pain from tennis elbow.

The most likely cause of tennis elbow is the repetitive rapid elongation of the forearm muscle from the initial shock wave of impact (Knudson, 2004). The combination of this repetitive micro-trauma, lack of adequate rest and individual susceptibility all contribute to many tennis players suffering from this injury. In theory, changes in racket properties could decrease the peak acceleration after ball impact, modifying muscular loading and potentially reduce injury risk. Increasing racket mass and I_S would provide greater resistance to the shock wave of impact and has been confirmed by experiments and modelling (Brody, 1979; Nesbit *et al.*, 2006). Off-axis impacts have the largest influence on the peak forces and vibrations transmitted to the player (Hennig, 2007; Knudson, 2004; Plagenhoef, 1982).

Increasing racket head size decreases the amplitude of post-impact frame vibration (Elliott *et al.*, 1980; Hennig *et al.*, 1992) compared to regular head rackets. The larger head allows the strings to absorb more of the energy of ball impact and the greater I_p value provides added resistance to off-axis impacts. The foundation work presented in these studies should be complemented by further research into the relationship between racket head size, string bed properties and impact loads applied to the player.

Decreasing the stiffness of the racket will also decrease the peak forces and accelerations transmitted to the body. Greater longitudinal compliance in the frame allows the strings and racket to deflect more and absorb more of the energy of impact than a stiff frame. Frame stiffness interacts with string tension, so players concerned about tennis elbow should also string their rackets at the lower end of the range of recommended string tensions. Simulation has shown impact forces between the ball and strings to decrease as string bed stiffness decreases (Allen *et al.*, 2009).

Damping properties of the racket materials and design also affect the energy transfer at impact. Rackets have been designed to try to isolate the impact energy from the body (e.g.

Wilson *Triad*) or store and damp out the energy of the shock and vibration of impact (e.g. Head *Intelligence*). The first generation of *Intelligence* frames were play-tested with players with a history of tennis elbow and appeared to reduce tennis elbow symptoms reported by the players (Kotze *et al.*, 2003). A subsequent double-blind 12-week study using a second-generation design (*Protector OS*) provided the first prospective evidence demonstrating that new racket technology can decrease the symptoms of tennis elbow compared to play with regular tennis rackets (Cottey *et al.*, 2006) with similar or slightly better racket power (Kawazoe *et al.*, 2010a). To the authors' knowledge, no other racket designs or materials have been rigorously tested for efficacy using blinded, prospective research designs.

Selecting a racket to decrease the risk of injury or reduce current symptoms of tennis elbow, like trying to optimize performance, is a complicated problem with many interacting factors. Designing rackets to minimize the risk of overuse injury is primarily based on theory due to the limit of basic science and prospective research in this area. Decreasing frame stiffness and string tension, as well as using rackets designed to damp out the energy transmitted to the body, might reduce symptoms of and risk of developing tennis elbow. More research is needed on the effectiveness of racket design parameters and damping technologies. Large prospective studies with uninjured players would go some way to establishing whether new racket designs actually decrease the incidence of tennis elbow in recreational tennis players.

Future developments in tennis racket design

The last three decades of technological development in tennis has changed the nature of the game considerably. New materials and manufacturing techniques have given rise to stiffer, lighter and larger rackets, which in turn have increased the speed and changed the style of play. While the modern game has its advocates and detractors, the role of technology and science is undeniable, but what more can it offer? While it can be tricky to predict the future and the effect of new technologies, there is a clue in the Babolat 'play and connect' prototype racket (as of summer 2012), which is able to track the motion of a player's swing. Modern, miniature sensors embedded in the racket measure motion during the swing and feed this information back to the player (or coach). The drop in size and price of sensing technology has made it possible to 'instrument' sports equipment for the consumer market. Sensors that measure rotations, accelerations and vibrations have the potential to provide immediate information to the player at all levels of ability. While this revolution in measurement technology could provide the user with a huge amount of information, there are also risks. The information might interfere with more meaningful inherent feedback or the player could be overwhelmed by excessive amounts of data. This potential measurement revolution in tennis is not only reliant on cheap, accurate and durable sensors, but also a meaningful and effective interpretation of the information this new technology provides. It is the role of the sports scientists and engineers to distill the collective knowledge of swing and impact mechanics into useful, easily understood metrics for the player and coach. Advanced construction, sensing and feedback technologies may be the keys to future improvements in tennis performance and lower risks of overuse injury.

Summary

This chapter has presented the racket and player as a complex system in which small changes can affect the equilibrium in unexpected ways. The modern player (at all levels) is concerned with performance, which is usually expressed as an increase in ball speed and/or spin or a greater degree of control over rebound angle. However, this increase in performance must be balanced with a need to control the risk of injury.

The sports engineer has explored this area using a combination of laboratory testing, modelling and measurements of tennis players in simulated and match-play conditions. Advances in the materials, design and construction of rackets has tended to increase frame stiffness and size and decrease mass. This evolution in racket properties has seen players adopt a variety of stroke techniques with more sequential joint coordination than in the past. Ball speeds and spins in match play have tended to increase along with this evolution in playing technique. If the modern player wants to minimize their risk of injury without affecting impact performance detrimentally, they should seek to increase frame mass and decrease string bed tensions. However, racket design parameters do interact with individual stroke biomechanics, particularly inertia properties.

The disconnect between racket performance in the laboratory and the performance of the complete player/racket system represents a fertile area for collaborative research in the future. Until more tennis-specific science and prospective data are available, most tennis players might select rackets that 'feel' good to them during play. A racket selected by a player based on 'feel' may not represent the mass, stiffness or head size that could maximize their performance. Racket designers should take into account player perception about racket 'feel', although preliminary research indicates that recreational players are not as consistent or sensitive to these variations as elite players.

Acknowledgements

The authors are grateful to several colleagues who we have collaborated with over the years. Several at the ITF Technical Department and the Centre for Sports Engineering at Sheffield Hallam University were particularly helpful in the writing of this chapter.

References

Allen, T., Haake, S. and Goodwill, S. (2009) 'Comparison of a finite element model of a tennis racket to experimental data', *Sports Engineering*, 12(2): 87–8.

Allen, T., Haake, S. J. and Goodwill, S. R. (2010a) 'Effect of friction on tennis ball impacts', *Proceedings of the Institution of Mechanical Engineers, Part P: Journal of Sports Engineering and Technology*, 224(3): 229–36.

Allen, T., Hart, J., Spurr, J., Haake, S. and Goodwill, S. (2010b) 'Validated dynamic analysis of real sports equipment using finite element: a case study using tennis rackets', *Procedia Engineering*, 2(2): 3275–80.

Allen, T. B., Haake, S. J. and Goodwill, S. R. (2011) 'Effect of tennis racket parameters on a simulated groundstroke', *Journal of Sports Sciences*, 29(3): 311–25.

Ariel, G. B. and Braden, V. (1979) 'Biomechanical analysis of ballistic vs. tracking movements in tennis skills', in J. Groppel (ed.), *Proceedings of a National Symposium on the Racquet Sports*, Champaign, IL: University of Illinois, pp. 105–24.

Arthur, C. (1992) 'Anyone for slower tennis?', *New Scientist*, 134(1819): 24–8.

Baker, J. A. W. and Wilson, B. D. (1978) 'The effect of tennis racket stiffness and string tension on ball velocity after impact', *Research Quarterly*, 49(3): 255–59.

Baker, J. A. W. and Putnam, C. A. (1979) 'Tennis racket and ball responses during impact under clamped and freestanding conditions', *Research Quarterly*, 50(2): 164–70.

Blanksby, B. A., Ellis, R. and Elliott, B. C. (1979) 'Selecting the right racquet: performance characteristics of regular-sized and over-sized tennis racquets', *Australian Journal of Health, Physical Education, and Recreation*, 86: 21–5.

Bower, R. and Sinclair, P. (1999) 'Tennis racquet stiffness and string tension effects on rebound velocity and angle for an oblique impact', *Journal of Human Movement Studies*, 37: 271–86.

Brody, H. (1979) 'Physics of the tennis racket', *American Journal of Physics*, 47(6): 482–7.

Brody, H. (1981) 'Physics of the tennis racket II: the sweet spot', *American Journal of Physics*, 49(9): 816–19.

Brody, H. (1987) 'Models of tennis racket impacts', *International Journal of Sport Biomechanics*, 3(3): 293–6.

Brody, H. (1997) 'The physics of tennis III: the ball-racket interaction', *American Journal of Physics*, 65(10): 981–7.

Brody, H. (2000) 'Player sensitivity to the moments of inertia of a tennis racket', *Sports Engineering*, 3(2): 145–8.

Brody, H. (2002) 'The tennis racket', in P. A. F. H. Renstrom (ed.), *Handbook of Sports Medicine and Science: Tennis*, Oxford: Blackwell Science, pp. 29–38.

Brody, H., Cross, R. and Lindsey, C. (2002) *The Physics and Technology of Tennis*, Solana Beach, CA: Racquet Tech Publishing.

Casolo, F. and Ruggieri, G. (1991) 'Dynamic analysis of the ball-racket impact in the game of tennis', *Meccanica*, 26(2–3): 67–73.

Choppin, S. B., Whyld, N.M., Goodwill, S.R. and Haake, S.J. (2005) '3D impact analysis in tennis', in A. Subic and S. Ujihashi (eds), *The Impact of Technology on Sport*, Tokyo: Australian Sports Technology Alliance, pp. 373–8.

Choppin, S., Goodwill, S. and Haake, S. (2010) 'Investigation into the effect of grip tightness on off-centre forehand strikes in tennis', *Journal of Sports Engineering and Technology*, 224(4): 249–57.

Choppin, S., Goodwill, S. and Haake, S. (2011) 'Impact characteristics of the ball and racket during play at the Wimbledon qualifying tournament', *Sports Engineering*, 13(4): 163–70.

Clerici, G. (1976) *Tennis*, London: Octopus Books.

Coe, A. (2000) 'The balance between technology and tradition in tennis', in S. J. Haake and A. Coe (eds), *Tennis Science & Technology*, Oxford: Blackwell Science, pp. 3–40.

Cottey, R., Kotze, J., Lammer, H. and Zirngibl, W. (2006) 'An extended study investigating the effects of tennis rackets with active damping technology on the symptoms of tennis elbow', in E. Moritz and S. Haake (eds), *Engineering of Sport 6*, New York: Springer, pp. 391–6.

Cross, R. (1998) 'The sweet spots of a tennis racquet', *Sports Engineering*, 1(2): 63–78.

Cross, R. (1999) 'Impact of a ball with a bat or racket', *American Journal of Physics*, 67(8): 692–702.

Cross, R. (2000) 'Flexible beam analysis of the effects of string tension and frame stiffness on racket performance', *Sports Engineering*, 3(2): 111–22.

Cross, R. (2001) 'Customising a tennis racket by adding weights', *Sports Engineering*, 4(1): 1–14.

Cross, R. (2010) 'The polar moment of inertia of striking implements', *Sports Technology*, 3(3): 215–19.

Cross, R. and Lindsey, C. (2005) *Technical Tennis*, Vista, CA: Racquet Tech Publishing.

Cross, R. and Bower, R. (2006) 'Effects of swing-weight on swing speed and racket power', *Journal of Sports Sciences*, 24(1): 23–30.

Cross, R. and Nathan, A. (2009) 'Performance versus moment of inertia of sporting implements', *Sports Technology*, 2(1–2): 7–15.

Davies, G., Rothberg, S. J., Jones, R. and Roberts, J. R. (2003) 'Player perception evaluation of "feel" in tennis ball impacts', in S. Miller (ed.), *Tennis Science and Technology 2*, London: International Tennis Federation, pp. 71–8.

Elliott, B. C. (1982) 'Tennis: the influence of grip tightness on reaction impulse and rebound velocity', *Medicine and Science in Sports and Exercise*, 14: 348–52.

Elliott, B. C. (1983) 'Spin and the power server in tennis velocity', *Journal of Human Movement Studies*, 9: 97–104.

Elliott, B. C. (1989) 'Tennis strokes and equipment', in C. L. Vaughn (ed.), *Biomechanics in Sport*, Boca Raton, FL: CRC Press, pp. 263–88.

Elliott, B. C. and Takahashi, K. (1997) 'The influence of grip position on upper limb contributions to racket head velocity in a tennis forehand', *Journal of Applied Biomechanics*, 13(2): 182–96.

Elliott, B. C., Blanksby, B. A. and Ellis, R. (1980) 'Vibration and rebound velocity characteristics of conventional and oversized tennis rackets', *Research Quarterly for Exercise and Sport*, 51(4): 608–15.

Elliott, B. C., Marsh, T. and Overheu, P. (1989) 'A biomechanical comparison of the multisegment and single unit topspin forehand drives in tennis', *International Journal of Sport Biomechanics*, 5(3): 350–64.

Furusho, J., Sakaguchi, M., Takesue, N. Sato, F., Naruo, T. and Nagao, H. (2001) 'Development of a robot for evaluating tennis rackets', *Journal of Robotics and Mechatronics*, 13(1): 74–9.

Gagen, L. M., Haywood, K. M. and Spaner, S. D. (2005) 'Predicting the scale of tennis rackets for optimal striking from body dimensions', *Pediatric Exercise Science*, 17(2): 190–200.

Glynn, J. A., King, M. A. and Mitchell, S. R. (2011) 'A computer simulation model of tennis racket/ball impacts', *Sports Engineering*, 13(2): 65–72.

Goodwill, S. and Haake, S. (2001). 'Spring damper model of an impact between a tennis ball and a racket', *Proceedings of the Institute of Mechanical Engineers. Part C Journal of Mechanical Engineering Scinece*, 215(11): 1331–41.

Goodwill, S. and Haake, S. (2003) 'Modelling of an impact between a tennis ball and racket', in S. Miller (ed.), *Tennis Science and Technology 2*, London: International Tennis Federation, pp.79–86.

Goodwill, S. R. and Haake, S. J. (2004) 'Ball spin generation for oblique impacts with a tennis racket', *Experimental Mechanics*, 44(2): 195–206.

Goodwill, S., Douglas, J., Miller, S. and. Haake, S. (2006) 'Measuring ball spin off a tennis racket', in F. Moritz and S. Haake (eds), *The Engineering of Sport 6, Vol. 1*, Sheffield: International Sports Engineering Association, pp. 379–84.

Goodwill, S., Capel-Davies, J., Haake, S. and Miller, S. (2007) 'Ball spin generation of elite players during match play', in S. Miller and J. Capel-Davies (eds), *Tennis Science and Technology 3*, London: International Tennis Federation, pp. 349–56.

Groppel, J. L, Shin, I., Thomas, J. and Welk, G. J. (1987) 'The effects of string type and tension on impact in midsized and oversized tennis racquets', *International Journal of Sport Biomechanics*, 3(1): 40–6.

Gruetter, D. and Davis, T. M. (1985) 'Oversized vs. standard racquets: does it really make a difference?', *Research Quarterly for Exercise and Sport*, 56:31-36.

Haake, S. J., Chadwidk, S. G., Dignall, R. J., Goodwill, S. and Rose, P. (2000) 'Engineering tennis – slowing the game down', *Sports Engineering*, 3(2): 131–43.

Haake, S., Choppin, S. and Goodwill, S. (2007) 'The evolution of the tennis racket and its effect on serve speed', in S. Mille and J. Capel-Davies (eds), *Tennis Science and Technology 3*, London: International Tennis Federation, pp. 257–71.

Haake, S., Allen. T., Jones, A., Spurr, J., Allen, T. and Goodwill, S. (2012) 'Effect of inter-string friction on tennis ball rebound', *Proceedings of the Institution of Mechanical Engineers, Part J: Journal of Engineering Tribology*, 226(7): 626–35.

Hatze, H. (1992) 'Objective biomechanical determination of tennis racket properties', *International Journal of Sport Biomechanics*, 8(4): 275–87.

Head, H. (1976) *Tennis Racket*, US Patent, 39999756.

Hennig, E. (2007) 'Influence of racket properties on injuries and performance in tennis', *Exercise and Sport Sciences Reviews*, 35(2): 62–6.

Hennig, E. M., Rosenbaum, D. and Milani, T. L. (1992) 'Transfer of tennis racket vibrations onto the human forearm', *Medicine and Science in Sports and Exercise*, 24(10): 1134–40.

ITF Technical Department (2012) *International Tennis Federation*, available at: www.itftennis.com/technical (accessed 1 March 2009).

Kamien, M. (1990) 'A rational management of tennis elbow', *Sports Medicine*, 9(3): 173–91.

Kawazoe, Y. (1997) 'Experimental identification of a hand-held tennis racket and prediction of rebound ball velocity in an impact', *Theoretical and Applied Mechanics*, 46: 177–88.

Kawazoe, Y. (2002) 'Mechanism of high-tech tennis rackets performance', *Theoretical and Applied Mechanics*, 51: 177–87.

Kawazoe, Y., Takeda, Y. and Nakagawa, M. (2010a) 'Performance prediction of active piezo fiber rackets in terms of tennis power', *Journal of System Design and Dynamics*, 4(1): 77–90.

Kawazoe, Y., Takeda, Y., Nakagawa, M., Casolo, F., Tomosue, R. and Yoshinari, K. (2010b) 'Prediction of impact shock vibrations at tennis player's wrist joint: comparison between conventional weight racket and light weight racket with super large head size', *Journal of System Design and Dynamics*, 4(2): 331–47.

Kelley, J., Goodwill, S., Capel-Davies, J. and Haake, S. (2008) 'Ball spin generation at the 2007 Wimbledon qualifying tournament', in M. Estivalet and P. Brisson (eds), *The Engineering of Sport 7, Vol. 1*, France: Springer, pp. 571–8.

Kentel, B. B., King, M. A. and Mitchell, S. R. (2011) 'Evaluation of a subject-specific, torque-driven, computer simulation model of one-handed tennis backhand ground strokes', *Journal of Applied Biomechanics*, 27(4): 345–54.

Kern, J. C. and Zimmerman, W. J. (1993) 'The effect of tennis racquet flexibility on rebound velocity', in J. Hamill, T. R. Derrick and E. H. Elliott (eds), *Biomechanics in Sports XI*, Amherst, MA: University of Massachusetts, pp. 193–5.

King, M. A., Kentel, B. B. and Mitchell, S. R. (2012) 'The effect of ball impact location and grip tightness on the arm, racquet, and ball for one-handed tennis backhand groundstrokes', *Journal of Biomechanics*, 45(6): 1048–52.

Knudson, D. (1989) 'Hand forces and impact effectiveness in the tennis forehand', *Journal of Human Movement Studies*, 17: 1–7.

Knudson, D. (1991a) 'Factors affecting force loading in the tennis forehand', *Journal of Sports Medicine and Physical Fitness*, 31: 527–31.

Knudson, D. (1991b) 'Forces on the hand in the tennis one-handed backhand', *International Journal of Sport Biomechanics*, 7: 282–92.

Knudson, D. (1997) 'Effect of grip models on rebound accuracy of off-center tennis impacts', in J. Wilkerson, K. Ludwig and W. Zimmerman (eds), *Biomechanics in Sports XV: Proceedings of the 15th International Symposium on Biomechanics in Sports*, Denton, TX: Texas Woman's University, pp. 483–7.

Knudson, D. (2004) 'Biomechanical studies on the mechanism of tennis elbow', in M. Hubbard, R. D. Mehta and J. M. Pallis (eds), *The Engineering of Sport 5: Vol. 1*, Sheffield: International Sports Engineering Association, pp. 135–9.

Knudson, D. (2006) *Biomechanical Principles of Tennis Technique*, Vista, CA: Racquet Tech Publishing.

Knudson, D. (2008) 'Biomechanical aspects of the tennis racket', in Y. Hong and R. Bartlet (eds), *Routledge Handbook of Biomechanics and Human Movement Science*, London: Routledge, pp. 248–60.

Knudson, D. and White, S. (1989) 'Forces on the hand in the tennis forehand drive: Application of force sensing resistors', *International Journal of Sport Biomechanics*, 5(3): 324–31.

Knudson, D. and Bahamonde, R. (2001) 'Effect of endpoint conditions on position and velocity at impact in tennis', *Journal of Sports Sciences*, 19(11): 839–44.

Knudson, D. and Elliott, B. (2004) 'Biomechanics of tennis strokes', in G. K. Hung and J. M. Pallis (eds), *Biomedical Engineering Principles in Sports*, New York: Kluwer Academic/Plenum Publishers, pp. 153–81.

Kotze, J., Lammer, H., Cottey, R. and Zirngibl, W. (2003) 'The effects of active piezo fibre rackets on tennis elbow', in S. Miller (ed.), *Tennis Science and Technology 2*, London: International Tennis Federation, pp. 55–60.

Li, L., Yang, S. H., Hwang, C. and Kim, Y. S. (2009) 'Effects of string tension and impact location on tennis playing', *Journal of Mechanical Science and Technology*, 23(11): 2990–7.

Liu, Y. K. (1983) 'Mechanical analysis of racket and ball during impact', *Medicine and Science in Sports and Exercise*, 15(5): 388–92.

McClusky, M. (2003) *Tennis Swaps Grace for Strength*, Wired News, available at: www.wired.com/news/technology/0,60177–0.html (accessed 21 November 2006).

Maffulli, N., Wong, J. and Almekinders, L. C. (2003) 'Types and epidemiology of tendinopathy', *Clinics in Sports Medicine*, 22(4): 675–92.

Miller, S. (2006) 'Modern tennis rackets, balls, and surfaces', *British Journal of Sports Medicine*, 40(5): 401–5.

Missavage, R. J., Baker, J. and Putnam, C. (1984) 'Theoretical modeling of grip firmness during ball-racket impact', *Research Quarterly for Exercise and Sport*, 55(3): 254–60.

Mitchell, S. R., Jones, R. and King, M. (2000) 'Head speed vs racket inertia in the tennis serve', *Sports Engineering*, 3(2): 99–110.

Nesbit, S. N., Elzinga, M., Herchenroder, K. and Serrano, M. (2006) 'The effects of racket inertia tensor on elbow loadings and racket behavior for central and eccentric impacts', *Journal of Sports Sciences and Medicine*, 5: 304–17.

Pellett, T. L. and Lox, C. L. (1997) 'Tennis racket length comparisons and their effect on beginning college player' playing success and achievement', *Journal of Teaching in Physical Education*, 16(4): 490–9.

Plagenhoef, S. (1982) 'Tennis racket testing', in J. Terauds (ed.), *Biomechanics in Sports*, Del Mar, CA: Research Center for Sports, pp. 411–21.

Reid, M. M., Campbell, A. C. and Elliott, B. C. (2012) 'Comparison of endpoint data treatment methods for the estimation of kinematics and kinetics near impact during the tennis serve', *Journal of Applied Biomechanics*, 28(1): 93–8.

Roberts, J. R., Jones, R., Harwood, C., Mitchell, S. R. and Rothberg, S. J. (2001a) 'Human perceptions of sports equipment under playing conditions', *Journal of Sports Sciences*, 19(7): 485–97.

Roberts, J. R., Jones, R. and Rothberg, S. J. (2001b) 'Measurement of contact time in short duration sports ball impacts: an experimental method and correlation with the perceptions of elite golfers', *Sports Engineering*, 4(4): 191–203.

Sakurai, S., Reid, M. and Elliott, B. (2012) 'Ball spin in the tennis serve: spin rate and axis of rotation', *Sports Biomechanics*, doi:10.1080/14763141.2012.671355.

Savage, N. and Subic, A. (2006) 'Relating grip characteristics to the dynamic response of tennis racquets', in E. F.Moritz and S. Haake (eds), *The Engineering of Sport 6: Vol. 2*, New York: Springer, pp. 155–60.

Seeley, M. K., Funk, M. D., Denning, W. M., Hager, R. L. and Hopkins, J. T. (2011) 'Tennis forehand kinematics change as post-impact ball speed is altered', *Sports Biomechanics*, 10(4): 415–26.

Sheets, A. L., Abrams, G. D., Corazza, S., Safran, M. R. and Andriacchi, T. P. (2011) 'Kinematics differences between the flat, kick, and slice serves measured using a markerless motion capture method', *Annals of Biomedical Engineering*, 39(12): 3011–20.

Sheridan, H. (2006) 'Tennis technologies: de-skilling and re-skilling players and the implications for the game', *Sport in Society*, 9(1): 32–50.

Sol, H. (1994) 'Computer aided design of rackets', in T. Reilly, M. Hughes and A. Lees (eds), *Science and Racket Sports*, London: E & FN Spon, pp. 125–33.

Tenner, E. (1996) *Why Things Bite Back: Technology and the Revenge of Unintended Consequences*, New York: Knopf.

Vallatta, A., Casolo, F. and Caffi, M. (1993) 'On the coefficients of restitution of tennis racquets', in J. Hamill, T. R. Derrick and E. H. Elliott (eds), *Biomechanics in Sports XI*, Amherst, MA: University of Massachusetts, pp. 196–200.

Watanabe, T. Y., Ikegami, Y. and Miyashita, M. (1979) 'Tennis: the effects of grip firmness on ball velocity after impact', *Medicine in Science in Sports*, 11(4): 359–61.

36

ROWING ERGOMETER DESIGN AND LUMBAR STRESS

Richard M. Smith, Michael H. Dickson and Floren Colloud

UNIVERSITY OF SYDNEY, SYDNEY

Introduction

Rowing is a physically and technically demanding skill that requires the back to act as a transfer for large forces and moments between the upper and lower extremities (Hagerman, 1984). Rowing is characterized by long-distance aerobic training sessions, which comprise 90 per cent of training volume and typically consist of rowing for 90–120 minutes at 18–20 strokes per minute, covering 20–25 km. Stroke rates during rowing training range from 15–40 strokes per minute and at race pace are typically 32–38 strokes per minute. Further, ergometer rowing is widespread in gyms for general purpose fitness training.

It is generally considered that the majority of rowing injuries are related to overuse. The most common type of injury in elite male rowers is the lower back (Hagerman, 1984; Hickey *et al.*, 1997; Reid and McNair, 2000). Lower back injury (LBI) has been reported to comprise 25–50 per cent of all rowing injuries that require medical attention (Goodman and Hooper, 2008; Wilson *et al.*, 2010; Winzen *et al.*, 2011).

Rowing injuries occur in various structures of the lumbar spine. The five main areas of injury diagnosis can be identified as mechanical, muscular, ligament strain, disc, pars and facet joint (Hickey *et al.*, 1997; Maurer *et al.*, 2011). Researchers have suggested different mechanisms to explain the various spinal structures at high risk of injury due to rowing. Suggested mechanisms include high volume training loads (Stallard, 1980; Teitz *et al.*, 2001), the rotational component of back motion during sweep rowing (Reid and McNair, 2000; Stallard, 1980), trunk muscle asymmetry, weakness and/or fatigability (Roy *et al.*, 1990), a large range of lumbar flexion at the catch and throughout the stroke (Caldwell *et al.*, 2003; Reid and McNair, 2000) and the introduction of new equipment such as ergometers and hatchet blades (Munro and Yanai, 2000; Strahan *et al.*, 2011).

About half of specific events causing rowing injuries occur off water (Hagerman, 1984). Some elite rowing training programmes include 10–15 per cent of total training time, off-water. The use of ergometers by elite rowers is now widespread, and ergometers are used for both testing and semi-specific muscular and technical training (Teitz *et al.*, 2001). As ergometer use has increased, coaches, rowers and researchers have expressed concern over possible ergometer-induced injuries. Rowing for more than 30 minutes on an ergometer was identified as a consistent predictor of lower back pain (LBP) in intercollegiate rowers (Teitz *et al.*, 2001).

The most commonly used types of ergometers can be classed as either fixed or sliding. On the fixed ergometer, the rower is positioned on a sliding seat and during the drive phase the rower is required to accelerate the entire body mass away from a stationary foot stretcher-flywheel complex. However, during on-water rowing, the rower and boat form a binary system characterized by a transfer of momentum between the rower and the boat. For the Olympic boat classes, the mass per rower of the boat plus oars (including the coxswain) range from 15.5 kg for a coxless four or a quadruple, to 21 kg for the eight. That is, although the velocity of the rower-oars-boat system may remain relatively constant, the individual masses of the rower and boat will move dependently about each other. In an attempt to more accurately simulate the dynamics of on-water rowing, sliding ergometers were developed. In addition to a sliding seat, the sliding ergometer has a foot stretcher-flywheel complex that is mounted on a slide. This allows a transfer of momentum between the rower and the sliding complex (Figure 36.1).

Rowers report the 'feel' of the sliding ergometer to more accurately simulate on-water rowing (Mahony *et al.*, 1999). Previous comparisons of fixed and sliding ergometers have focused on physiological and external force variables. While physiological responses appear similar (Mahony *et al.*, 1999), differences in external force profiles have been reported at the handle, seat and foot stretcher (Kleshnev and Keshneva, 1995; Colloud *et al.*, 2006). It has been suggested that these differences result from the need to overcome larger inertial forces on the fixed ergometer (Kleshnev and Keshneva, 1995; Colloud *et al.*, 2006).

The different inertial requirements of the fixed and sliding ergometers may result in changes in mechanical stress at the lumbar spine during the drive as well as the recovery phases. Specific mechanical stresses of the lumbar spine have been identified as risk factors of lower back pain and injury (McGill, 2002). More specifically, estimations of mechanical compressive forces have been used to indicate lumbar stresses involved with physical activity.

Biomechanical modelling has been used extensively in an attempt to further the understanding of mechanical stresses involved in the lower back (McGill, 2002). Ergometer rowing requires motion predominantly in the flexion-extension plane and as such can be modelled in the sagittal plane only, although (Wilson *et al.*, 2012) found a small 4.7–8.8° range of motion in the frontal plane at L3. Motion analysis and 2D modelling for sagittal plane lifting tasks has been used by Dennis and Barrett (2002). Previous rowing studies have also employed 2D motion analysis and 2D biomechanical modelling in ergometer and on-water rowing (Kyröläinen and Smith, 1999; Morris *et al.*, 2000; Steer *et al.*, 2006). The use of 3D motion analysis will allow for more accurate determination of body segment motion (dynamic accuracy < 2.0 mm; Richards, 1999).

It is the aim of this study to accurately estimate the spinal compressive forces in elite rowers during the drive phase, while using Concept2 Fixed rowing ergometer (C2F), Concept2 Sliding rowing ergometer (slides fitted to front and rear stands, C2S) and Rowperfect (RP) rowing ergometers. It is hypothesized that due to increased inertial requirements, lumbar compressive forces will be greater when rowing on the C2F, compared to the C2S and RP ergometers during the drive phase.

Materials and methods

Subjects

Elite male rowers (*n* = 15) volunteered to participate in this study. Their mean age (± SD) was 25.2 ± 4.4 years, height 1.915 ± 0.072 m and body mass 91.0 ± 7.4 kg. The subjects were both elite heavyweight and lightweight rowers made up of Olympic and international representatives ($n = 10$) and national, state and university competitors ($n = 5$). Their average Concept2 2,000 m test performance was 6 minutes 9 seconds ± 13 seconds, with a range of 5 minutes 46 seconds to 6 minutes 34 seconds. There were four specialist scullers, six sweep oar rowers and five who trained for both sweep rowing and sculling. The frequency of training sessions ranged from 7–11 per week.

Subjects were required to be injury free and have no current, or history of, serious lower back injury. The subjects were fully informed of the risks associated with the experiment and gave written consent to participate. The Human Ethics Review Committee of the University of Sydney approved this study.

Experimental design

The experiment was a multivariate repeated measures design with three within subject factors: ergometer (three levels: C2F, C2S, RP); stroke rate (three levels: 20 strokes min^{-1}, 32 strokes min^{-1}, race pace); stroke (10 levels: 10 strokes); and two primary (maximum lumbar compressive forces, catch lumbar compressive forces) and seven secondary (stroke rate, handle force, average external power output, trunk acceleration, trunk-pelvis angle, hip movement, drive time) dependent variables. The external forces acting on the rower and the 3D motion of the rowing stroke were recorded during the three ergometer conditions. All three ergometers consisted of an air-braked flywheel connected to a handle via a recoiling chain. They were the stationary Concept2 Model C Indoor Rower (Concept2 Inc., Morrisville, VT, USA) (C2F), the Concept2 Model C with slides fitted to the front and rear stands (C2S) and the RowPerfect ergometer (RP), with free-floating stretcher mechanism (Rowperfect Australia) (Figure 36.1). The C2F, C2S and RP ergometer conditions were presented on the same day for each subject. The order of presentation was balanced to reduce carry-over effects.

Three different stroke rate conditions were tested on each ergometer to reflect normal training and racing. The stroke rates chosen for testing were 20 strokes per minute (to simulate training), 32 strokes per minute (an easily reproducible high stroke rate) and a Race Pace (RA) stroke rate (self-determined 2,000 m mid-race simulation). The three stroke rate conditions were presented in an incremental order (beginning with 20 strokes per minute) to minimize the effects of fatigue.

For the C2F and C2S trials, flywheel resistance was set on level 4 (used for heavyweight testing of Australian National Team rowers) and for the RP, the largest wind disc (400 mm diameter) was used (a setting commonly used by elite rowers). The rower was provided with visual information feedback of stroke rate via a digital display mounted on all ergometers (Speed Coach, Nielsen-Kellerman, Marcus Hook, PA, USA). The rowers were instructed to perform their usual rowing technique, especially in terms of stoke length and stroke rhythm.

All subjects had previous experience with all three ergometer conditions. Familiarization of 5-minute warm-up rowing on each ergometer was conducted immediately prior to testing. Subjects then performed 1 minute of rowing at each stroke rate, with a 1-minute rest period between stroke rate trials. The subjects were asked to row at 80 per cent maximal propulsive power for each stroke rate. This was a compromise between maximal and mid-race power per stroke as reported 2,000 m mid-race propulsive power is 60–70 per cent of maximal. The race pace condition was a self-determined 2,000 m mid-race stroke simulation. A rest period of 5 minutes was given between ergometer conditions, the ergometers were changed over and then familiarization and stroke rate trials were repeated. Total rowing time on each ergometer was approximately 8 minutes.

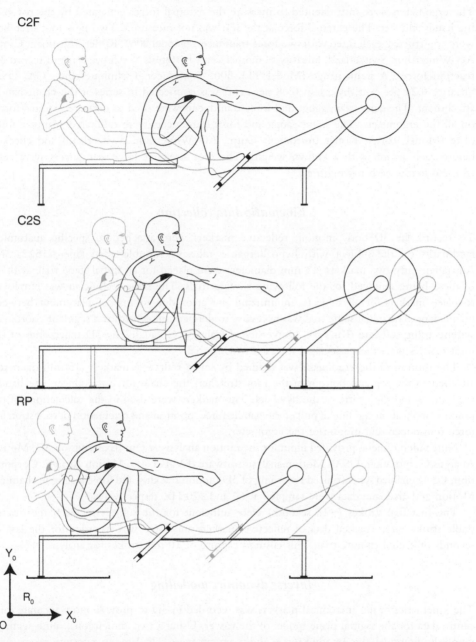

Figure 36.1 Representation of the Concept2 Fixed (C2F), Concept2 Sliding (C2S) and RowPerfect (RP) rowing ergometers and the interaction between rower and ergometer motions in the laboratory reference frame ($R_0 = (O, X_0, Y_0)$. Catch and finish positions of the rowing cycle are indicated by solid and broken lines, respectively.

Force data collection

The ergometers were instrumented to measure the external forces generated by the rower at the hands and feet. The external force at the seat was not measured. Two new foot stretchers were constructed, each fitted with two force transducers (Model 9067, Kistler Instrument Corp., AG Winterthur, Switzerland, linearity ≤ 0.5 per cent, hysteresis ≤ 0.5 per cent) to record 3D reaction forces. A strain gauge (Model TLL-500, Transducer Techniques Inc., CA, USA, linearity 0.24 per cent, hysteresis 0.08 per cent) was connected in series at the chain-handle attachment. The same strain gauge and force transducers were used to measure external forces on all the ergometers. The strain gauge and force transducers were calibrated against a force plate (Model 9281A, Kistler Instrument Corp., AG Winterthur, Switzerland) and checked before each session with a known weight. The foot stretcher force transducers were reset (zeroed) before each rowing trial.

Kinematic data collection

To record the 3D body motion, reflective markers were attached to specific anatomical landmarks on the subject with hypoallergenic adhesive (double-sided tape #1522, 3M, Australia). Fifty-two markers (15 mm diameter) were placed for an initial static trial, with 12 of these being removed for the following rowing trials. The same technician was employed to place markers for all subjects, minimizing the error due to marker placement between technicians. The initial static trial was necessary to define joint centres and segment coordinate systems using software (KinTrak, University of Calgary, Canada). The 3D trajectories of the joint centres were then calculated for each rowing trial.

The motion of the ergometer was defined by seven reflective markers (15 mm diameter) attached to the top and bottom of the foot stretcher, the chain force transducer, the handle extremities and the centre of the flywheel. The markers were used in the calculations of the point of application and line of pull of the handle force, position and orientation of foot stretcher force transducers and motion of the ergometer.

Nine video cameras provided input for the motion analysis system (Expertvision 3D, Motion Analysis Corporation, USA). Motion analysis software (EVaRT 4.0, Motion Analysis Corporation, USA) enabled synchronized recording of 3D motion tracking and force analogue channels. Motion and analogue data were sampled at 60 and 120 Hz, respectively.

The first five strokes (~ 15 seconds) were sufficient for the subject to reach the desired stable stroke rate. Tracked data of reflective markers and force was recorded for the last 45 seconds of each 1-minute trial. This ensured capture of 10 full strokes for analysis.

Inverse dynamics modelling

The kinematics of the anatomical markers was recorded in 3D to provide more accurate joint centre data for the sagittal plane model of the rower. Using a two-dimensional, nine-segment whole-body model, the net joint forces and moments were calculated in a custom programme based on the inverse dynamics method described by Winter (1979). An exception was that the sliding of the shoulder was also modelled, resulting in 19° of freedom. Air resistance was neglected.

The average position of the left and right limb joint centres and stretcher forces were calculated for the two-dimensional model. Segment masses were estimated using parameters from Kreighbaum and Barthels (1985) and the position of segment centre of mass and moment of inertia properties from Winter (1979), except for the trunk segment centre of mass, which was from Zatsiorsky (2002). The spectra of position and force data were analysed to determine optimum cut-off frequencies for the raw data according to the method of Giakas and Baltzopoulos (1997). The outcome of this analysis was a second-order Butterworth filter with a cut-off frequency of 5 Hz for position and 10 Hz for force data.

To determine the 2D mechanical actions of the pelvis on the trunk (i.e. net resultant force $\mathbf{F_{Trunk}}$ and net flexion moment M_{Trunk}), the inverse dynamics process started from the handle force, extending through the upper limb and down the trunk. The trunk segment, with embedded reference frame $\mathbf{R_T}$, was defined as a rigid body running from C7 along the spinal longitudinal axis to $O_{L4/L5}$. The inter-vertebral disc (IV disc) centroid, $O_{L4/L5}$, was estimated using the iliac crest at the most lateral part of the torso as the caudal level and mid-distance between the anterior and posterior skin surface along the iliac line, as the anterior-posterior coordinate (McGill, 2003; McGill et al., 1988) (Figure 36.2). The trunk-pelvis angle was defined as the anterior included angle between the trunk and pelvis segments.

A separate inverse dynamics calculation was initiated starting from the foot stretcher force; this extended up the lower limb to estimate the net hip moment. The calculation from the handle-down previously used to calculate the net lumbar mechanical actions was continued to also estimate the net hip moment. The root mean square difference (RMS difference) between the two estimates was used as an accuracy estimate of the inverse dynamics method.

Spinal modelling

The current study used a sagittal model of the lumbar spine to partition $\mathbf{F_{Trunk}}$ and M_{Trunk} into extensor muscle force ($\mathbf{F_{ES}}$) and resultant bone-on-bone force at L4/L5 ($\mathbf{F_{L4/L5}}$) (Figure 36.2). All these vectors were expressed in $\mathbf{R_T}$. The lumbar extensor muscles were considered to act as a common extensor group about $O_{L4/L5}$ with a common moment arm of 0.0623 m (d_{ES}). The muscle moment arm and muscle line of action used, was that reported by McGill et al. (1993), α being the angle between the line of muscle action and the longitudinal axis of $\mathbf{R_T}$, with a cosine of 0.949. Intra-abdominal pressure was considered to make no contribution to M_{Trunk} in the current model. The extension moment due to intra-abdominal pressure may be very small or cancelled out by the compression force produced by contraction of the abdominal muscles, and would become even less in a flexed position (McGill and Norman, 1986). The current model can only account for compressive forces due to an extension moment. During a flexion moment, the anterior musculature of the abdomen needs to be considered to accurately estimate lumbar spinal forces. Accordingly, the net lumbar moment was considered to be solely due to $\mathbf{F_{ES}}$ acting at d_{ES} from $O_{L4/L5}$ in $\mathbf{R_T}$ (Eqn. 1). This allowed determination of $\mathbf{F_{ES}}$ (Eqn. 3). $\mathbf{F_{L4/L5}}$ was resolved into a compressive (F_{Comp}) component. Positive F_{Comp} was defined

Table 36.1 Equations for spinal compressive (F_{Comp}) force calculations

M_{Trunk}	$=$	$\lVert \mathbf{F_{ES}} \rVert \cdot d_{ES}$		(1)
$\lVert \mathbf{F_{ES}} \rVert$	$=$	$((F_{ESX})^2$	$+\ (F_{ESY})^2)^{1/2}$	(2)
$\lVert \mathbf{F_{ES}} \rVert$	$=$	$-M_{Trunk} / d_{ES}$		(3)
F_{TrunkY}	$=$	F_{Comp}	$-\ F_{ESY}$	(4)
F_{ESY}	$=$	$\lVert \mathbf{F_{ES}} \rVert \cdot \cos \alpha$		(5)
F_{Comp}	$=$	F_{TrunkY}	$+\ \lVert \mathbf{F_{ES}} \rVert \cdot \cos \alpha$	(6)

Vectors are considered from the pelvis acting on the trunk expressed in the frame embedded in the trunk segment ($\mathbf{R_T}$).

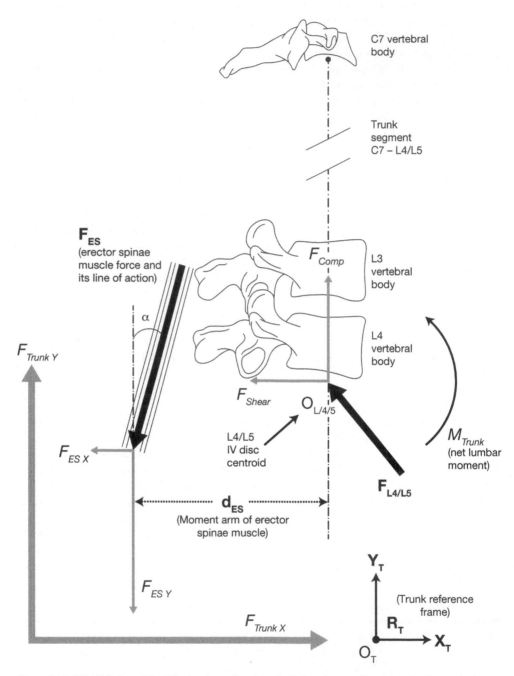

Figure 36.2 Simplified model of the lumbar spine for calculating shear and compressive forces during the rowing action. Vectors are considered from the pelvis acting on the trunk expressed in the trunk frame ($R_T = O_T$, X_T, Y_T).

as the inferior force acting parallel to the trunk segment through the spinal axis. F_{Comp} was determined by the sum of the trunk axial component ($F_{Trunk\ Y}$) of the resultant joint force and the extensor trunk axial component ($||\ \mathbf{F_{ES}}\ ||\ \cdot\cos\alpha$) of the muscle force (Eqn. 6).

Handle external power output was computed as the dot product of force on and velocity of the handle. The product of horizontal force on and velocity of the stretcher realized the stretcher external power output. Average total external power was calculated by summing the instantaneous handle and the stretcher power and taking the mean value over each stroke.

Analysis of results

Ten full strokes were analysed from each rowing trial. These rowing stokes were defined by the absolute handle displacement relative to ergometer position, beginning at the catch when the handle begins its negative horizontal displacement and finishing at the completion of a full stroke (Figure 36.1). Then, each stroke was normalized to 100 per cent stroke and force-time stroke profiles were constructed for desired variables. Ensemble force-time stroke profiles represent the mean of all subjects and strokes for one condition, 95 per cent confidence intervals were included to indicate variability across subjects. Variable-time profiles were constructed for compressive force, handle force, lumbar moment, lumbar angle, trunk acceleration and net hip moment.

Discrete mean values represented the ensemble mean of all subjects and strokes for the desired variable. Mean discrete variables included compressive forces at the catch, maximum compressive and handle forces, timing of maximum compressive and handle forces, joint angle at maximum spinal forces, stroke characteristics and RMS difference between net hip moment calculations.

Statistical analysis

Multivariate analysis of variance with repeated measures (SPSS for Windows, SPSS Inc., USA) was used to test the significance of any observed differences in the means. The degrees of freedom were adjusted (Huyn-Feldt) if the data failed Mauchly's test of sphericity. A priori contrasts (simple for ergometer and stroke rate, polynomial for stroke) and post hoc pairwise comparisons were used. A Bonferroni adjustment was made for pairwise comparisons and multiple dependent variables.

Results

The rowing stroke can be separated into two phases, drive and recovery. The drive phase begins at the catch and ends at the finish position. The recovery phase begins at the finish position and ends at the catch for the following stroke (Figure 36.1).

Comparison of stroke profiles between stroke rates revealed similar patterns for all variables. Differences between stroke profiles due to stroke rate were observed in the magnitude of forces and proportional changes in the time taken for the whole rowing stroke. Stroke profiles for higher stroke rates exhibited larger magnitude of forces in both maxima and minima of the curves. For the lower stroke rates, stroke profile changes in the proportion of drive and recovery time resulted in the curve for the drive phase being compressed to the left, followed by an extended recovery curve.

Drive and recovery phases of the rowing stroke are separated on the figure (Figure 36.3) by lines indicating the catch, finish and catch for the following stroke. As the patterns were similar across stroke rates, the stroke profiles chosen for presentation are the ensemble means for the race pace condition.

Rowing consistency was evidenced by the lack of any effect of stroke on any of the tested variables or interaction with ergometer or stroke rate.

Lumbar compressive forces

Force-time stroke profiles

The pattern of the net lumbar moment stroke profile closely matched the curve of the compressive force stroke profile. Values of maximum extension moment at race pace were 250–300 Nm. Only compressive (Figure 36.3a) forces due to a lumbar extension moment (positive forces in stroke profiles) are considered relevant as during a lumbar flexion moment the anterior musculature of the abdomen may contribute to spinal forces and have not been included in the current spinal model.

Compressive force was high at the catch and during early drive phase, increasing to reach a peak at mid drive phase. For the remainder of the drive phase, compressive force declined sharply, reaching zero at about 35–40 per cent stroke. During the recovery, compressive force gradually increased, from zero at ~ 60 per cent stroke, returning to high values at the new catch.

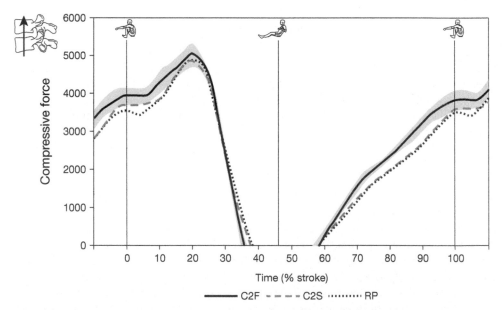

Figure 36.3a Stroke profile of ensemble mean compressive force at race pace for the three ergometer conditions. The C2F ergometer condition is shown as a solid line with the shading representing the 95 per cent confidence interval. Rower figures indicate stages of the stroke: catch, finish and new catch positions. A positive value indicates a force acting to compress L4 onto L5.

The compressive force stroke profile was similar for all subjects as indicated by the 95 per cent confidence intervals. The RP and C2S ergometers have very similar compressive force profiles and all ergometers have similar peak compressive force at mid drive phase (21 per cent stroke). The C2F curve shows compressive force on the fixed ergometer to be significantly greater than the two sliding ergometers during early drive phase (0–13 per cent stroke) and again in recovery (66–100 per cent stroke) ($p > 0.05$).

Lumbar compressive forces at the catch

Ensemble mean lumbar compressive forces were analysed at the catch and at maximum values during the drive phase. Compressive forces increased with increased stroke rate for all conditions ($p < 0.001$) and showed distinct differences between ergometer conditions.

Lumbar compressive force at the catch was significantly different between all ergometer conditions ($p < 0.001$) (Table 36.2). C2F produced the largest compressive force at the catch, followed by C2S and RP produced the least. Effect size for interaction due to ergometer was large and differences in means (for all stroke rates) ranged from 150 N (C2F versus C2S) to 435 N (C2F versus RP). At race pace C2F, compressive force was 6 per cent larger than C2S and 9 per cent larger than RP (as per cent of C2F). Compressive force at the catch on C2F was 77 per cent of compressive force at maximum and slightly less (~ 70 per cent) for both the sliding ergometers.

Maximum lumbar compressive forces

Maximum compressive forces for each ergometer and stroke rate condition are presented in Table 36.2.

There were no differences observed in maximum compressive force between C2S and both RP and C2F. Mean maximum compressive force was greater when rowing on the C2F ergometer compared to the RP ergometer ($p < 0.01$). While this was a significant difference the effect size was not large (Eta^2 = 0.334) and at race pace the difference between mean values represented a 3 per cent increase in compressive force on the C2F (166 N).

Average compressive forces were calculated as the mean of the positive curve during drive phase. At race pace, average drive phase compressive forces were C2F: 3,675 N for C2S: 3,373 N and RP: 3,361 N. During the drive phase, the fixed ergometer produced 8–9 per cent larger compressive force compared to the sliding ergometers.

Trunk motion

Trunk acceleration

Figure 36.3b shows the ensemble mean absolute horizontal acceleration of the trunk segment centre of gravity (COG) throughout the stroke. The two sliding ergometers have very similar trunk acceleration profiles. The C2F has much greater trunk acceleration when compared to the RP and C2S ergometers. C2F trunk acceleration ranges from a negative peak in early drive phase of -7.9 m.s^{-2}, to a positive peak in late drive phase of 7.3 m.s^{-2}, a range of 15.2 m.s^{-2}. Both the sliding ergometers require much less trunk acceleration, a range of 9.2 m.s^{-2} (-5.6–3.6 m.s^{-2}, which represents about 60 per cent of C2F range).

Table 36.2 Mean and SD for all variables, comparisons between ergometer conditions, power and effect size.

Stroke rate	C2F	C2S	RP	Comparison over all stroke rates (pair)	Sig.	For the effect of ergometer	
						Power	Effect size
	Maximum Lumbar Compressive Force						
20	4290 ± 103	4210 ± 109	4010 ± 124	C2F versus C2S	0.167	0.898	0.334
32	4770 ± 96	4630 ± 100	4610 ± 108	C2F versus RP	0.008		
RA	4980 ± 128	4820 ± 99	4820 ± 111	C2S versus RP	0.394		
	Maximum Lumbar Shear Force						
20	2040 ± 44	2040 ± 59	2000 ± 64	C2F versus C2S	0.954	0.138	0.042
32	2310 ± 39	2270 ± 47	2330 ± 49	C2F versus RP	1.000		
RA	2430 ± 54	2370 ± 51	2440 ± 54	C2S versus RP	0.862		
	Catch Lumbar Compressive Force						
20	3300 ± 93	2970 ± 85	2790 ± 80	C2F versus C2S	0.000	1.000	0.818
32	3670 ± 114	3380 ± 88	3220 ± 78	C2F versus RP	0.000		
RA	3790 ± 120	3550 ± 89	3440 ± 84	C2S versus RP	0.000		
	Stroke Rate						
20	20.9 ± 0.13	21.1 ± 0.25	21.2 ± 0.19	C2F versus C2S	0.043	0.947	0.440
32	31.6 ± 0.22	32.2 ± 0.20	32.0 ± 0.23	C2F versus RP	0.003		
RA	34.8 ± 0.46	36.2 ± 0.63	37.0 ± 0.64	C2S versus RP	0.298		
	Maximum Handle Force						
20	887 ± 23	860 ± 32	861 ± 32	C2F versus C2S	0.001	0.948	0.424
32	1010 ± 21	946 ± 23	980 ± 26	C2F versus RP	0.131		
RA	1070 ± 25	977 ± 26	1010 ± 27	C2S versus RP	0.141		
	Drive Time						
20	1.02 ± 0.02	0.98 ± 0.02	0.98 ± 0.02	C2F versus C2S	0.009	0.972	0.453
32	0.83 ± 0.01	0.81 ± 0.01	0.81 ± 0.01	C2F versus RP	0.007		
RA	0.79 ± 0.01	0.76 ± 0.01	0.75 ± 0.01	C2S versus RP	1.000		
	External Power						
20	278 ± 10	280 ± 13	269 ± 10	C2F versus C2S	0.520	0.511	0.168
32	467 ± 15	473 ± 14	476 ± 13	C2F versus RP	0.167		
RA	526 ± 23	551 ± 22	581 ± 24	C2S versus RP	0.855		

20: 20 strokes per minute; 32: 32 strokes per minute; RA: race pace; C2F: Concept2 fixed ergometer; C2S: Concept2 sliding ergometer; RP: RowPerfect ergometer.

Trunk-pelvis angle

Trunk-pelvis angle throughout the stroke followed a similar pattern for all stroke rates. However, there was substantial variability between subjects for the trunk-pelvis stroke profile. The most consistent feature was an increased flexion from ~ 20–30 per cent of the stroke. Mean trunk-pelvis angle at the catch for the race pace condition was ~ 146° on C2F and ~ 148° on both C2S and RP. Trunk-pelvis angles at the catch were generally greater than at the time of maximum spinal force production (corresponds to 22 per cent of stroke, detailed below).

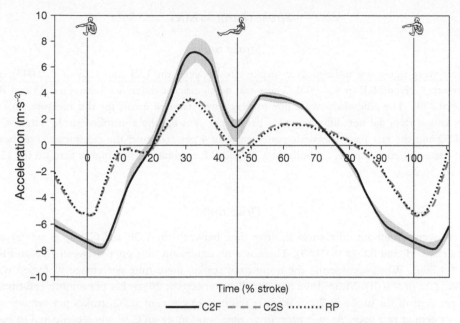

Figure 36.3b Stroke profile of ensemble mean horizontal acceleration of trunk segment COG at race pace for the three ergometer conditions. Positive values represent anterior acceleration. The C2F ergometer condition is shown as a solid line with the shading representing the 95 per cent confidence interval. Rower figures indicate stages of the stroke: catch, finish and new catch positions.

Table 36.3 Ensemble mean RMS error for ergometer and stroke rate conditions

	Mean RMS error (± SD)		
	Concept2 Fixed	Concept2 Sliding	RowPerfect
20 strokes per minute	24.3 ± 9.6	32.1 ± 22.8	45.3 ± 37.8
32 strokes per minute	29.6 ± 9.3	27.9 ± 10.1	49.5 ± 39.9
Race pace	36.4 ± 19.5	32.7 ± 12.3	48.0 ± 35.5

Inverse dynamics validation

The net hip moments calculated from the 'handle-down' and from the 'stretcher-up' were compared to provide validation for the inverse dynamics approach. The two different calculations gave similar hip moments within stroke rate and ergometer conditions. Mean RMS difference between the net hip moments of the stretcher-up and handle-down inverse dynamics methods provided good validation of the moment calculation at ~ 5 per cent of the peak-to-peak amplitude of the hip joint moment (Table 36.3).

Stroke characteristics

Stroke rate

There were significant differences in stroke rate between the C2F and C2S (p = 0.043) and between C2F and RP (p = 0.003). There was no significant difference between C2S and RP (p = 0.298). The differences were due to very small standard errors for this measure. In fact the strokes rates did not differ by more than 1 per cent for the controlled stroke rates of 20 and 32 and the race pace was within an average of 4 per cent over the ergometer conditions. Self- determined race pace, on both the C2S and RP ergometers, was higher than on the C2F (Table 36.2).

Drive time

There were significant differences in drive time between the C2F and C2S (p = 0.009) and between C2F and RP (p = 0.007). There was no significant difference between C2S and RP (p = 1.000). When considering the normalized stroke, drive time percentage increased with stroke rate (p < 0.01). Mean drive time for all ergometers at 20 strokes per minute constituted 35 per cent of the stroke at 20 strokes per minute, 43 per cent at 32 strokes per minute and 46 per cent at race pace. At race pace, drive time was longer on C2F when compared to both the sliding ergometers. This difference represented 1–2 per cent of total stroke time.

Handle force

Handle force profile was similar for all stroke rate conditions. Handle force increased with stroke rate for all conditions. There was a significant difference in handle force between the C2F and C2S (p = 0.001) but not between C2F and RP (p = 0.131) or between C2S and RP (p = 0.141). Maximum handle force was higher on C2F compared to C2S by 63 N (~ 6 per cent of maximum handle force) at race pace (Table 36.2).

A consistent feature of the handle force stroke profiles was the difference in onset time of handle force between the ergometer conditions. Onset of handle force was similar on C2S and RP, however, on C2F the lag in application of handle force was almost double (1.8 times the RP or C2S lag).

Timing of peak handle force was different for the fixed and sliding ergometers. However, the differences were only 1–2 per cent of total stroke time. Mean maximum handle force on the C2F ergometer was consistently later than both the sliding ergometers. The RP ergometer reached peak handle force earlier than both the Concept2 ergometers. The ensemble mean time to maximum handle force for the race pace condition was 22.2 ± 2.3 per cent of stroke (mean of C2F, C2S and RP).

External power

The mean average external powers across ergometers were 275 W (20 strokes per minute), 472 W (32 strokes per minute) and 553 W (race pace). There were no significant differences in the comparisons between the ergometers (Table 36.2). The actual differences among the means were limited to 1.6, 0.7 and 3.4 per cent, respectively.

Discussion

Compressive forces

Compressive force profiles, for the fixed and both the sliding ergometer conditions, indicate that the lumbar spine is under considerable stress during ergometer rowing. The most significant differences between ergometers were observed at the catch. The C2F ergometer produced consistently larger compressive forces at the catch, when compared to the C2S and RP ergometers.

Differences in lumbar stress between the fixed and sliding ergometers at the catch cannot be attributed to differences in handle force profiles as the handle force is zero at the catch. When no force is applied to the handle, the force produced by the rower is used only to accelerate the stretcher complex and the body mass (in opposite directions). As the stretcher is stationary on the fixed ergometer, all force produced by the rower at the catch is used to accelerate the rower COG. In comparison to the sliding ergometers, the C2F exhibits far greater horizontal trunk acceleration at the catch. As the handle force is zero, the net lumbar moment at the catch is determined largely by the required acceleration of the trunk, head and arms. Therefore, at the catch, the significantly larger compressive forces produced are the result of the larger body mass acceleration requirements of the fixed ergometer.

In contrast to the scenario at the catch, differences in maximum compressive force may be related to handle force. Maximum compressive force and maximum handle force occur simultaneously, at ~ 21–22 per cent of stroke. At this time, horizontal trunk acceleration is close to zero on all ergometers. Horizontal trunk acceleration is not a complete measure of the inertial contributions to the net lumbar moment. However, it gives a good indication of the magnitude and direction of upper body mass acceleration and the differences between fixed and sliding ergometers. Accordingly, when trunk acceleration is minimal, net lumbar moment is predominantly determined by the magnitude of handle force.

The C2F ergometer tended to produce higher maximum handle force. These handle force differences, rather than the effects of body COG acceleration, are the most likely contributors to the increased maximum compressive force observed on the C2F. These differences in maximum compressive force were not large. However, the combination of acceleration effects and handle force differences in early drive phase, result in a consistently greater compressive force produced on the C2F ergometer, for a large proportion of the stroke (~ 45 per cent).

Risks of injuries

Mean maximum compressive forces exceeded the National Institute for Occupational Safety and Health (NIOSH) manual handling recommendations (1994) for safe lifting (3,400 N) during all stroke rate and ergometer conditions (Munro and Yanai, 2000; National Institute for Occupational Safety and Health, 1994). The vertebral body is the most likely to be injured by a purely compressive load and this recommended maximum compressive force is based on cadaver experiments of vertebral breaking limits. However, this limit considers only static lifting situations. For the trunk, rowing can be considered as a repetitive, dynamic, flexion-extension movement. Repetitive dynamic movements, with large inertial force components, may place structures other than just the vertebral body at risk of injury.

Most resistance to flexion comes from the IV ligaments (~ 70 per cent). A comprehensive review of mechanical risks of damage to the lumbar spine (Adams and Dolan, 1995) identifies IV ligaments as the most likely structure to be damaged by forward bending movements. As tension increases in these ligaments, there is also an increased compression force on the IV discs. Compression forces at full flexion can increase by up to 100 per cent. Adams and Dolan (1995) also suggest that compressive forces > 3,000 N, for repetitive movements involving a large range of lumbar flexion, place the IV disc at risk of gradual prolapse injury.

Caldwell *et al.* (2003) reported a large range of flexion in the lumbar spine. At the catch they found 74–89 per cent of maximal static lumbar flexion. Compressive force at the catch, in the current study, exceeded 3,000 N at 32 strokes per minute and race pace, on all ergometers. This threshold was also exceeded on C2F at 20 strokes per minute, a stroke rate typical for long distance aerobic training sessions. At this stroke rate, both C2S and RP kept below this limit with 10 and 15 per cent lower compressive force, respectively, at the catch than C2F.

Spinal stress due to a flexed loaded posture has been considered a mechanical risk of LBI during rowing for many years (Stallard, 1980). The extensor muscles of the back are described by Hagerman (1984) as being anatomically weak during rowing, especially at the catch. Increased lumbar flexion at the catch has been suggested to place substantial stress on the passive structures of the lumbar spine (Caldwell *et al.*, 2003; Reid and McNair, 2000). When the lumbar region is flexed at > 75 per cent of maximum, considerable tension is distributed among the non-contractile tissues (Adams *et al.*, 1994). These include the lumbodorsal fascia, intervertebral ligament (IV ligaments), IV discs and the non-contractile components of spinal extensor muscles. Muscle activation of the back extensors has been shown to be low during the catch (~ 20–30 per cent MVC) (Kyröläinen and Smith, 1999; Caldwell *et al.*, 2003). Accordingly, a large proportion of the net lumbar moment must be supported by the passive structures of the lumbar spine.

Trunk-pelvis angle

The trunk-pelvis angle presented in this study is difficult to compare to previously reported values. Flexion of the lumbar spine has been reported by Caldwell *et al.* (2003) and some studies report the absolute angle of the trunk and pelvis segments, but not the interaction between the two.

Bull and McGregor (2000) found that the absolute angle, of both the trunk and pelvis, tends to extend throughout the drive phase. However, in an attempt to characterize normal lumbo-pelvic technique, only a large variability between subjects ($n = 6$) was reported. Similar results were observed in the current study. The absolute angles of the trunk and pelvis segments followed similar trends of extension during the drive phase. Trunk-pelvis angle, between the segments, varied considerably. This variability may be explained by individual anatomical variations. Differences in body structure require the application of different techniques to achieve maximum effectiveness for the individual.

Interestingly, the trunk-pelvis angle indicated that, in the catch position, the rower's trunk and pelvis were relatively extended. Caldwell *et al.* (2003) found a large range of lumbar flexion at the catch, in secondary school rowers. Lumbar flexion at the catch was considered an important factor in lumbar tissues stress during ergometer rowing. These authors suggest that if pelvis could be held in a more anteriorly rotated posture at the catch, this may help reduce the range of lumbar flexion and resulting passive tissue stress. It is possible that as the subjects in the current study were elite, international class oarsmen, the extended trunk-pelvis angle observed may be due to technical adaptation. The inclusion criteria of the study limited volunteers to those without history of serious LBP. It is possible that non-elite rowers exhibit different patterns of lumbar-pelvic motion. At this very elite level, it is possible that the oarsmen, who have survived the years of training and competition without serious LBI, may have developed technical skills to deal with the lumbar stress challenge of rowing, while maintaining performance.

The most consistent feature of trunk–pelvis angle between subjects was an increased flexion through the mid to late drive phase (~ 20–30 per cent of stroke). This is possibly a result of the peaking of handle force. If the trunk–pelvis angle can be considered indicative of lumbar flexion, then it seems that the lower back is held in substantial flexion throughout the propulsive phase of the stroke. This rounded position of the lower back is technically advantageous, as it minimizes the vertical movement of the body mass throughout the drive phase. This position may also provide considerable resistance to compressive force as Adams *et al.* (1994) suggest that moderate flexion of the lumbar spine is the optimal posture for safe resistance of large compressive loads.

It seems that despite individual anatomical and technical variability, there are several observations regarding technique. A posture at the catch of increased anterior rotation of the pelvis may help reduce stress on the lumbar spine. During the drive phase, a moderately flexed lumbar posture may be suited to optimal compressive force resistance and technical effectiveness.

Inverse dynamic validation

Comparison of the net hip moments calculated by the two different inverse dynamics approaches was used as a measure of validity of the inverse dynamics calculations. Average difference for C2F and C2S was 15 and 20 Nm, respectively, and was less than the average error on RP of 36 Nm. A similar inverse dynamics comparison for a sagittal plane lifting task found a correlation of $r = 0.99$ for net lumbar moments calculated by both models with an average difference of 4–9 Nm (de Looze *et al.*, 1992). While these results are considerably more accurate than our own, this is most likely due to differences in the body segment accelerations in rowing compared to the lifting task.

Conclusions

At the catch, rowing on the C2F ergometer produced consistently larger compressive loading of the lumbar spine, compared to the C2S and RP ergometers. This was due to the large body acceleration requirements of the stroke while rowing on the fixed ergometer.

Maximum compressive force was related to handle force production and exceeded recommendations for safe loading in both static and repetitive activities. This maximum compression force may place the vertebral body at risk, while the large compressive force produced during repetitive flexion at the catch, may lead to injuries of the IV ligaments and discs in particular during long distance aerobic training.

It is possible that these elite male rowers have found a safe posture for the lumbar spine at the time of maximum compressive loading. Further research into trunk–pelvic motion, posture and range of lumbar flexion is needed to determine technique contribution to risk of LBI. Differences in females and sub-elite rowers are also of interest.

It seems that at the catch, differences in compressive forces can be attributed to the effects of upper body acceleration which, in turn, depend on the ratio of body mass to ergometer/fan assembly mass. Even greater differences may be obtained if the mass of the instrumentation for the stretcher could be reduced. During mid drive phase, differences in maximum compressive force can be explained by different handle force production. While these results emphasize the significant mechanical stress on the lower back during ergometer rowing, similar research is needed during on-water rowing. Additional components of on-water rowing, such as rotation of the trunk during the sweep, may contribute to lower back stress.

Nomenclature

α	Angle between the line of muscle action and the longitudinal axis of R_T (cosine of this angle is 0.949)
catch	Event in the rowing stroke that separates the recovery phase from the drive phase
d_{ES}	Moment arm from L4/L5 IV disc centroid to $\mathbf{F_{ES}}$
drive phase	Propulsive part of the rowing stroke, begins at the catch and ends at the finish
drive time	The time done from catch to finish during the rowing stroke
ES	Common extensor muscle group acting at $O_{L4/L5}$
F_{Comp}	Vertical component of $\mathbf{F_{L4/L5}}$ expressed in R_T
$\|\ \mathbf{F_{ES}}\ \|$	Modulus of the resultant force $\mathbf{F_{ES}}$
$\mathbf{F_{ES}}$	Resultant force of L5 acting on L4 due to extensor muscles of the lumbar spine expressed in R_T
$F_{ES\,X}$	Horizontal component of $\mathbf{F_{ES}}$ expressed in R_T
$F_{ES\,Y}$	Vertical component of $\mathbf{F_{ES}}$ expressed in R_T
finish	Event in the rowing stroke that separates the drive phase from the recovery phase
$\mathbf{F_{L4/L5}}$	Resultant bone-on-bone force acting at L4/L5
F_{Shear}	Horizontal component of $\mathbf{F_{L4/L5}}$ expressed in R_T
$\mathbf{F_{Trunk}}$	Resultant joint force acting on the trunk expressed in R_T
$F_{Trunk\,X}$	Horizontal component of $\mathbf{F_{Trunk}}$
$F_{Trunk\,Y}$	Vertical component of $\mathbf{F_{Trunk}}$
handle force	Absolute forces exerted by the handle on the rower
IV disc	Inter-vertebral disc
IV ligament	Inter-vertebral ligament
M_{Trunk}	Net moment of the pelvis acting on the trunk expressed in $O_{L4/L5}$ and projected in R_T
O	Origin of R_0
$O_{L4/L5}$	Centre of the L4/L5 IV disc
O_T	Origin of R_T
R_0	The laboratory reference frame
RA	Self determined 2,000 m mid-race stroke rate
R_T	The reference frame embedded in the trunk segment
recovery time	The time done from finish to catch during the rowing stroke
stretcher force	Absolute forces exerted by the stretcher on the rower
stroke length	Absolute horizontal displacement of the handle relative to the stretcher from catch to finish
stroke rate	Number of strokes performed by the rower during 1 minute (strokes per minute)
θ	Angle between the line of pull of the handle and the horizontal axis X_0
trunk acceleration	Absolute horizontal acceleration of the COG of the trunk

trunk-pelvis angle	The anterior included angle formed by the trunk and pelvis segments
X_0	Horizontal component of R_0
X_T	Horizontal component of R_T
Y_0	Vertical component of R_0
Y_T	Vertical component of R_T

Acknowledgements

Floren Colloud was granted by a Bourse Lavoisier from the French Foreign Office. We wish to thank the subjects who gave their time and effort to participate as well as coaches of NSWIS, Sydney University Boat Club and UTS Boat Club for helping with recruiting subjects. Thanks to Ray Patton, Professional Officer and laboratory manager, Exercise Health and Performance Research Group, The University of Sydney, for his technical assistance throughout this project.

References

Adams, M. A. and Dolan, P. (1995) 'Recent advances in lumbar spinal mechanics and their clinical significance', *Clinical Biomechanics*, 10(1): 3–19.

Adams, M. A., McNally, D. S., Chinn, H. and Dolan, P. (1994) 'Posture and the compressive strength of the lumbar spine', *Clinical Biomechanics*, 9(1): 5–14.

Bull, A. M. J. and McGregor, A. H. (2000) 'Measuring spinal motion in rowers: the use of an electromagnetic device', *Clinical Biomechanics*, 15(10): 772–6.

Caldwell, S. J., McNair, P. J. and Maynard, W. (2003) 'The effects of repetitive motion on lumbar flexion and erector spinae muscle activity in rowers', *Clinical Biomechanics*, 18(8): 704–11.

Colloud, F., Bahaud, P., Doriot, N., Champely, S. and Chèze, L. (2006) 'Fixed versus free-floating stretcher mechanism in rowing ergometers: mechanical aspects', *Journal of Sports Sciences*, 24: 479–93.

de Looze, M. P., Kingma, I., Toussaint, H. M. and Bussmann, J. B. J. (1992) 'Validation of a dynamic linked segment model to calculate joint moments in lifting', *Clinical Biomechanics*, 7(3): 161–9.

Dennis, G. J. and Barrett, R. S. (2002) 'Spinal loads during individual and team lifting', *Ergonomics*, 45(10): 671–81.

Giakas, G. and Baltzopoulos, V. (1997) 'Optimal digital filtering requires a different cut-off frequency strategy for the determination of the higher derivatives', *Journal of Biomechanics*, 30(8): 851–5.

Goodman, N. and Hooper, I. (2008) *2007 Australian Rowing Teams: A Discussion of Illness and Injury Statistics*, Canberra: Rowing Australia.

Hagerman, F. C. (1984) 'Applied physiology of rowing', *Sports Medicine*, 1(4): 303–26.

Hickey, G. J., Fricker, P. A. and McDonald, W. A. (1997) 'Injuries to elite rowers over a 10-yr period', *Medicine and Science in Sports Exercise*, 29(12): 1567–72.

Kleshnev, V. and Keshneva, E. (1995) 'Biomechanical features of rowing on devices with mobile or stationary workplace', *Proceedings of the XVth Congress of the International Society of Biomechanics*, Jyvaskyla: University of Jyvaskyla, pp. 482–3.

Kreighbaum, E. and Barthels, K. M. (1985) *Biomechanics: A Qualitative Approach for Studying Human Movement*, 2nd edn, Minneapolis, MN: Burgess Pub. Co.

Kyröläinen, H. and Smith, R. (1999) 'Mechanical power output and muscle activities during maximal rowing with different stroke rates', *Journal of Human Movement Studies*, 36(2): 75–94.

McGill, S. M. (2002) *Low Back Disorders: Evidence-based Prevention and Rehabilitation*, Champaign, IL: Human Kinetics.

McGill, S. M. (2003) Personal correspondence.

McGill, S. M., Patt, N. and Norman, R.W. (1988) 'Measurement of the trunk musculature of active males using CT scan radiography: implications for force and moment generating capacity about the L4/L5 joint', *Journal of Biomechanics*, 21(4): 329–41.

McGill, S. M. and Norman, R. W. (1986) 'Partitioning of the L4-L5 dynamic moment into disc, ligamentous, and muscular components during lifting', *Spine*, 11(7): 666–78.

McGill, S. M., Santaguida, L. and Stevens, J. (1993) 'Measurement of the trunk musculature from T5 to L5 using MRI scans of 15 young males corrected for muscle fibre orientation', *Clinical Biomechanics*, 8(4): 171–8.

Mahony, N., Donne, B. and O'Brien, M. (1999) 'A comparison of physiological responses to rowing on friction-loaded and air-braked ergometers', *Journal of Sports Sciences*, 17(2): 143–9.

Maurer, M., Soder, R. B. and Baldisserotto, M. (2011) 'Spine abnormalities depicted by magnetic resonance imaging in adolescent rowers', *The American Journal of Sports Medicine*, 39(2): 392–7.

Morris, F. L., Smith, R. M., Payne, W. R., Galloway, M. A., and Wark, J. D. (2000) 'Compressive and shear force generated in the lumbar spine of female rowers', *International Journal of Sports Medicine*, 21: 519–23.

Munro, C. and Yanai, T. (2000) 'Forces on the lower back during rowing performance in a single scull', *Proceedings of XVIII International Symposium on Biomechanics in Sports*, Hong Kong: The Chinese University of Hong Kong, pp. 186–9.

National Institute for Occupational Safety and Health (1994) *Applications Manual for the Revised NIOSH Lifting Equation*, Atlanta, GA: National Institute for Occupational Safety and Health.

Reid, D. A. and McNair, P. J. (2000) 'Factors contributing to low back pain in rowers', *British Journal of Sports Medicine*, 34(5): 321–2.

Richards, J. G. (1999) 'The measurement of human motion: a comparison of commercially available systems', *Human Movement Science*, 18: 589–602.

Roy, S. H., De Luca, C. J., Snyder-Mackler, L., Emley, M. S., Crenshaw, R. L. and Lyons, J. P. (1990) 'Fatigue, recovery, and low back pain in varsity rowers', *Medicine and Science in Sports Exercise*, 22(4): 463–9.

Stallard, M. C. (1980) 'Backache in oarsmen', *British Journal of Sports Medicine*, 14(2–3): 105–8.

Steer, R. R., Mcgregor, A. H. and Bull, A. M. J. (2006) 'A comparison of kinematics and performance measures of two rowing ergometers', *Journal of Sports Science and Medicine*, 5: 52–9.

Strahan, A. D., Burnett, A. F., Caneiro, J. P., Doyle, M. M., O'Sullivan, P. B. and Goodman, C. (2011) 'Differences in spinopelvic kinematics in sweep and scull ergometer rowing', *Clinical Journal of Sport Medicine*, 21(4): 330–6.

Teitz, C. C., O'Kane, J., Lind, B. K. and Hannafin, J. A. (2001) 'Back pain in intercollegiate rowers', *American Journal of Sports Medicine*, 30(5): 674–9.

Wilson, F., Gissane, C., Gormley, J. and Simms, C. (2010) 'A 12-month prospective cohort study of injury in international rowers', *British Journal of Sports Medicine*, 44(3): 207–14.

Wilson, F., Gormley, J., Gissane, C. and Simms, C. (2012) 'The effect of rowing to exhaustion on frontal plane angular changes in the lumbar spine of elite rowers', *Journal of Sports Sciences*, 30(14): 1481–9.

Winter, D. A. (1979) *Biomechanics of Human Movement*, 1st edn, New York: Wiley Interscience.

Winzen, M., Voigt, H. F., Hinrichs, T. and Platen, P. (2011) 'Injuries of the musculoskeletal system in German elite rowers', *Sportverletzung-Sportschaden*, 25(3): 153–8.

Zatsiorsky, V. M. (2002) *Kinetics of Human Motion*, Champaign, IL: Human Kinetics.

37

PROTECTIVE HEADGEAR IN SPORTS

Kevin Laudner[1] and Robert C. Lynall[2]

[1]ILLINOIS STATE UNIVERSITY, NORMAL
[2]UNIVERSITY OF NORTH CAROLINA AT CHAPEL HILL, CHAPEL HILL

Introduction

Several studies have investigated the biomechanics of head impacts among various levels of American football players. Studies conducted on collegiate-level American football players have reported mean linear head acceleration values ranging from 21 to 32 g, with some of the peak accelerations reaching 173 g (Brolinson *et al.*, 2006; Duma *et al.*, 2005). Another study investigating these impact forces among high school American football players reported the mean linear acceleration value was approximately 25.1 g (Broglio *et al.*, 2010). During the course of the study, 13 concussions were reported, with the highest linear acceleration value reported to be 146 g. Based on these studies and the potential long-term repercussions of traumatic brain injuries sustained from multiple football-related impacts (Gavett *et al.*, 2011; Guskiewicz *et al.*, 2003, 2005, 2007), a substantial amount of research and grant dollars have been used to target innovations in American football helmet design. However, American football is not the only sport at risk. Reports have shown that head injuries account for 30 per cent of all injuries sustained by cyclists, 13 per cent among football (soccer) players, 44 per cent among cricket players and 21 per cent among rugby players (Finch *et al.*, 1998). Although research data are limited for sports such as baseball/softball, field hockey and basketball, these athletes are also at risk of head injuries. Overall, researchers estimate that 1.6–3.8 million sport-related traumatic brain injuries occur each year (Langlois *et al.*, 2006).

Due to the high incidence of head injuries among athletes, the use of protective headgear has been strongly recommended in various sporting activities that have a reasonable chance of head trauma. Headgear for each sport has various designs and is constructed with different materials based on the impact forces and the needs of the individual athletes. Helmets have been shown to significantly decrease head impact forces sustained during sports such as cycling (Thomas *et al.*, 1994; Thompson *et al.*, 1996), American football (Lewis *et al.*, 2001), ice hockey (McIntosh and Janda, 2003), lacrosse (Caswell and Deivert, 2002), cricket and baseball (McIntosh and Janda, 2003).

Helmet construction

The first documented use of an American football helmet occurred in 1893 during an inter-collegiate game. Unfortunately, helmets were not made mandatory by the National Collegiate

Athletic Association (NCAA) until 1938 and by the National Football League (NFL) until 1940. Early forms of headgear were constructed of leather with a chin strap and designed to cover essentially the dome of the head, as well as the ears, while the face and even much of the posterior skull were left completely exposed.

Over time, advances were made in shell size and shell materials, leading to a decrease in the number of different helmet models available (National Operating Committee on Standards for Athletic Equipment (NOCSAE), 2011e). These advancements in helmet shell design and construction were employed with the purpose of allowing for more shell deformation and gradual head deceleration. Modern day helmets are reportedly 2.7 times heavier, 4.3 cm longer, 7.6 cm higher and 4.9 cm wider than helmets developed in the 1970s (Viano et al., 2012).

As helmet technology progressed, manufacturers began constructing headgear out of plastics and metal alloys to provide increased protection (Daneshvar et al., 2011). Polyurethane covers were developed and placed over the existing exterior shell of a helmet to provide further protection. However, research has shown little difference in the occurrence of concussions while wearing this type of helmet cover (Torg et al., 1999). Similar devices have been constructed to be added to the interior of helmets, as well as barriers that can be attached to non-protective headgear, such as hats; although, no independent, peer-reviewed research has investigated the effectiveness of these devices.

Foam padding was added to the interior of helmets and eventually progressed to various sizes, designs and placements, as well as pocket filled materials including both fluid and air (Daneshvar et al., 2011; Krzeminski et al., 2011; McIntosh et al., 2004). Various types of foam with different absorptive properties have been used and include ethyl vinyl acetate and polyvinyl chloride nitrile rubber (Daneshvar et al., 2011). Suspension helmets were implemented and use a web-based system to create a small amount of space between the interior shell of the helmet and the athlete's head in an attempt to 'cradle' the head. Bishop et al. (1984) investigated the effects of different helmet interior cushion (liner) systems and found that padded helmets were significantly more effective in absorbing impacts than pure suspension helmets. Similar results were reported by Myers et al. (1993), who showed that pneumatic or combination pneumatic-foam padding systems were more effective at dissipating impact force than suspension type helmets.

In 1951, a single metal bar was added to football helmets to cover the mouth area of a player. Over time, this face protection transformed into two bars, widening the protective coverage, and eventually into multiple bars for an even greater area of protection. Face shields were produced to prevent trauma to the eye region where smaller objects were able to pass between the face bars. In 1996, the American Academy of Pediatrics and American Academy of Ophthalmology recommended that these shields be mandatory for functionally one-eyed athletes (worse than 20/40 with best correction in the worse eye) (American Academy of Pediatrics Committee on Sports Medicine and Fitness and American Academy of Ophthalmology Committee on Eye Safety and Sports Ophthalmology, 1996). These shields are made out of extremely strong polycarbonate and are reported to endure typical impacts produced during football competition (Baker et al., 2008).

In 2002, the Revolution® helmet by Riddell® was introduced, which included an exterior shell that protruded more anteriorly and distally with respect to the mandible compared to traditional football helmets. The Revolution helmet also had a greater distance between the interior shell surface and the players head, as well as a different interior liner design. These design differences were implemented with the intent of greater impact absorption at the side of the head and face. As a result, high school football players wearing the Revolution helmet reported significantly less concussions compared to those wearing traditional style helmets.

Furthermore, there was a 31 per cent decreased relative risk of sustaining a concussion among players wearing the Revolution helmet (Collins *et al.*, 2006). Despite the recognized benefit of this helmet, only 25 per cent of NFL players wore the Revolution helmet during the 2008–9 competitive season (Viano *et al.*, 2012).

The Xenith Shock Bonnet® football helmet was designed with the intent of being able to adapt to an impact (Xenith LLC, 2012). According to the manufacturer, this helmet is equipped with shock absorbers that adapt to the energy of the hit regardless of severity, providing superior protection compared to traditional padded helmets. These shock absorbers are stated to compress and vent air as an impact occurs, thereby decreasing the magnitude of the force. Krzeminski *et al.* (2011) investigated the effectiveness of a single shock absorber to attenuate impact forces. The results of this study support manufacturer claims of the effectiveness of the shock absorber to attenuate impact forces effectively at impact speeds up to 3.0m.s^{-1}. Unfortunately, no current data are available detailing the efficiency of the Shock Bonnet helmet specifically in attenuating impact forces.

Although helmet construction can play a large role in the distribution of forces and therefore the occurrence of a concussion, it is not the only factor. In the 1960s, coaches taught their athletes to put their face into the number of the jersey of the opposing player during a block or tackle (Mueller and Blyth, 1987). However, in 1967, the American Medical Association Committee on Medical Aspects of Sports reported that this type of technique was not always being executed or taught correctly (Heck *et al.*, 2004). Rather than keeping the face up, athletes were dropping their head, which resulted in the top of the head making the initial contact. This method of using the crown of the head to make contact was termed 'spearing' and has been reported to increase the risk of cervical spine injuries and subsequent permanent quadriplegia (Torg *et al.*, 1979). In 1975, the NCAA and NFL outlawed players from using the crown of their head as the initial point of contact during blocking and tackling manoeuvres. The implementation of this rule significantly decreased the risk of cervical spine injuries among American football players, with the rates of occurrence falling from 34 in 1976 to only five in 1984 (Torg, 1985). Clinicians also recommended that subsequent sports such as diving, rugby, ice hockey and gymnastics should also limit this type of head contact to minimize catastrophic neck injuries (Torg, 1985). In 2004, the National Athletic Trainers' Association released a position statement recommending players, coaches and officials be educated on the dangers of spearing. This association also recommended an increase in practice time that targets correct tackling, ball carrying and blocking techniques, and to increase efforts in the enforcement of spearing penalties (Heck *et al.*, 2004).

Testing standards

In 1969, the National Operating Committee on Standards for Athletic Equipment (NOCSAE) was established with the goal of assisting injury reduction research, with a primary interest in American football helmets (NOCSAE, 2011e). In 1970, NOCSAE began standardizing football helmet construction and maintenance, and in 1973 a standardized helmet testing system was established (NOCSAE, 2011e). In 1978, all NCAA helmets had to be certified by NOCSAE, with the National Federation of State High School Associations soon following in 1980 (NOCSAE, 2011e). Currently, NOCSAE continues to publish updated testing standards, but does not approve, disapprove, certify or recertify any athletic equipment itself (NOCSAE, 2012j). Instead, independent companies test equipment, basing their decision to certify or not on the performance of the headgear within the guidelines published by NOCSAE.

Currently, NOCSAE provides certification guidelines and testing standards for various types of equipment in multiple sports. For example, in American football NOCSAE publishes equipment standards for not only helmets, but also facemasks and hand coverings (e.g. hand pads, gloves). Along with American football, NOCSAE publishes standards for equipment in baseball/softball, hockey, lacrosse, polo and football (NOCSAE, 2011e).

While the testing varies slightly between helmets of various sports, several factors remain constant. Headform impacts are measured via a triaxial accelerometer mounted at the centre of gravity of the headform. This accelerometer must provide measurements in three orthogonal axes and be able to provide appropriate measurements at severity index (SI) levels of ± 2 per cent across a range of 600–2,500. Severity index is a measure of the severity of impact with respect to the instantaneous acceleration detected by the headform during a collision. In order to calculate SI, the following formula is applied: $SI = {}_0^T\!\int A^{2.5}dt$, where 'A' is equal to instantaneous resultant acceleration and 'dt' are time increments in seconds with the integration carried out over the essential duration of the acceleration pulse (NOCSAE, 2012j). The helmet must fit the headform in accordance with the helmet manufacturers' specifications. Drop tests are conducted in various helmet locations after the equipment has been exposed to several temperatures, including ambient laboratory temperature of 22 ± 3°C and a high temperature environment in which the equipment is conditioned for a minimum of 4 hours at a temperature of 46 ± 3°C. Each piece of equipment has standard drop test impact velocities, ranging from 3.46 m.s^{-1} to 5.46 m.s^{-1}, which must be achieved in order for the test to be considered valid (NOCSAE, 2012j). Standards also exist to test headgear against projectiles, such as a baseball, softball, or hockey puck. Projectile velocities for these tests range from 24.6 m.s^{-1} to 28 m.s^{-1} (NOCSAE, 2012a, 2012c). These standards are similar to the drop testing in that the headgear is exposed to impacts at various velocities and in multiple locations at both an ambient and high temperature condition.

In order for the headgear to become certified, it must meet certain testing criteria set forth by NOCSAE. The peak SI of any single impact may not exceed 1,200. At the slowest impact velocity, the SI must not exceed 300. Although repositioning of the headgear on the headform during the testing is appropriate, the headgear must survive all tests 'substantially intact and ready for use' (NOCSAE, 2012a, 2012b, 2012c, 2012d, 2012e).

Proper fit and maintenance

Although manufacturers spend millions of dollars and an extensive amount of time designing innovative headgear, even the best helmets are relatively useless without proper fit and maintenance. Coaches, parents and athletes should be routinely educated on how to properly fit a helmet to allow for a minimal amount of movement on the head and good visibility. Gieck and McCue (1980) reported that with a properly fit helmet, when unstrapped, the helmet should not move excessively in the transverse or sagittal planes of motion when grabbed and pulled by the facemask. The authors also note that there should be approximately 1–2 fingers width between the top of the players' eyebrows and the inferior border of the anterior aspect of the helmet. Spacers of varying thickness can be added to improve this fit. Finally, during cervical extension the posterior aspect of the helmet should not restrict motion as it contacts the spine.

Along with proper fit, headgear should be frequently monitored for signs of fatigue. Bishop *et al.* (1984) reported that suspension liners were inferior to padded helmet liners, speculating that the webbing of suspension helmets stretched over time, thereby decreasing the efficiency of absorbing impact. Similar concerns have been reported regarding repeated use among lacrosse helmets (Caswell and Deivert, 2002) and rugby headgear (Knouse *et al.*, 2003), which may have decreased force absorption abilities following repeated impacts. Other concerns include the repeated exposure of helmet face shields to ultraviolet light, which may degrade the polycarbonate, thereby decreasing its flexibility (Zimmerman *et al.*, 2011). Thus, researchers have recommended that face shields be frequently replaced to minimize the risk of this material fatigue (Zimmerman *et al.*, 2011). Gieck and McCue (1980) recommended that headgear be routinely checked prior to and throughout the competitive season for signs of cracks, loosening fit, bent facemasks, failing interior liners and missing hardware.

Along with guidelines for certifying new helmets, NOCSAE publishes testing standards and recertification guidelines for used equipment that are very similar to that of the new equipment. Testers must select a sample size that is 'adequate and representative' of the overall group of equipment being tested. NOCSAE does not specify a certain number or percentage of the group be tested, but leaves it up to the tester to determine appropriate sample size (NOCSAE, 2011a, 2011b, 2011c, 2011d). The recertification process varies slightly between different types of equipment, but several conditions must be met in order for any equipment to be recertified. The tested equipment must survive all tests 'intact and ready for subsequent use', must be free from cracks and the peak SI of any impact may not exceed 1,200 (1,500 for helmets manufactured prior to 1 January 1997) (NOCSAE, 2012f, 2012g, 2012h, 2012i).

Effectiveness of headgear

Numerous changes have been implemented in American football helmet design since its introduction in the late 1800s. Viano *et al.* (2012) conducted a study investigating the effectiveness of modern design football helmets used in 2010 compared to those used in the early 1990s. These authors reported mixed results comparing the various helmet designs of different eras, with some of the modern helmets performing better in certain grading criteria and others performing worse, while other grading criteria showed no significant differences between helmets. Overall, only four (Schutt™ DNA Pro, Riddell Revolution®, Riddell Revolution® IQ, Riddell Revolution® Speed) of the 17 modern style helmets tested showed better impact absorption compared to the older style helmets. The improved performance of these modern day helmets may be partially explained by the increased weight and size of the helmets, as well as the increased padding compared to older models (Viano and Halstead, 2012). Furthermore, these helmets have been reported to produce 10–20 per cent less concussions among National Football League players (Viano *et al.*, 2006).

Although American football has been reported to have the highest number of concussions, ice hockey (combined concussions reported among both men's and women's ice hockey) has shown the highest rate of concussions per athlete exposure (Hootman *et al.*, 2007). This may be partially explained by the limited efficiency of ice hockey helmets to attenuate impacts. Youth ice hockey helmets have been shown to provide adequate protection during low impacts of 2 m.s^{-1} and 4 m.s^{-1} (Hoshizaki *et al.*, 2012); however, the efficiency of the same helmets to provide adequate protection significantly decreased at impact speeds of 6 m.s^{-1} and 8 m.s^{-1}. Similar results have been shown among cricket helmets, which are reported to provide good protection at relatively low ball speeds (19 m.s^{-1}), moderate protection at slightly faster ball speeds (27 m.s^{-1}) and poor protection at more realistic ball speeds (36 m.s^{-1} and 45 m.s^{-1}) (McIntosh and Janda, 2003). In regard to face protection, researchers suggest that full face protection ice hockey helmets decrease the risk of head and face injuries compared to partial face protection and no face protection style helmets (Asplund *et al.*, 2009). In a study investigating the effectiveness of rugby headgear, McIntosh *et al.* (2004) reported a significant increase in protection when the thickness of the padding was increased from 10 to 16 mm.

Football also poses the risk of head trauma caused by the accumulation of forces during heading the ball. Football is the only sport that purposefully uses the head to control the ball, which at times can be travelling at speeds exceeding 88.5 km.h^{-1} (Kirkendall *et al.*, 2001). The head also can make contact with various other implements during play including opposing players' elbows and heads, as well as the ground and goal posts. In an effort to protect football players, headgear has been constructed with designs ranging from a padded headband to a full helmet. Unfortunately, the efficiency of this headgear has been met with mixed results. Some research has reported that there are no differences in impact with or without the headgear (Naunheim *et al.*, 2003; Withnall *et al.*, 2005). Conversely, Delaney *et al.* (2008) reported that youth football players were more likely to suffer a concussion when not wearing headgear. These conflicting results among current research add to the confusion surrounding the best methods for decreasing head injuries among football players.

Major League Baseball pitchers often throw balls between 38 m.s^{-1} and 45 m.s^{-1}, highlighting the need for batters, catchers and umpires to wear helmets. Although research has shown benefits for players wearing helmets while batting (McIntosh and Janda, 2003; Nicholls *et al.*, 2004), there is currently little research investigating the effects of catchers and umpires using helmets. When comparing impact characteristics of a headform wearing a facemask versus a headform with no facemask, one study reported that impacts to the facemask reduced head linear acceleration by as much as 85 per cent (Shain *et al.*, 2010). Beyer *et al.* (2012) used real game video footage to recreate several concussion-causing impacts to umpires and catchers in the laboratory. In 10 recreated impacts, the authors reported ball velocity as it crossed home plate to range between 31.6 and 39.2 m.s^{-1}. When the impacts were recreated at a ball speed of 27 m.s^{-1}, headform linear acceleration values ranged from 9 to 28 g, with the highest values reported at the lateral nose impact location and the lowest values reported at the lateral forehead position. At impact ball speeds of 38 m.s^{-1}, the authors report headform linear acceleration values ranged from 26 to 42 g, with the largest values recorded at the chin impact location and the lowest values at the eyebrow location.

Unfortunately, numerous cases have been reported of catchers forced to retire early due to repeated head trauma from ball-to-helmet contact. In 2006, former San Francisco Giants catcher Mike Matheny took multiple foul tips off his mask and was unable to finish the season, forcing him to retire the following February (Ortiz, 2007). Shortly after, then Los Angeles Dodgers athletic trainers Stan Conte and Dave Groeschner conducted an unpublished survey of 261 professional catchers (Ortiz, 2007). These clinicians found that approximately 20–25 per cent of catchers reported some concussion symptoms from foul tips to the mask or helmet. Former St. Louis Cardinals catcher Jason LaRue was also forced to retire when persistent symptoms, such as headaches and nausea, continued following repeated concussions (ESPN.com News Services, 2010). LaRue stated his position as a catcher left him exposed to repeated blows to the head, something he was not willing to risk. LaRue estimated he has had close to 20 concussions since his days as a high school athlete. LaRue stated, 'As a catcher you're so vulnerable to getting another [concussion]. All it takes is a foul ball to the head. Even as a backup that happened [3 to 5] times last year. It's not a question of if it would happen again, it's when'.

Summary

Sport-related headgear design and construction have made extensive advances since the first helmet was introduced in the late 1800s. However, due to the recognized seriousness of traumatic brain injuries and other facial pathologies, there continues to be a weighted interest in advancing headgear innovations. These innovations do not just apply to sports that require headgear, such as American football, ice hockey, and lacrosse, but also to sports that typically do not wear headgear, such as football and baseball pitchers. As such, it is imperative that research continues to investigate the effectiveness of helmet design and construction innovations, as participation in various sports continues to rise.

References

American Academy of Pediatrics Committee on Sports Medicine and Fitness and American Academy of Ophthalmology Committee on Eye Safety and Sports Ophthalmology (1996) 'Protective eyewear for young athletes', *Pediatrics*, 98(2/1): 311–13.

Asplund, C., Bettcher, S. and Borchers, J. (2009) 'Facial protection and head injuries in ice hockey: a systematic review', *British Journal of Sports Medicine*, 43(13): 993–9.

Baker, K. R., Zimmerman, A., Grzybowski, D. M., McLaughlin, W. R., Katz, S. E., Pfriem, D. B. and Good, G. W. (2008) 'Optical quality and impact resistance comparisons of 2 football helmet faceshields', *Optometry*, 79(8): 455–63.

Beyer, J., Rowson, S. and Duma, S. (2012) 'Concussions experienced by Major League Baseball catchers and umpires: field data and experimental baseball impacts', *Annals of Biomedical Engineering*, 40(1): 150–9.

Bishop, P. J., Norman, R. W. and Kozey, J. W. (1984) 'An evaluation of football helmets under impact conditions', *American Journal of Sports Medicine*, 12(3): 233–6.

Broglio, S., Schnebel, B., Sosnoff, J., Shin, S., Fend, X., He, X. and Zimmerman, J. (2010) 'Biomechanical properties of concussions in high school football', *Medicine and Science in Sports and Exercise*, 42(11): 2064 71.

Brolinson, P. G., Manoogian, S., McNeely, D., Goforth, M., Greenwald, R. and Duma, S. (2006) 'Analysis of linear head accelerations from collegiate football impacts', *Current Sports Medicine Reports*, 5(1): 23–8.

Caswell, S. and Deivert, R. (2002) 'Lacrosse helmet designs and the effects of impact forces', *Journal of Athletic Training*, 37(2): 164–71.

Collins, M., Lovell, M., Iverson, G., Ide, T. and Maroon, J. (2006) 'Examining concussion rates and return to play in high school football players wearing newer helmet technology: a three-year prospective cohort study', *Neurosurgery*, 58(2): 275–86.

Daneshvar, D. H., Baugh, C. M., Nowinski, C. J., McKee, A. C., Stern, R. A. and Cantu, R. C. (2011) 'Helmets and mouth guards: the role of personal equipment in preventing sport-related concussions', *Clinics in Sports Medicine*, 30(1): 145–63.

Delaney, J. S., Al-Kashmiri, A., Drummond, R. and Correa, J. A. (2008) 'The effect of protective headgear on head injuries and concussions in adolescent football (soccer) players', *British Journal of Sports Medicine*, 42(2): 110–15.

Duma, S., Manoogian, S., Bussone, W., Brolinson, P.G., Goforth, M., Donnenwerth, J., Greenwald, R., Chu, J. and Crisco, J. (2005) 'Analysis of real-time head accelerations in collegiate football players', *Clinical Journal of Sport Medicine*, 15(1): 3–8.

ESPN.com News Services (2010) *Jason LaRue Retiring from Baseball*, available at: http://sports. espn.go.com/mlb/news/story?id=5592023 (accessed 21 December 2012).

Finch, C., Valuri, G. and Ozanne-Smith, J. (1998) 'Sport and active recreation injuries in Australia: evidence from emergency department presentations', *British Journal of Sports Medicine*, 32(3): 220–5.

Gavett, B., Stern, R. and McKee, A. (2011) 'Chronic traumatic encephalopathy: a potential late effect of sport-related concussive and subconcussive head trauma', *Clinics in Sports Medicine*, 30(1): 179–88.

Gieck, J. and McCue, F. C. III (1980) 'Fitting of protective football equipment', *American Journal of Sports Medicine*, 8(3): 192–6.

Guskiewicz, K., McCrea, M., Marshall, S., Cantu, R., Randolph, C., Barr, W., Onate, J. and Kelly, J. (2003) 'Cumulative effects associated with recurrent concussion in collegiate football players: the NCAA Concussion Study', *The Journal of the American Medical Association*, 290(19): 2549–55.

Guskiewicz, K., Marshall, S., Bailes, J., McCrea, M., Cantu, R., Randolph, C. and Jordan, B. (2005) 'Association between recurrent concussion and late-life cognitive impairment in retired professional football players', *Neurosurgery*, 57(4): 719–26.

Guskiewicz, K., Marshall, S., Bailes, J., McCrea, M., Harding, H., Matthews, A., Mihalik, J. and Cantu, R. (2007) 'Recurrent concussion and risk of depression in retired professional football players', *Medicine and Science in Sports and Exercise*, 39(6): 903–9.

Heck, J. F., Clarke, K. S., Peterson, T. R., Torg, J. S. and Weis, M. P. (2004) 'National athletic trainers' association position statement: head-down contact and spearing in tackle football', *Journal of Athletic Training*, 39(1): 101–11.

Hootman, J., Dick, R. and Agel, J. (2007) 'Epidemiology of collegiate injuries for 15 sports: summary and recommendations for injury prevention initiatives', *Journal of Athletic Training*, 42(2): 311–19.

Hoshizaki, B., Vassilyadi, M., Post, A. and Oeur, A. (2012) 'Performance analysis of winter activity protection headgear for young children', *Journal of Neurosurgery. Pediatrics*, 9(2): 133–8.

Kirkendall, D. T., Jordan, S. E. and Garrett, W. E. (2001) 'Heading and head injuries in soccer', *Sports Medicine*, 31(5): 369–86.

Knouse, C., Gould, T., Caswell, S. and Deivert, R. (2003) 'Efficacy of rugby headgear in attenuating repetitive linear impact forces', *Journal of Athletic Training*, 38(4): 330–5.

Krzeminski, D. E., Goetz, J. T., Janisse, A. P., Lippa, N. M., Gould, T. E., Rawlins, J. W. and Piland, S. G. (2011) 'Investigation of linear impact energy management and product claims of a novel American football helmet liner component', *Sports Technology*, 4(1–2): 65–76.

Langlois, J., Rutland-Brown, W. and Wald, M. (2006) 'The epidemiology and impact of traumatic brain injury: a brief overview', *The Journal of Head Trauma Rehabilitation*, 21(5): 375–8.

Lewis, L. M., Naunheim, R., Standeven, J., Lauryssen, C., Richter, C. and Jeffords, B. (2001) 'Do football helmets reduce acceleration of impact in blunt head injuries?', *Academic Emergency Medicine*, 8(6): 604–9.

McIntosh, A. S. and Janda, D. (2003) 'Evaluation of cricket helmet performance and comparison with baseball and ice hockey helmets', *British Journal of Sports Medicine*, 37(4): 325–30.

McIntosh, A., McCrory, P. and Finch, C. F. (2004) 'Performance enhanced headgear: a scientific approach to the development of protective headgear', *British Journal of Sports Medicine*, 38(1): 46–9.

Mueller, F. O. and Blyth, C. S. (1987) 'Fatalities from head and cervical spine injuries occurring in tackle football: 40 years' experience', *Clinics in Sports Medicine*, 6(1): 185–96.

Myers, T. J., Yoganandan, N., Sances, A., Jr, Pintar, F. A., Reinartz, J. and Battocletti, J. H. (1993) 'Energy absorption characteristics of football helmets under low and high rates of loading', *Bio-medical Materials and Engineering*, 3(1): 15–24.

National Operating Committee on Standards for Athletic Equipment (2011a) *Laboratory Procedural Guide for Recertifying Baseball/Softball Batter's and Catchers Helmets*, DOC (ND) 028-07m11, Overland Park, KS: NOCSAE.

National Operating Committee on Standards for Athletic Equipment (2011b) *Laboratory Procedural Guide for Recertifying Football Helmets*, DOC (ND)005-96m11a, Overland Park, KS: NOCSAE.

National Operating Committee on Standards for Athletic Equipment (2011c) *Laboratory Procedural Guide for Recertifying Hockey Helmets*, DOC (ND) 033-04m11, Overland Park, KS: NOCSAE.

National Operating Committee on Standards for Athletic Equipment (2011d) *Laboratory Procedural Guide for Recertifying Lacrosse Helmets*, DOC (ND) 044-04m11, Overland Park, KS: NOCSAE.

National Operating Committee on Standards for Athletic Equipment (2011e) *Homepage of National Operating Committee on Standards for Athletic Equipment*, available at: http://nocsae.org (accessed 17 December 2012.)

National Operating Committee on Standards for Athletic Equipment (2012a) *Standard Performance Specification for Newly Manufactured Baseball/Softball Batter's Helmets*, DOC (ND) 022-10m12, Overland Park, KS: NOCSAE.

National Operating Committee on Standards for Athletic Equipment (2012b) *Standard Performance Specification for Newly Manufactured Football Helmets*, DOC (ND) 002-11m12, Overland Park, KS: NOCSAE.

National Operating Committee on Standards for Athletic Equipment (2012c) *Standard Performance Specification for Newly Manufactured Hockey Helmets*, DOC (ND) 030-11m12, Overland Park, KS: NOCSAE.

National Operating Committee on Standards for Athletic Equipment (2012d) *Standard Performance Specification for Newly Manufactured Lacrosse Helmets with Faceguard*, DOC (ND) 04-11m12, Overland Park, KS: NOCSAE.

National Operating Committee on Standards for Athletic Equipment (2012e) *Standard Performance Specification for Newly Manufactured Polo Helmets*, DOC (ND) 050-11m12, Overland Park, KS: NOCSAE.

National Operating Committee on Standards for Athletic Equipment (2012f) *Standard Performance Specification for Recertified Baseball-Softball Batters and Catchers Helmets*, DOC (ND) 026-11m12, Overland Park, KS: NOCSAE.

National Operating Committee on Standards for Athletic Equipment (2012g) *Standard Performance Specification for Recertified Football Helmets*, DOC (ND) 004-11m12, Overland Park, KS: NOCSAE.

National Operating Committee on Standards for Athletic Equipment (2012h) *Standard Performance Specification for Recertified Hockey Helmets*, DOC (ND) 032-11m12, Overland Park, KS: NOCSAE.

National Operating Committee on Standards for Athletic Equipment (2012i) *Standard Performance Specification for Recertified Lacrosse Helmets*, DOC (ND) 043-11m12, Overland Park, KS: NOCSAE.

National Operating Committee on Standards for Athletic Equipment (2012j) *Standard Test Method and Equipment Used in Evaluating the Performance Characteristics of Protective Headgear/Equipment*, DOC (ND) 001-11m12, Overland Park, KS: NOCSAE.

Naunheim, R. S., Ryden, A., Standeven, J., Genin, G., Lewis, L., Thompson, P. and Bayly, P. (2003) 'Does soccer headgear attenuate the impact when heading a soccer ball?', *Academic Emergency Medicine: Official Journal of The Society for Academic Emergency Medicine*, 10(1): 85–90.

Nicholls, R., Elliott, B. and Miller, K. (2004) 'Impact injuries in baseball: prevalence, aetiology and the role of equipment performance', *Sports Medicine*, 34(1): 17–25.

Ortiz, J. L. (2007) *Baseball Taking Note of Concussions*, available at: www.usatoday.com/sports/baseball/2007–06–18-focus-concussions_N.htm (accessed 21 December 2012).

Shain, K., Madigan, M., Rowson, S., Bisplinghoff, J. and Duma, S. (2010) 'Analysis of the ability of catcher's masks to attenuate head accelerations on impact with a baseball', *Clinical Journal of Sport Medicine*, 20(6): 422–7.

Thomas, S., Acton, C., Nixon, J., Battistutta, D., Pitt, W. R. and Clark, R. (1994) 'Effectiveness of bicycle helmets in preventing head injury in children: case-control study', *British Medical Journal*, 308(6922): 173–6.

Thompson, D. C., Rivara, F. P. and Thompson, R. S. (1996) 'Effectiveness of bicycle safety helmets in preventing head injuries. A case-control study', *Journal of The American Medical Association*, 276(24): 1968–73.

Torg, J. S. (1985) 'Epidemiology, pathomechanics, and prevention of athletic injuries to the cervical spine', *Medicine and Science in Sports and Exercise*, 17(3): 295–303.

Torg, J. S., Quedenfeld, T. C., Burstein, A., Spealman, A. and Nichols, C. III (1979) 'National football head and neck injury registry: report on cervical quadriplegia, 1971 to 1975', *American Journal of Sports Medicine*, 7(2): 127–32.

Torg, J. S., Harris, S. M., Rogers, K. and Stilwell, G. J. (1999) 'Retrospective report on the effectiveness of a polyurethane football helmet cover on the repeated occurrence of cerebral concussions', *The American Journal of Orthopedics*, 28(2): 128–32.

Viano, D. and Halstead, D. (2012) 'Change in size and impact performance of football helmets from the 1970s to 2010', *Annals of Biomedical Engineering*, 40(1): 175–84.

Viano, D., Pellman, E., Withnall, C. and Shewchenko, N. (2006) 'Concussion in professional football: performance of newer helmets in reconstructed game impacts – part 13', *Neurosurgery*, 59(3): 591–606.

Viano, D. C., Withnall, C. and Halstead, D. (2012) 'Impact performance of modern football helmets', *Annals of Biomedical Engineering*, 40(1): 160–74.

Withnall, C., Shewchenko, N., Wonnacott, M. and Dvorak, J. (2005) 'Effectiveness of headgear in football', *British Journal of Sports Medicine*, 39(1): i40–8.

Xenith LLC (2012) *Xenith Innovation*, available at: www.xenith.com/football/innovation/ (accessed 21 December 2012).

Zimmerman, A. B., Good, G. W., McLaughlin, W. R. and Katz, S. E. (2011) 'Intercollegiate usage schedule and the impact resistance of used football helmet faceshields', *Journal of the American Optometric Association*, 82(5): 274–83.

SECTION 9

Modelling and simulation in sports and exercise

38

MODELLING AND SIMULATION IN SPRINGBOARD DIVING

Pui Wah Kong

NANYANG TECHNOLOGICAL UNIVERSITY, SINGAPORE

Introduction

Springboard diving is an aesthetic aquatic sport and is part of the Olympic Games. A dive comprises the approach and hurdle, the take-off from the springboard, the airborne movement and the entry into water (Figure 38.1). Biomechanically, the three main objectives of springboard diving are: (1) to generate sufficient angular momentum to execute somersaults and twists; (2) to obtain height during flight and thus time in the air; and (3) to travel safely but not excessively away from the board (Miller and Munro, 1985). In order to score high in competitive diving, close attention must also be paid to the aesthetic components of a dive such as adopting a tight shape during somersaulting, keeping the toes pointed throughout the dive and minimizing the splash at the entry.

The take-off from the springboard

The dive height and horizontal distance travelled in flight, as well as the angular momentum required to execute somersaults and twists are all determined at the take-off from the springboard. Once the diver is in the air, he or she can only control the speed of rotation by altering body shape. Thus, many studies have used computer simulation models to understand the mechanics of the take-off in terms of generating both linear and angular momentum.

Modelling the springboard

Attempts have been made to model the springboard either alone or in concert with the diver to reflect the extreme complexity of the system. Kuipers and van de Ven (1992) applied linear field equations to examine the torsional force exerted on the springboard during unilateral contact. Kooi and Kuipers (1994) used a continuous method to develop a lumped-parameter model. It is conceptually appealing but difficult to implement modelling the board as a continuous system with the fundamental parameters distributed throughout. Complex methods require intensive computation, making it difficult to integrate with a full-body human model of a diver. Thus, there is a need for a simplified model with reasonable accuracy.

471

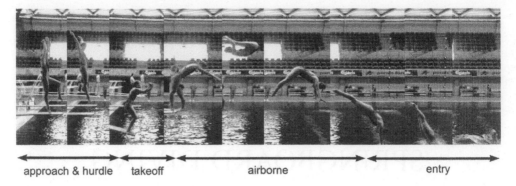

approach & hurdle   takeoff   airborne   entry

Figure 38.1 A dive comprises the approach and hurdle, the take-off from the springboard, the airborne movement and the entry into the water.

Sprigings *et al.* (1989) modelled the Duraflex board using two different approaches: a finite element analysis and a simplified mass-spring model. The mass-spring model consists of a lumped mass connected to a parallel arrangement of a linear spring and a dashpot (Figure 38.2a). They compared the resulting parameters calculated from the two approaches and concluded that the linear mass-spring model could reasonably represent the dynamic behaviour of the springboard. Even though Kooi and Kuipers (1994) further proposed a single degree-of-freedom (DOF) 'bar model', the linear mass-spring model was generally accepted to represent the complex springboard system in diving research (Boda, 1992; Cheng and Hubbard, 2004; Jiang *et al.*, 2000a, 2000b, 2001; Liu and Wu, 1989; Wu and Liu, 1989). While the mass-spring model is superior for its simplicity and the direct method for determining model parameters, it only represents the vertical behaviour of the springboard and thus the vertical reaction force acting on the diver. It should be noted that the springboard deflects in a curve, providing also a horizontal reaction force that plays an important role in the generation of angular momentum

(a)   **(b)**

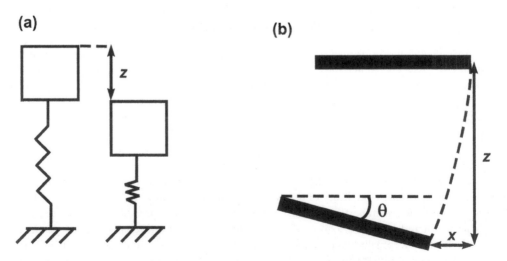

Figure 38.2 (a) A linear mass-spring model of the springboard with one degree of freedom (DOF): vertical movement (z) is commonly used in a diver-springboard system. (b). A 3-DOF rod model of the springboard allows vertical (z), horizontal (x) and rotational (θ) movement (Yeadon *et al.*, 2006).

and board clearance. In addition, the springboard rotates as it deflects and the board rotation influences the diver's orientation.

To overcome the limitations of a simple mass-spring model, Yeadon *et al.* (2006) developed a 3-DOF springboard model, which represents the vertical (z), horizontal (x) and rotational (θ) behaviour of the springboard (Figure 38.2b). The vertical movement of the springboard was modelled as a linear mass-spring system with no damping, and the stiffness was allowed to increase with the distance of the foot from the springboard tip (Sprigings *et al.*, 1989):

$$k_s = m(d + 0.15) + c \tag{1}$$

where k_s is vertical springboard stiffness, m is the slope, d is the distance from the toes to the tip of the springboard and c is a constant. The springboard stiffness was defined by the two parameters m and c and their input values were determined via optimization procedures in matching simulations (m = 7,551 N.m^{-2} and c = 3,597 N.m^{-1} for a fulcrum number of 7.5). Two regression equations were obtained from experimental data to relate the horizontal ($x = -0.194\ z^2$, R^2 = 0.98, SE = 4.8 mm) and angular displacements ($\theta = -28.599\ z$, R^2 = 0.96, SE = 1.7°) to the vertical displacement of the springboard tip. This new method enabled the horizontal and angular displacement, velocity, and acceleration to be computed from the vertical displacement time history. This 3-DOF rod model has been successfully evaluated to accurately reflect the springboard behaviour (Yeadon *et al.*, 2006) and had been used in a diver-springboard system to optimize performance (King *et al.*, 2009).

Fulcrum setting

Divers can adjust the fulcrum setting of the springboard to regulate the amount of stiffness. Boda (1992) modelled the springboard and the diver as an oscillating system. Oscillation frequencies of individual divers during a standing backward take-off on a springboard and on a force plate were measured. With the objective of gaining maximal height, a regression equation was derived to predict the optimal fulcrum number based on preferred fulcrum number, oscillation rate on land and body weight. This equation may provide some general guidelines for novice divers but may not be applicable to elite divers since factors such as strength, training and technique were not considered. Using a rotational mass-spring model proposed by Kooi and Kuipers (1994) with a four-segment model of a diver, Cheng and Hubbard (2005) investigated the influence of fulcrum setting on jump height during a standing backward jump. It was concluded that larger fulcrum numbers (more compliant) are beneficial for taller/heavier divers due to the more time allowed for joint extensions.

The armswing

Sprigings and Watson (1985) used a two-segment model of the diver together with a linear mass-spring model of the springboard to search for the optimal timing of the armswing during take-off. It was found that the upward acceleration of the arms with respect to the shoulders should commence at the moment of board contact. Sprigings *et al.* (1986) later modified the model to three segments to investigate the timing of the relative force patterns of the arms, torso and legs during take-off. The authors suggested that modification should only be made to the timing but not the already learned movement pattern.

Optimizing take-off technique

There are two types of take-off from the springboard, the running take-off and the standing take-off. A running take-off involves an approach (usually 3–4 steps) and a hurdle step prior to the take-off phase. Divers use the running take-off for the forward (forward travel, forward rotation) and the reverse (forward travel, backward rotation) dive groups. In a standing take-off, divers stand at the tip of the springboard with their back facing the water. This take-off position is used for the backward (backward travel, backward rotation) and inward (backward travel, forward rotation) dive groups. Twisting dives can be performed using the standing or running take-off.

For running take-offs, Sprigings and Miller (2004) used a planar five-segment diver model with joint torque generators to optimize the take-off technique in dives from the reverse group. Their simulation results suggested that divers should delay the most forceful extension of their lower extremities until just before maximum board depression. Also, tilting the lower leg forward during the board recoil phase plays an important role in establishing angular momentum for reverse rotation. The knee kinematics of their simulation did not, however, match well with previous experimental data on elite divers. Nevertheless, this study was the pioneer work in optimizing diving take-off techniques using a torque-driven simulation model.

To optimize forward somersaulting dives, Kong *et al.* (2005) developed an eight-segment torque-driven model with a 3-DOF board model to simulate a forward two-and-one-half somersault in a pike position. It was found that by changing the activation pattern alone without an increase in strength, the diver could generate substantially more forward angular momentum during the take-off to improve the dive with sufficient time to prepare for the entry (Figure 38.3). The optimized take-off technique for this dive was characterized by a faster knee extension, a faster and increased hip extension before a rapid hip flexion towards the end of the take-off phase. Using the same model to simulate also the reverse dive group, it was found that a more complex activation profile is needed in order to generate the forward travel and backward rotation required in this dive group (Kong *et al.*, 2006a). To produce reverse somersaulting dives, the diver needs to flex the knees towards the end of the take-off phase in combination with hip hyper-extension to generate backward angular momentum and to move the mass centre forward to ensure forward travel away from the board.

In searching for optimal jumping strategies during a standing backward take-off, Cheng and Hubbard (2005) found that the joint torque activation patterns for maximizing jump height differed between springboard take-off and rigid-surface jumping. The springboard take-off strategies include partial extension, slight flexion and maximal extension activation of the lower extremities timed around maximal board depression. The same researchers did another simulation study to examine the effect of armswing on generating maximal angular momentum for backward somersaulting (Cheng and Hubbard, 2008). It was found that the arm contributed nearly 60 per cent of the total angular momentum and that more joint work (except at the knee) could be done with an armswing. The amount of angular momentum, however, will be largely reduced in order to produce sufficient horizontal velocity for the diver to travel safely away to clear the board.

In summary, the computer simulation model has been shown to be a promising tool to gain insight of springboard diving take-off techniques and to optimize diving performance. Previous modelling studies have investigated the take-off in the forward, backward and reverse dive groups in terms of maximizing dive height and angular momentum, but no studies have examined the inward or twisting dive take-offs. Future modelling studies should also consider imposing realistic anatomical constraints and including robustness to activation timing

(a) original performance

(b) optimised simulation

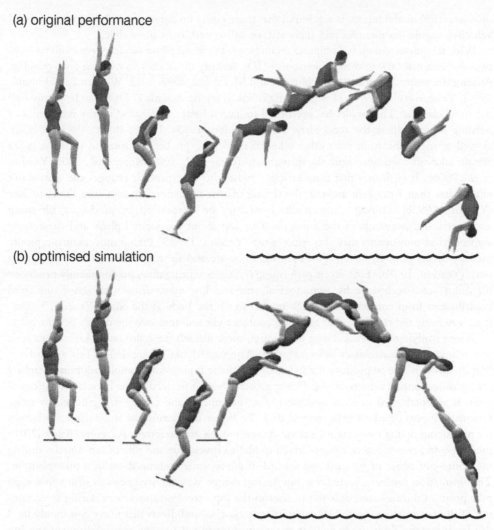

Figure 38.3 Graphical comparisons of an (a) original performance of a forward two-and-a-half somersault in a pike position performed by a diver; and (b) optimized simulation with increased angular momentum for forward rotation.

perturbations in the optimization procedures in order to ensure some consistency of performance (Kong *et al.*, 2006b).

The diver in the airborne phase

The aerial technique of diving has been studied extensively with the use of simulation models. Miller (1970) was one of the earliest sports biomechanics researchers to use computer simulation as a research tool. She studied the airborne phase of non-twisting dives and limited her model to four segments. Since then, many other planar flight phase models of a diver were developed to examine the aerial techniques of somersaulting dives. For example, Figgen (1989) used an eight-segment diver model to investigate pike and tuck multiple somersaulting dives. Based on theoretical model inputs, it was found that there could be different combinations of vertical velocity, angular momentum and angle at take-off to perform a good dive.

With the advancement in computer technology, the aerial phase models have evolved from two-dimensional (2D) to three-dimensional (3D), making the studies on twisting dives possible. Among the many 3D models (Koschorreck and Mombaur, 2009, 2012; Wooten and Hodgins, 1996), Yeadon et al.'s (1990) 11-segment rigid linked segments with 17 DOF can be considered the most classical. This model has been used to gain a better understanding the mechanics of twisting somersaults in the aerial phase alone (Yeadon, 1993a, 1993b, 1993c, 1993d, 1993e), as well as in combination with other take-off models to predict the rotation in flight given certain take-off conditions from the springboard (King et al., 2009; Kong et al., 2005; Yeadon et al., 2006). It is shown that introducing a twist into a somersault changes the somersault rate by less than 1 per cent and that the timing of arm adduction can influence the twist rate (Yeadon, 1993b). During a somersault, twist may be introduced by producing tilt using asymmetrical movements of the arms, chest or hip about the sagittal plane and these same asymmetrical movements may also remove tile (Yeadon, 1993c). Piking movements, typically used by divers prior to the entry of twisting dives, are also shown to be effective in stopping twist (Yeadon, 1993b). Elite divers performing multiple twisting dives predominantly produced tilt using aerial technique by asymmetrical arm and hip movements with about one-third contribution from contact twist, which tended to tilt the body at the entry (Yeadon, 1993e). It is, however, not clear whether reducing contact twist will improve the diver's performance.

When studying the aerial diving techniques, most models were driven by kinematics such as the angle time histories of different joints. The underlying assumption of this approach is that the diver is able to produce the specified kinematic inputs; for example, adopting a tighter pike position during somersaulting. This approach, though neglecting the human physiological limit, is acceptable for slow to moderately fast movements and can be strengthened by using kinematic inputs based on experimental data. To better understand the muscular contribution for producing diving movements, kinetic-driven models are preferred. Recently, Kong (2010) used a planar, two-segment torque-driven model to investigate the role of hip muscles during the come-out phase of forward and inward multiple somersaulting dives in a pike position. The simulation results indicated that hip flexion torque was required both to maintain a rigid pike position during somersault and to control the hip extension movement during the come-out of the fast rotating dives. This study informs coaches and divers that many commonly used dry-land exercise drills producing hip extension movement by concentric actions of the hip extensor muscles do not replicate the neuromuscular control during the actual come-out when the diver is in the air.

The entry into the water

While the take-off and aerial phase of diving have been widely studies, much less is known about the diver-water interaction during the entry. A 'rip' entry, a water entry with little splash and a sound as if someone has ripped a piece of paper, is a key to obtaining high scores from the judges in competitive diving. Over the years, various underwater techniques have been developed for different dive groups in order to minimize splash and to maintain a vertical orientation of the body throughout the entire entry phase. Examples of such underwater techniques include swimming the arms, rolling for forward somersaulting entry, scooping the back for back somersaulting entries and flexing the knees for over-rotated back somersaulting entries. There are many variations within each technique, and their contribution to a good entry is not clear. From an injury prevention perspective, the impact force and joint loading on the diver are of great interest since divers reach the water level at high velocities. To date, very limited theoretical or experimental studies have addressed the issues related to diving water entry.

A recent breakthrough is the study by Qian *et al.* (2010), which used a finite element model to simulate the splash control during the initial phase of the water entry. The human body was modelled as a wedged solid object and the water as an ideal fluid. By investigating the relationship between hand patterns and splash height, they found a squared object as the ideal shape for water entry and advised divers to internally rotate the arms to form a flat impact surface. Despite the many limitation of this simple model, it is exciting to see this pioneer piece of work on modelling the diving entry. Hopefully, more future work will be done on this area in order to advance our understanding of the mysterious 'rip' entry as well as the impact loading on the divers.

Conclusion

In summary, considerable effort and advancement have been made to understand the mechanics of the take-off and aerial techniques in springboard diving. Although not commonly practised, there is a high potential to apply computer simulation modelling to optimize performance for individual divers and to invent new dives. More future work can be expected in modelling the diver-water interaction during the entry. Such work may enhance diving performance by searching for optimal underwater techniques during the entry and contribute to injury prevention by quantifying of the impact loading on the diver.

References

Boda, W. (1992) 'Modelling the springboard and diver as an oscillating spring system', unpublished doctoral dissertation, University of Massachusetts.

Cheng, K. B. and Hubbard, M. (2004) 'Optimal jumping strategies from compliant surfaces: a simple model of springboard standing jump', *Human Movement Science*, 23(1): 35–48.

Cheng, K. B. and Hubbard, M. (2005) 'Optimal compliant-surface jumping: a multi-segment model of springboard standing jumps', *Journal of Biomechanics*, 38(9): 1822–9.

Cheng, K. B. and Hubbard, M. (2008) 'Role of arms in somersaulting from compliant surfaces: a simulation study of springboard standing dives', *Human Movement Science*, 27(1): 80–95.

Figgen, M. (1989) 'Computer simulation of the two-dimensional flight phase of an athlete', *Proceedings of the XII International Congress of Biomechanics*, Los Angeles, CA: University of California, p. 274.

Jiang, Y., Li, J., Shu, T. and Zhang, Z. (2000a) 'A study on selected factors affecting takeoff height in three-meter springboard diving', *Proceedings of the XVIII International Symposium on Biomechanics in Sports II*, Hong Kong: Chinese University of Hong Kong, pp. 529–32.

Jiang, Y., Shu, T. and Li, J. (2000b) 'The standard control function of take-off phase in springboard diving', *Proceedings of the XVIII International Symposium on Biomechanics in Sports II*, Hong Kong: Chinese University of Hong Kong, pp. 533–6.

Jiang, Y., Zhu, S., Li, J. and Shen, Z. (2001) 'Optimization of human-board system with elastics', *Journal of Biomathematics*, 16(1): 1–8.

King, M. A., Kong, P. W. and Yeadon, M. R. (2009) 'Determining effective subject-specific strength levels for forward dives using computer simulations of recorded performances', *Journal of Biomechanics*, 42(16): 2672–7.

Kong, P. W. (2010) 'Hip extension during the come-out of forward and inward multiple pike somersaulting dives is controlled by eccentric contraction of hip flexors', *Journal of Sports Sciences*, 28(5): 537–43.

Kong, P. W., Yeadon, M. R. and King, M. A. (2005) 'Optimisation of takeoff techniques for maximum forward rotation in springboard diving', *Proceedings of the XXIII International Symposium on Biomechanics in Sports*, Beijing: The China Institute of Sport Science, pp. 569–72.

Kong, P. W., Yeadon, M. R. and King, M. A. (2006a) 'Modelling the muscle activation in springboard diving takeoffs', *Journal of Biomechanics*, 39(1): S184.

Kong, P. W., Yeadon, M. R. and King, M. A. (2006b) 'Constraints and robustness considerations in the optimisation of springboard diving takeoff technique', *Proceedings of the XXIV International Symposium on Biomechanics in Sports*, Salzburg: International Society of Biomechanics in Sports, pp. 1–8.

Kooi, B. W. and Kuipers, M. (1994) 'The dynamics of springboards', *Journal of Applied Biomechanics*, 10(4): 335–51.

Koschorreck, J. and Mombaur, K. (2009) 'Optimisation of somersaults and twists in platform diving', *Computer Methods in Biomechanics and Biomedical Engineering*, 12(1): 157–9.

Koschorreck, J. and Mombaur, K. (2012) 'Modelling and optimal control of human platform diving with somersaults and twists', *Optimization and Engineering*, 13(1): 29–56.

Kuipers, M. and van de Ven, A. A. F. (1992) 'Unilateral contact of a springboard and a fulcrum', *Journal of Applied Mechanics: Transactions of the ASME*, 59: 682–4.

Liu, T. and Wu, X. (1989) 'Best instant of take-off from springboard', *Proceedings of the XII International Congress of Biomechanics (Abstract 23)*, Los Angeles, CA: University of California.

Miller, D. I. (1970) 'A computer simulation model of the airborne phase of diving', unpublished doctoral dissertation, The Pennsylvania State University.

Miller, D. I. and Munro, C. F. (1985) 'Greg Louganis' springboard takeoff: I: temporal and joint position analysis', *International Journal of Sport Biomechanics*, 1(3): 209–20.

Qian, J., Zhang, S. and Jin, H. (2010) 'Computer simulation of "splash control" and research of the rip entry technique in competitive diving', *International Journal of Sports Science and Engineering*, 4(3): 165–73.

Sprigings, E. J. and Watson, L. G. (1985) 'A mathematical search for the optimal timing of the armswing during springboard diving take-offs', in D. A. Winter, R. W. Norman, R. P. Wells, K. C. Hayes and A. E. Patla (eds), *Biomechanics IX B*, Champaign, IL: Human Kinetics, pp. 389–94.

Sprigings, E. and Miller, D. I. (2004) 'Optimal knee extension timing in springboard and platform dives from the reverse group', *Journal of Applied Biomechanics*, 20(3): 275–90.

Sprigings, E. J., Watson, G., Haseganu, E. and Derby, D. (1986) 'A model for optimizing the timing of the relative force patterns of the arms, torso, and legs during springboard diving take-offs', *Proceedings of the North American Congress on Biomechanics*, Montreal: Canadian Society for Biomechanics, pp. 39–40.

Sprigings, E. J., Stilling, D. S. and Watson, L. G. (1989) 'Development of a model to represent an aluminium springboard in diving', *International Journal of Sport Biomechanics*, 5(3): 297–307.

Wooten, W. L. and Hodgins, J. K. (1996) 'Animation of human diving', *Computer Graphics Forum*, 15(1): 3–13.

Wu, X. and Liu, T. (1989) 'The mechanics of take-off from springboard', *Proceedings of the XII International Congress of Biomechanics (Abstract 24)*, Los Angeles, CA: University of California.

Yeadon, M. R. (1993a) 'The biomechanics of twisting somersaults. Part I: rigid body motions', *Journal of Sports Science*, 11(3): 187–98.

Yeadon, M. R. (1993b) 'The biomechanics of twisting somersaults. Part II: contact twist', *Journal of Sports Science*, 11(3): 199–208.

Yeadon, M. R. (1993c) 'The biomechanics of twisting somersaults. Part III: aerial twist', *Journal of Sports Science*, 11(3): 209–18.

Yeadon, M. R. (1993d) 'The biomechanics of twisting somersaults. Part IV: partitioning performances using the tilt angle', *Journal of Sports Science*, 11(3): 219–25.

Yeadon, M. R. (1993e) 'Twisting techniques used by competitive divers', *Journal of Sports Science*, 11(4): 337–42.

Yeadon, M. R., Atha, J. and Hales, F. D. (1990) 'The simulation of aerial movement – IV. A computer simulation model', *Journal of Biomechanics*, 23(1): 85–9.

Yeadon, M. R., Kong, P. W. and King, M. A. (2006) 'Parameter determination for a computer simulation model of a diver and a springboard', *Journal of Applied Biomechanics*, 22(3): 167–76.

39

MODELLING IN ROWING

Luisa Consiglieri

R. TOMÁS DA FONSECA 26, PATEO CENTRAL, 1600–256 LISBOA

Introduction

Rowing is a sport consisting of a continuous cyclical movement, which demands efficiency and accurate coordination of the full body to maximize performance. The rowing cycle is formed by the rower sliding back and forth along a monorail through the action of cyclical extension and flexion of the lower limbs. This general concept refers to different sports; for instance, the sport where the subject pulls one oar (in boat or indoor) and the ergometer rowing. In the ergometer rowing, the subject pulls a handle, which is connected to the flywheel that generates the rowing resistance. In recent years, this rowing motion has become a new competitive sport, a training for on–water race-pace rowers or simply an indoor exercise for healthy purposes. A statistical analysis describing motion and load characteristics of ergometer rowing is used to test the hypothesis that rowing stroke technique is associated with the incidence of low back pain (see O'Sullivan *et al.*, 2003). Indeed, the use of the values obtained for the torques may improve performance and prevent injuries such as chronic back pain (Bartlett and Bussey, 2011).

The forces generated by the biomechanical system have been evaluated by analysis of experimental data for the rowing exercise (see Pudlo *et al.*, 2005, and the references therein). Non-invasive techniques cannot estimate muscle forces accurately, and mathematical models are required to predict such forces. Using the multi-body based methodology, the anatomical segments of a human subject are considered to be rigid bodies interconnected by kinematical joints (Bresler and Frankel, 1950). The knowledge of experimental recorded data (spatial positions and orientations) of each body segment is sufficient to calculate resultant joint moments by the inverse dynamics method. In spite of the uncertainty, due to inaccuracies of the testing equipment (Riemer *et al.*, 2008; Robert *et al.*, 2007, and the references therein), of the anthropometric and kinematic input data needed for the inverse dynamics procedure, it is crucial that a correct model exists in order to evaluate the internal moments about the various body joints. The development of computational methods in the last few decades produced a large impact in the assessment of theoretical models. Moreover, the explicit ordinary differential equations (ODE) provide friendly numerical simulations (i.e. with negligible computational cost). Our objective is to determine an analytical expression that models the way in which each torque exerted about the joints cooperates to produce a measured movement when this

479

movement is taken into account. Effectively, the main goal is to predict moments of force for both pathological and sport exercise performances.

We deal with a mathematical model to a linked multi-segmented human body in order to apply the inverse analysis dynamics. The need for adoption of non-linear behaviours is indisputable (Gordon, 2003). The system of ordinary differential equations, formulated for angles and for the displacement of the body's centre of mass in the biomechanical model, describes the motion of the referred activity. An elementary multi-body mechanical system is used as an example to discuss the assumptions and procedures adopted. Since motion analysis does not identify the cause of errors, it is imperative to present as much as possible the number of unknown variables describing the motion by continuous methods, and to delineate their magnitude, timing and phasic relationships. In our rigid segment assumptions, the shoulder and elbow joints have three rotational degrees of freedom, and the others joints are represented by hinges with one degree of freedom in flexion and extension in the sagittal plane. All the corresponding kinematic and kinetic data are acquired from the literature and they are examined in order to determine the torques at the joints generated to maintain the movement, and consequently to establish the best performance during ergometer rowing.

In previous works, an algorithm for a 2D inverse problem was presented (for instance, see Hahn *et al.*, 2005). A simple 2D model for rowing seems to be adequate when the study is restricted to the performance of the legs in a planar configuration. Despite the existent research on rowing over the last decade (Baudouin and Hawkins, 2004; Découfour *et al.*, 2008; Fothergill *et al.*, 2008; Nevill *et al.*, 2010; Sforza *et al.*, 2012), no one model is widely accepted, and much remains to be learned with regard to the biomechanics of even ergometer rowing.

Mathematical model

The equations of motion can be derived by means of the Lagrange method. The problem is defined by the lagrangian motion equations ($k = 1, \ldots, n$):

$$\frac{d}{dt}\left(\frac{\partial L}{\partial \dot{q}_k}\right) - \frac{\partial L}{\partial q_k} = F_k \tag{1}$$

where $q = (q_1, \ldots, q_n)$ are the generalized variables, F denotes a non-conservative force and L denotes the Lagrangian operator, which represents the algebraic difference of the kinetic and the potential energies. Here, the superposed dot and d/dt both denote the derivative with respect to time, and $\partial/\partial y$ is the partial derivative with respect to y.

The approach used to state the final system of ODE consists in introducing the displacement of the centre of mass of each segment of the body.

Kinematic coordinates

The human skeleton can be modelled as a set of linked segments. For instance, the foot, the shank, the thigh, the hand, the arm, the forearm, the head and the trunk, which can be decomposed into the pelvis (L4-L5 to trochanter), the lumbar segment (L1 to L4-L5), the lower thoracic segment (T10L1), and the upper two thoracic segments (T4T7, T7T10), or even more bony segments. This 3D articulated linkage has its rigid body segments joined together by frictionless hinges (one-dimensional rotational points).

The rowing cycle consists of two stroke phases: drive and recovery. The drive phase represents the phase of force application, also known as the propulsion phase. This phase begins

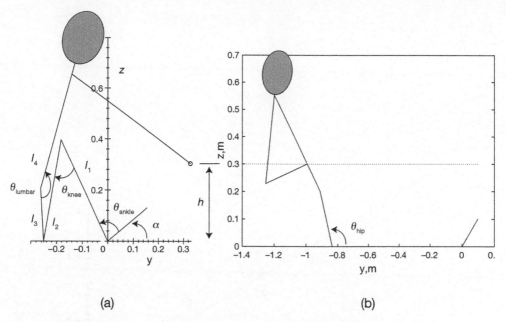

(a)   (b)

Figure 39.1 Schematic representations of the catch position (a), and of the final position of the drive phase, which coincides with the initial position of the recovery phase (b).

at the catch position (i.e. full flexion of the lower limb and lumbar joints and full extension of the upper limb joints, see Figure 39.1a) and ends when the configuration characterized by full extension of the lower limb and lumbar joints and full flexion of the upper limb joints is reached (see Figure 39.1b). The recovery phase, during which the rower glidingly returns to the initial position of the next cycle, ends when the catch position is reached.

The symmetry of rowing, due to the facts that the feet are in symmetrical foot-stretcher and the sliding seat moves on the track, was usually used for the study in sagittal plane (see, for instance, Colloud *et al.*, 2006). This reflects the rowing motion on ergometer in which the rower grips the handle symmetrical with both hands (see Figure 39.2). However, the rowing in boat is not completely symmetric to the sagittal plane due to different oar motion.

In the rowing performance, the feet are placed firm and flat upon the stretcher. Thus, the multi-segmented human body model can be described by comprising eight segments (the shank, the thigh, the pelvis, the head-trunk, two upper arms and the two forearms including the hands). The origin of the three-dimensional Cartesian reference frame is considered to be located at the ankle articulation (Figure 39.1) and the position of each centre of mass is denoted by (x_i, y_i, z_i) where $i = 1, \ldots, 6$ correspond, respectively, to the segments: shank (1), thigh (2), pelvis (3), head-trunk (4), right upper arm (5) and right forearm-hand (6). Since the movement is assumed to have a bilateral symmetry at any instant of time $t > 0$, the centres of mass of the left arm and forearm are positioned at $(-x_5, y_5, z_5)$ and $(-x_6, y_6, z_6)$, respectively. The angles formed by the four first segments are denoted by θ_{ankle}, θ_{knee}, θ_{hip}, and θ_{lumbar} (see Figure 39.1). For each $i = 1, \ldots, 6$, m_i denotes the mass of segment i, r_i the distance between the centre of mass of each segment and the distal end and l_i the length of segment i from the distal to the proximal end. Notice that m_1, m_2, m_5 and m_6 are the masses of the two shanks, thighs, upper arms and forearms, respectively. Since the hands are closed, they are assumed to be without length.

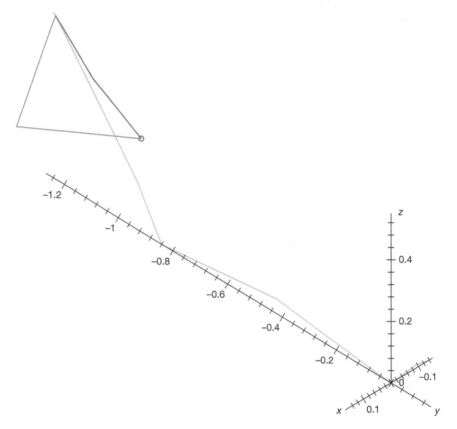

Figure 39.2 Schematic representation of an intermediate position.

Both lower limbs are assumed to be in the sagittal plane ($x = 0$) and their movement can be considered to take place in the plane $0yz$. The centre of mass of the shank is given by:

$$\begin{cases} x_1 = 0 \\ y_1 = r_1 \cos q_1 \ , \quad q_1 = \alpha + \theta_{\text{ankle}} \ , \\ z_1 = r_1 \sin q_1 \end{cases}$$

where α is the angle made by the back of the stretcher and the horizontal axis $0xx$ and it may vary from 43 to 53° (technically, the raked angle). Here we use 45°.

The centre of mass of the thigh is given by:

$$\begin{cases} x_2 = 0 \\ y_2 = l_1 \cos q_1 - r_2 \cos q_2 \ , \quad q_2 = q_1 - \theta_{\text{knee}} \ . \\ z_2 = l_1 \sin q_1 - r_2 \sin q_2 \end{cases}$$

Rowing is performed in a seated position. This position yields the following constraint, which is introduced by the position of the hip at the horizontal level $z = 0$ and the fixed lengths of the thigh and the shank:

$$l_1 \sin q_1 = l_2 \sin q_2. \tag{2}$$

This last equation lowers the problem's dimension by one unit, but also poses some difficulties to the calculations. So q_2 will be kept as an unknown variable and only z_3 and z_4 are simplified in the following kinematic equations.

The trunk is decomposed into the pelvis and the thorax and care is taken of their interaction (the lumbar angle). The centre of mass of the pelvis is taken as:

$$\begin{cases} x_3 = 0 \\ y_3 = l_1 \cos q_1 - l_2 \cos q_2 + r_3 \cos q_3 \; , \quad q_3 = q_2 - \theta_{\text{hip}} \; . \\ z_3 = r_3 \sin q_3 \end{cases}$$

The kinematic equations of the centre of mass of the head-trunk are:

$$\begin{cases} x_4 = 0 \\ y_4 = \displaystyle\sum_{i=1}^{3} (-1)^{i+1} l_i \cos q_i + r_4 \cos q_4 \; , \quad q_4 = q_3 - 180° + \theta_{\text{lumbar}} \; . \\ z_4 = l_3 \sin q_3 + r_4 \sin q_4 \end{cases}$$

We emphasize that for each $i = 1, \ldots, 4$, q_i is the measured angle with respect to the horizontal in the sagittal plane.

The shoulder-elbow-wrist/hand complex has a 3D characterization (see Figure 39.2). The position (x_5, y_5, z_5) of the centre of mass of the right upper arm is given, as a function of the spherical coordinates q_5 and q_6, by:

$$\begin{cases} x_5 = r_5 \sin q_5 \sin q_6 \\ y_5 = \displaystyle\sum_{i=1}^{3} (-1)^{i+1} l_i \cos q_i + l_4 \cos q_4 + r_5 \sin q_5 \cos q_6 \; . \\ z_5 = l_3 \sin q_3 + l_4 \sin q_4 - r_5 \cos q_5 \end{cases}$$

similarly, the position (x_6, y_6, z_6) of the centre of mass of the right forearm is given as a function of the spherical coordinates, q_7 and q_8, by:

$$\begin{cases} x_6 = l_5 \sin q_5 \sin q_6 + r_6 \sin q_7 \sin q_8 \\ y_6 = \displaystyle\sum_{i=1}^{3} (-1)^{i+1} l_i \cos q_i + l_4 \cos q_4 + l_5 \sin q_5 \cos q_6 + r_6 \sin q_7 \cos q_8 \; . \\ z_6 = l_3 \sin q_3 + l_4 \sin q_4 - l_5 \cos q_5 - r_6 \cos q_7 \end{cases} \tag{3}$$

Also, the stroke phases may be determined according to the movement of the handle in the horizontal direction. The motion of the handle backward, away from the flywheel, represents the drive phase, while the recovery phase is determined as the handle motion in the opposite direction. If we consider that (x_7, y_7, z_7) is the wrist-hand complex position, which coincides with the handle displacement, then $x_7 = 0$ so that the movement is symmetrically executed. Since the wrist-hand positioned at $(0, y_7, z_7)$ belongs to the spherical surface centred at the elbow, articulation with radius l_6, the right forearm segment is constrained by that position, that is:

$$
\begin{cases}
x_6 = \left(1 - \dfrac{r_6}{l_6}\right) l_5 \sin q_5 \sin q_6 \\[3mm]
y_6 = \left(1 - \dfrac{r_6}{l_6}\right)\left(\displaystyle\sum_{i=1}^{3}(-1)^{i+1} l_i \cos q_i + l_4 \cos q_4 + l_5 \sin q_5 \cos q_6\right) + \dfrac{r_6}{l_6} y_7 \\[3mm]
z_6 = \left(1 - \dfrac{r_6}{l_6}\right)\left(l_3 \sin q_3 + l_4 \sin q_4 - l_5 \cos q_5\right) + \dfrac{r_6}{l_6} z_7 \ .
\end{cases}
\tag{4}
$$

Although this constraint also lowers another dimension to the problem, q_7 and q_8 are kept as unknown variables in order to simplify the calculations.

Notice that the shoulder-elbow-wrist/hand complex is well defined by either the angles q_5, q_6, q_7, and q_8 according to (3) or the angles q_5 and q_6 and the wrist-hand position $(0, y_7, z_7)$ according to (4). Therefore, a different choice of the generalized coordinates will give a different explicit expression to L (cf. (5)).

Motion equations

With $q = (q_1, \ldots, q_8)$ and (x_i, y_i, z_i), $i = 1, \ldots, 6$, as above, let I_i be the moment of inertia of segment i about its centre of mass. Let us consider the Lagrangian operator:

$$
L(q) = \frac{1}{2}\sum_{i=1}^{6} m_i\left((\dot{x}_i)^2 + (\dot{y}_i)^2 + (\dot{z}_i)^2\right) + \sum_{i=1}^{8} I_i(\dot{q}_i)^2 - g\sum_{i=1}^{6} m_i z_i \ ;
\tag{5}
$$

with g denoting the acceleration constant due to gravity, and the non-conservative force:

$$
F = \begin{bmatrix}
T_1 - T_2 + r_0\left(F_{1z}\cos\alpha - F_{1y}\sin\alpha\right) \\
T_2 - T_3 - \left(l_2\cos q_2 - l_1\cos q_1\right)F_{\text{seat}} \\
T_3 - T_4 - \left(l_2\cos q_2 - l_1\cos q_1\right)F_{\text{seat}} \\
T_4 - T_5 \\
T_5 - T_7 \\
T_6 - T_8 \\
T_7 + y_7 F_{7z} - z_7 F_{7y} \\
T_8
\end{bmatrix}_{8\times1},
$$

where each T_k denotes the k-th joint torque in the x-direction ($k = 1, \ldots, 5$), T_6 the 5-th joint torque in the z-direction, and T_7 and T_8 the 6-th joint torque in the x and z-directions, respectively, which are assumed constant and independent of the angular displacement of the joint. The vector $(0, 0, F_{\text{seat}})$ denotes the vertical force applied by the sliding seat on the rower ischia, and $F_{\text{handle}} = (0, F_{7y}, F_{7z})$ represents the external force generated by the flywheel's mechanism and the air resistance transmitted to the two hands. It is assumed that the friction forces generated at the sliding seat as well as the air resistive force during the rowing cycle are minimal and are thus neglected. The reaction force at the feet stretcher, $F_{\text{stretcher}} = (0, F_{1y}, F_{1z})$, is assumed to be located at the centre of mass of the feet, and r_0 denotes the distance between the centre of mass of the foot and the distal end.

After some calculations, the Lagrangian operator L can be rewritten as:

$$L(q) = \frac{1}{2}\sum_{i,j=1}^{8}\dot{q}_i I_{ij}\dot{q}_j - g\sum_{i=1}^{6}m_i z_i$$

with $I(q) = [I_{ij}]_{i,j=1,\dots,8}$ representing the inertia mass matrix.

Observing that the inertia mass matrix I is symmetric, it is possible from (1) to obtain the following matrix form of the problem under study:

$$I(q)\ddot{q} = B(q,\dot{q}) + G(q) + T ,\qquad(6)$$

where $B(q, \dot{q}) = [B_i]_{i=1,\dots,8}$ represents the Coriolis and centrifugal effects, $G(q)$ represents the gravitational and external effects, and T the internal moments of force. Explicit expressions are given in detail by Consiglieri and Pires (2009).

The system (6) can be analysed by two forms: direct or inverse dynamics (Winter, 1990). Direct dynamics analysis is concerned with obtaining the response over time of the multi-body system when driven by loads. It is supposed to be known the moments of force that are realized across each biomechanical joint, and one looks up to calculate the angles that determine the motion, through the resolution of the system of ordinary differential equations of the second order. This resolution of mathematical interest has no such interest on the clinical point of view, because the amplitudes of the angles can be measured by non-invasive methods whereas the same does not happen with the moments of force. The objective of the inverse dynamics analysis is to calculate the moments of force that result from the muscle activity about the joints, which is responsible by the performed motion. For the determination of the moments of force, the angles are supposed to be known, as well as respective velocities and accelerations, which determine the given trajectories. Then, the necessary muscle control can be identified. Effectively, the direct resolution is useful to create a standard of reference with which the physiatrists or the physiotherapists can compare and determinate the disorders. Consequently, this analysis may be valuable in the diagnostic of pathologies and, in particular, the clinical state of determinate organ.

To simplify the description of the methodology, the model presented here is only inverse dynamically analysed. For this purpose, the knowledge of kinematic and kinetic data is required, namely the motion of the biomechanical system and all external applied forces. With this interpretation, the moment of forces $T_1, \dots, T_8$ can be stated as:

$$\begin{bmatrix} T_1 \\ T_2 \\ \vdots \\ T_8 \end{bmatrix}_{8\times1} = \begin{bmatrix} 1 & 1 & 1 & 1 & 1 & 0 & 1 & 0 \\ 0 & 1 & 1 & 1 & 1 & 0 & 1 & 0 \\ 0 & 0 & 1 & 1 & 1 & 0 & 1 & 0 \\ 0 & 0 & 0 & 1 & 1 & 0 & 1 & 0 \\ 0 & 0 & 0 & 0 & 1 & 0 & 1 & 0 \\ 0 & 0 & 0 & 0 & 0 & 1 & 0 & 1 \\ 0 & 0 & 0 & 0 & 0 & 0 & 1 & 0 \\ 0 & 0 & 0 & 0 & 0 & 0 & 0 & 1 \end{bmatrix} \cdot \left(I(q)\ddot{q} - B(q,\dot{q}) - G(q) \right) .\qquad(7)$$

After the data input, the torques $T_1, \dots, T_8$ are directly obtained from the above system.

Kinematic and kinetic data

The collected data is reduced to verify and update the mathematical model, and to enable the inverse dynamics analysis. The inertial properties associated with each anatomical segment are mass, moment of inertia, anthropometric segment length and the distance of its centre of mass from the proximal point.

The movement is formed by the trajectories of the joints in the Cartesian space. The pattern of extension/flexion of each joint is precisely described by the trajectories of the intrasegmental angles. We find explicit functions, by polynomial interpolation, to define the trajectory curves (as functions of time percentage of the total cycle duration).

The initial positions that correspond to the beginning of each stroke phase can be completely described in the plane Oyz (Figure 39.1). At the initial instant, the vertical coordinate of the wrist-hand complex position is known as $z_7(0)=h$, and this value should remain constant and equal to h during the whole rowing cycle for the exercise to be correctly performed. At the initial position of the recovery phase, the handle touches the chest of the subject. Indeed, the hands earlier bring the handle firmly home to the chest.

The trajectories can be explored via examination, that is, the trajectories can be obtained while performing the predetermined task. Each angular displacement can be approximated by the Taylor formula:

$$\theta_i\left(t\right)=\sum_{k=0}^{N}\theta_i^{(k)}\left(0\right)\frac{t^k}{k!} \quad \text{for} \ N \in IN , \tag{8}$$

with $\theta_i^{(k)}$ being the derivative of order k of θ_i. Taking into account that $\dot{\theta}_i(0) = \ddot{\theta}_i(0) = 0$, the terms of order 1 and 2 of the polynomial function in (8) vanish. Clearly, the remaining terms are constants obtained from experiments. The accuracy of this approximated formula depends on the number of the physiological values considered. The velocities and the accelerations can be obtained by differentiation of the polynomial functions in (8).

Figure 39.3 shows the profiles of θ_{ankle} and θ_{knee} performed by the lower limbs, and the profiles of θ_{hip} and θ_{lumbar} performed by the trunk (in the percentage of time). For instance, the ankle angle can be determined as (for $N = 5$):

$$\theta_{\text{ankle}}\left(t\right)=\begin{cases} 70+65\left(\dfrac{10}{35^3}t^3-\dfrac{15}{35^4}t^4+\dfrac{6}{35^5}t^5\right) & \text{if } \ t<35 \\[2mm] 180 \ \text{if} \ 35\leq t\leq 45 \\[2mm] 70+65\left(\dfrac{10}{55^3}\left(100-t\right)^3-\dfrac{15}{55^4}\left(100-t\right)^4+\dfrac{6}{55^3}\left(100-t\right)^5\right) & \text{if } \ t<35 \end{cases}$$

.

Hence, q_1 holds and, therefore, q_2 follows from (2).

Body-swing and slide-back move back in unison, and they practically end together (respectively, $t = 40$ per cent and $t = 35$ per cent). Simultaneously with the knees coming firmly down, the elbows pass the sides, while the shoulders still continue moving back and downwards. Body-swing and slide-forward move slower, with the duration according to the body's rest, and end at the same percentage of time ($t = 100$ per cent). As they end, the arms are perfectly straight from shoulder to wrist. An ideal cycle begins its swing-back without the loss of a fraction of time.

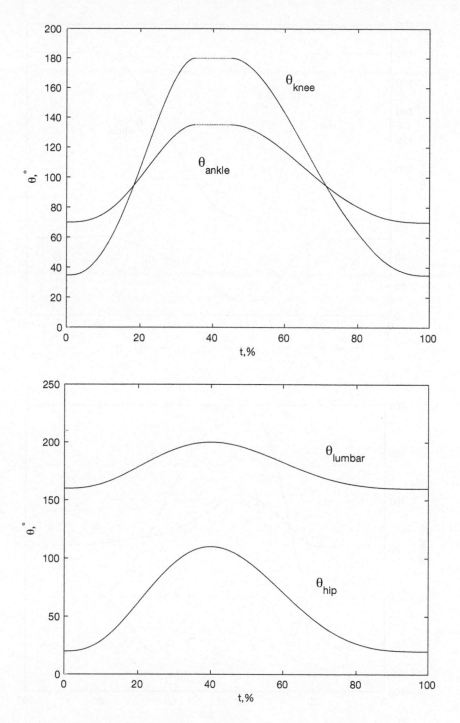

Figure 39.3 Example of phasic angular displacement patterns normalized in time as % of the cycle of the ergometer rowing. (a) Lower limbs: ankle angle $\theta_{ankle} = q_1 - \alpha$ and knee angle $\theta_{knee} = q_1 - q_2$; (b) trunk: hip angle $\theta_{hip} = q_3 - q_2$, and lumbar angle $\theta_{lumbar} = q_4 - q_3 + 180°$ (graphs were adapted from Bull and McGregor, 2000; Nowicky *et al.*, 2005).

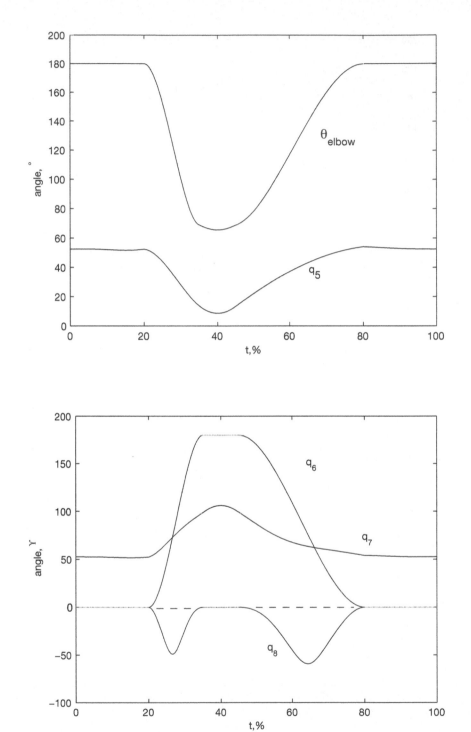

Figure 39.4 Profiles of (a) q_5, and the elbow angle (θ_{elbow}); and (b) the remaining spherical coordinates (q_6, q_7 and q_8), while the cycle of the ergometer rowing is performed during the time duration (0–100 per cent).

Moreover, once the angle measured at the elbow between the two segments (θ_{elbow}, Figure 39.4a displays one profile of the elbow angle) is known, the handle displacement y_7 is well determined by the following formula:

$$\left(Y_4(t) - y_7(t)\right)^2 + \left(Z_4(t) - h\right)^2 = l_5^2 + l_6^2 - 2l_5l_6\cos\theta_{elbow}(t) ,$$

where $(0, Y_4, Z_4)$ denotes the 3D position of the shoulder articulation:

$$\begin{cases} Y_4 = \sum_{i=1}^{3}(-1)^{i+1} l_i \cos q_i + l_4 \cos q_4 \\ Z_4 = l_3 \sin q_3 + l_4 \sin q_4 \end{cases}.$$

Consequently, under the above constraint and with the knowledge of one q_i ($i = 5, 6, 7, 8$), it is possible to obtain the other three (Figure 39.4).

At the initial period of the drive phase (0–20 per cent), both upper limbs are fully extended ($\theta_{elbow} = 180$, and $q_5 = q_7$), and located at the sagittal plane ($q_6 = q_8 = 0$, i.e. $x = 0$).

Figure 39.5 shows the external forces during a single cycle. The contributions of the external applied forces at each joint are essential in order to provide an accurate model of the multi-body system. The forces are mathematically represented by a vector with three components: vertical, anterior-posterior and lateral.

The anterior-posterior handle force has a bell-shaped profile (see Figure 39.5a) with a rapid increase in the magnitude of the force until a peak is reached, followed by a decrease. After this decrease, a constant value is reached, which is found to be equal to the traction force provided by the elasticity of the self-recoiling system. The vertical handle force also shows a reverse bell shape in the propulsion phase (see Figure 39.5a).

The force of reaction on the seat is a response of the muscular actions as well as of the weight of the body transmitted by the hip. The anterior-posterior component is neglected because it evaluates the horizontal friction due to the seat track. Then, the force of reaction is confined to the vertical component. The sliding seat load has a bell shape (see Figure 39.5b), reaching its maximum when the lower limbs and trunk are fully extended. Finally, Figure 39.5b also illustrates the non-linear behaviour of the two components of the stretcher force. Their values indicate how much the feet pressure forwards (F_{1y}) or downwards (F_{1z}) against the stretcher, as the slide moves. The weight of the subject is distributed on the seat slider, and on the feet stretcher.

Illustrative relations

The main objective of this section is to provide a better understanding of the correlation between the human skeletal data, and the torques imposed on the joints. The contribution of each joint torque from the action of the muscles is obtained by the calculation of the whole system (7). In order to record the torques, we use the Taylor formula (8) to obtain the angles related with the ankle, the knee, the hip, the lumbar and shoulder-elbow-wrist/hand complex as recorded in Figures 39.3 and 39.4.

In this application, the full cycle for the exercise in a rowing ergometer was constructed by assuming bilateral symmetry. At the early drive phase (0–20 per cent) and late recovery phase (80–100 per cent), the rower cycle is performed at the sagittal plane ($q_6 = q_8 = 0$) with the upper limbs fully extended ($\theta_{elbow} = 180$, and $q_5 = q_7$, cf. Figure 39.4). The profiles obtained for the torques are as predicted: the maximum and minimum values occur at the same instants

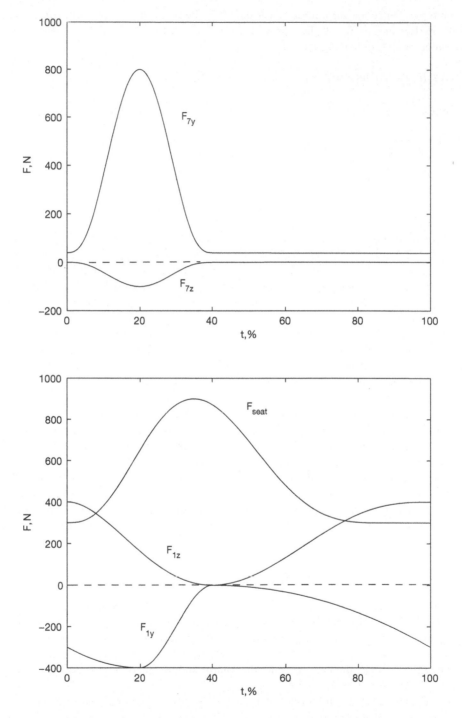

Figure 39.5 (a) Antero-posterior and vertical handle forces (F_{7y} and F_{7z}, respectively) as functions of percentage of time; (b) vertical seat force (F_{seat}), and antero-posterior and vertical stretcher forces (F_{1y} and F_{1z}, respectively) as functions of percentage of time (graphs were adapted from Hase *et al.*, 2002; Pudlo *et al.*, 2005).

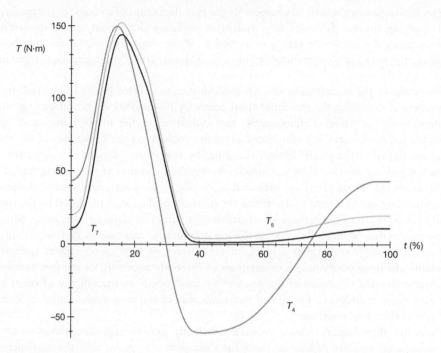

Figure 39.6 The joint torques T_4, T_5 and T_7 corresponding to the lumbar, shoulder and elbow joints, respectively, in the x-direction.

as the peaks of the external forces (see Figure 39.6). Indeed, for the joints of the upper body, the peaks of T_4, T_5 and T_7 match the ones of the handle forces, and the anterior-posterior stretcher force (see Figure 39.5). No significant values in magnitude are revealed in the remaining patterns of T_5 and T_7 during the recovery phase. This predicts no significant activity, as expected. The profile of T_4 corresponds to the range of lumbar-joint motion experienced during rowing. The sign change during the late recovery phase is consistence with the existence of the countermovement (i.e. the muscles are preparing themselves to stop the movement in order to prevent hyperextension).

These results are consistent with the muscle activity patterns of experienced rowers on the Concept 2C (cf. Nowicky *et al.*, 2005), and they support the hypothesis of a minimum-metabolic energy in rowing.

Conclusions

This model for the analysis of rowing motion is characterized by the system of equations of motion describing body-segmental dynamics. The equations of motion of the constrained biomechanical system are assembled using rigid bodies describing the anatomical segments interconnected by ideal joints. The Lagrange method is applied to define the mathematical model by the ODE system. The comparison with the classical Newton-Euler recursive procedure makes it possible to assess the simplicity of this method (for instance, see Cerne *et al.*, 2011; Consiglieri and Pires, 2007). The resultant methodology will assist the work of professionals of orthopedics and sports medicine in the determination of the torques at the joints generated to maintain the movement.

This model presents several advantages: (1) the easy deduction of torques from experimental data, applying inverse dynamics to a system of ordinary differential equations describing simultaneously the motion of each part as well as of the entire system; (2) the possibility of extending the model to a more complex linked multi-body; and (3) its negligible computational cost.

The study of the contribution of each individual muscle force is not considered. Indeed, the process of modelling the musculoskeletal geometry has its own shortcomings (e.g. muscle moment arms and paths). Consequently, the evaluation of the forces transmitted by the individual joint structures still constitutes an open problem via the evaluation of the muscle forces developed at the joints. Notwithstanding, by the inverse dynamics analysis the joint torques, which are developed by the muscles during the execution of the predetermined task, can be predicted. These forces are evaluated according to the continuous system of equations of motion. The model is used to determine the moment of the forces produced by the muscles about each joint, from quantitative observations of a particular trajectory (motion). Although the current analysis strongly depends on the input kinematic data and on their availability, for instance, the correct trajectories depend on the efficacy of high speed camera systems that determine changing positions and orientations of the body segments, or the measurement of the magnitudes and directions of the reaction forces depends on the efficacy of strain gauge or piezoelectric transducers, the aim of this work was to improve mathematical models that may contribute to new software.

Here, the physiological data are assumed sufficiently smooth neglecting the eventual jerks caused by temporary loss of balance, since the main goal is to prove how the new method is useful and of low computational cost. More sophisticated simulations can be performed with other physiological data. Moreover, the present analytical model can be applied to a large number of rower performances since the main assumptions correspond to the seat sliding along the central bar, and the two hands of the rower grasping the handle that is attached by a chain to the flywheel (which in turn puts a fan in motion).

Only the bilateral symmetry of the rowing movement and the correctness of the horizontal trajectory of the handle were additionally assumed in order to simplify the presentation. Also the data taken from the literature have these same characteristics corresponding to the stable base of the ergometer. Notice that these two limitations can be removed with the obvious implication of having to deal with a more complex model. Future work should exclude these two limitations in order to provide a complete study on the relation between involuntary inaccurate movements and lumbar pains (see Pudlo *et al.*, 2005, and the references therein). Indeed, the 3D model may be asymmetric according to the rowing in water in which the oarman is subjected to different loads. Nevertheless, a major decomposition of the trunk will help the investigation of the occurrence of spine injury in rowers.

The present theoretical model was numerically studied by solving two examples (Consiglieri and Pires, 2009), where a comparison between the appropriate initial position of the upper limbs and the torques is examined. We believe that the ability to predict the internal moments is particularly important because it offers the possibility of investigating the impacts of the coordination and function of the movements on the human structure. The results obtained with different sets of data can lead to improvements in the procedures for the correction of joint performances and in the prevention of injuries.

From the fact that the human body always attempts to spend a minimal energy, some compensations are due to appear at unaffected organs when malfunctions arise. To avoid these compensations, the study of muscle coordination is imperative and still remains an open problem.

References

Bartlett, R. and Bussey, M. (2011) *Sports Biomechanics: Reducing Injury Risk and Improving Sports Performance*, 2nd edn, London: Routledge.

Baudouin, A. and Hawkins, D. (2004) 'Investigation of biomechanical factors affecting rowing performance', *Journal of Biomechanics*, 37(7): 969–76.

Bresler, B. and Frankel, J. P. (1950) 'The forces and moments in the leg during level walking', *Transactions of the American Society of Mechanical Engineers*, 72: 27–36.

Bull, A. M. J. and McGregor, A. H. (2000) 'Measuring spinal motion in rowers: the use of an electromagnetic device', *Clinical Biomechanics*, 15(10): 772–6.

Cerne, T., Kamnik, R. and Munih, M. (2011) 'The measurement setup for real-time biomechanical analysis of rowing on an ergometer', *Measurement*, 44(10): 1819–27.

Colloud, F., Bahuaud, P., Doriot, N., Champely, S. and Chèze, L. (2006) 'Fixed versus free-floating stretcher mechanism in rowing ergometers: mechanical aspects', *Journal of Sports Sciences*, 24(5): 479–93.

Consiglieri, L. and Pires, E. B. (2007) 'Analytical approach for the evaluation of the torques using inverse multibody dynamics', *Multibody System Dynamics*, 18(3): 471–83.

Consiglieri, L. and Pires, E. B. (2009) 'An analytical model for the ergometer rowing: inverse multibody dynamics analysis', *Computer Methods in Biomechanics and Biomedical Engineering*, 12(4): 469–79.

Découfour, N., Barbier, F., Pudlo, P. and Gorce, P. (2008) 'Forces applied on rowing ergometer concept2®: a kinetic approach for development (P94)', in M. Estivalet and P. Brisson (eds), *The Engineering of Sport 7, Vol. 1*, Paris: Springer-Verlag, pp. 483–90.

Fothergill, S., Harle, R. and Holden, S. (2008) 'Modeling the model athlete: automatic coaching of rowing technique', *Lecture Notes in Computer Science, Structural, Syntactic, and Statistical Pattern Recognition*, 5342: 372–81.

Gordon, S. (2003) 'A mathematical model for power output in rowing on an ergometer', *Sports Engineering*, 6(4): 221–34.

Hahn, D., Schwirtz, A. and Huber, A. (2005) 'Anthropometric standardisation of multiarticular leg extension movements: A theoretical study', *Isokinetics and Exercise Science*, 13(2): 95–101.

Hase, K., Kaya, M., Yamazaki, N., Andrews, B. J., Zavatsky, A. B. and Halliday, S. E. (2002) 'Biomechanics of rowing: I. a model analysis of musculo-skeletal loads in rowing for fitness', *JSME International Journal. Series C, Mechanical Systems, Machine Elements and Manufacturing*, 45(4): 1073–81.

Nevill, A. M., Beech, C., Holder, R. L. and Wyon, M. (2010) 'Scaling concept II rowing ergometer performance for differences in body mass to better reflect rowing in water', *Scandinavian Journal of Medicine and Science in Sports*, 20(1): 122–7.

Nowicky, A. V., Burdett, R. and Horne, S. (2005) 'The impact of ergometer design on hip and trunk muscle activity patterns in elite rowers: an electromyographic assessment', *Journal of Sports Science and Medicine*, 4: 18–28.

O'Sullivan, F., O'Sullivan, J., Bull, A. M. J. and McGregor, A. H. (2003) 'Modelling multivariate biomechanical measurements of the spine during a rowing exercise', *Clinical Biomechanics*, 18(6): 488–93.

Pudlo, P., Pinti, A. and Lepoutre, F. X. (2005) 'Experimental laboratory apparatus to analyze kinematics and 3D kinetics in rowing', *Sports Engineering*, 8(1): 39–46.

Riemer, R., Hsiao-Wecksler, E. T. and Zhang, X. (2008) 'Uncertainties in inverse dynamics solutions: a comprehensive analysis and an application to gait', *Gait and Posture*, 27(4): 578–88.

Robert, T., Chèze, L., Dumas, R. and Verriest, J. P. (2007) 'Validation of net joint loads calculated by inverse dynamics in case of complex movements: application to balance recovery movements', *Journal of Biomechanics*, 40(11): 2450–6.

Sforza, C., Casiraghi, E., Lovecchio, N., Galante, D. and Ferrario, V. F. (2012) 'A three-dimensional study of body motion during ergometer rowing', *The Open Sports Medicine Journal*, 6: 22–8.

Winter, D. A. (1990) *Biomechanics and Motor Control of Human Movement*, 2nd edn, New York: John Wiley & Sons.

40

HEAD-BRAIN-SAS BIOMECHANICS AND TBI IN SPORTS AND ACCIDENTS

Parisa Saboori[1] and Ali M. Sadegh[2]

[1]MANHATTAN COLLEGE, NEW YORK
[2]CITY UNIVERSITY OF NEW YORK, NEW YORK

Traumatic brain injury (TBI) is mainly due to automotive accidents, contact sports, falls or blunt impacts to the head. It has been shown that subarachnoid space (SAS) trabeculae play an important role in damping and reducing the relative movement of the brain with respect to the skull, thereby reducing traumatic brain injuries (TBI) (Zoghi-Moghadam and Sadegh, 2010). However, the histology, architecture and mechanical properties of the SAS are not well established in the literature. Previous investigators have oversimplified the complex architecture of the SAS trabeculae and have employed soft solid materials for the SAS, which may lead to unreliable results.

In this chapter, the mechanotransduction of head impacts to the brain with the emphasis on the role of material modelling of the subarachnoid space is presented. The 2D and 3D local and global models of the SAS and the head were created, validated and the effect of SAS material properties on transferring the external load to the brain was investigated. It was concluded that the trabeculae can be simulated as tension elements since they buckle with minimal compressive load. The results indicated that the elastic modulus of E = 1,150 Pa is a realistic value for SAS. The effect of the different types of material modelling of SAS on transferring the load to brain was studied and was compared with the experimental study of Feng *et al.* (2010). Finally, the 3D head model was subjected to a series of impact velocities, and the strain in the brain as a function of applied velocity impact was determined. It has been conclude that, for the impact velocity range of 17–20 MPH, the strain in the brain varied 10–13 per cent. The results reveal that the material properties of the SAS play a significant role in determining the strain in the brain and therefore understanding different types of the head/brain and TBI injuries.

Introduction

Traumas involving vehicular collisions, falls or contact sports such as football, hockey and boxing could cause relative motion between the brain and the skull leading to Traumatic Brain Injury. In recent years, it has been reported that exposure to a blast from and improvised explosive device (IED) can cause TBI. Based on *Centers for Disease Control and Prevention* (CDC) report, TBI is a major public health problem in the US, especially among male young people, adults ages 15–24, and elderly people of 75 years and older. Children age 5 and younger are also at high risk for TBI (CDC).

Traumatic brain injury (TBI) is generally caused by contact (blunt head impact) or non-contact (angular acceleration) to the head. Symptoms of TBI can be mild, moderate, or severe, depending on the extent of the damage to the brain. CDC reports further indicate that each year about 1.7 million people experience a type of TBI in the USA. Approximately 52,000 people die from head injuries and about 1.365 million, nearly 80 per cent, of head injured people are treated in hospital emergency rooms. TBI is a major contributing factor to a third (30.5 per cent) of all injury-related deaths in the United States (Faul *et al.*, 2010). About 75 per cent of TBIs that occur each year involve concussions or other forms of mild TBI. Therefore, in recent years, head and brain biomechanics have been attracted the attention of many investigators.

Anatomically, the human brain is encased in the skull and is suspended and supported by a series of fibrous tissue layers, dura mater and the three layers: arachnoid, trabeculae and pia mater, known as the meninges. In addition, cerebrospinal fluid (CSF) located in the space between the arachnoid and pia mater known as subarachnoid space (SAS) stabilizes the position of the brain during head movements, as shown in Figure 40.1. Blunt head impacts and/or non-contact angular accelerations of the head cause relative motion between the brain and the skull. This increases the normal and shear stresses in the skull/brain interface region, which leads to the rupture of cerebral blood vessels and in particular bridging veins. This may also increase the strain in the brain which causes TBI. Subarachnoid space (SAS) trabeculae play an important role in damping and reducing this relative movement of the brain with respect to the skull, thereby reducing traumatic brain injuries.

To explain the likely injury process of the brain and to quantify the response of the human head to blunt impacts, investigators have employed experimental, analytical and numerical methods. Many researchers have used the finite element (FE) method to study head/brain injuries (Al-Bsharat, 1999a, 1999b; Feng *et al.*, 2010; Gupta *et al.*, 2009; Moss *et al.*, 2009; Ruan *et al.*, 1993; Takhounts *et al.*, 2008; Zhang *et al.*, 2001b, 2001c, 2002).The complicated geometry and architecture of the SAS and trabeculae makes it impossible to model all the details of the region. Thus, in these studies and other similar studies, the meningeal layers and the subarachnoid region have been simplified as a soft elastic material or in some cases as water (i.e. soft solid having bulk modulus of water and very low shear modulus) (Kleiven and Hardy, 2002; Zhang *et al.*, 2001c, 2002). That is, the hydraulic damping (i.e. the fluid solid interaction) and the mechanical role of the fibrous trabeculae and the cerebrospinal fluid (CSF) in the

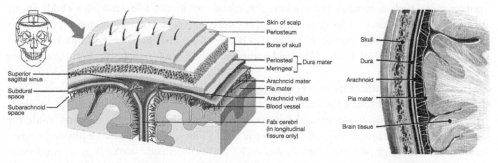

Figure 40.1 Sagittal and lateral views of meninges layer (with kind permission from Addison Wesley Longman Inc.)

subarachnoid space (SAS) were ignored. These simplifications, which are due to the complex architecture and random orientation of the trabeculae, could make the result unreliable.

In addition to the simplified models, the mechanical properties of SAS are not well established in the literature. A few studies (Jin *et al.*, 2006; Zhang *et al.*, 2001a, 2002), have reported a wide range of elastic modulus of trabeculae up to three orders of magnitudes. This wide range of the reported elastic modulus (from E = 59.81 × 10^3 Pa (Jin *et al.*, 2006) to E = 21.5 × 10^6 Pa (Zhang *et al.*, 2002)) questioning the validity of these data.

The SAS that includes CSF and the trabeculae has a complex structure. This is due to abundance of trabeculae, which are in the form of rods (fibres), thin transparent plates, and tree-shaped that is extended from the arachnoid (subdural) to the pia mater. The pia mater adheres to the surface of the brain and follows all the brain contours including the folds of the cerebral and cerebella cortices. This gives the subarachnoid space a highly irregular shape and makes the flow of CSF around the brain non-laminar and complicated. This interaction between the CSF and the trabeculae suggests that their functions are not independent. The interaction between the fluid and solid phase mechanically support the brain.

While the functionality of the SAS is understood, the histology and biomechanics of this important region has not been fully investigated. It is understood, however, that the arachnoid is a thin vascular layer composed of layers of fibroblast cells interspersed with bundles of collagen. The trabecula is also a collagen based structure. Only the histology of the trabeculae of the optical nerves has been studied (Killer *et al.*, 2003). The histology of the human brain trabeculae has not been addressed in the literature, however Saboori (2011) investigated the histology and architecture of the SAS trabeculae.

In this chapter, the mechanotransduction of the head impacts to the brain with the emphasis on the role of material modelling of the subarachnoid space as it relates to Traumatic Brain Injuries (TBI) is presented. This leads to the establishment of a criterion for the range of external impacts to the head, which causes concussion or TBI. This investigation was achieved through two steps. First, the 2D and 3D local and global models of the SAS and the head were created, validated and the effect of SAS material properties on transferring the external load to the brain was investigated. Second, the 3D head model was subjected to a range of impacts and the effect of impacts on the brain, leading to traumatic brain injury was studied.

Traumatic brain injury

Traumatic brain injury (TBI) is a major public health problem, especially among young male people, adults ages 15–24, and elderly people of 75 years and older. Children aged 5 and younger are also at high risk for TBI. TBI is a complex from of brain injury that is generally caused by contact sports such as football and hockey, automobile accidents, falls, shaking a child, or any type of accident or medical procedures. In recent years, it has been reported that exposure to a blast from an improvised explosive device (IED) can cause TBI. Each year, about 1.7 million people experience a TBI in the USA and approximately 52,000 people die from head injury accidents.

During an impact the brain moves in an oscillatory motion with respect to the skull, which causes a shear wave through the brain. TBI can be classified based on the severity of accident. In severe head trauma, an intracranial haemorrhage occurs, where there is bleeding inside the skull due to the rupture of a blood vessel in the skull. This could be due to a physical trauma such as head injury or non-traumatic causes such as a haemorrhagic stroke (e.g. an aneurysm).

Depending on the severity of the impact, an injured patient with a mild TBI may remain conscious or may experience a loss of consciousness for a few seconds or minutes. Different symptoms of mild TBI may include headache, confusion, lightheadedness, dizziness, blurred vision or tired eyes, and trouble with memory.

Different types of TBI

Concussion

Concussion is the most common type of head injury and may be defined as the loss of consciousness immediately following a trauma. Concussion is also included in the broad category of 'Closed Head Injury' (CHI). A major defining characteristic of concussion that helps to distinguish it from other types of TBI is the absence of a post-trauma 'waiting period'. In general, the severity of a concussion is characterized by the duration of loss of consciousness (LOC). Concussions and other brain injuries are fairly common. About every 21 seconds, someone in the United States has a serious brain injury. One of the most common reasons people sustain concussions is through sports injuries such as football, boxing and hockey, even with the use of protective headgear.

Contusion

Contusion refers to a bruising of part of the brain, frequently on the cortex (outer layer). It may result from either head contact, or head acceleration without contact, and a secondary contusion may result from brain movement within the skull due to a trauma. Contusions occur primarily in the cortical tissue, especially under the site of impact. The brain may be contused when it collides with bony protuberances on the inside surface of the skull. Because contusions involve structural brain damage, they are more serious than concussions.

Severe contusions lead to swelling in the brain, which can cause additional brain damage (i.e. memory loss, attention problems, emotional disturbances, loss of ability to understand or express speech). The prognosis for contusion depends upon the severity of the injury. Mild contusions are able to heal on their own with no medical intervention, while extremely severe contusions can cause herniation of the brain, and eventually coma.

Coma

Coma is a state of unconsciousness that can last for more than 6 hours when a person cannot be awakened and fails to respond normally to painful stimuli, light or sound, and does not initiate voluntary actions. In order for a patient to maintain consciousness, two important neurological components, the cerebral cortex, which is the grey matter covering the outer layer of the brain, and reticular activating system (RAS or ARAS), located in the brainstem, must function perfectly. Injury to either or both of these components is sufficient to cause a patient to experience a coma.

Coup-countercoup injury

A contusion may occur at the point of impact (coup) or at the opposite site of initial impact (or injury), in which case it is referred to as 'countercoup'. This kind of trauma occurs when the force impacting the head is not only great enough to cause a contusion at the site of impact, but is also able to rebound the brain and cause it to slam into the opposite side of the skull, which causes the additional contusion. A cerebral contusion is different than cerebral haemorrhage as it combines vascular and tissue damages. It occurs directly beneath the site of the impact at the coup site but it also occurs on the contralateral site of the impact, the counter-coup site.

Literature review

Experimental, analytical and numerical methods, and in particular finite element (FE) methods, have been employed by investigators to explain the likely injury process of the brain and to quantify the response of the human head to blunt impacts (Al-Bsharat *et al.*, 1999a, 1999b; Kleiven and Hardy, 2002; Ruan *et al.*, 1993; Zhang *et al.*, 2001b, 2001c, 2002). The complicated geometry of the SAS and trabeculae makes it impossible to model all the details of the region. Thus, in these studies and other similar studies, the meningeal layers and the subarachnoid region have been simplified as a soft elastic material or in some cases as water (i.e. soft solid having bulk modulus of water and very low shear modulus) (Kleiven and Hardy, 2002; Zhang *et al.*, 2001b, 2002). The shortcoming of these approaches is that the hydraulic damping (i.e. the fluid solid interaction) and the mechanical role of the fibrous trabeculae and the cerebrospinal fluid (CSF) in the subarachnoid space (SAS) were ignored. In addition to the simplified models, the mechanical properties of SAS are not well established in the literature. There have been a wide range of young modulus for pia arachnoid complex (PAC), from 21.5×10^6 Pa (Zhang *et al.*, 2002), to 11.18×10^3 Pa (Jin *et al.*, 2006), up to three orders of magnitudes. Only Zoghi-Moghadam and Sadegh (2010) determined the damping characteristics of SAS region by using the experimental study of Hardy *et al.* (1997). This was done by determining the damping coefficient of the brain/skull system and relating it to the hydraulic resistance of the CSF in the SAS region. The study of brain biomechanics are divided into two categories: experimental and analytical studies.

Experimental studies

In the animal (pig) experimental study by Meaney *et al.* (1995), diffuse axonal injury (DAI) of brain injury was investigated. They found that a diffuse axonal injury occurred when the brain tissues are subjected to a strain of 20 per cent. This threshold value is taken as a reference in most of the mechanical studies about TBI. In their cadaveric experiment study, Nahum *et al.* (1977) applied initial velocity of the impact and measured intracranial pressures, duration of the applied load and the impactor's mass. They also measured the input force, changes in skull acceleration and *in vivo* intracranial pressure with time during the impact. Hardy *et al.* (2001) and Al-Bsharat *et al.* (1999a, 1999b) measured the relative motion of the brain with respect to skull in human cadaver heads using neutral density technology and high-speed biplanar X-ray. They observed that the brain undergoes displacement relative to skull on the order of ± 5 mm when impacted with an angular speed of 17–22 rad.s^{-1}.

The histology of the trabeculae in the optical nerves has been studied by Killer *et al.* (2003). Their TEM and SEM studies of trabeculae in the optic nerve revealed pillars, septa and plate-like structures. Sabet *et al.* (2008) and Bayly *et al.* (2005) used tagged MRI and studied the brain deformation of adult volunteers subjected to a mild (non-traumatic and safe) angular acceleration ranging from 250 to 300 rad.s^{-2} and a rapid deceleration. They observed brain strain ranging between 2 and 5 per cent. Rowson and Duma (2011) studied the football helmet performance by integrating player head impact exposure and risk of concussion.

Analytical and numerical studies

The Wayne State University brain injury model (WSUBIM) has been developed and improved over the last several years (Al-Bsharat *et al.*, 1999a, 1999b; Jin *et al.*, 2006; Ruan *et al.*, 1993;

Zhang et al., 2001a, 2001b, 2001c; Zhou et al., 1995). The 3D FEM model of the human head has been validated by experimental data published by Nahum et al. (1977). The model was improved to be used for direct and indirect impact combined with translational and rotational acceleration. The main advantages of this model are the simulations of bone fractures in the face and skull.

National Highway Traffic Safety Administration (NHTSA) created a very sophisticated head model to be used for computer simulation study of TBI, the result of which is reported in Takhounts et al. (2008) as SIM Model. The material properties for different section of the model were base on previous study of study of Takhounts et al. (2003a, 2003b). They also used the football player helmet example to indicate the real impact force to the head. They concluded that the angular injury criteria better predicts traumatic brain injury. Feng et al. (2010) studied a human subject's head that was dropped on its own gravity approximately 2 cm. They concluded that the rotation and the displacement of the specific locations in the brain relative to the skull is approximately 2–3 mm.

Material properties

Material properties of the SAS are an important factor in modelling and finite element analyses of the SAS, when its histology and functionality is known. The second significant factor in the modelling is to accurately identify the type of tissue and the material for each segment of the SAS as it transfers the load to the brain. A wide range of material properties for the SAS region has been addressed in literature. In this chapter, we briefly explain the material properties that are used for each part of the head/brain analyses.

Brain

The brain material properties are relatively established in the literature. While a wide range of material properties are reported in the literature, depending on the type of the study, different material properties can be used. Fallenstein et al. (1969), Galford and McElhancy (1969), Holbourn (1945) and Koeneman (1966) used simple linear elastic material properties for their constitutive brain tissue. Arbogast and Margulies (1997), Bilston et al. (1998), Estes and McElaney (1970) and Miller and Chinzei (1997) used linear and quasi-linear viscoelastic. Darvish and Stone (2001) and Takhounts et al. (2003b) applied fully non-linear Green-Rivlin for their model. Nicolle et al. (2004) used Ogden Rubber with linear viscoelastic and Takhounts et al. (2008) used linear viscoelastic model. Atomic Force Microscope Indentation (AFM) was used to measure the mechanical property of the brain and, more specifically, in the hippocampus of the rat (Elkin et al., 2007). Zhang et al. (2001a, 2001b, 2001c, 2002) also used linear viscoelastic material properties for the brain tissue.

The extensive variety of the brain material properties reported in the literature make the decision rather complicated. Takhounts et al. (2008) performed simple shear displacement test on the 1 × 1 × 1 cube and studied the effect of different material properties, and the strain field was compared with the existing experimental study (e.g. Hardy et al., 2001). They conclude that the linear viscoelastic model will be fitted in most of the analyses and it is a suitable model for brain/head impact analysis. Summary of different material properties used for simple shear displacement are given on Table 40.1.

The subarachnoid space (SAS)

The histology, architecture and material properties of the subarachnoid space trabeculae have not been fully addressed in the literature. However, Killer et al. (2003) studied the structure

Table 40.1 Tissue material properties of the brain as a linear viscoelastic model, used in this study

Brain tissue	
Shear modulus at t = 0 (G_0) (Pa)	10.0×10^3
Shear modulus at t = ∞ (G_∞) (Pa)	2.0×10^3
Bulk modulus at t = 0 (K_0) (Pa)	5.0×10^7
Bulk modulus at t = ∞(K_∞) (Pa)	5.0×10^7
Relaxation time (λ) (s^{-1})	16
Density (ρ) (kg/m3)	1.04×10^3

of the trabeculae in the human optic nerve. They found that the structure of the trabeculae varies along the optic nerve.

While the trabeculae are collagen based, their material properties are not explicitly reported in the literature. However, it has been reported that the trabecula is a soft connective tissue containing 50 per cent collagen and 50 per cent water (Alcolado *et al.*, 1986). Because of the softness and elastic membrane characteristics of the trabeculae, the combination of the CSF and the trabeculae absorbs head impacts and protects the brain. Therefore, for the modelling and FE analysis of the head/brain, biomechanics investigators substitute and approximate the dura mater and the meninges including the CSF by a soft elastic material. We believe that this approximation compromises the mechanism and magnitude of the external load transfer to the brain. Nevertheless, Jin *et al.* (2006) experimentally measured some mechanical properties of pia arachnoid complex (PAC) as 59.81×10^3 Pa where it was stretched in the tangential direction (with respect to the head) and not in the radial direction. Previously, Zhang *et al.* (2001a, 2001b, 2001c) reported the mechanical properties for arachnoid trabeculae (as 11.5×10^6 Pa). As one can compare the two reported properties, they are three orders of magnitude different. The material properties of SAS used in this study are shown in Table 40.2.

Dura mater, skull and skin

The material property of the dura mater, skull and the scalp are fully addressed in the literature and they are considered to be soft elastic material, the skull also modelled as a rigid region with young modulus of 12.2 x 10^9 Pa (Takhounts *et al.*, 2003a, 2003b). Table 40.2 tabulates the material properties of the human head model.

Finite element modelling

One of the motivations of the SAS experimental study was to create more accurate models for computer simulations (Saboori, 2011). The highly inhomogeneous and dense SAS, which was found in the experimental studies of Saboori (2011), made it impossible to create a true global model for the SAS. Several 2D and 3D models were created using the experimental studies. Functionality of the SAS was one of main reasons to investigate the SAS material properties using FE analysis.

2D model

To further estimate material properties of the trabeculae, a two-dimensional (2D) transverse model of the head was created using the magnetic resonance imaging (MRI) of a subject (see

Table 40.2 Material properties of the head/brain model

Tissues	Variables	Values
Skin	Young's modulus (E) (Pa)	5.67×10^3
	Poisson's ratio (υ)	0.48
	Density (ρ) (kg/m³)	1.06×10^3
Skull	Young's modulus (E) (Pa)	12.2×10^9
	Poisson's ratio (υ)	0.22
	Density (ρ) (kg/m³)	2.12×10^3
Dura mater	Young's modulus (E) (Pa)	31.5×10^6
	Poisson's ratio (υ)	0.45
	Density (ρ) (kg/m³)	1.13×10^3
SAS	Young's modulus (E) (Pa)	1.15×10^3
	Poisson's ratio (υ)	0.48
	Density (ρ) (kg/m³)	1.13×10^3
Muscles	Young's modulus (E) (Pa)	1.00×10^7
	Poisson's ratio (υ)	0.38
	Density (ρ) (kg/m³)	$1.01 \times \star 10^3$
Neck	Young's modulus (E) (Pa)	6.04×10^9
	Poisson's ratio (υ)	0.38
	Density (ρ) (kg/m³)	1.18×10^3

Source: Adapted from Takhounts (2003a, 2003b).

Figure 40.2a). The FE model consists of the scalp, skull, dura mater, SAS and the brain, as shown in Figure 40.2b.

The FE model was created using the MRI images from an adult female patient (age 50s); all the dimensions were directly taken from the MRI. Abaqus 9.6-2 were used as pre processors, the details of the geometry and the dimensions were determined using eRAD/Image Medical Practice builder 1-2-3 software and were imported into Abacus sketch module. The model was then meshed using tetrahedral elements. The same boundary conditions as the experimental study of Sabet *et al.* (2008) were used. To simulate the experiment of Sabet *et al.* (2008), the model was subjected to the same boundary conditions as the experimental study and the same loading (i.e. a mild angular acceleration of 100 rad.s^{-2} to the head). Abaqus multi point constrain (MPC) was used to control the centre point. General contact was defined as an interface boundary condition between the SAS and dura mater. Abaqus explicit dynamic analysis was performed.

To estimate the material properties of the SAS, as soft solid, 12 different cases were studied. The results of the strain in the brain were determined and were compared with the 2–6 per cent strain of the experimental study of Sabet *et al.* (2008) and Bayly *et al.* (2005). The results revealed that for the Young modulus range of 1,000–1,500 Pa the strain range is within the range reported by Sabet *et al.* (2008). The middle range of 1,150 Pa was selected for our analyses since it was the closest range to experimental results (Saboori, 2011).

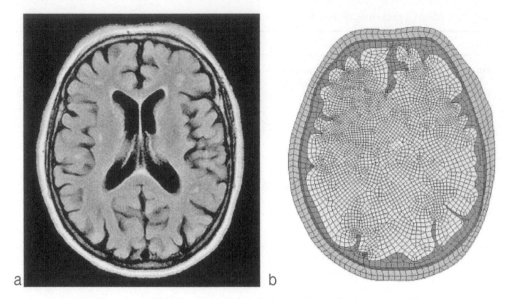

Figure 40.2 (a) MRI image of the transverse plane of a human head; (b) the FE model.

Also, three different materials for SAS were proposed. The material properties of each material type (i.e. soft solid, fluid and porous material) were analysed and compared with study of Sabet *et al.* (2008). The strain in the brain for each material type was compared with the experimental study. The result indicated that the strain in the brain for all three SAS material models was in good agreement with the experiment. That is, if one decides to use soft solid, fluid or porous materials to model the SAS, in local or global FE analyses, the properties found in this study are appropriate for modelling investigations (Saboori, 2011; Saboori and Sadegh, 2010, 2011a, 2011b, 2011c, 2011d; Saboori *et al.*, 2010).

3D model

The 3D head-neck model was created using the MRI images of a female adult patient in her 50s. The details of the geometry and the dimensions were determined using eRAD/Image Medical Practice builder 1-2-3 software. To create 3D model of the head, initially transverse, sagittal and lateral planes of the head were defined. Several cross-sections from each plane were imported into the Abaqus/CAE sketch modulus, each cross-section was measured and the data were used to create the same section in the Abaqus/CAE. Different layers of the head were assembled together to create a completed head model (Figure 40.3).

Validation of the 3D head model

The model was validated against the experimental study of Feng *et al.* (2010). In their study, a human subject's head dropped on its own gravity approximately 2 cm and came in contact with a rubber band that is used as a stopper. Displacement data were then obtained from this mild frontal head angular acceleration of the head and the impact with the rubber band. A tagged magnetic resonance imaging method was used to measure *in vivo* relative displacement between the brain and the skull of three adult male human subjects. Their study provides an

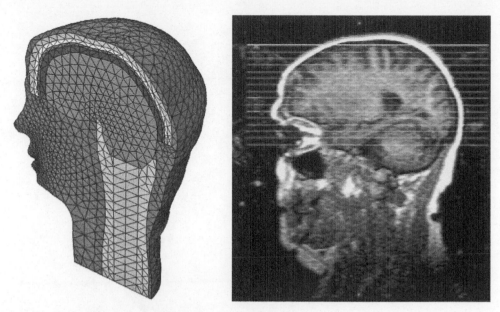

Figure 40.3 The MRI and the FEM model of the head/brain.

important set of displacement measurements in the human brain during the mild frontal skull impact. The result of Feng *et al.* (2010) shows that, at the four specific locations of the brain, the rotation and the displacement of these points relative to the skull is approximately 1–3 mm.

The 3D head model was subjected to the same displacement of 2 cm and boundary condition of the experiment. The displacements of different sections of the brain were compared to the four material locations (a, b, c and d) corresponding to the experimental study as shown in Figure 40.4.

Figures 40.5 and 40.6 depicts the comparison of the relative displacements between the skull and the brain in location 'a' and 'b' of the experimental study.

Note that the experimental curve of Feng *et al.* (2010) shown in Figures 40.5 and 40.6 indicate two peaks during the 168 ms period of the study. The first peak, which occurs at about 40–60 ms, is due to the moment when the head has its maximum angular acceleration. This moment is when the head of the subject hits the rubber band. Once the elastic rubber band is stretched, it creates a rebound force pushing the head upward. Then the head of the subject separates from the rubber band fallowed by dropping down on its own gravity. This is the moment when the second peak occurs. Note that in our model, we did not consider the rebound force of the rubber band as it refers to the second peak. It is important to indicate that the time lag after the first peak between experiment and our FEM results is due to the secondary force of the rubber that is not considered in our FE model.

Figure 40.5 and reveal that for the Young's modulus of 1,000 Pa, the relative displacement between the brain and the skull is in good agreement with the 1–2 mm range of the displacement in subject 2 of the experimental study of Feng *et al.* (2010). That is, the proposed young modulus of 1,000 Pa for the SAS is a reliable and appropriate value. The proposed range of E, also suggest that the SAS material is soft and absorbs the brain movements. This confirms our hypothesis on the functionality of the SAS that act as damper and shock absorber of the brain. This model could be used for computer simulation of TBI.

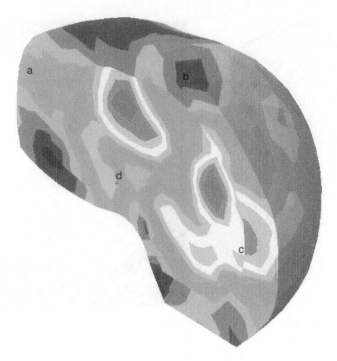

Figure 40.4 Four material locations in the 3D head model.

The blunt head impact

The 3D head model was used to study the strain in the brain when the head is subjected to a wide range of impacts. The duration of typical blunt impacts are known to be approximately between 30–50 ms (Hardy *et al.*, 2001; Zhang *et al.*, 2001a, 2001b, 2001c). The displacement curve of these typical impacts is approximately a sine curve (Hardy *et al.*, 2001). Considering these data, we established a series of curves for each case of the velocity impacts where the amplitude of the sine velocity curve correspond the 2.5–27 mph velocity impact. These impacts were applied to the frontal region of the head of the 3D model. The inferior section of the neck of the model was restrained. Half symmetric boundary conditions were applied on the sagittal plane of symmetry of the model.

The maximum value of the strain in the brain corresponding to each case was determines and the maximum strain-velocity curve was plotted in Figure 40.7. This figure shows that if the applied impact velocity to the head varies from 2.5 to 27 mph, the maximum strain increase from 2 to 17 per cent. This figure reveals that as the impact speed increases, the strain in the brain also increases with a profound peak values.

In their studies, Meaney *et al.* (1995) and Bayly *et al.* (2005) indicated that different types of the TBI occur if the axon of the neuron nerve in the brain stretches more than 10–15 per cent. That is, the myelin sheath around the axon nerve will be damaged and, in that case, these nerve tissues are not able to recover and heal themselves. This usually is the stage when TBI will occur in severe cases. As shown in Figure 40.7, these analyses reveal that the velocity impact on the frontal head is proportional with the maximum strain in the brain (i.e. with the increase in velocity of the impact, the likelihood of TBI is increased).

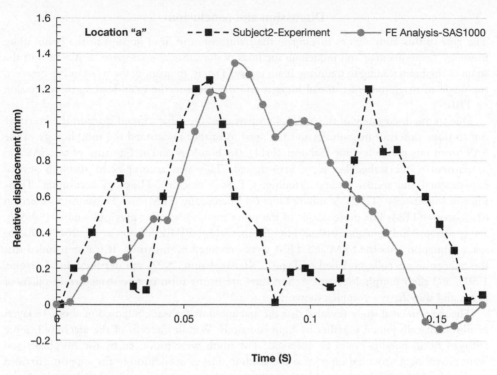

Figure 40.5 Relative displacement between the skull and the brain at the location 'a'.

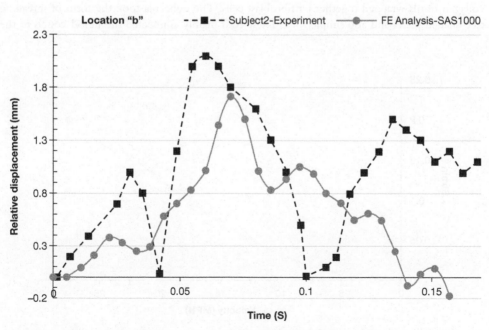

Figure 40.6 Relative displacement between the skull and the brain at the location 'b'.

Discussion and conclusion

The goal of this study was to investigate the transmission of head impacts to the brain, using histology (experimental) and modelling methods of the subarachnoid space, as it relates to the strain in the brain leading to traumatic brain injury. That is, to quantify the relationship between the range of magnitude of external impacts and the strain in the brain leading to concussion or TBI.

Due to the discrepancy of the material properties of the subarachnoid space in the literature (up to three orders of magnitude) and the need to further understand the morphology of the SAS, from our previous study (Saboori, 2011), the histology and architecture of the SAS and in particular, the trabeculae were investigated. This was accomplished through several experimental and animal studies including, CT Scan machine, Histology sectioning, Two-Photon Microscopy (TPM), Scanning Electron Microscopy (SEM) and Transmission Electron Microscopy (TEM) For more details of the other methods see our previous studies (Saboori, 2011; Saboori and Sadegh, 2010, 2011a, 2011b, 2011c, 2011d; Saboori *et al.*, 2010). Due to space limitation only the SEM and TEM were presented in this study. It was concluded that the trabeculae are collagen based of Type I (Kierszenbaum, 2007; van der Rest and Garrone, 1991), and their morphology and architectures are in the form of tree shaped rods, pillars or plates and they have a complex network.

The experimental study revealed that the arachnoid mater was composed of about 10 layers of fibroblast cells joined together by tight junctions. Within the cells of the arachnoid, some collagen fibrils bundles could be observed. The fibrils were produced by the fibroblasts and were providing a structural support to the arachnoid layer in addition to the support provided by the fibroblasts. The arachnoid layer appeared to be permeable on the TEM results. Some fluid was observed in the spaces between the fibroblasts. The layer at the junction with the SAS was spreading at some locations and was forming a descending trabecula from arachnoid to the pia mater in the tree-shaped architecture. This trabecula mainly consisted of bundles of collagen fibrils wrapped together by fibroblast cells. The trabecula took the form of spreading tree-shaped plates and also simple rods. These rods mainly connected the blood vessels to the

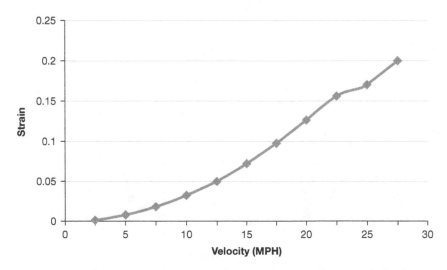

*Figure 40.*7 Variation of the strain in the brain as a function of impact velocity to the head.

arachnoid/pia mater. The trabeculae were commonly connecting the external layer of fibroblasts of the blood vessels to the arachnoid or pia mater. While these results are for rat, it is believed that the human brain has the same architecture.

One of the motivations of the SAS experimental study was to create more accurate models for computer simulations. The highly inhomogeneous and dense SAS that was found during our experimental study made it impossible to create true global model for the SAS. Several 2D and 3D models were created using our experimental studies. Functionality of the SAS was one of main reasons to investigate the SAS material properties using FE analysis.

As the first part of this study and to understand our previous results in a more global sense, a three-dimensional (3D) model of the head-neck using magnetic resonance imaging (MRI) and Abaqus/CAE sketch modulus was created. The 3D head model was validated against the experimental study of Feng *et al.* (2010). The validated 3D head model is a convenient tool to study the effect of the different types of the impacts to the brain. The nodal solution of the strain in the brain was plotted in the material location 'a' and 'b' and the relative displacement between the skull and the brain was compared with the experimental study of Feng *et al.* (2010).

In the experimental study of Feng *et al.* (2010), a human subject's head is dropped on its own gravity approximately 2 cm and the forehead comes in contact with a rubber band that is used as a stopper. Displacement data were then obtained from this mild frontal head angular acceleration of the head and the impact with the rubber band. A tagged magnetic resonance imaging method was used to measure *in vivo* relative displacement between the brain and the skull of three adult male human subjects. Their experimental study provides an important set of displacement measurements in the human brain during the mild frontal skull impact. The result of Feng *et al.* (2010) shows that at the four specific locations of the brain, the rotation and the displacement of these points relative to the skull is approximately 1–3 mm.

The experimental result of Feng *et al.* (2010) shown in Figures 40.5 and 40.6 indicate two peaks during the 168 ms period of the study. The first peak, which occurs at about 40–60 ms, is due to the time when the head has its maximum angular acceleration. This is when the forehead of the subject hits the rubber band (see Figures 40.5 and 40.6). Once the elastic rubber band is stretched, it creates a rebound force, pushing the head upward. Then the head of the subject separates from the rubber band fallowed by dropping down on its own gravity. This is the moment when the second peak occurs. Note that in our 3D head model, we did not consider the rebound force of the rubber band as it refers to the second peak. It is important to indicate that the time lag after the first peak, between experiment and our FEM results, is due to the secondary force of the rubber that is not considered in our FE model.

The result of 3D head model validation indicates that the proposed young modulus of 1,000 Pa for the SAS is a reliable and appropriate value. Note that in our 2D model, which was validated with the experimental work of Sabet *et al.* (2008), the optimum value of the young modulus was 1,150 Pa. Therefore, a range of 1,000–1,150 Pa for the young modulus is proposed. The proposed value of E also suggests that the SAS material is soft and absorbs the brain's movement. This confirms our hypothesis about the functionality of the SAS, which acts as a damper and a shock absorber of the brain.

At the last step, the 3D head model was subjected to the wide range of velocity impacts and the relationship between the applied velocities and the strain in the brain was analysed. Previous research indicated that different types of the TBI occur if the axon of the neuron nerve in the brain stretches more than 10–15 per cent (Bayly *et al.*, 2005; Meaney *et al.*, 1995). That is, the myelin sheath around the axon nerve will be damaged, and in that case these nerve tissues are not able to recover and heal themselves. This usually is the stage when TBI will occur in severe cases.

These analyses reveal that the velocity impact on the frontal head is proportional with the maximum strain in the brain and thereby different type of TBI. It has been concluded that 10–13 per cent of the strain in the brain, which corresponds to the velocity impacts of 17–20 mph, is less than the 20 per cent threshold of brain injury (TBI) addressed in the literature (Bayly *et al.*, 2005; Meaney *et al.*, 1995). It is concluded that if the head is subjected to an impact velocity of less than 17 mph, the strain in the brain is below the threshold of TBI.

References

Al-Bsharat, A. S., Hardy, W. N., Yang, K. H., Khalil, T. B., Tashman, S. and King, A. I. (1999a) *Brain/Skull Relative Displacement Magnitude Due to Blunt Head Impact: New Experimental Data and Model*, SAE technical paper No. 99SC22, Warrendale, PA: SAE International.

Al-Bsharat, A. S., Zhou, C., Yang, K. H., Khalil, T. B. and King, A. I. (1999b) 'Intracranial pressure in the human head due to frontal impact based on a finite element model', *Proceedings of the 1999 Bioengineering Conference*, Big Sky: American Society of Mechanical Engineers, pp. 113–4.

Alcolado, J. C., Moore, I. E. and Weller, R. O. (1986) 'Calcification in the human choroid plexus, meningiomas and pineal gland', *Neuropathology and Applied Neurobiology*, 12(3): 235–50.

Arbogast, K. B. and Margulies, S. S. (1997) *Regional Differences in Mechanical Properties of the Porcine Central Nervous System*, SAE technical paper No. 973336, Warrendale, PA: SAE International.

Bayly, P. V., Cohen, T. S., Leister, E. P., Ajo, D., Leuthardt, E. and Genin, G. M. (2005) 'Deformation of the human brain induced by mild acceleration', *Journal of Neurotrauma*, 22(8): 845–56.

Bilston, L. E., Liu, Z. and Phan-Thien, N. (1998) 'Linear viscoelastic properties of bovine brain tissue in shear', *Biorheology*, 34(6): 377–85.

Darvish, K. and Stone, J. (2001) 'Relationship of decreased brain tissue viscoelasticity to traumatic axonal injury following traumatic brain injury', *Proceedings of the 7th International Neurotrama Synposium*, Adelaide: Medimond.

Elkin, B. S., Azeloglu, E. U., Costa, K. D. and Morrison, B. III (2007) 'Mechanical heterogeneity of the rat hippocampus measured by AFM indentation', *Journal of Neurotrauma*, 24(5): 812–22.

Estes, M. S. and McElaney, J. H. (1970) *Response of Brain Tissue of Compressive Loading*, ASME, No. 70-BHF-13, New York: American Society of Mechanical Engineers.

Fallenstein, G. T., Hulce, V. D. and Melvin, J. W. (1969) 'Dynamic mechanical properties of human brain tissue', *Journal of Biomechanics*, 2(3): 217–26.

Faul, M., Xu, L., Wald, M. M. and Coronado, V. G. (2010) *Traumatic Brain Injury in the United States: Emergency Department Visits, Hospitalizations, and Deaths*, Atlanta, GA: Centers for Disease Control and Prevention, National Center for Injury Prevention and Control.

Feng, Y., Abney, T. M., Okamoto, R. J., Pless, R. B., Genin, G. M. and Bayly, P. V. (2010) 'Relative brain displacement and deformation during constrained mild frontal head impact', *Journal of the Royal Society*, 7(53): 1677–88.

Galford, J. E. and McElhaney, J. H. (1969) 'A viscoelastic study of scalp, brain, and dura', *Journal of Biomechanics*, 3(2): 211–21.

Gupta, S., Soellinger, M., Boesiger, P., Poulikakos, D. and Kurtcuoglu, V. (2009) 'Three-dimensional computational modeling of subject-specific cerebrospinal fluid flow in the subarachnoid space', *Journal of Biomechanical Engineering*, 131(2): 021010.

Hardy, W. N., Foster, C. D., King, A. I. and Tashman, S. (1997) 'Investigation of brain injury kinematics: Introduction of a new technique', *Crashworthiness, Occupant Protection and Biomechanics in Transportation Systems*, 225: 241–54.

Hardy, W. N., Foster, C. D., Mason, M. J., Yang, K. H., King, A. I. and Tashman, S. (2001) 'Investigation of head injury mechnisms using neutral density technology and high-speed biplaner X-ray', *Stapp Car Crash Journal*, 45: 337–68.

Holbourn, A. H. S. (1945) 'The mechanics of brain injury', *Brithish Medical Bulletin*, 3(6): 147–9.

Jin, X., Lee, J. B., Leung, L. Y., Zhang, L., Yang, K. H. and King, A. I. (2006) 'Biomechanical response of the bovine pia-arachnoid complex to tensile loading at varying strain-rates', *Stapp Car Crash Journal*, 50: 637–49.

Kierszenbaum, L. A. (2007) *Histology and Cell Biology: An Introduction to Pathology*, 2nd edn, Mosby: Elsevier Health Sciences.

Killer, H. E., Laeng, H. R., Flammer, J. and Groscurth, P. (2003) 'Architecture of arachnoid trabeculae, pillars, and septa in the subarachnoid space of the human optic nerve', *The British Journal of Ophthalmology*, 87(6): 777–81.

Kleiven, S. and Hardy, W. N. (2002) 'Correlation of an FE model of the human head with local brain motion-consequences for injury protect', *Stapp Car Crash Journal*, 46: 123–44.

Koeneman, J. B. (1966) 'Viscoelastic properties of brain tissue', unpublished master's thesis, Case Institute of Technology.

Meaney, D. F., Smith, D. H., Shreiber, D. I., Bain, A. C., Miller, R. T., Ross, D. T. and Gennarelli, T. A. (1995) 'Biomechanical analysis of experimental diffuse axonal injury', *Journal of Neurotrauma*, 12(4): 689–95.

Miller, K. and Chinzei, K. (1997) 'Constitutive modeling of brain tissue: experiment and theory', *Journal of Biomechanics*, 30(11–12): 1115–21.

Moss, W. C., King, M. J. and Blackman, E. G. (2009) 'Skull flexure from blast waves: a mechanism for brain injury with implications for helmet design', *Physical Review Letters*, 103(10): 108702.

Nahum, A. M., Smith, R. and Ward, C. C. (1977) *Intracranial Pressure Dynamics During Head Impact*, SAE technical paper No. 770922, Warrendale, PA: SAE International.

Nicolle, S., Lounis, M. and Willinger, R. (2004) 'Shear properties of brain tissue over a frequency range relevant for automotive impact situations: new experimental results', *Stapp Car Crash Journal*, 48: 239–58.

Rowson, S. and Duma, S. M. (2011) 'Development of the STAR evaluation system for football helmets: integrating player head impact exposure and risk of concussion', *Annals of Biomedical Engineering*, 39(8): 2130–40.

Ruan, J. S., Khalil, T. B. and King, A. I. (1993) *Finite Element Modeling of Direct Head Impact*, SAE technical paper No. 933114, Warrendale, PA: SAE International.

Sabet, A. A., Christoforou, E., Zatlin, B., Genin, G. M. and Bayly P. V. (2008) 'Deformation of the human brain induced by mild acceleration', *Journal of Biomechanics*, 41(2): 307–15.

Saboori, P. (2011) 'Mechanotransduction of head impacts to the brain leading to TBI: histology and architecture of subarachnoid space', unpublished doctoral thesis, The City University of New York.

Saboori, P. and Sadegh, A. (2010) 'The effect of SAS materials and modeling in transferring impact loads to the brain', *Proceedings of the International Mechanical Engineering Congress and Exposition (IMECE)*, Vancouver: American Society of Mechanical Engineers, pp. 187–90.

Saboori, P. and Sadegh, A. (2011a) 'Architecture and histology of the sub arachnoid space trabeculae in the brain', *Proceedings of Biomedical Engineering Society 2011 Annual Meeting*, Hartford, CT: Biomedical Engineering Society.

Saboori, P. and Sadegh, A. (2011b) 'Effect of trabecular architecture on transferring load/impact to the brain: a local model of single trabecula', *Proceedings of 2011 Biomedical Engineering Society Meeting*, Farmington, NM: American Society of Mechanical Engineers.

Saboori, P. and Sadegh, A. (2011c) 'Mechanotransduction of external load to the brain: the effect of trabecular architecture', *Proceedings of ABS 2011*, Long Beach, CA: American Biomedical Society.

Saboori, P. and Sadegh, A. (2011d) 'Brain subarachnoid space architecture: histological approach', *Proceedings of ASME 2011 International Mechanical Engineering Congress and Exposition*, Denver, CO: American Society of Mechanical Engineers, pp. 89–94.

Saboori, P., Germanier, C. and Sadegh, A. (2010) 'Mechanics of CSF flow through trabecular architecture in the brain', *Proceedings of the 26th Southern Biomedical Engineering Conference (SBEC)*, College Park: Springer Berlin Heidelberg, pp. 440–3.

Takhounts, E. G., Eppinger, R. H., Campbell, J. Q., Tannous, R. E., Powe, E. D. and Shook, L. S. (2003a) 'On the development of the SIMon finite element head model', *Stapp Car Crash Journal*, 47: 107–33.

Takhounts, E. G., Crandall, J. R. and Darvish, K. K. (2003b) 'On the importance of nonlinearity of brain tissue under large deformation', *Stapp Car Crash Journal*, 47: 79–92.

Takhounts, E. G., Ridella, S. A., Hasija, V., Tannous, R. E., Campbell, J. Q., Malone, D., Danelson, K., Stitzel, J., Rowson, S. and Duma, S. (2008) 'Investigation of traumatic brain injuries using the next generation of simulated injury monitor (SIMon) finite element head model', *Stapp Car Crash Journal*, 52: 1–31.

van der Rest, M. and Garrone, R. (1991) 'Collagen family of proteins', *FASEB Journal: Official Publication of the Federation of American Societies for Experimental Biology*, 5(13): 2814–23.

Zhang, L., Yang, K. H., Dwarampudi, R., Omori, K., Li, T., Chang, K., Hardy, W. N., Khalil, T. B. and King, A. I. (2001a) 'Recent advances in brain injury research: a new human head model development and validation', *Stapp Car Crash Journal*, 45: 369–94.

Zhang, L., Yang, K. H. and King, A. I. (2001b) 'Biomechanics of neurotrauma', *Neurological Research*, 23(2–3): 144–56.

Zhang, L., Yang, K. H. and King, A. I. (2001c) 'Comparison of brain responses between frontal and lateral impacts by finite element modeling', *Journal of Neurotrauma*, 18(1): 21–30.

Zhang, L., Bae, J., Hardy, W. N., Monson, K. L., Manley, G. T., Goldsmith, W., Yang, K. H. and King, A. I. (2002) 'Computational study of the contribution of the vasculature on the dynamic response of the brain', *Stapp Car Crash Journal*, 46: 145–64.

Zhou, C., Khalil, T. B. and King, A. I. (1995) *A New Model Comparing Impact Responses of the Homogeneous and Inhomogeneous Human Brain*, SAE technical paper No. 952741, Warrendale, PA: SAE International.

Zoghi-Moghadam, M. and Sadegh, A. (2010) 'Equivalent fluid model for CSF and SAS trabeculae using head/brain damping', *International Journal of Biomedical Engineering and Technology*, 4(3): 195–210.

41

MODELLING
AND SIMULATION IN
DISCUS THROW

Mikhail P. Shestakov

TRAINING CENTER OF RUSSIAN NATIONAL TEAMS, MOSCOW

Introduction

Development and refinement of sports training methods is the only valid possibility to improve sport results. Effective sports training calls for correct organization and science-based control. It is pointless to analyse training programmes of elite athletes and introduce their 'secrets' into training plans developed for other athletes. It is very difficult to control sports training, because a coach has no possibility to exert direct influence on sport performance, except for providing a training programme and requiring its strict execution, in particular adjustment of movement technique (Zatsiorsky, 1998).

A coach and an athlete interact with each other and the environment. To control a process of athletic training, a coach needs information concerning:

- target requirements for the development of morphological structures and changes in related test results;
- criteria (or levels) of technique mastery, which determine ways of reaching the final goal.

Technique of discus throw

A discus throw can be performed in a standing position, but higher performance is achieved when the discus is thrown following a turn. Detailed analysis of the throwing technique allows us to divide the discus throw into five phases: preparation – a double support phase; entry – a single support phase on the left foot; airborne phase (after the left foot breaks contact with the support); transition – a single support phase on the right foot (which ends as the left foot touches the ground) and delivery – a double support phase, which ends at release of the discus.

From the initial position at the rear of the ring with feet about shoulder width apart, the thrower brings the discus as far back as he or she can (after preliminary swings). The forward swing of the right arm to the left is followed by slight rotation of the thrower's body counterclockwise and minor transfer of the body weight to the left foot. When the right arm with the discus swings to the right, and the athlete transfers his or her body weight to the right foot, the left foot touches the ground by the ball of the foot. The shoulders are relaxed and follow the movement of the right arm.

The turn helps gain the speed when the athlete moves within a limited area – the ring. During the turn, the thrower: (1) develops the maximal speed of movement that is later transferred into the final effort; and (2) creates the most advantageous conditions for the delivery phase.

The entry consists of two phases: (1) transfer of the body weight to the rotating left foot; and (2) push off by the left foot in the direction of the throw and a wide swing by the right leg. In the first phase, the thrower transfers his or her body weight from the right foot to the left one by pushing off the right foot and rotating the pelvis. In the second phase, the thrower pushes off the right leg, swings the right leg in a wide arc and steps in the direction of the throw. Consequently, left rotation of the trunk slows down. Preliminary stretching of thigh flexors and adductors permits the thrower to achieve high speed during the swing. The throwing arm moves in the same direction with the right foot. When the thrower bends the left knee, he or she slightly lowers the hand with the discus, but then raises it high again.

The airborne phase starts with the left foot breaking contact with the support and finishes with the right foot landing. The thrower has to make the airborne phase as short as possible not to lose contact with the support and stretch muscles of the shoulder girdle and the trunk. To shorten the airborne phase, elite throwers push off the left foot immediately before landing on the right foot. The thrower lands on the right foot about 10 cm in front of the centre of the ring with the throwing hand brought well back and right at the shoulder level, the trunk bent at the waist and the left hand in front of the chest. The shoulder girdle is rotated to the right relative to the pelvis.

When the right foot lands on the support, the athlete is ready for the final effort. At this moment, the discus is at the maximal distance from the point of delivery. The thrower plants the left foot near the front edge of the ring, brings the left arm across the body (so that the axis of the shoulder girdle becomes perpendicular to the axis of the pelvis), keeping the body weight on the right foot.

The final effort starts from rotation and extension of the legs. Rotation and extension of the right leg straightens the trunk and moves in the direction of the throw. At the same time, the left leg blocks any further movement, and the thrower brings the discus in the lowest position by the widest possible swing. The maximal acceleration of the discus in the double support phase is achieved due to well-coordinated legwork, stretching of the chest muscles, and whipping motion of the throwing arm. In the delivery phase, the thrower rotates the shoulder girdle, brings the left arm forward at the chest level in order to stretch muscles and contribute to the vertical vector of the discus speed. When the discus is released, the axis of the shoulder girdle and the axis of the pelvis should be in the same plane.

Technique development in discus throw

The essence of technique learning in coaching consists in elaboration of a training programme in accordance with actual goals, state of the athlete's organism, and mechanisms of its functioning and development. A necessary condition of any training is stable and well-balanced development of an athlete throughout the training process. Sports training affects main morphological structures of the athlete's body and therefore cannot be efficiently controlled without comprehensive estimation of its possible effects on the athlete. Correct approach to coaching means that at each stage of training the coach forms a training plan in his or her mind, estimates potential results and risks, makes necessary adjustments, and only then offers it to the athlete.

Until recently, algorithms of mental activity or, in other words, algorithms of decision-making (Ladenko, 1987) were created exclusively on the ground of personal experience and professional intuition. In recent years, this problem has been solved with the help of computing machinery that allowed scientists to simulate development of decision-making algorithms. Mathematical models of biological objects were developed (Drus, 1976) and used by scientists as theoretical representation of the objects and phenomena being studied. In biological studies, intrinsic complexity of a living organism as a simulation object (a human being, an animal, or a plant) requires division of the whole object into subsystems corresponding to various systems and subsystems of the organism (Bloom, 1976; Levashov, 1989; Panayotis, 1987).

In pedagogy, the theory of motor skills learning and technique improvement leans upon the theory of movement control and modelling and simulation of movements in biological objects. Until now, models that were used for studies in this field did not incorporate integral features of any biological object (such as memory, mentality, and self-development), and therefore could not provide complete description of the object. We may state that at present there is no theoretical basis for synthesis of knowledge accumulated in biology (in particular, biomechanics) and sport pedagogy (in particular, learning movements).

Simulation modelling has become one of the most commonly used methods in studies related to investigation of biological objects. Model theory assumes the possibility for high complexity of models based on involvement of maximal number of various parameters (Blauberg and Yudin, 1973). However, in the field of biomechanics, including too many parameters into the model might make it excessively complicated. A simple 'black box' real-time model is often more useful in scientific studies than complicated models, which produce results after hours-long calculations. Validity of a biomechanical model consists in its ability to reflect the real-world process accurately. A simulation model is considered valid, if results of simulation modelling conform to real experimental data.

Simulation modelling has been widely used for examination of control mechanisms in human movements. Simulation technologies provide means for quantitative assessment of internal structure of a motor action (range of movements, torques, angular momentum vectors) and external manifestation of muscular activity (force and velocity in the centres of mass of various body segments).

Issues of technique development are related to examination of flexibility and stability of motor programmes. All movements performed by an athlete are based on execution of certain programmes of actions, each corresponding to a motor programme. A programme of action is a model of a forthcoming activity. It is based on the development of logic, algorithm and functional structure of the motor action in the human brain. It leans upon: (1) previous experience that is stored in the memory with probability equal to '1'; and (2) actual conditions, which include both constantly changing environment and the actual physical condition of the athlete's body. When planning a motor action, an athlete has to foresee possible changes, which may be happening in an unpredictably changing environment. An ability to execute a voluntary movement means that a man can control purposeful movements of his body or body parts more or less precisely. This concept might be related to formation of biomechanisms (Seluyanov and Shalmanov, 1995).

Biomechanism

Biomechanism is an independent combination of movements of a few body parts that converts energy from one form into another and changes location and speed of the centre of body mass of an athlete while executing a motor action (Seluyanov and Shalmanov, 1995). If the athlete is able to consciously perceive a task solved with the help of a biomechanism, he or she can voluntary control and change the biomechanisms he or she uses.

Simulation modelling in biomechanical studies uses models, which consist of ideal elements of various biomechanisms (i.e. muscles, bones, joints and the control block):

1   skeletal muscles:
  • convert chemical energy into mechanical energy;
  • transmit energy from other energy sources;
  • store and release energy due to their elastic components;
  • damp external impacts due to their resilient components;
2   bones serve as:
  • levers for force and energy transfer;
  • pendulums for energy conversion;
  • rods for support and counteraction to external impacts;
3   joints serve as:
  • hinges to join bones into kinematic chains;
  • hinges to limit dislocation of interconnected bones;
4   the control block's task is to take control of motor actions. For the purpose of our studies, we assumed that the control block is a 'black box' with a few entries and one (or more) exit. To model the control block, we used an artificial neural network.

Pre-programmed muscle activity patterns are formed in the athlete's mind before he or she starts the movement itself. To introduce changes in the movement technique, an athlete has to make alterations in the motor programmes, which control the activity of muscles involved in execution of the movement.

Neural networks

Processing of large-scale data arrays in biomechanical studies requires adequate mathematical tools. Lack of sufficient information, a large amount of multifactor parameters and fuzzy rules of calculations make any statistical data manipulation extremely complicated. The neural networks help to solve these tasks. The main feature of this approach consists in self-learning (or self-adjustment) of the mathematical apparatus. The first artificial neural networks were developed when scientists attempted to simulate behaviour of living organisms, which were able to perceive external impacts and learn from their experience (Lippman, 1987).

An artificial neural network can adapt its behaviour to external conditions. Any alteration in input signals enables the process of self-adjustment within the network to generate an adequate response (Rumelhart *et al.*, 1986). After learning, the artificial neural network becomes insusceptible to minor changes in the input signals. The ability to recognize an image in conditions of noise and artifacts is vital for image identification in real world (Hopfield, 1982).

Most contemporary theorists agree that principal properties of the brain are determined by the topological structure of the brain neural network and dynamics of pulse propagation in it (Rose, 1995). To understand how the brain works, we should connect elementary neural elements in organizational structures topologically similar to the brain (Hecht-Nielsen, 1988). In his work, Hecht-Nielsen (1988) supposed that different zones of the brain work according to a uniform principle – the principle of image identification. Hebb (1949) assumed that all psychic functions (memory, emotions, thinking, etc.) are determined by the activity of neural ensembles, which consist of nervous cells connected into specific networks. In his work on organization of behaviour, Hebb (1949) hypothesized that memory traces might be results of synapse modification.

Artificial neural networks have been induced by biological studies: they learn by experience, apply acquired 'knowledge' in unfamiliar situations, obtain important data from an information flow (Levashov, 1989). A neural network in mathematics is a multilayer net structure, which consists of rather simple single-type processor elements – neurons. Neurons are connected between each other to form layers (as a rule, two or three layers), an input layer and an output layer being present in any network. Neurons of the input layer get information about the actual situation, and the output layer indicates possible response of the system. To work correctly, the neural network needs specific adjustment (referred to as 'learning') when many sample tasks are assigned to the network. If the network responds inadequately (i.e. the state of the output layer differs from the desirable one), the internal structure of the network is modified to minimize the error. As a rule, the modification concerns 'weights of inter-connections'. After 'learning', the network must work with minimal total error.

Artificial neural networks are commonly used in researches related to categorization, scientific prognostication and non-linear relationships. For some time past, a neurobionic approach suggested by Averkin *et al.* (1992) has been taken in studies with the use of neural networks. Biocyberagogics has become a new scientific trend and served a theoretical basis for our experimental and model studies (Shestakov, 2000).

Example of a simple model

An attempt was made to use an artificial neural network to improve vertical jump technique. To model a vertical jump, we used a two-dimensional model consisting of six links: foot – shank – thigh – trunk with head – arm – forearm with hand. The six links were connected by cylindrical hinges with no friction, the muscles being attached to the links of the upper and lower extremities (Figure 41.1).

The goal of the vertical jump was to lift the body's centre of mass to the maximal height. The motor action included two biomechanisms: (1) legs and trunk straightening; and (2) swinging links. The neural network had three input parameters: the biomechanism of legs and trunk straightening (X1), the biomechanism of swinging links (X2) and the level of physical fitness (X3); and a single output parameter – a result in the vertical jump (Y1). The level of physical fitness was estimated according to absolute strength in knee and hip joint extensors measured with the help of the Biodex System 3 dynamometer (Biodex Medical Systems, Inc., Shirley, New York, USA).

To obtain 'input-output' pairs and 'teach' the neural network, a pedagogical experiment was held. Ninety-three students of the Russian Academy of Physical Education participated in the experiment. After learning, the matrix had an rms-error of 0,067 that was considered satisfactory.

Then a group of the students ($n = 8$) completed a training programme (3 weeks, 15 workouts) intended for improvement of jumping technique and based on using training exercises with extra weight (3 kg dumb-bells). Learning curves for both simulated (a) and real (b) training processes are shown in Figure 41.1. Comparison of the learning curves showed that the neural network correctly simulated the real training process, taking into account its specific features. This experiment proved that biomechanisms and artificial neural networks were effective tools for simulation of sport technique development, optimization and individualization of sports training.

Three biomechanisms are commonly singled out in the delivery phase of the discus throw:

- pivoting
- leg straightening, and
- whipping movement.

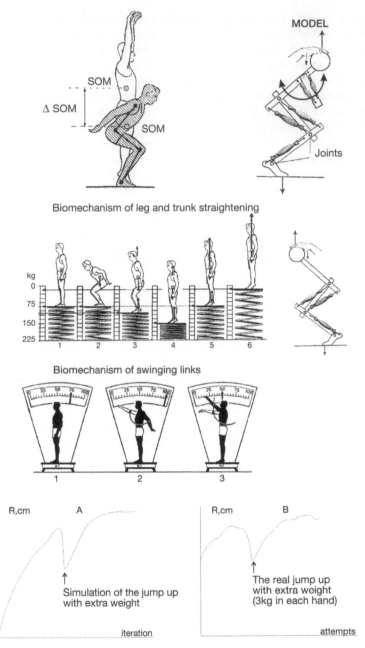

Figure 41.1 Curves of 'learning' in simulated (a) and real (b) training aimed at improvement of vertical jump technique.

The biomechanisms of pivoting and leg straightening are easy to define and describe. The biomechanism of whipping movement requires special attention, because it increases final acceleration and plays significant role in all throws.

It is generally accepted that most of 'relocating' movements comprise the final 'whipping' mechanism. This idea was supported by studies held in various sports: handball (Petracheva,

1995), tennis (Agashin and Zaitseva, 1972), shot-put and javelin throw (Godik *et al.*, 1993), and javelin throw (Bartonietz, 2000). 'Whipping' technique in throws is based on successive acceleration and deceleration of body parts in a kinematic chain (i.e. temporal relation of maximal values of linear and angular speed in adjacent kinematic links), which continuously grows from proximal to distal sections. Lanka and Shalmanov (1982) and Popov (1993) have both shown that optimal temporal relation between maximal speeds in adjacent kinematic links is more important than their absolute values. However, the mechanism of arm-whipping is effective only when used in combination with the other biomechanisms. Further studies will show, if the 'whipping' movement plays the most important role in reaching maximal acceleration of the throwing hand.

The effect of physical fitness on motor skills development

Interrelation between physical fitness and motor skills changes with age and level of sport performance.

Model experiment

We verified this idea by empirical investigation with the help of a simulation model of the discus throw. In the model experiment, we used an adjusted neural network for investigation of the effect of changes in physical qualities of discus throwers on throwing technique. The input parameters for the neural network included: characteristics of physical fitness; contribution of the biomechanism of pivoting (P); contribution of the biomechanism of whipping (W); and contribution of the biomechanism of leg and trunk straightening (LTS). The result in discus throw was the output. The neural network was 'instructed' with the use of data measured in a pedagogical study. Twenty-three elite discus throwers ($n = 23$) participated in this study; methods of tensodynamography, polydynamography and cinecyclography were used.

An adjusted matrix of the neural network permitted to establish the range of adequate output values (i.e. results in discus throw). This helped to determine critical values of the 'level of physical fitness' (one of the neural network inputs), which caused considerable decrease in the output parameter – the 'result' in discus throw. Experimental data are presented in Figure 41.2.

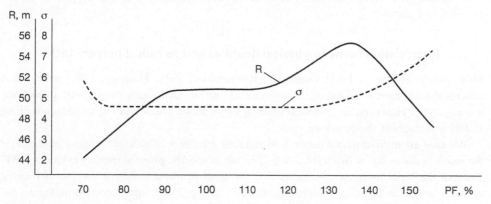

Figure 41.2 The effect of changes in the input X3 characterizing the level of physical fitness (PF) (simulation data).

The results permit to estimate conformity of physical development to technique improvement in discus throwers. It is clearly seen that either increase, or decrease in the input parameter X3 (physical fitness) has negative effect on the final result. It is important that the R (the output) decreases without any significant changes in σ. When the value X3 grows, the accuracy of the neural network operation decreases. The reason might be that the neural network operation is stable only when the input parameters do not exceed certain limits.

This permits to suppose that adequate execution of a motor programme largely depends on proportion (congruence) between a set of parameters, which determine success of the given motor action. Either an insufficient level of physical fitness, or its disproportional growth have negative effect on the quality of movements. Thus, the principle of congruence defines the necessary and sufficient level of physical fitness for successful development of sport technique.

Pedagogical experiment

The results of simulation modelling were verified in a pedagogical experiment that lasted 6 months. Twenty-three discus throwers were divided into three groups according to their results: group A – R (result) = 53.4 ± 2.6 m (n = 6), group B – R = 56.4 ± 4.8 m (n = 8), group C – R = 55.4 ± 3.6 m (n = 9), the last one (C) being the control group. The athletes in the control group completed a conventional training programme and did not take into account the results of the simulation experiment. Each athlete involved in the experimental groups completed an individual physical training programme based on the results of simulation modelling. The training programme in group A was focused primarily on improvement of the biomechanism of pivoting, while athletes in group B paid more attention to whipping movements.

Results of the pedagogical study proved positive effect of individualized training plans on the throwing technique. The athletes in groups A and B managed to increase the contribution of the target biomechanisms in the throwing result (pivoting in the group A – + 6.1 per cent (p < 0.05), whipping movement in the group B (+ 4.1 per cent, p < 0.05)). Strength and velocity grew insignificantly in both experimental groups (+ 0.9 per cent, p > 0.05). Contribution of the biomechanism of leg and trunk straightening increased in the control group C due to focused strength and velocity development (lot of exercises with extra weight) on the background of insufficient technique improvement. All the athletes improved their sport results (p > 0.05), the increase in the throw distance being slightly greater in the experimental groups.

Interrelation between physical qualities and technical preparedness

Most authors (Matveev, 1991; Osolin and Khomenkov, 1974; Platonov, 1986) believe that athletes should improve technique of movements and simultaneously throughout a year-long training cycle. However, no common opinion exists about peculiarities of technique training at different stages of the year-long cycle.

We used an artificial neural network to simulate the effect of different training methods on the result in discus throw (see Table 41.1). The use of specific physical training exercises (SPT) changed the input parameter, characterizing the level of physical fitness; the use of training exercises aimed at technique improvement (TT) changed the inputs corresponding to the biomechanisms of LTS, R and whipping movement.

Table 41.1 Results of simulation modelling of different training programmes

Training programme	Duration of 'training', simulation (iteration)	$\Delta R,$ cm	σ
Consecutive use of SPT and TT	565	8.3	4.5
Simultaneous use of SPT and TT	916	4.2	4.8
	600	3.7	2.1
Only TT	382	2.8	2.4
Only SPT	286	2.9	1.9

The simulation demonstrated that consecutive use of SPT and TT in neural network 'training' gave the best results. This means that improvement of the motor programme required sufficient level of physical qualities development for its realization (the 'principle of congruence'). Any disproportion in physical training is undesirable. The principle of congruence and a conventional cyclic character of the training process call for the use of SPT by portions (quantization of the total volume of SPT) (i.e. technique development should be always preceded by a portion of SPT). The simulation modelling results agree with empirical data published by Verkhoshanskiy (1977).

Effect of changes in anthropometric parameters on sport movement technique

Organization of the long-term training technique is affected largely by biological changes in the growing organism of an athlete, the most evident being changes in the body mass and body proportions. As the skeleton and muscles grow, physical strength increases. In other words, formation of the structure precedes development of the function. The common pattern may be described as follows: growth of muscles – development of strength – coordination improvement. This is particularly important for coordinated activity of different groups of muscles.

Therefore, when the level of special physical fitness remains constant, changes in distribution of the body mass may have either positive or negative effects on the efficacy of biomechanisms in motor activity.

Simulation modelling

We used a simplified model consisting of a pivot fixed at one end. An adjusted neural network controlled the model by sending signals to two elastic antagonistic structures (Figure 41.3). The length (L) and mass (m) of the pivot both had effect on the control moment (Mr) that was taken into account in the equation. Simulation modelling results are summarized in Table 41.2.

Table 41.2 Accuracy of the neural network operation (σ) depending on the pivot's length and mass

| | Increase in mass-inertia indices | | | | | | | | |
	0%	0.5%	1%	1.5%	2%	2.5%	3%	3.5%	4%
Pivot length L.m	0.8	0.8	0.8	1.3	1.8	5.0	6.1	7.9	12.1
Pivot mass m.kg	0.8	0.8	0.8	0.8	1.0	1.2	4.3	4.9	8.3

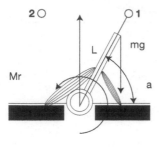

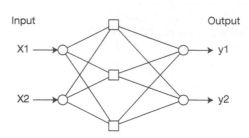

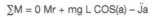

$$\sum M = 0 \ Mr + mg \ L \ COS(a) - \ddot{J}a$$

Figure 41.3 Control of pivot's displacement from position 1 to position 2 with the help of the adjusted neural network. Elements: pivot, hinge, base, control moment. L – pivot's length; m – pivot's mass; J – inertia moment; a – angle of inclination. Mr = f(i,a,á), where Mr is the control moment that depends on the activation of elastic structure (force), speed changes in elastic structure length (viscosity and Hill's law). Neural network: X1 – a motor programme; X2 – intensity of the movement; y1 – 'muscle activity' of the agonist; y2 – 'muscle activity' of the antagonist.

After the network learned to recognize an image '2' (displacement of the pivot from position '1' to position '2' by 'muscular activity' of both agonist and antagonist), the input X1 (the motor programme) was changed. The change consisted in alteration in the length (L) and mass (m) of the pivot (in per cent). Simulation modelling demonstrated that the 2.5 per cent (and greater) increase in the length of the pivot and the 3 per cent increase in its mass caused significant deterioration in the network's operation that could be caused by disturbances in agonist-antagonist coordination.

It appears probable that a threshold exists, after which any alteration in one of the inputs results in changes in the output and significant deterioration in the operation of the network. To restore normal operation, the network needs additional learning. Simulation modelling has shown that mass-inertia characteristics do not have linear relationship with the output parameters, and a spurt-like change takes place in the pattern of the output function after a certain threshold.

Pedagogical experiment

To estimate contribution of each biomechanism in discus throw, we examined standing throws performed by athletes of different ages.

Methods

Dynamic values of vertical and horizontal components of the ground reaction force were recorded with the use of a force platform PD-3, while kinematic characteristics were assessed with the help of video filming. Electrical activity of the right gastrocnemius muscle, the biceps muscle of the left thigh, the left oblique muscle of the abdomen and the right greater pectoral muscle was recorded with the help of a 'Medicor' Electromyographer (with an inter-electrode distance of 20 mm). Special software was used in data processing. Fifty-seven male discus throwers (13–19 years of age) took part in the experiment.

Results and discussion

The results demonstrated that athletes of different age and qualification had typical patterns of the registered parameters.

The results showed that novice athletes performing a throw primarily used the muscles of the shoulder girdle. Advanced throwers performed the throw by non-simultaneous movements of the lower extremities and the shoulder girdle. Elite throwers demonstrated a clear movement pattern: after the successive straightening of the right knee joint and the right hip joint, the oblique abdomen muscles were activated, and finally the muscles of the shoulder joint of the throwing arm were involved in the movement.

Profound analysis of the experimental data permitted to estimate contribution of the main biomechanisms into the throw performed by the athletes of different age according to speed achieved in the system 'thrower-discus' in separate phases of the throw. It was revealed that just the use of the biolmechanism of 'whipping' permitted athletes to achieve best results in throwing. The group of 14–15-year-old athletes was of special interest, because we found significant intragroup spread in the contribution of the whipping biomechanism in this group.

We divided the group of 14–15-year-old throwers into two subgroups according to the rate of annual increase in mass-inertia characteristics (MIC) (Table 41.3).

The values in the Table 41.3 clearly show lesser contribution of the whipping biomechanism in athletes with rapidly increasing mass-inertia characteristics. To study the issue we used simulation modelling. Inputs for the neural network included: mass-inertia characteristics (MIC) and contribution (in per cent) of each biomechanism; the output was the release speed of the discus.

Simulation modelling has shown that gradual increase in MIC caused an increase in the output. However, if MIC growth exceeded 7.5 cm per year, the output values abruptly decreased. Simulation modelling has shown that in the period of rapid growth, it is advisable to learn and improve the biomechanisms of rotation and leg straightening separately. These data permitted to develop a special training programme for young athletes in the period of fast morphofunctional development, which helped to improve throwing technique on the ground of physical qualities development. This programme included various simulation drills for technique adjustment, as well as physical exercises based on the involvement of either the biomechanism of rotation, or the biomechanism of leg and trunk straightening.

Conclusion

Simulation modelling has proved to be an effective method for developing generalized concepts of technique improvement in sports training, because it is based on the fundamental laws of pedagogy, biomechanics and physiology. In our researches, we managed to simulate transition of a biomechanical model from its initial state to a predetermined state with the help of a self-learning neural network. The suggested pedagogical principles of sport technique adjustment

Table 41.3 Contribution of different biomechanisms in discus throw in the group of 14–15-year-old athletes

Contribution of biomechanisms, %	Biomechanism of rotation	Biomechanism of legs straightening	Biomechanism of whipping
Group A, increase in MIC < 5 cm/year	30	30	40
Group B, increase in MIC > 7.5 cm/year	50	25	25

permit to solve complex tasks of technique development and meet the highest requirements to contemporary level of sports results.

The strategy of long-term sports training should be based on the correspondence of special physical fitness of an athlete to motor tasks he or she has to solve at each stage of training. To perform a motor action successfully, an athlete has to develop an adequate motor programme, its adequacy being dependent on proportionality of few parameters, which determine its execution. The lack of physical fitness, as excessive development of some physical qualities, has a negative effect on sport movement technique. The 'principle of congruence' determines the necessary and sufficient level of different physical qualities for successful technique improvement. Simulation modelling involved in our researches has shown that the consecutive use of special physical exercises and technique adjustment drills produced best results in neural network 'training'. According to the principle of quantization, technique improvement must always be preceded by special physical development.

References

Agashin, F. K. and Zaitseva, L. S. (1972) 'Muscle work in tennis players', *Theory and Practice of Physical Education*, 8: 25–8.

Averkin, A. N., Gaase-Rappoport, M. G. and Pospelov, D. A. (1992) *Artificial Intelligence. Defining Dictionary*, Moscow: Radio i Svyaz.

Bartonietz, K. (2000) 'Javelin throwing: an approach to performance development prevention', in V. M. Zatsiorsky (ed.), *Biomechanics in Sport: Performance Enhancement and Injury Prevention*, International Olympic Committtee, pp. 401–34.

Blauberg, I. V. and Yudin, Y. G. (1973) *Formation and Essence of Systems Approach*, Moscow: Nauka.

Bloom, B. S. (1976) *Human Characteristics and School Learning*, New York: McGraw-Hill.

Drus, V. A. (1976) *Simulation of Training Process*, Kiev: Zdorovie.

Godik, M. A., Ramesh, P., Poltorapavlov, N. V. and Shalmanov, A. A. (1993) 'Comparative research in kinematics of shot-put and javelin throw in decathlon competitors and track-and-field throwers', *Theory and Practice of Physical Education*, 5–6: 1–7.

Hebb, D. O. (1949) *The Organization of Behavior. A Neuropsychlogical Theory*, New York: Wiley & Sons.

Hecht-Nielsen, R. (1988) 'Neurocomputing: picking the human brain', *IEEE, Spectrum*, 3: 36–41.

Hopfield, J. J. (1982) 'Neural network and physical systems with emergent collective computational abilities', *Proceedings of the National Academy of Sciences*, 79: 2554–8.

Ladenko, I. S. (1987) *Intelligent Systems in Target-oriented Control*, Novosibirsk: Nauka.

Lanka, Y. E. and Shalmanov, A. A. (1982) *Biomechanics of Shot Put*, Moscow: Phisicheskaya kultura i Sport.

Levashov, O. V. (1989) 'Simulating models of sensory systems', *Itogy nauky i techniky. VINITI/Bionics. Biokibernetics. Bioengineering*, 6: 3–152.

Lippman, R. P. (1987) 'An introduction to computing with neural nets', *IEEE ASSP Magazine*, 4(2): 4–22.

Matveev, L. P. (1991) *Theory and Practice of Physical Pducation: IPhE Students' Manual*, Moscow: Phisicheskaya kultura i sport.

Osolin, N. G. and Khomenkov, L. S. (1974) *Controlling of Training Process in Track&Field: Track&Field Coach's Manual*, Moscow: Phisicheskaya kultura i sport.

Panayotis, E. M. (1987) 'Improvement without computer assistance of the graphically estimated parameters of the linear one-compartment open model', *Biopharmaceutics and Drug Disposition*, 8: 387–94.

Petracheva, I. V. (1995) *Efficacy of Handball Throw in Players of Different Performance Level*, Moscow: RGAFK.

Platonov, V. N. (1986) *Training of Top Athletes*, Moscow: Phiskultura i sport.

Popov, G. I. (1993) 'Coordination changes in javelin throw technique: model and experimental estimation', *Theory and Practice of Physical Education*, 1: 7–13.

Rose, S. (1995) *The Making of Memory from Molecules to Mind*, Moscow: Mir.

Rumelhart, D. E., Hinton, G. E. and Williams, R. J. (1986) 'Leaning representations by back-propagation errors', *Nature*, 323: 533–6.

Seluyanov, V. N. and Shalmanov, A. A. (1995) 'Biomechanisms as the basis of biomechanics of human movements in sport', *Theory and Practice of Physical Education*, 7: 6–10.

Shestakov, M. P. (2000) 'Artificial intelligence in sport science of XXI centure', *Theory and Practice of Physical Education*, 7: 8–14.

Verkhoshanskiy, Y. V. (1977) *Fundamentals of Special Strength Training in Sport Athletes*, Moscow: Phiskultura i sport.

Zatsiorsky, V. M. (1998) *Kinematics of Human Motion*, New York: Human Kinetics.

42

THREE-DIMENSIONAL MUSCULOSKELETAL MODELLING OF RESISTANCE TRAINING EXERCISES

Kim Nolte

UNIVERSITY OF PRETORIA, PRETORIA

Training exercises and training exercise equipment

The general publics' growing awareness of the importance of exercise and wellness has led to an exercise-fitness revolution. Enthusiasm for exercise and fitness is at unprecedented levels with millions of people spending countless hours and substantial amounts of money on sport and exercise (Prentice, 2003). Increased mechanization and the incidence of hypokinetic diseases are two important factors that have contributed to the emphasis on fitness. With increased mechanization, many tasks that once required physical work and a considerable amount of time can now be accomplished very quickly by pushing a button or setting a dial (Hockey, 1996). Consequently, the exercise equipment manufacturing industry has rapidly expanded over the past few years, largely due to the amplified eagerness for exercise and fitness and thus equipment demand. Not only have sales of conventional exercise equipment grown enormously but there has also been an escalation in the number of new exercise equipment being designed and marketed. According to Beachle and Earle (1994), the machine age is upon us, and we have a wide variety of exercise devices to choose from, depending on our likes and dislikes. The two primary categories of exercise training equipment include cardiorespiratory and resistance training equipment. This chapter will focus on computer-assisted modelling of exercising on resistance training equipment, although most of the principles can also be applied to other types of exercise equipment.

Resistance training

Resistance training refers to a method of conditioning designed to overload the musculoskeletal system, leading to accelerated enhancement of muscle strength (Fleck and Kraemer, 1997). The term resistance training encompasses a wide range of resistive loads and a wide variety of training modalities, including, free weights (barbells and dumbbells), weight machines, elastic tubing, medicine balls, stability balls and body weight (Howley, 2007).

The current popularity of resistance training is so extraordinary that only those who were alert to such facts as the growing use of weights for sports, the changing attitudes about strength as an aspect of femininity and the increasing interest in fitness could have foreseen what has now come to pass (Pearl and Moran, 1986). Traditionally, resistance training was used primarily by adult athletes to enhance sport performance and increase muscle size. Today, resistance training is recognized as a method of enhancing the health and fitness of men and women of all ages and abilities (Howley, 2007). The popularity of resistance training is clearly evidenced by the extensive growth of fitness centres and sales of resistance exercise equipment for home use. The increased popularity of, and participation in, body-building competitions worldwide is also indicative of the level of interest in the benefits derivable from resistance training (Vaughn, 1989).

Although new pieces of exercise equipment are continuously being designed and produced, the 'core' pieces of resistance training equipment such as the chest press and leg extension machines have not changed significantly since their inception. It does, however, appear as if the future trends of resistance training equipment will be towards sleeker designs and user friendliness, as well as the incorporation of the computer or electronic technology. From a biomechanics perspective, some machines are more sound than others and the quality of machines can vary widely (Beachle and Earle, 1994). Equipment design must be regenerative in nature. Designers have not only an obligation to comply with the regulations of appropriate governing bodies, but also the responsibility for the safety and comfort of the users. Unfortunately, these guidelines mainly address equipment used by various sporting codes, with little or no enforceable guidelines for resistance training equipment. Mandatory regulations

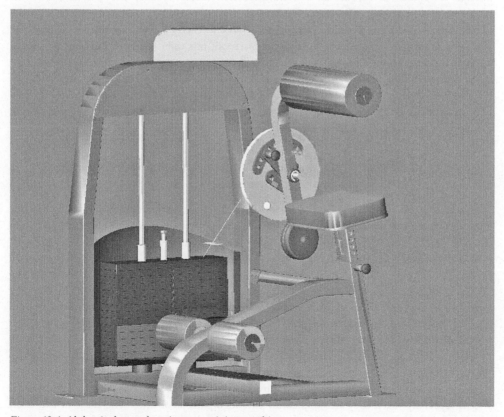

Figure 42.1 Abdominal crunch resistance training machine.

would enhance the quality of fabrication, as well as augmenting the enjoyment of users, secure in the knowledge that real injury risks in the sport or recreation of their choice have thereby been reduced (Reilly and Lees, 1984).

Three-dimensional musculoskeletal modelling

Conceptual, physical and mathematical models have all proven useful in biomechanics. Mathematical models range from the extreme simplicity of some models, to the complexity of models that represent numerous body segments and muscles, or elaborate bone shapes (Alexander, 2003). There are two approaches to studying the biomechanics of human movement: inverse dynamics and forward dynamics. The aim of such models is to estimate or predict muscle forces, joint moments and/or joint kinematics (Buchanan et al., 2004). The most widely used digital human modelling software systems, such as Jack and Safework, lack built-in inverse-dynamics capability. However, newer software packages such as LifeModeler™, AnyBody, SIMM and OpenSIMM are making these computations available for ergonomics applications (Wagner et al., 2007).

Connected multi-body systems, such as a person training on a piece of exercise equipment, exhibit notoriously complex behaviour when driven by external and internal forces and torques. The problem of reconstructing internal forces and/or torques from movements and known external forces is called the 'inverse dynamics problem', whereas calculating motion from known internal forces and/or torques and resulting reaction forces is called the 'forward dynamics problem' (Otten, 2003). Therefore, the inverse dynamics analysis produces estimates of the joint torques required to perform a specified movement, each of which represents the resultant action of all muscles crossing the joint. Dynamic motion is then achieved (forward dynamics) via activation of the muscles, which subsequently produces force and in turn, move the joints in a controlled fashion to accomplish the predetermined task, in this case the movement of the piece of exercise training equipment. Quite often, these tasks are also required to take place against the action of external forces such as gravity and the resistance of the weights on the exercise machine (Erdemir et al., 2007).

Three-dimensional (3D) musculoskeletal modelling of resistance training exercises

Mathematical and computer modelling is suitable for a wide variety of applications such as the design, production and alteration of medical equipment (prostheses, orthopaedic and orthodontic devices), as well as sports and training equipment (Alexander, 2003; Kazlauskiené, 2006). With the capability to simulate musculoskeletal human models interacting with mechanical systems many questions concerning the effects of the training equipment on the body can be studied. In addition, computer simulation models permit the study of the complex interactions between biomechanical variables (Kenny et al., 2005). Various kinematic and kinetic data can be obtained from most 3D musculoskeletal modelling simulations, and this information could then be used to assess the exercise (Table 42.1).

When exercising, it is important to train using correct form and technique in order to obtain maximum benefits from the exercise and to reduce the risk of injury. Unfortunately, when exercising, people may adopt unhealthy postures that put strain on their musculoskeletal system especially when they are adopted for extended periods of time. The cause of exercisers adopting unhealthy postures may be the result of a number of factors, namely:

Table 42.1 Data which can be obtained from most 3D musculoskeletal modelling software packages

Body motion data for each body segment (kinematics)	Position
	Velocity
	Acceleration
	Angular acceleration
Soft tissue data (kinematics and kinetics)	All muscle force and contraction histories
Joint data (sagittal, transverse and frontal planes)	Torque
(kinematics and kinetics)	Angle
Contact forces (kinetics)	Contact forces

Source: Biomechanics Research Group (2006).

- the design of the exercise equipment (limitations in the equipment design that does not allow adjustability to accommodate the appropriate range of anthropometric variances);
- limited knowledge regarding correct exercise technique and/or posture;
- fatigue; and
- overloading (i.e. trying to lift excessive resistance).

When designing equipment to promote appropriate exercise posture, anthropometric data should be considered a key resource. It is important that exercise equipment accommodates a range of anthropometric dimensions that is suited to the population group (end-user population) that will make use of the equipment. 3D musculoskeletal modelling simulations may thus be used to assess whether the exercise training equipment's engineered adjustability accommodates individuals of differing anthropometric dimensions appropriately (Figure 42.2).

Other variables can be assessed to determine musculoskeletal injury risk during exercise training such as maximal muscle tensions. Muscle tensions near or higher than maximum calculated capacity or above realistic measurements for the muscle group could indicate risk for musculoskeletal injuries. It is also possible to compare safe loading limits of joints with recorded values during the 3D musculoskeletal modelling simulations. The limitation of this approach is that limited safe loading joint limit values are available and the most readily available are those for the spine. The vulnerable joints during a particular exercise vary according to the requirements of the movement and the joints involved in the movement however in most exercises the spinal column remains a commonly injured area (acute or chronic) of the body, and therefore it is useful to assess these values (Calhoon and Fry, 1999; Lavallee and Balam, 2010).

There are three load types: compression, tension and shear. Tensile loads tend to pull the ends of a body apart, compressive loads tend to push the ends together, and shear loads tend to produce horizontal, or parallel, sliding of one layer over another (Whiting and Zernicke, 2008). In terms of risk assessment of musculoskeletal injury during exercise, it may be valuable to evaluate the compression and anterior/posterior (A/P) shear forces of the cervical, thoracic and lumbar spine due to the fact that the back is a common area injured during exercise. In addition, research regarding the maximum recommended limits when performing various tasks exists, thus making comparisons between recorded values and recommended limits possible. It is important to bear in mind when performing and applying such analyses that the spine of the default models of most modelling software often does not consist of all the individual vertebrae but rather of various segments that represent the different regions of the vertebral column with joints between these segments. Individualized vertebra and corresponding joints might produce different results, and therefore data should be cautiously interpreted.

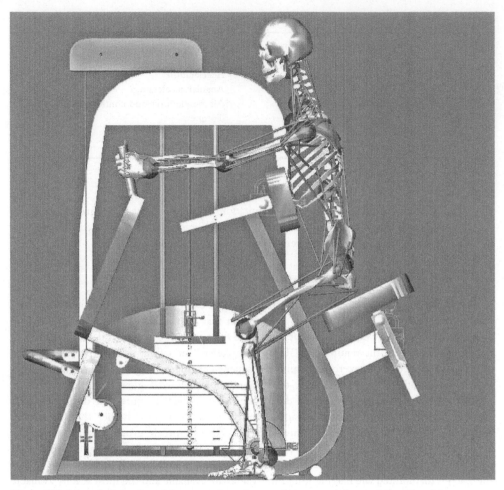

Figure 42.2 Musculoskeletal model representing a large male on a seated row resistance training machine.

The following information exists regarding joint loading limits of the spine that can be used for the comparisons and interpretation of the results of 3D musculoskeletal simulations while training on a specific piece of exercise equipment. Research from the American National Institute for Occupational Safety and Health (1997) recommends that spinal compression forces should not exceed 3,400 N to avoid injury. However, there is a very real threat of musculoskeletal injury before this failure limit value has been reached (Cooper and Ghassemieh, 2007; Knapik and Marras, 2009; Snook and Ciriello, 1991). British standards (British Standards Institute, 2002) recommend 600 N as the cut-off point for carrying masses; no further recommendations except 'time of exposure needs to be minimized' and 'a preferred system requires optimal ergonomic position with reduced back bending posture' are made. The most commonly cited spine tolerance is 1,000 N for shear force as stipulated by McGill (1996).

A few additional aspects need to be considered when comparing the results of the 3D musculoskeletal simulations and the recommended joint loading limits such as the activities used to determine the safe joint loading limits, as well as training status and core musculature of the exerciser. Most of the activities used to determine safe joint loading limits are during occupational activities or activities of daily living and not during exercising. In addition, modelling does not take into consideration varying training status or muscular strength and endurance of individuals that could either increase or decrease their risk for injury depending on which side of the continuum they find themselves. Core musculature also plays an important role in protecting exercisers, especially the spine, during training, which is also not taken into account. The core can be defined as the lumbo-pelvic-hip complex. The core is where the centre of gravity is located and where all movement begins (Prentice, 2010a). The core operates as an integrated functional unit whereby the entire kinetic chain works synergistically to produce force, reduce force and dynamically stabilize against abnormal force. In an efficient state, each structural component distributes weight, absorbs force and transfers ground reaction forces (Prentice, 2010b).

In terms of exercise efficacy, muscle force production values obtained during 3D musculoskeletal modelling of a training exercise can be analysed. Does the exercise train the muscles it was supposed to and does the exercise manage to isolate the relevant muscle groups or not? For example, an exercise that is supposed to train the abdominal muscles (rectus abdominis, internal and external obliques and transversus abdominis muscles) should have as little contribution from the hip flexor muscles (iliacus and psoas major muscles) as possible. Ideally, different exercises that are supposed to train similar muscle groups should be compared in order to determine how effective the exercises are with regards to training relevant muscle groups.

Approaches to 3D musculoskeletal modelling of resistance training exercises

There are various approaches to 3D musculoskeletal modelling of training exercises. The process described in this text is only one possible approach that could be used. There are advantages and disadvantages to each approach, and one needs to consider these before an approach is chosen. For example, the process described does not make use of video motion capture data of the exercise, and it is important to understand when motion capture is appropriate. Furthermore, steps can be added, removed or adjusted as required depending on the objectives or outcomes of the modelling simulation.

Here is a summary of possible processes or steps to be used for the modelling of a resistance training exercise:

1 Gather anthropometric data and corresponding functional strength data.
2 Import or create a human body model.
3 Create the relevant soft tissues.
4 Merge a computer-aided design (CAD) model of the training machine with the human body model.
5 Position the human body model on the exercise training machine.
6 Add the applicable constraints to the model.
7 Add motion agents to the model.
8 Run an equilibrium simulation.
9 Run an inverse-dynamics simulation.
10 Prepare the model for dynamic simulation.
11 Run a parametric analysis.
12 Complete a literature search on the relevant resistance training exercise as well as relevant literature on safe loading limits.
13 Interrogate the results.
14 Conclude findings.

Slight variations in the modelling procedure may be necessary in order to complete the protocol successfully for the piece of training equipment.

Equipment

A 3D musculoskeletal full body model must be created using digital human modelling software and incorporated into a multi-body dynamics model of the exercise machine modelled. A default model as generated by the software may be used or a more detailed model can be created depending on the exercise and aims of the modelling project. When creating a musculoskeletal model various active muscle types can usually be selected depending on the modelling software being used; for example, open or closed loop and simple or Hill-based muscles. Open loop muscles fire via a user-defined activation curve over a certain period of time. Closed loop muscles contain proportional-integral-differential (PID) controllers. The PID controller algorithm uses a target length/time curve to generate the muscle activation, and the muscles follow this curve. Simple muscles fire with no constraints except for the physiological cross-sectional area (pCSA), which designates the maximum force a muscle can exert. As a result, graphs of simple muscle activation curves will generally peak at a flat force ceiling value. Hill-based muscles operate on the traditional combination of an active contractile element (CE) and a passive parallel elastic element (PE). The contractile element contains a muscle activation state that controls the active muscle force capability, while the parallel elastic element exerts opposing forces that more accurately simulate the movement and force exertion of real muscles (Biomechanics Research Group, 2006; Nolte *et al.*, 2011).

Musculoskeletal full body human and resistance training machine computer-aided design (CAD) models

Various anthropometric cases can be created for each exercise to be modelled. The anthropometric cases should correspond with the user population of the exercise equipment. It is recommended that the anthropometric cases created represent the smallest, average and largest individual that will used the exercise machine. One possible solution for the purpose of building these biomechanical models, is to assume a correlation between body mass index (BMI) and functional body strength. Similar assumptions have previously been made in biomechanics full body model simulations (Rasmussen *et al.*, 2005). A study by Annegarn *et al.* (2007) also verified scaled modelling strengths against actual functional body strengths and correlations ranged from 0.64 to 0.99. Body form variances described by principle components (PCs) analysis can also be considered in the modelling process. This technique will identify positive and negative boundary cases of each PC, representing the boundary conditions to be accommodated in design (Gordon and Brantley, 1997).

Design variables can be created using the software in which the multi-body dynamics model of the exercise machine is modelled in order to adjust variables such as the external resistance (as selected by the amount of weights when using a selectorized resistance training machine) and to specify the radius of the cam over which the cable of an actual exercise machine would run in order to lift the selected resistance. A special contact force (solid to solid) could be created between the weights being lifted and the remainder of the weight stack during the simulation. A coupler joint could be created to link the revolute joint (driver) of the lever arm attached to the handlebars or part of the exercise training machine to be moved by the exerciser, depending on which exercise is to be simulated with the translational joint of the weight stack. Lastly, such a design variable created for the radius of the cam must then be referenced as the scale of the coupled joint (translational joint at weights). The design variable created for the mass of the weights can then be adjusted according to the predetermined resistance for each anthropometric case.

The external resistance applied in the models should be based on normative strength data that is available for the particular exercise. Unfortunately, normative data for strength values may not always be available and an alternative method may need to be used. In a study by Nolte *et al.* (2011), the external resistance used for the seated biceps curl resistance training exercise simulation was based on data obtained from RSA-MIL-STD 127, Vol. 5 (RSA Military Standards Steering Committee, 2001). This database consists of a range of human functional strength measurement variables for the South African National Defence Force males and females. Due to its representivity this standard is considered an accurate representation of the functional body strength of the South Africa population (RSA Military Standards Steering Committee, 2001). Furthermore, functional strength data was used from activities that most closely resembled the movements of the exercise as well as the muscle groups used during such movement. Depending on the objectives of the 3D musculoskeletal modelling an appropriate resistance for the anthropometric case should then be selected (percentage of one repetition maximum (1-RM)), as well as the number of repetitions to be performed determined.

Simulation

Extreme care should be taken with the positioning of the musculoskeletal model onto the exercise training machine to ensure technique, posture and positioning are correct and according to best exercise principles if video motion capture is not to be used. Furthermore, total manufacturer adjustability of the exercise machine should be used in order to ensure the best possible positioning for each of the anthropometric cases on the piece of exercise equipment.

It is important that steps be taken in order to ensure realistic kinematics are achieved during the inverse dynamics simulations such as: (1) positioning of the human model on the exercise equipment; (2) adjustment of the posture to allow for the human machine interface to be created; (3) creating the constraints between the human and machine; (4) prescribing the motion of the repetitions; (5) evaluation of the resultant kinematics; and (6) adjustment of joint positions until inverse dynamics results in a realistic exercise movement. Bushing elements and spherical joints can be used to secure relevant body parts to the exercise training machine. Bushing elements are preferred to fixed joint elements because it allows for limited translational and rotational motion. In addition, the amount of motion can be controlled by changing stiffness and damping characteristics in all three orthogonal directions.

The inverse dynamics – forward dynamics method can then be applied during the simulations. During the inverse dynamics simulation, a rotational motion is applied to the revolute joint of the lever arm in order to generate the required movement of the resistance training machine. This movement should replicate the concentric and eccentric phase of the exercise. The time set for the concentric phase can be slightly shorter than that of the eccentric phase in order to mimic conventional resistance training technique in which the downward phase is more deliberate to prohibit the use of momentum. Furthermore, a step function can also be included in the concentric phase in order to ensure a gradual start to the movement. Thus, the muscles of the model are trained during the inverse dynamics simulation in order to calculate the changes in muscle lengths to result in the required machine movement.

After the inverse dynamics simulation is performed, the rotational motion should be removed from the rotational joint of the lever arm of the resistance training machine. The recorded muscle length changes and resulting joint movements can then be used to drive the model during the forward dynamics simulation in the manner as developed through the inverse dynamics simulation. During the forward dynamics simulation, the model is guided by the internal forces (muscle length changes resulting in joint angulations and torques) and influenced by external forces (gravity, contact and determined exercise resistance). It is important to note it may be necessary to make changes to the default model (if a default model is being used) to solve the models with plausible kinematics during the forward dynamics simulations depending on the complexity of exercise or movement. Changes that may be necessary include the manipulation of specific muscle origins and insertions, increasing the pCSA of relevant muscles and decreasing the joint stiffness in the forward dynamics simulations. It is important that any changes made are realistic or plausible.

Data analysis

The anthropometric dimensions and exercise postures of the musculoskeletal human models can be visually assessed in relation to the dimensions and adjustability of the resistance training equipment in order to determine if the relevant anthropometric cases representative of the end-user population can comfortably be accommodated on the resistance training machine. Key aspects included start and end exercise posture, as well as maintaining correct exercise technique throughout the exercise during the simulation. Correct technique can be assessed in terms of limited compensatory movements and performing the exercise through the full range of motion as determined by the inverse dynamics.

The kinematic and kinetic data from the simulations should be analysed specifically in terms of peak muscular force production of the prime movers of the exercise. Therefore, does the equipment exercise the muscles it was designed to exercise? And have any of the muscles reached peak muscle force production, which could allude to possible injury risk for the muscles involved? Furthermore, the risk of injury to the musculoskeletal system of the exerciser can be ascertained by comparison of measured forces with safe loading limits for the relevant joints found in the literature.

Conclusion

3D musculoskeletal modelling is able to highlight some interesting design elements and flaws as well as biomechanical and anthropometrical limitations of specific training exercises. However, there are limitations that have to be taken into consideration, especially when using the default model of particular modelling software.

The following problems or limitations can be encountered with the modelling process of training exercises:

- The primary limitation of the default model of most modelling software is that it lacks adequate bio-fidelity.
- The modelling can be a fairly time-consuming process, requiring a process of many iterations to be able to provide plausible results.
- Caution should be taken when using default models and not assume that a matching anthropometry will result in reliable muscle strength capabilities; this is further complicated by the significant variance in muscular strength between subjects of similar anthropometry due to differences in conditioning levels.
- To truly evaluate exercise efficacy, all the important muscles that contribute to the movement should be present. It is sometimes possible to add muscles to default models

and then assess their relative contribution to the produced force (as a percentage of their maximal force-generating capacity).

- It is important to bear in mind when evaluating spine loads that the spine of default models do not always consist of all the individual vertebrae, but often rather of various segments that represent the different regions of the vertebral column with joints between these segments. Thus, individualized vertebra and corresponding joints might produce different results.
- It appears that more complex, multi-joint or compound exercises pose problems for default models, and therefore models with more detailed musculature may be required to solve the forward dynamics simulations sufficiently.

To conclude, in order to get significant value from 3D modelling of training exercises, it is imperative that the researcher or individual doing the simulations has adequate training and in-depth knowledge of the software that will be used, as well as biomechanical and functional anatomy expertise. Despite the challenges involved with the modelling process in comparison to other methods, it is a relatively simple, inexpensive and safe means for evaluating training exercises. It is, however, important at the beginning of the process to set clear objectives, the relevant research on the particular exercise is completed and the appropriate approach is selected for the 3D musculoskeletal modelling of the training exercise.

Acknowledgements

My appreciation and thanks to both Prof. Schalk Els and Prof. Ernst Krüger for sharing with me their expertise and advice. To Dr Heinrich Nolte, my grateful thanks for his endless support and belief invested in me. To Mrs Yvonne De'Ath my sincere thanks for the arduous task of proofreading.

References

Alexander, R. M. (2003) 'Modelling approaches in biomechanics', *Philosophical Transactions of the Royal Society*, 358(1437): 1429–35.

American National Institute for Occupational Safety and Health. (1997) Musculoskeletal disorders and workplace factors: a critical review of epidemiologic evidence for work-related musculoskeletal disorders of the neck, upper extremity, and low back, Cincinnati, OH: National Institute for Occupational Safety and Health Division of Biomedical of Behavioural Science.

Annegarn, J., Rasmussen, J., Savelberg, H. H. C. M., Verdijk, L. B. and Meijer, K. (2007) 'Strength scaling in human musculoskeletal models', *Proceedings of the European Workshop on Movement Sciences*, Amsterdam: VU University Amsterdam.

Beachle, T. R. and Earle, R. W. (1994) *Essentials of Strength Training and Conditioning*, Champaign, IL: Human Kinetics.

Biomechanics Research Group (2006) *LifeMOD Biomechanics Modeler Manual*, San Clemente, CA: Biomechanics Research Group, Inc.

British Standards Institute (2002) BS EN 1005-3: 2002, Safety of machinery – human physical performance – part 3: Recommended force limits for machinery operations, London: British Standards Institute.

Buchanan, T. S., Lloyd, D. G., Manal, K. and Besier, T. F. (2004) 'Neuromuscular modelling: estimation of muscle forces and joint moments and movements from measurements of neural command', *Journal of Applied Biomechanics*, 20(4): 369–95.

Calhoon, G. and Fry, A. C. (1999) 'Injury rates and profiles of elite competitive Olympic weightlifters', *Journal of Athletic Training*, 34(3): 232–8.

Cooper, G. and Ghassemieh, E. (2007) 'Risk assessment of patient handling with ambulance stretcher systems (ramp/ winch), easy-loader, tail-lift using biomechanical failure criteria', *Medical Engineering & Physics*, 29(7): 775–87.

Erdemir, A., McLean, S., Herzog, W. and van den Bogert, A. J. (2007) 'Model-based estimation of muscle forces exerted during movements', *Clinical Biomechanics*, 22(2): 232–54.

Fleck, W. J. and Kraemer, S. J. (1997) *Designing Resistance Training Programs*, Champaign, IL: Human Kinetics.

Gordon, C. C. and Brantley, J. D. (1997) 'Statistical modelling of population variation in the head and face', *Proceedings of the Design and Integration of Helmet Systems International Symposium*, Massachusetts.

Hockey, R. V. (1996) *Physical Fitness. The Pathway to Healthful Living*, 8th edn, Missouri: McGraw-Hill.

Howley, E. T. (2007) *Fitness professional's handbook*, 5th edn, Champaign, IL: Human Kinetics.

Kazlauskiené, K. (2006) 'Design and research of biomechanical models of human with joint replacements', unpublished doctoral thesis, Kaunas University of Technology.

Kenny, I. C., Wallace, E. S., Brown, D. and Otto, S. R. (2005) *Validation of a full-body computer simulation of the golf drive for clubs of differing length*, University of Ulster: R & A Limited.

Knapik, G. G. and Marras, W. S. (2009) 'Spine loading at different lumbar levels during pushing and pulling', *Ergonomics*, 52(1): 60–70.

Lavallee, M. E. and Balam, T. (2010) 'An overview of strength training injuries: acute and chronic', *Current Sports Medicine Reports*, 9(5): 307–13.

McGill, S. M. (1996) 'Searching for the safe biomechanical envelope for maintaining healthy tissue', *Proceedings of the Pre-Meeting Workshop, International Society for the Study of the Lumbar Spine: The Contribution of Biomechanics to the prevention and treatment of low back pain*, Vermont: International Society for the Study of the Lumbar Spine.

Nolte, K., Krüger, P. E. and Els, P. S. (2011) 'Three dimensional musculoskeletal modelling of the seated biceps curl resistance training exercise', *Sports Biomechanics*, 10(2): 146–60.

Otten, E. (2003) 'Inverse and forward dynamics: models of multi-body systems', *Philosophical Transactions of the Royal Society: Biological Sciences*, 29(358): 1493–500.

Pearl, B. and Moran, G. T. (1986*) Getting Stronger: Weight Training for Men and Women*, Bolinas, CA: Shelter Publications.

Prentice, W. E. (2003) *Fitness and Wellness for Life*, 7th edn, St Louis, MO: McGraw-Hill.

Prentice, W. E. (2010a) *Rehabilitation Techniques for Sports Medicine and Athletic Training*, New York: McGraw-Hill.

Prentice, W. E. (2010b) *Essentials of Athletic Injury Management*, 8th edn, New York: McGraw-Hill.

Rasmussen, J., de Zee, M., Damsgaard, M., Christensen, S. T., Marek, C. and Siebertz, K. (2005) 'A general method for scaling musculo-skeletal model', Paper presented at the *10th International Symposium on Computer Simulation in Biomechanics*, Ohio, 28–30 July.

Reilly, T. and Lees, A. (1984) 'Exercise and sports equipment: Some ergonomics aspects', *Applied Ergonomics*, 15(4): 259 –79.

RSA Military Standards Steering Committee. (2001) RSA-MIL-STD-127, Vol. 5, Ergonomic design: Biomechanics – specific functional body strength data standard, Pretoria: RSA Military Standards Steering Committee.

Snook, S. H., and Ciriello, V. M. (1991) 'The design of manual handling tasks: revised tables of maximum acceptable weights and forces', *Ergonomics*, 34(9): 1197–213.

Vaughn, C. L. (1989) *Biomechanics of Sport*, Boca Raton, FL: CRC Press.

Wagner, D., Rasmussen, J. and Reed, M. (2007) 'Assessing the importance of motion dynamics for ergonomic analysis of manual materials handling tasks using the AnyBody modelling system', *Proceedings of the 2007 Digital Human Modelling for Design and Engineering Conference*, Seattle, WA: SAE International, pp. 2007–01–2504.

Whiting, W. C. and Zernicke, R. F. (2008) *Biomechanics of Musculoskeletal Injury*, 2nd edn, Champaign, IL: Human Kinetics.

Measurement in adapted sports and exercise

43

BIOMECHANICS OF VERTICAL JUMP PERFORMANCE IN UNILATERAL TRANS-TIBIAL AMPUTEES

Siobhán Strike,[1] Ceri Diss[1] and Marlene Schoeman[2]

[1]UNIVERSITY OF ROEHAMPTON, LONDON
[2]UNIVERSITY OF THE FREE STATE, BLOEMFONTEIN

Introduction

Vertical jumping is a closed skill that is fundamental to numerous recreational activities and training strategies (Davis *et al.*, 2003). It is easily controlled and consists of clear phases, each with its own underlying performance criterion for successful execution (Spagele *et al.*, 1999). This makes it a valuable experimental model in biomechanical research to assess the cause and effect of human movement strategies for different population groups (Challis, 1998; Kakihana and Suzuki, 2001; Strike and Diss, 2005). The fundamental objective is to achieve the greatest vertical velocity ($v_{(z)}$) at take-off in order to reach maximum height ($s_{(z)}$) of the centre of mass (*CoM*) during flight (Dowling and Vamos, 1993). The height is determined by the biomechanics in the preceding phases that are required to generate vertical impulse. Therefore, $s_{(z)}$ is related to the ability of the jumper to produce power at the joints and to coordinate the inter-joint coupling. Inter-joint coordination is a measure of the capacity of the neuromuscular system to organize itself to enable the successful execution of complex skills. Coordination in jumping is dependent on the sequential proximal-distal peak activation of the muscles, which has been shown to be the most effective in accelerating the body given the anatomical and geometric constraints of the musculo-skeletal system (Bobbert and van Ingen Schenau, 1988). Transtibial amputees are defined by the absence of the lower leg, ankle joint and foot segment. The biarticular plantarflexors have been severed, and so ineffective co-contraction with the knee extensors, in combination with the loss of the most distal joint in the proximal-distal sequencing, may result in altered coordination of the movement.

Typically, lower leg prostheses consist of a socket, which fits over the residual limb, a pylon that replaces the shank of the lower leg and a prosthetic foot. The role of lower limb prostheses is to replace the missing ankle and enable interaction of the residual limb with the ground for the transmission of action and reaction ground forces (Jones *et al.*, 2006; Pitkin, 1997). Lower leg prostheses also aim to provide adequate shock absorption for the prevention of proximal joint injuries and residual limb skin breakdown (Pitkin, 1995). Patellar tendon-bearing sockets are most commonly used and designed to distribute the load placed on the residual limb away from the tibial condyles to the patellar tendon (Selles *et al.*, 2005).

In the foot, the keel is designed to provide stability and balance while accommodating flexibility (Klute *et al.*, 2001; Pitkin, 1995). Unlike the human foot, however, the keel is fabricated with a single stiffness profile that cannot adapt to function across a spectrum of activity levels and functional demands (Klute *et al.*, 2001). Therefore, the prosthesis is limited in its mechanical functionality when the dynamic movement changes, resulting in movement-specific compensatory mechanisms at the residual joints and the intact limb. Compression of the keel resembles dorsiflexion at the prosthetic ankle and enables the storage of energy. Resistive compliance of the keel replaces the eccentric contraction of the plantarflexors, and the recoil of the keel resembles concentric contraction of the plantarflexors to bring about 'plantarflexion' and returns the stored energy to assist in propulsion.

Previous work examining the biomechanics of transtibial amputees in producing the movements associated with the vertical jump take-off has indicated that the joint moments and overall work done on the intact and prosthetic sides was reduced at the knee and that the ranges of motion at the knee and ankle joints were restricted (Schoeman *et al.*, 2012; Strike and Diss, 2005). Restricted ankle motion when wearing figure skating skates has been shown to significantly reduce the knee joint range of motion, and although the proximal-distal joint moment coordination was not altered while squat jumping, the delay between hip and knee extension increased while it was reduced between the knee and ankle (Haguenauer *et al.*, 2006). In an able-bodied (AB) sample group, the contributions of knee strength and hip-knee coordination were independent and significantly correlated to $s_{(v)}$, suggesting that both strength and coordination are necessary to attain height (Tomioka *et al.*, 2001). The sequencing and timing of the joint rotations and the manner of the inter-segmental joint coupling has not previously been assessed for lower limb amputees. In multi-articular movements, the interjoint coordination can be described as the relationship of angular displacement of two adjacent joints. The technique is common in determining the coupling mechanisms of the lower limb in running (Chang *et al.*, 2008) and in determining the efficacy of training drills to sport performance (Wilson *et al.*, 2009).

Therefore, the aim of this research was to determine if the joint coordination on the intact and residual sides are affected by the presence of a lower limb amputation. It was suggested that the joint coupling pattern at the hip-knee and the knee-ankle would be different between the prosthetic (AMP-P) and intact (AMP-I) sides for amputees and compared to AB limbs.

Methods

Participants

Six unilateral transtibial amputee (AMP) participants (5 male and 1 female) and 10 AB participants (9 male and 1 female) of the same age range (18–50 years) with no pathology participated in the study. All AMPs were more than 12 months post-surgery with no secondary pathology and the amputation was as a result of trauma. All participants had to be able to ambulate independently and be recreationally active without being specifically trained in a sporting activity involving jumping. The typical grade of the AMPs participating in the research was K3, which is defined as '. . . a typical community ambulator with the ability to traverse most environmental barriers and may have vocational, therapeutic, or exercise activity that demands prosthetic use beyond simple locomotion' (Rosenberger, 2000). All the AMPs wore patellar tendon-bearing sockets with rigid pylons and their own prosthesis (Table 43.1).

Table 43.1 Amputee participant characteristics

Participant	Height (m)	Body mass (kg)	Amputated limb	Prosthetic foot	
AMP1	1.91	87	L	Esprit®	
AMP2	1.86	71	R	Elite Foot®	
AMP3	1.82	83	L	Vari-flex®	
AMP4	1.92	101	L	Spring Lite®	
AMP5	1.88	70	R	Modullar III™	
AMP6	1.79	100	R	Mobis®₁D₁₀	

One AMP (6) was the only participant not to wear a dynamic elastic response (DER) prosthesis. However, as the purpose of the research was to determine the joint coordination patterns rather than the energy stored at the prosthesis, it was considered possible to include this participant. All participants signed an informed consent form and the research was approved by the University and the National Health Services' Ethics Committees.

Data collection

Data were collected in a single session. Anthropometric measurements were recorded and 34 reflective markers attached to the participants according to Vicon requirements for full body modelling (Vicon™, Oxford UK; Davis *et al.*, 1991). Following a 5-minute warm-up on a treadmill at a self-selected fast walking velocity, the participants were given the opportunity to practise and familiarize themselves with the jumping criteria and laboratory conditions. Ten maximal effort bilateral countermovement jumps were performed with hands on hips and 1 minute's rest was given between each trial. The instruction given was to jump as high as possible. The jumps were performed from an initial position where each foot was placed on a separate force plate. Trials were excluded if the participants used their arms or if they missed the force plates during landing. Data were collected using two Kistler (model 9581C, sampling at 1,080 Hz) force plates synchronized with a nine-camera infrared system (Vicon™, Oxford, UK, model 612, sampling at 120 Hz). The trial with the greatest $s_{(v)}$ was analysed for each participant since the biomechanics that underpin maximal performance would give greater insight into joint coordination patterns rather than examining a variety of jump performances.

Data analysis

Kinematic data were smoothed using a Woltring quintic spline (MSE = 15 mm^2) algorithm. The Vicon whole body model was run to produce coordinate data for the *CoM*. The Davis *et al.* (1991) model was run to produce sagittal plane coordinate data for the hip, knee and ankle. The sagittal plane was chosen as movement in this plane is predominant in producing the jumping movement as displayed by previous three-dimensional studies (Nagano *et al.*, 2007). The $s_{(z)}$ was determined by the *CoM*'s vertical displacement (maximum vertical position less vertical position at take-off). The AB right leg was used for comparison against the AMP-P and AMP-I sides.

The initiation of the jump was defined as the time when the *CoM* displaced vertically in the downward direction, which also marked the start of the countermovement phase. Amortization, the time when the *CoM* was at its minimum vertical displacement, occurred during the transition between the countermovement and propulsion phases. The propulsion phase ended at take-off. Take-off was defined by the vertical force under each foot being < 10N. The take-off phase was time-normalized from seconds to 100 per cent stance, from the initiation of the countermovement to the end of propulsion.

The joint coordination was quantified using sagittal plane relative joint motion (angle-angle) of the hip-knee and knee-ankle, and a modified vector coding technique (Heiderscheit *et al.*, 2002). The angle-angle plots were created with the proximal joint on the abscissa (Figures 43.1a and 43.1c). Thereafter, the coupling angle was determined by finding the subtended angle of the resultant vector between two successive time points and the right horizontal. By defining location in each of the four quadrants, and by converting the angle from radians to degrees, the coupling angle ranged from 0 to 360° (Chang *et al.*, 2008; Wilson *et al.*, 2009).

The coupling angle indicates the coupling pattern for the movement (Chang *et al.*, 2008). Eight coupling strategies were identified and are illustrated in Figure 43.1. They were: in-phase flexion (22.5–67.4°); in-phase extension (202.5–247.4°); anti-phase distal extension (112.5–157.4°); anti-phase proximal extension (292.5–337.4°); proximal flexion (0–22.5 and 337.5–359.9°); proximal extension (157.5–202.4°); distal flexion (67.5–112.4°) and distal extension (247.5–292.4°).

The mean coupling angle at each time instance during the jump was determined for the AMP and AB groups using circular statistics where appropriate (Chang *et al.*, 2008). Due to the emergence of different mechanisms to produce the results, the research design was underpowered and statistical analysis was not appropriate. To determine the difference in the

Coupling Angle definition							
Hip Flexion	In-Phase Flexion	Knee Flexion	Anti-Phase	Hip Extension	In-Phase Extension	Knee Extension	Anti-Phase
0-22.5 & 337.5-359.5°	22.5-67.4°	67.5-112.4°	112.5-157.4°	157.5-202.4°	202.5-247.4°	247.5-292.4°	292.5-337.4°

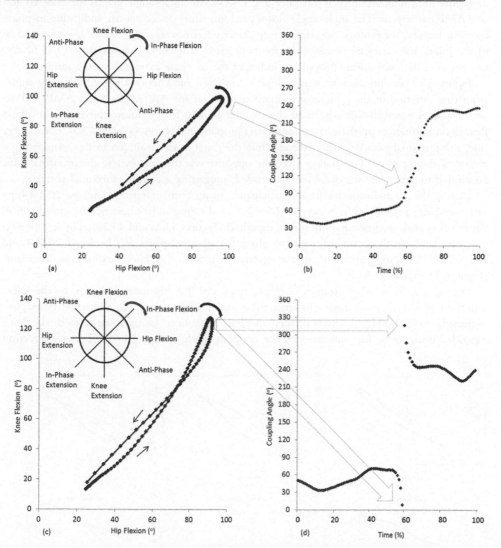

Figure 43.1 Calculation of the coupling angle. The angle–angle plot for the hip–knee (a and c) is used to calculate the coupling angle (b and d). The angle subtended by the vector between successive points in the angle–angle plot defines the coordination pattern, and eight patterns are defined.

coupling angle over the take-off phase between the AB, AMP-P and AMP-I, the root mean squared difference (RMSD) was calculated.

Results

The AMPs jumped lower than the AB participants performing a mean $s_{(z)}$ (± standard deviation) of 0.16 m (± 0.06) compared to 0.31 m (± 0.04), respectively.

Figure 43.2 illustrates typical hip-knee and knee-ankle angle-angle graphs for one AB and one AMP participant. The angle-angle plot is predominantly on a diagonal, indicating in-phase motion. Initally, the positive diagonal during the countermovement indicates in-phase flexion of the joints, then transition enables the joints to move from flexion to extension and finally, the negative diagonal during propulsion indicates the in-phase extension of the joints.

Figure 43.3 presents the instantaneous mean hip-knee and knee-ankle joint coupling angles from the initiation of the countermovement to take-off for AB, AMP-P and AMP-I. Two key strategies emerged that related to the manner in which the countermovement in-phase flexion transitioned to in-phase extension during propulsion (Figures 43.1 and 43.3). For strategy one, the proximal joint began to extend while the distal joint continued to flex, suggesting a proximal-distal pattern. For strategy two, the opposite was the case, where the proximal joint continued to flex while the distal joint extended, suggesting a distal to proximal pattern.

During the countermovement, all participants, using both strategies, demonstrated a hip-knee coupling angle that was between 22.5–67.4°, indicating an in-phase flexion coordination pattern (i.e. both the knee and hip flexed together) (Figures 43.3a and 43.3b). The knee-ankle coupling angle in the countermovement phase for all participants was between 0–22.4 and 337–359.4°, indicating a knee flexion coordination pattern (i.e. knee flexion was dominant) (Figures 43.3c and 43.3d).

During transition, when strategy one was employed, the hip extended prior to the knee, indicated by the coupling angle changing in an anticlockwise direction about the polar plot, increasing to 202–247.5°, which defined in-phase extension. Using strategy two, the knee extended prior to the hip, indicated by the coupling angle changing in a clockwise direction

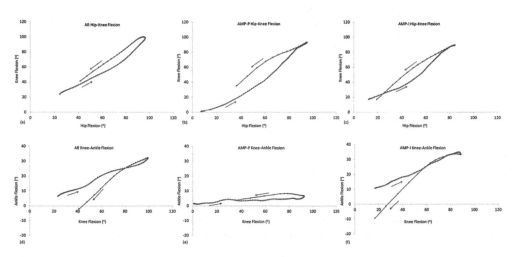

Figure 43.2 Typical angle-angle plots for the hip-knee (a–c) and knee-ankle (d–f) joints over the course of the take-off phase for AB (a and d), AMP-P (b and e) and AMP-I (c and f). The angle-angle plot was used to determine the coupling angle.

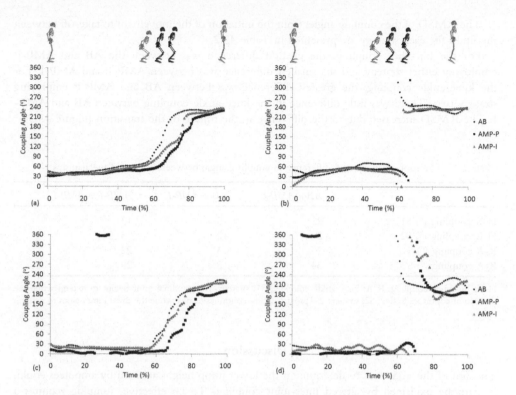

Figure 43.3 Mean coupling angle for the AB(◆) AMP-P(■) and AMP-I(▲). The hip-knee coupling angle (a and b) and the knee-ankle coupling angle (c and d) for strategy 1 (a and c) and strategy 2 (b and d) indicate the coordination pattern. Two strategies were identified to enable the transition from countermovement (~ 0–60 per cent take-off phase) to propulsion (~ 80–100 per cent take-off phase). Strategy 1 (a and c) proceeded anti-clockwise around the polar plot, indicating proximal joint extension occurred while the distal joint continued to flex. Strategy 2 (b and d) proceeded clockwise around the polar plot, indicating distal joint extension occurred while the proximal joint continued to flex.

about the polar plot to in-phase extension, crossing 360° and decreasing to 202–247.5°. Using both strategies, the transition began earlier for AB compared to AMP-I and AMP-P, though the coupling angles were similar (Figures 43.3a and 43.3b). The transition was very rapid for AMP-I, indicating a very ballistic change from countermovement to propulsion (Figure 43.3b). For the knee-ankle coupling transition, employing strategy one, the knee extended prior to the ankle, with the AB and AMP-I transitioning before AMP-P (Figure 43.3c). Utilizing strategy two, the ankle extended prior to the knee, which occurred earlier for AB compared to AMP-P and AMP-I (Figure 43.3d).

During propulsion, all participants, using both strategies, demonstrated a hip-knee coupling angle that was between 202.5 and 247.4°, indicating an in-phase extension coordination pattern (i.e. both the knee and hip simultaneously extended) (Figures 43.3a and 43.3b). The knee-ankle coupling angle during propulsion was affected by the presence of the prosthesis and was strategy dependent. Using strategy one, the AB and AMP-I adopted an in-phase extension pattern while the AMP-P adopted a knee extension pattern (Figure 43.3 c). Utilizing strategy two, AB adopted an in-phase extension pattern while AMP-I and AMP-P adopted a knee extension pattern, with a coupling angle between 157.5 and 202.4° (Figure 43.3d).

The RMSD of the coupling angles from the initiation of the movement to take-off between the limbs for each strategy are presented in Table 43.2.

For the hip-knee coupling, the greatest difference was between the AB and AMP-P employing either strategy and the smallest difference was between AMP-P and AMP-I. For the knee-ankle coupling, the greatest difference was between AB and AMP-P employing strategy two. There was little difference in the knee-ankle coupling between AB and AMP-I. The RMSD increased due to the difference in the timing of the transition (Figure 43.3).

Table 43.2 The root mean squared difference in coupling angle between limbs and mechanisms

	AB v AMP-P	*AB v AMP-I*	*AMP-P v AMP-I*
H-K coupling (°) S1	28	15	13
H-K coupling (°) S2	28	12	5
K-A coupling (°) S1	20	3	22
K-A coupling (°) S2	34	5	29

H-K: hip-knee coupling; K-A: knee ankle coupling; S1: strategy 1 – proximal joint begins to extend while the distal joint continues to flex; S2: strategy 2 – proximal joint continues to flex while the distal joint begins to extend.

Discussion

The aim of the study was to determine if the lower jump height attained by amputees could, in part, be explained by altered inter-joint coupling. To be effective, jumping requires a countermovement followed by a rapid transition to propulsion. This is a relatively complex multi-joint task, which may be compromised due to the presence of a prosthesis. The anatomy of the amputee is altered due to a prosthetic joint, which is not as flexible or responsive as the human joint. A two-legged vertical jump is predominantly a symmetrical activity where functioning of the contralateral segments is influenced by the constraints from the proximal fixed pelvis and the distal side-by-side positioning of the feet. Hence, it is likely that any changes that occur as a result of amputation on the prosthetic side will affect the intact side. We chose to analyse the patterns on both the AMP-P and AMP-I, and to compare them to each other and to AB participants with similar experience in jumping.

The AMPs did not jump as high as the AB participants, which previous work has indicated is related to the reduced work done at selected joints (Schoeman *et al.*, 2012). Achieving a maximum jump is also dependent on the coordination and correct sequencing and timing of the joints' angular motions (Hudson, 1986). The segmental joint angles and the associated coupling angles can detail the joint coordination patterns and strategies adopted to produce a maximal jump. The vector-coding method has been used previously to identify changes in the coordination of the rearfoot with the forefoot in injured runners (Chang *et al.*, 2008; Hamill *et al.*, 1999; Heiderscheit *et al.*, 2002) and in determining the efficacy of triple jump training drills (Wilson *et al.*, 2009). Vector-coding has shown to be a useful tool to determine coordination patterns but it has not been used previously for amputees or for vertical jump analysis.

In the countermovement phase, there was a clear overall in-phase flexion coupling between the hip and knee joints and a knee flexion coupling between the knee and ankle joints. These coupling patterns were adopted by all participants and were not influenced by the presence of the prosthesis for AMP-P or AMP-I (Figure 43.3).

In the propulsion phase, the hip-knee coupling was consistently in-phase extension, which was adopted by all participants and was not influenced by the presence of the prosthesis (Figures 43.3a and 43.3b). However, the knee-ankle coupling was affected by the presence of the prosthesis. The AB and AMP-I adopted an in-phase extension pattern, while the AMP-P adopted a knee extension pattern (Figures 43.3c and 43.3d). Possibly, the altered pattern was used to compensate for the reduced ankle joint range of motion and the lack of active response at the inert prosthesis.

The vector-coding technique identified two distinct strategies for transitioning from the countermovement to the propulsion phases. As both AMP and AB participants adopted either of the two strategies, the level of experience of the participants rather than the amputation was the likely reason for the variation. The majority of participants used strategy one in the hip-knee coupling. In this strategy, the hip began to extend while the knee continued to flex until both joints came into in-phase extension, suggesting a proximal-distal joint coupling. This is consistent with previous research, which has found that an anterior trunk lean during the countermovement is accompanied by a delay in knee extension onset during the transition (Nagano *et al.*, 2007) to avoid further anterior rotation of the trunk and the consequential loss in balance (Bobbert and Van Zandwijk, 1999). Bobbert and van Ingen Schenau (1988) found that, shortly after the end of the countermovement, the hip extensor muscles initiated the backward rotation of the trunk and the activation of the biarticular muscles about the hip and the knee delayed knee extension. The presence of the prosthesis served to cause a delay in this transition, which may influence the overall jump performance (Figure 43.3a). The development of an active state within the muscle contractile elements and the lengthening of the series-elastic elements (reflected in the depth of the countermovement) should be coordinated in order for the stored elastic energy to be utilized effectively. Since the knee and the hip are the main contributors to the total work done in a countermovement jump (Fukashiro and Komi, 1987; Hubley and Wells, 1983; Jacobs *et al.*, 1996; Vanezis and Lees, 2005), enhanced work through a countermovement can be attributed mainly as a result of active state development within the contractile elements (Arakawa *et al.*, 2010), at least for the AB population. Since the AMP participants do not have a complete functional lower leg and therefore cannot rely on the development of an active state and muscular functioning, they are dependent on the storage of elastic energy in the passive prosthetic keel to be released in propulsion. Therefore, as far as the contribution to total work from the lower leg and prosthesis is concerned, the countermovement serves to manifest the concept of elastic potentiation seen in the stretch-shortening cycle and the delay in the transition from countermovement to propulsion suggests an inefficient mechanism.

In contrast to strategy one, when using strategy two, the knee began to extend while the hip continued to flex, until both joints came into an in-phase extension. This is suggestive of a distal-proximal coupling between the knee and the hip (Figurer 43.3b). This strategy is indicative of poor coordination. Vanrenterghem *et al.* (2008) found a decrease in anterior trunk lean resulted in decreased jumping performances, mainly due to the subsequent decrease in hip power. However, they also found that a more upright trunk resulted in an increase in maximum knee power (Vanrenterghem *et al.*, 2008). Strategy two may be a way of optimizing the coordination pattern with relative joint strength at the hip and the knee.

Two strategies were also used at the knee-ankle coupling in transition from the counter-movement to the propulsion phases (Figures 43.3c and 43.3d). Again, most participants chose strategy one, which involved extending the knee while the ankle continued to dorsiflex until both joints came into in-phase extension/plantarflexion coupling. This strategy is indicative of a proximal-distal coordination strategy. Bobbert and van Ingen Schenau (1988) determined that a timely activation of the plantarflexors was needed for the transfer of powers generated at the knee to assist in the plantarflexion later in the propulsion phase. Again, the later timing of the transition by the AMP-P side (Figure 43.3c) suggests the timing of the return of elastic energy stored in the prosthesis during countermovement may impinge on an effective coordination pattern. This, in conjunction with the knee extension (rather than an in-phase extension) pattern in propulsion, suggests a compensation as a consequence of the lack of response at the prosthetic ankle. The subsequent effect on the knee may be a further reason for the reduced jump height by the amputees.

In contrast to strategy one, strategy two involved plantarflexion of the ankle joint prior to extension of the knee (Figure 43.3d). The lowest AB jumpers utilized this strategy, indicating that it is unlikely to be a successful strategy. The AMPs who selected strategy two for the knee-ankle coupling did not select strategy two at the hip-knee. This indicates an ankle, hip, knee kinematic chain was developed. All three performed the vertical jump at varying heights, which suggests that the strategy is not necessarily related to the height jumped on the prosthetic side and may be related to the other factors such as the nature of the prosthesis and the stability in loading. Schoeman *et al.* (2012) found reduced knee extensor moments for amputees when performing a vertical jump and has shown that amputees maintain an upright knee to ensure stability at the joint. Therefore, strategy two may be adopted on the AMP-P side in order to stabilize the joint (Markolf *et al.*, 1978; Vanezis and Lees, 2005). Reorganization of coordination is consistent for findings for older people with reduced ankle capacity (Haguenauer *et al.*, 2005).

The loss of a limb and its replacement by a prosthesis can cause some disruption to the coordination pattern from the initiation of the movement to take-off as evidenced by the RMSD (Table 43.2). We had anticipated that the hip-knee coupling would be similar between the limbs and that the knee-ankle coupling would be affected due to the presence of the prosthesis. The greatest difference in the RMSD was between the AB and the AMP-P side for the knee-ankle coupling when using strategy two, and the least was between the AB and the AMP-I side at the knee-ankle coupling using strategy one. It would appear that although the prosthesis affects the intact joint motion (Schoeman *et al.*, 2012), the coupling pattern between the AMP-I side and the AB participants' knee-ankle coupling is resistant to change and symmetry in the coupling between AMP-P and AMP-I is sacrificed. Although the countermovement and propulsion phases had similar coupling patterns (Figure 43.3), the timing of the transition was quite different between the AB participants and the AMP-P side, which appears to be the primary cause of the increased RMSD.

Wilson *et al.* (2009) found significant differences in joint coupling angles between drills and triple-jumps in the middle 20 per cent of contact, which coincided with the transition from braking to propulsion, and that this phase also coincided with the greatest variation in coordination patterns between jumpers. Our identification of different strategies to achieve this transition suggests that grouping participant data in this phase without first interrogating the individual data for transition strategies should be avoided, as the different strategies will alter the average coupling angle and increase the perceived variability.

Upward translation of the *CoM* is brought about by rotation of the lower limb joints through concentric contraction of the associated muscle groups (Bobbert and van Soest, 2001). The timing of the extensor moment has been shown to be most effective when a proximal-distal coordination pattern is used (Bobbert and van Ingen Schenau, 1988). Previous research on older people (Haguenauer *et al.*, 2005) and figure skaters (Haguenauer *et al.*, 2006) has suggested that the timing and sequencing of the joint extensions are altered by the lack of motion or strength at the ankle plantarflexors. Here, we analysed coordination of the joint coupling rather than the joint moments to determine if the presence of the prosthesis altered the coordination pattern. Future research should integrate the kinematic chain as determined by the joint coupling with the timing of the peak moments in order to determine how the moments and coupling are related and how these relate to jump height.

Conclusions

Since a specific proximal-distal coordination pattern is essential for the optimal execution of a complex motor task such as jumping (Bobbert and van Ingen Schenau, 1988), the altered coordination patterns presented by the AMPs helps to explain the reduced flight heights compared to the AB participants. Not all of the participant groups illustrated a proximal-distal coupling pattern, and it would appear that non-trained individuals have not yet mastered the most effective movement pattern. The timing of the transition from countermovement to propulsion was consistently delayed for the AMP-P side compared to AB. The knee extension strategy during propulsion was the only consistent difference to the AMP-I side and the AB participants. Further work is required to understand the factors that may influence strategy choice, including experience, strength and flexibility, both for AB and AMP participants. Thereafter, further work is required on determining the effect of coordination on the achievement of jump height.

References

Arakawa, H., Nagano, A., Yoshioka, S. and Fukashiro, S. (2010) 'Interaction between elastic energy utilization and active state development within the work enhancing mechanism during countermovement', *Journal of Electromyography and Kinesiology*, 20(2): 340–7.

Bobbert, M. F. and van Ingen Schenau, G. J. (1988) 'Coordination in vertical jumping', *Journal of Biomechanics*, 21(3): 249–62.

Bobbert, M. F. and van Soest, A. J. (2001) 'Why do people jump the way they do?', *Exercise and Sport Sciences Reviews*, 29(3): 95–102.

Bobbert, M. F. and Van Zandwijk, J. P. (1999) 'Dynamics of force and muscle stimulation in human vertical jumping', *Medicine and Science in Sports and Exercise*, 31(2): 303–10.

Challis, J. H. (1998) 'An investigation of the influence of bi-lateral deficit on human jumping', *Human Movement Science*, 17(3): 307–25.

Chang, R., Van Emmerik, R. and Hamill, J. (2008) 'Quantifying rearfoot-forefoot coordination in human walking', *Journal of Biomechanics*, 41(14): 3101–5.

Davis, D. S., Briscoe, D. A., Markowski, C. T., Saville, S. E. and Taylor, C. J. (2003) 'Physical characteristics that predict vertical jump performance in recreational male athletes', *Physical Therapy in Sport*, 4(4): 167–74.

Davis, R. B., Ounpuu, S., Tyburski, D. and Gage, J. R. (1991) 'A gait analysis data collection and reduction technique', *Human Movement Science*, 10(5): 575–87.

Dowling, J. J. and Vamos, L. (1993) 'Identification of kinetic and temporal factors related to vertical jump performance', *Journal of Applied Biomechanics*, 9(2): 95–110.

Fukashiro, S. and Komi, P. V. (1987) 'Joint moment and mechanical power flow of the lower limb during vertical jump', *International Journal of Sports Medicine*, 8 (Suppl 1): 15–21.

Haguenauer, M., Legreneur, P. and Monteil, K. M. (2005) 'Vertical jumping reorganization with aging: a kinematic comparison between young and elderly men', *Journal of Applied Biomechanics*, 21(3): 236–46.

Haguenauer, M., Legreneur, P. and Monteil, K. M. (2006) 'Influence of figure skating skates on vertical jumping performance', *Journal of Biomechanics*, 39(4): 699–707.

Hamill, J., Van Emmerik, R. E. A., Heiderscheit, B. C. and Li, L. (1999) 'A dynamical systems approach to lower extremity running injuries', *Clinical Biomechanics*, 14(5): 297–308.

Heiderscheit, B. C., Hamill, J. and Van Emmerik, R. E. A. (2002) 'Variability of stride characteristics and joint coordination among individuals with unilateral patellofemoral pain', *Journal of Applied Biomechanics*, 18(2): 110–21.

Hubley, C. L. and Wells, R. P. (1983) 'A work-energy approach to determine individual joint contributions to vertical jump performance', *European Journal of Applied Physiology*, 50(2): 247–54.

Hudson, J. L. (1986) 'Coordination of segments in the vertical jump', *Medicine and Science in Sports and Exercise*, 18(2): 242–51.

Jacobs, R., Bobbert, M. F. and Van Ingen Schenau, G. J. (1996) 'Mechanical output from individual muscles during explosive leg extensions: the role of biarticular muscles', *Journal of Biomechanics*, 29(4): 513–23.

Jones, S. F., Twigg, P. C., Scally, A. J. and Buckley, J. G. (2006) 'The mechanics of landing when stepping down in unilateral lower-limb amputees', *Clinical Biomechanics*, 21(2): 184–93.

Kakihana, W. and Suzuki, S. (2001) 'The EMG activity and mechanics of the running jump as a function of takeoff angle', *Journal of Electromyography and Kinesiology*, 11(5): 365–72.

Klute, G. K., Kallfelz, C. F. and Czerniecki, J. M. (2001) 'Mechanical properties of prosthetic limbs: adapting to the patient', *Journal of Rehabilitation Research and Development*, 38(3): 299–307.

Markolf, K. L., Graff-Radford, A. and Amstutz, H. C. (1978) 'In vivo knee stability. A quantitative assessment using an instrumented clinical testing apparatus', *The Journal of Bone and Joint Surgery*, 60(5): 664–74.

Nagano, A., Komura, T. and Fukashiro, S. (2007) 'Optimal coordination of maximal-effort horizontal and vertical jump motions: a computer simulation study', *Biomedical Engineering Online*, 6: 20.

Pitkin, M. R. (1995) 'Mechanical outcomes of a rolling-joint prosthetic foot and its performance in the dorsiflexion phase of transtibial amputee gait', *Journal of Prosthetics and Orthotics*, 7(4): 114–23.

Pitkin, M. R. (1997) 'Effect of design variants in lower-limb prostheses on gait synergy', *Journal of Prosthetics and Orthotics*, 9(3): 113–22.

Rosenberger, B. (2000) *Medicare O & P reimbursement: Part 3 of 3: Can I have a Cadillac?*, available at: www.amputee-coalition.org/inmotion/sep_oct_00/medic.html (accessed 18 August 2010).

Schoeman, M., Diss, C. E. and Strike, S. C. (2012) 'Kinetic and kinematic compensations in amputee vertical jumping', *Journal of Applied Biomechanics*, 28(4): 438–47.

Selles, R. W., Janssens, P. J., Jongenengel, C. D. and Bussmann, J. B. (2005) 'A randomized controlled trial comparing functional outcome and cost efficiency of a total surface-bearing socket versus a conventional patellar tendon-bearing socket in transtibial amputees', *Archives of Physical Medicine and Rehabilitation*, 86(1): 154–61.

Spagele, T., Kistner, A. and Gollhofer, A. (1999) 'Modelling, simulation and optimisation of a human vertical jump', *Journal of Biomechanics*, 32(5): 521–30.

Strike, S. C. and Diss, C. (2005) 'The biomechanics of one-footed vertical jump performance in unilateral trans-tibial amputees', *Prosthetics and Orthotics International*, 29(1): 39–51.

Tomioka, M., Owings, T. M. and Grabiner, M. D. (2001) 'Lower extremity strength and coordination are independent contributors to maximum vertical jump height', *Journal of Applied Biomechanics*, 17(3): 181–7.

Vanezis, A. and Lees, A. (2005) 'A biomechanical analysis of good and poor performers of the vertical jump', *Ergonomics*, 48(11–14): 1594–603.

Vanrenterghem, J., Lees, A. and Clercq, D. D. (2008) 'Effect of forward trunk inclination on joint power output in vertical jumping', *Journal of Strength and Conditioning Research*, 22(3): 708–14.

Wilson, C., Simpson, S. and Hamill, J. (2009) 'Movement coordination patterns in triple jump training drills', *Journal of Sports Sciences*, 27(3): 277–82.

44

THREE-DIMENSIONAL PUSHRIM FORCES DURING DIFFERENT RACING WHEELCHAIR PROPULSION SPEEDS

Weerawat Limroongreungrat[1] and Yong Tai Wang[2]

[1]MAHIDOL UNIVERSITY, BANGKOK
[2]GEORGIA STATE UNIVERSITY, ATLANTA

Introduction

Wheelchair racing is one of the most popular sports among persons with locomotors disabilities. Wheelchair racing competition can range from 100 m, in a short distance event, to 42,000 m in a marathon event. With an increase in the number of wheelchair athletes participating in these competitions, there is an increasing occurrence of sports-related injuries and overuse syndromes, which may result from various factors, including training techniques, pattern and use of protective equipment, and flexibility, strength and amount of time in training of the athletes (Ferrara and Davis, 1990; Taylor and Williams, 1995).

The relationship between the kinematics of racing wheelchair propulsion (RWP) and propulsion speeds has been studied by several researchers (O'Connor *et al.*, 1998; Walsh *et al.*, 1986; Wang *et al.*, 1995). Walsh (1987) investigated the effects of different propulsion frequencies on speed during the last 40 m of a 60 m wheelchair sprint. The authors suggested that to increase sprinting velocity, athletes should execute the recovery phase of the propulsion cycle as quickly as possible by keeping the hands in close proximity to the pushrims. This recommendation was later supported by the studies of Wang *et al.* (1995) and O'Connor *et al.* (1998).

Wang *et al.* (1995) examined three-dimensional (3D) kinematics of wheelchair propulsion across four different racing propulsion velocities (90, 70, 50 and 30 per cent of the peak velocities). The results showed that as speed increased from 30 to 90 per cent of peak velocities, the cycle time decreased from 1.09 to 0.9 seconds. Greater trunk flexion and elbow flexion at the initial contact angle were found at higher velocities. A similar result was reported by O'Connor *et al.* (1998), who investigated both physiologic principles and biomechanics of RWP. They also found that wrist and elbow linear velocities increased as speed increased, which implies the use of a punching technique in RWP.

It has been found that propulsion speeds can affect pushrim forces in conventional wheelchair propulsion (Boninger *et al.*, 1997; Koontz *et al.*, 2002). However, the effect of speed on pushrim forces during RWP is still limited at present. This information is very useful since it can enhance our understanding of the kinetics of RWP and may result in training that is more appropriate; thereby, it may help to reduce potential injuries for racing wheelchair athletes. To the authors' knowledge, only Goosey-Tolfrey *et al.* (2001) reported pushrim forces during RWP; however, the force-instrumented system used in the study was only capable of registering two force components: tangential and medio-lateral. Although radial force does not contribute to forward motion during RWP, it provides useful information on frictional forces between the hand and pushrim. The force instrumented system developed for the present study was specifically designed to measure 3D pushrim force components during RWP. Therefore, the purpose of this study was to investigate 3D pushrim forces during three different speeds of RWP.

Method

Participants

Five experienced male wheelchair racers, mean age (SD) of 28.4 (± 6.87) years old, volunteered for this study. The athletes read and signed consent forms that followed the guidelines of the Institutional Review Board at Georgia State University. The inclusion criteria were: (1) wheelchair athletes who classified as T52–T54 classification; and (2) no shoulder pain or upper extremity pain. General information such as age, years of wheelchair racing experience and body mass were recorded before the experiment and are presented in Table 44.1.

Instrumentation

Kinetic data were obtained from a force instrumented wheel system (IWS), which consisted of a six-dimensional JR-3 force/torque transducer (Model 45E15A-U760, JR-3 Inc., Woodland, CA) attached to the hub of the racing wheelchair. The JR-3 force/torque transducer has a full mechanical load rating of 1,125 N for *x* and *y* axes, and 2,250 N for the *z* axis with a 127 Nm torque rating for all three dimensions. The details of the instrumented wheel system and its validity have been described elsewhere (Limroongreungrat *et al.*, 2009).

The IWS was mounted on the right axle of 27-in standard racing rear wheel. The standard pushrim was used in the study (0.905 cm in tube diameter and 40.64 cm pushrim diameter). Pushrim force and moment data were collected at a sampling rate of 600 Hz.

The voltage outputs were recorded in the range of ± 10 V. Kinematic data were collected with a six-120 Hz Peak Performance optical camera system and were digitized and reduced

Table 44.1 Physical and disability characteristics of the five participants

Athlete	Disability	Classification	Age (years)	Years of participation in sport	Body mass (kg)
1	Bilateral knee amputee	T54	27	5	71.2
2	Arthrogryposis	T54	36	20	88.0
3	C6-7	T52	33	11	80.3
4	T12 incomplete SCI	T53	18	13	40.8
5	T12 incomplete SCI	T54	28	8	75.3

with Peak Motus motion analysis software version 8.2.0 (Peak Performance Technologies, Inc., Englewood, CO). Kinematic data were selected to coincide with the propulsion phase, which was defined by the kinetic data (moment about JR-3 force/transducer z axis). The propulsion phase was defined as the period when the M_z deviated ± 5 per cent from baseline, until it once again returned to baseline. This eliminated the need to estimate from the kinematic data whether the hand is in contact with the pushrim (Cooper *et al.*, 1997).

The kinematic and kinetic systems were connected to an A/D interface unit attached to the Peak Performance system (Peak Performance Technologies, Inc., Englewood, CO), by connecting to a 12-bit resolution DT3010 data acquisition board (Data Translation, Inc, Marlboro, MA). Both systems were synchronized via a 5 V transistor-transistor logic synchronization pulse.

Determinations of pushrim forces and propulsion efficiency

Three pushrim forces, tangential force (F_t), radial force (F_r) and axial force (F_z), were determined from the following equations (Figure 44.1).

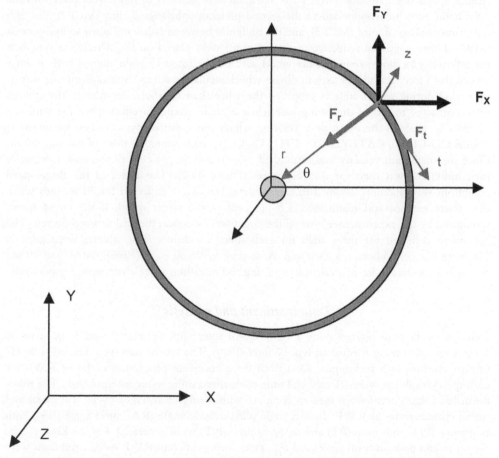

Figure 44.1 Global (X, Y, Z) and pushrim (*t, r, z*) coordinate systems. The force components are converted to the three pushrim forces: tangential force (F_t), radial force (F_r) and axial force (F_z).

$$F_t = F_X \sin \theta \cos \beta - F_Y \sin \theta \cos \beta + F_Z \sin \theta \sin \beta \qquad (1)$$

$$F_z = F_Z \sin \beta \qquad (2)$$

Since $F_{total}^2 = F_X^2 + F_Y^2 + F_Z^2 = F_t^2 + F_r^2 + F_z^2$, then F_r can be determined as

$$F_r = \sqrt{F_{total}^2 - F_t^2 - F_z^2} \qquad (3)$$

where F_X, F_Y and F_Z are forces in global coordinate system and β is a camber angle (these details are described elsewhere; Limroongreungrat *et al.*, 2009).

Racing wheelchair propulsion mechanical efficiency (F_{FEF}) was determined from the ratio between the square of tangential force (F_t) and the square of total force component (F_{total}) (Boninger *et al.*, 1997).

Experimental procedure

The standard racing wheelchair was secured to a platform containing a stationary roller system (Eagles Sports, Inc., Atlanta, GA). Three retroreflective markers (8 mm) were placed on the right hand, which corresponded to the second metacarpophalangeal joint (MCP2), the fifth metacarpophalangeal joint (MCP5), and the midpoint between radial and ulnar styloid process (MW). Three additional reflective markers (8 mm) were placed on the wheelchair system at the following locations: centre of the wheel, and on the interface plate aligned with x and y axis of JR-3 force transducer axes to obtain wheel angular positions. After a 5-minute warm-up period during which athletes propelled the wheelchair on the roller system, the athletes were instructed to propel the racing wheelchair at their maximum effort speed for 1 minute in order to establish the mean peak velocity, which was captured by a cordless speedometer (model CC-CL200, CATEYE, CO, LTD., Osaka, Japan) mounted in front of the wheelchair. Once the maximum velocity was established, 90, 70 and 50 per cent of the peak velocity of each individual was used for data collection (Figure 44.2). The order of the three speed conditions was randomly assigned to each athlete. Data were collected for 30 seconds when the athlete reached and maintained ±5 per cent of the target speed. If the target speed, monitored by the experimenter, was off the target for 5 seconds, the trial was recollected. The data were collected for three trials for each speed condition. The athletes were given a 2-minute rest period between each trial. According to Wang *et al.* (1995), the 90 and 70 per cent speed conditions are equivalent to sprinting and marathon wheelchair racing, respectively.

Data treatment and analysis

Kinematic data were filtered using a Butterworth filter with optimal cut-off frequencies of 6 Hz determined using residual analysis (Winter, 1990). The kinetic data were filtered at 30 Hz utilizing Butterworth techniques. Data from three complete propulsion cycles of RWP for each speed condition were selected and time-normalized using spline interpolation. The time-normalized data curves were used to compute within subject averaged cycle. Temporal and spatial characteristics of RWP: contact angle (CA), release angle (RA), push angle (PA), push frequency (PF), push time (PT) and recovery time (RT) were generated. For the kinetic data, the mean and peak pushrim forces and F_{FEF} ratio during different RWP speed conditions were calculated. The statistical package SPSS version 12.0 (SPSS, Chicago, IL) was used to analyse all statistical procedures. A Freidman test was used to identify differences of mean and peak

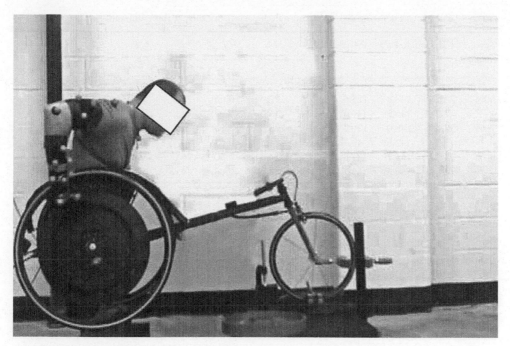

Figure 44.2 Experimental set-up

pushrim forces between speed conditions since a Kolmogorov-Smirnov test revealed non-normal distribution of the data (p < 0.05). Wilcoxon signed rank test was used for post hoc analysis if there were statistically significant changes within group.

Results

The temporal and spatial characteristics of RWP during three different speed conditions are presented in Table 44.2. The mean CA and RA among the three propulsion speed conditions are very similar. The mean CA ranged from 23.2 to 27.4°, while the RA ranged from 144.7 to 148.8°. As the propulsion speeds increased from 50 to 90 per cent, the average PT and RT decreased but the PF increased from 69.7 to 90.9 cycles per minute.

The mean and peak force data of pushrim forces at 50, 70 and 90 per cent of maximum speed are shown in Table 44.3. All pushrim forces, the tangential, radial and axial forces, increased as the speed of propulsion increased. However, no statistical differences between the three speeds were found (*p > 0.05*). The mean F_{FEF} was approximately 38 per cent and remained stable as speed increased.

Discussion

Wheelchair propulsion kinematics

The purpose of this study was to investigate 3D pushrim forces during different racing wheelchair propulsion speeds. The mean CA in this study ranged from 23.2 to 27.4°, which were similar to previous reports (Goosey-Tolfrey *et al.*, 2001; Wang *et al.*, 1995), but the RA

Table 44.2 Mean values of spatial and temporal characteristics during three different speed conditions

Speed conditions	CA (°)	RA (°)	PA (°)	PT (s)	%	RT (s)	%	CT (s)	PF (push/ min)	Speed ($m.s^{-1}$)
50%	23.2	148.8	125.6	0.23	27.0	0.63	73.0	0.87	69.7	2.37
	(7.2)	(45.8)	(40.3)	(0.05)	(5.2)	(0.07)	(5.2)	(0.07)	(6.7)	(0.35)
70%	27.4	148.0	120.7	0.19	25.2	0.56	74.8	0.75	80.7	3.32
	(3.7)	(42.8)	(40.7)	(0.03)	(4.1)	(0.07)	(4.1)	(0.08)	(8.7)	(0.35)
90%	24.1	144.7	123.6	0.16	24.0	0.50	76.0	0.66	90.9	4.27
	(4.8)	(36.5)	(33.7)	(0.04)	(4.6)	(0.08)	(4.6)	(0.05)	(6.9)	(0.45)

CA: contact angle; RA: release angle; PA: push angle; PT: propulsion time; RT: recovery time; CT: cycle time; PF: push frequency.

Table 44.3 Mean (SD) of mean and peak values for the pushrim forces and mean F_{FEF} during propulsion phase at three different speed conditions

Force characteristics	Speed conditions		
	50%	*70%*	*90%*
F_t mean (N)	52.9	57.9	63.0
	(15.4)	(16.3)	(17.2)
F_t peak (N)	89.1	102.3	114.3
	(14.8)	(18.9)	(21.0)
F_r mean (N)	62.5	68.0	72.7
	(21.0)	(21.6)	(21.7)
F_r peak (N)	104.6	123.5	136.0
	(17.2)	(18.8)	(20.4)
F_z mean (N)	22.9	24.7	28.2
	(8.3)	(8.4)	(7.0)
F_z peak (N)	58.3	70.3	85.0
	(20.6)	(21.1)	(27.1)
mean F_{FEF} (%)	38.05	38.3	38.8
	(11.8)	(11.4)	(11.1)

and PA were different. The PA in the present study ranged from 120.7 to 125.6°, whereas previous studies reported ranges between 170 and 180° (Wang et al., 1995). These differences may be due to different sitting positions that the participants used in this study. Since the standard racing wheelchair and pushrims were used in the current study rather than the athletes' own competitive racing wheelchairs, all athletes in this study had to use the upright position. Different disability levels of the athletes, the control of the upper body and anthropometric characteristics of athletes may have contributed to the different CA and RA (Chow et al., 2000).

As the speed increased from 50 to 90 per cent of the maximum propulsion speed, the CT decreased from 0.87 to 0.66 seconds. The PT decreased from 27 to 24 per cent while the RT increased from 73 to 76 per cent. These results were consistent with the previous study of Wang *et al.* (1995), who reported that both propulsion phase time and recovery phase time decreased as speed increased; however, the propulsion phase time decreased at a faster rate than the recovery phase time. Wang *et al.* (1995) concluded that it was more important to execute the propulsion phase at the faster rate than the recovery phase in order to obtain maximum velocity of pushing when speed increased.

Pushrim forces and propulsion efficiency

In general, all pushrim forces (F_t, F_r and F_z) increased as propulsion speeds increased. The pushrim forces were compared to the work of Goosey-Tolfrey *et al.* (2001), who reported the mean and peak tangential (F_t) and axial forces (F_z) of six wheelchair racers at two different propulsion speeds: 4.70 and 5.64 m.s^{-1}. Goosey-Tolfrey *et al.* (2001) found the mean F_t and F_z at the speed of 4.7 m.s^{-1} were 75 and 53 N, respectively. These forces are found to be higher than the mean F_t and F_z in the present study, which were 63 and 28.2 N at the 90 per cent of maximum speed condition (4.27 m.s^{-1}). The differences of these forces may be due to propulsion speeds, sitting positions and the testing racing wheelchair. Nevertheless, the magnitudes of F_z during RWP are much greater than the F_z reported during CWP (Boninger *et al.*, 1997). The greater magnitude of F_z confirms that RWP involves a 'punching' technique as opposed to the grasping technique of the pushrim seen in everyday use (Goosey-Tolfrey *et al.*, 2001; Vanlandewijck *et al.*, 1994). In addition, this F_z is very important in order to maintain contact with the pushrim and prevent the hand from slipping during the propulsion. The magnitude of the F_z is directly related to the coefficient of friction of the hand and the pushrim. As a result, in order to prevent slipping, some racing wheelchair athletes attempt to increase the friction between the hand and pushrim by using sticky tape, formulated rubber or synthetic racing gloves.

Since the instrumented wheel system in the study of Goosey-Tolfrey *et al.* (2001) was only capable of recording 2D pushrim forces, no F_r was reported. The peak F_r in the current study ranged from 104.6 to 136.9 N as the speed increased from 50 to 90 per cent. One interesting finding is that both mean and peak F_r in this study were higher than both mean and peak F_t in all speed conditions. This result differs from our expectation that F_t would be greater than F_r during RWP due to the better propulsion efficiency. The higher F_r could possibly be due: to (1) the results of misdirected forces adopted by the wheelchair athletes; or (2) the use of an upright racing position causing the change of their propulsion techniques. Nonetheless, the greater F_r or F_t during wheelchair propulsion in conventional wheelchair studies is also inconclusive. Boninger *et al.* (1997) reported pushrim forces of six traumatic spinal cord injured participants during conventional wheelchair propulsion and found the peak F_t and F_r to be 62.1 and 47.4 N, respectively. However, in their subsequent study with the larger sample size (34 wheelchair users), they found that the F_r (72.6 N) is higher than F_t (43.7 N) (Boninger *et al.*, 1999). As a result, future research is needed to investigate the force application strategy of RWP with a larger sample size.

The F_{FEF} ratio of the present study cannot be compared to the study of Goosey-Tolfrey *et al.* (2001) since the total force in the previous study did not consider the F_r. As a result, the ratio of the tangential force to total measured force from the previous study was much greater than the present study. However, the F_{FEF} ratio remained stable for both studies as the propulsion speed increased. This may imply that even if the speed increases, the wheelchair athletes may use the same force applications strategy, executed at a faster rate. For the propulsion test, the peak F_t and F_z are found to be lower than the results of Goosey-Tolfrey *et al.* (2001), who reported the peak of F_t and F_z during RWP at the speed of 5.64 m.s^{-1} to be 158 and

82 N, respectively. The discrepancy of forces may be due to several factors, such as different pathologies among athletes, poor individual optimization of the racing wheelchair and propulsion speed.

It seems clear that the wheelchair-athlete interface is very important in the optimization of wheelchair racing performance. Adjusting the wheelchair to the physical and functional capacity of the individual athlete is probably the most challenging. However, this is also the most complex task in performance optimization. Using a standard racing wheelchair and pushrims may not be suitable for athletes and influence propulsion technique. Therefore, future researchers need to evaluate racing wheelchair propulsion on the athlete's own racing wheelchair and comfortable pushrim sizes in order to obtain an individual's natural propulsion technique.

References

Boninger, M. L., Cooper, R. A., Robertson, R. N. and Shimada, S. D. (1997) 'Three-dimensional pushrim forces during two speeds of wheelchair propulsion', *American Journal of Physical Medicine and Rehabilitation*, 76(5): 420–6.

Chow, J. W., Millikan, T. A., Carlton, L. G., Chae, W. and Morse, M. I. (2000) 'Effect of resistance load on biomechanical characteristics of racing wheelchair propulsion over a roller system', *Journal of Biomechanics*, 33(5): 601–8.

Cooper, R. A., Robertson, R. N., VanSickle, D. P., Boninger, M. L. and Shimada, S. D. (1997) 'Methods for determining three-dimensional wheelchair pushrim forces and moments: a technical note', *Journal of Rehabilitation Research and Development*, 34(2): 162–70.

Ferrara, M. S. and Davis, R. W. (1990) 'Injuries to elite wheelchair athletes', *Paraplegia*, 28(5): 335–41.

Goosey-Tolfrey, V. L., Fowler, N. E., Campbell, I. G. and Iwnicki, S. D. (2001) 'A kinetic analysis of trained wheelchair racers during two speeds of propulsion', *Medical Engineering and Physics*, 23(4): 259–66.

Koontz, A. M., Cooper, R. A., Boninger, M. L., Souza, A. L. and Fay, B. T. (2002) 'Shoulder kinematics and kinetics during two speeds of wheelchair propulsion', *Journal of Rehabilitation Research and Development*, 39(6): 635–49.

Limroongreungrat, W., Wang, Y. T., Chang, L., Geil, M. D. and Johnson, J. T. (2009) 'Technical note: an instrumented wheel system for measuring 3-D pushrim kinetics during racing wheelchair propulsion', *Research in Sports Medicine*, 17(3): 182–94.

O'Connor, T. J., Robertson, R. N. and Cooper, R. A. (1998) 'Three-dimensional kinematic analysis and physiologic assessment of racing wheelchair propulsion', *Journal of Adapted Physical Activity Quarterly*, 15(1): 1–14.

Taylor, D. and Williams, T. (1995) 'Sports injuries in athletes with disabilities: wheelchair racing', *Paraplegia*, 33(5): 296–9.

Vanlandewijck, Y. C., Spaepen, A. J. and Lysens, R. J. (1994) 'Wheelchair propulsion efficiency: movement pattern adaptations to speed changes', *Medicine and Science in Sports and Exercise*, 26(11): 1473–81.

Walsh, C. (1987) 'The effect of pushing frequency on speed in wheelchair sprinting', *Sports 'n Spokes*, 13(1), 13–14.

Walsh, C. M., Marchiori, G. E. and Steadward, R. D. (1986) 'Effect of seat position on maximal linear velocity in wheelchair sprinting', *Canada Journal of Applied Sport Science*, 11(4): 186–90.

Wang, Y. T., Deutsch, H., Morse, M., Hedrick, B. and Millikan, T. (1995) 'Three dimensional kinematics of wheelchair propulsion across racing speeds', *Journal of Adapted Physical Activity Quarterly*, 12(1): 78–89.

Winter, D. A. (1990). *Biomechanics and motor control of human movement*, 2nd edn, New York: John Wiley & Sons, Inc.

45

DEVELOPMENT AND APPLICATION OF WHEELCHAIR TENNIS FITNESS TEST FOR IMPROVING COMPETITIVENESS

Kayoko Ando[1] and Shinji Sakurai[2]

[1]RIKKYO UNIVERSITY, NIIZA
[2]CHUKYO UNIVERSITY, TOYOTA

History of disability sport

Sir Ludwig Guttmann launched the disability sport movement at Stoke Mandeville Hospital in the United Kingdom in 1944 as a form of rehabilitation for young soldiers injured in World War II (Thomas and Smith, 2009).

Guttmann held an archery contest for persons with spinal cord injuries on the day of the Opening Ceremony of the London Olympics on 29 July 1948. Sixteen archers participated. This contest, held annually thereafter, had blossomed by 1952 into the Stoke Mandeville Games, a bi-national event with 130 participants (Brittain, 2010).

The first Paralympic Games were held in Rome several weeks after the 1960 Olympics in that city. Four hundred athletes from 21 countries participated (Brittain, 2010). By 2012, it had grown to the Paralympic Games in London in which 4,250 athletes from 164 countries participated in 20 events (International Paralympic Committee, 2012).

The term 'Paralympics' originally meant 'paraplegics and Olympics', but now, as an international athletic event that includes other disabilities, is said to derive from the Greek preposition 'para', meaning 'next to', giving a meaning of parallel or next to the Olympic Games (Brittain, 2010).

History of wheelchair tennis

Wheelchair sport is appropriate for people with a wide range of disabilities in lower extremities, including amputations, spinal cord injuries, cerebral palsy and spina bifida (Goosey-Tolfrey, 2010). Wheelchair sport events include wheelchair basketball, rugby, tennis, racing, archery, fencing and table tennis. Wheelchair tennis is an internationally developing sport.

Originating in 1976 by American Brad Parks, the game has developed from a recreational activity to a professional sport (International Tennis Federation (ITF), 2012). Parks and several other disabled athletes began playing and promoting wheelchair tennis in numerous exhibitions and clinics in the United States. The sport quickly grew as a result of this high exposure level, and in 1977 the first wheelchair tennis tournaments were held (ITF, 2012).

On 1 January 1998, the International Wheelchair Tennis Association (IWTA) was fully integrated into the ITF (ITF, 2012). This marked the first time an association for disabled athletes was integrated into an international association for able-bodied athletes (Pluim and Safran, 2004).

Paralympic wheelchair tennis competition was introduced in the 1988 Seoul Paralympics, and became an official event in the 1992 Barcelona Games (ITF, 2012). One hundred and sixty other international wheelchair tennis competitions are held in 42 countries, which demonstrates the sport's growing popularity internationally. Wheelchair tennis tournaments are held concurrently and in the same venues as the four Grand Slam tournaments: the Australian Open, the French Open, Wimbledon, and the US Open.

Wheelchair tennis in Japan

Wheelchair tennis began in Japan in 1983. What is now the Japan Wheelchair Tennis Association (JWTA) was formed in 1989 to coincide with the launch of the International Wheelchair Tennis Association (IWTA) in 1988. The JWTA works with the ITF/IWTA to engage in various international activities promoting the sport in Asia. Japan is currently thought to have about 1,000 active wheelchair tennis athletes. Around 400 of these athletes participate competitively. Japan's men's team victory at the 2002 World Team Cup in Switzerland was the beginning of a great run for Japanese wheelchair tennis. At the 2008 Beijing Paralympics, Japanese athlete Shingo Kunieda claimed the men's singles gold medal and, together with Satoshi Saida, the men's doubles bronze medal. Kunieda successfully defended his gold in men's singles at the 2012 London Paralympics.

Wheelchair tennis and disability classes

Wheelchair tennis is played on a regulation tennis court under rules identical to regular tennis, except that players can return the ball after up to two bounces (ITF, 2012). Competition is divided into men's, women's, quads and junior classes. The quads class is open to quadriplegics and other severely disabled persons of both sexes. Persons under 18 years of age participate in the junior class (ITF, 2012). Apart from the quads and junior classes, wheelchair tennis is only divided according to sex, thus not intricately divided into various disability categories in contrast to basketball and athletics.

Disability types and injury levels are known to have a large impact on physical fitness level and thus competitiveness in sports performance. Yabe (2003) states that persons with a cervical spinal cord injury have very poor motor function of the upper and lower limbs, but that persons with lumbar spinal injury have upper limb motor function comparable to able-bodied individuals, as evidenced by more than 1-hour difference between world record of wheelchair marathon races for various disability levels ($1°20'14''$: T53/54 class, $1°40'07''$: T52 class, $2°23'08''$: T51 class). In terms of training, persons with lower spinal injuries reportedly gain the same benefit from aerobic training as their able-bodied peers (Barfield *et al.*, 2009). Investigating maximal oxygen uptake, Lin *et al.* (1993) found that persons with higher (T1–5) injuries had lower, but not significantly different, uptake from persons with mid-level (T6–10) injuries, while persons with lower injuries (T11 and below) had significantly higher uptake than the other two groups. Comparing the strength of the shoulder muscles of wheelchair tennis athletes, Bernard *et al.* (2004) found that persons with lower spinal injuries had more strength than those with higher spinal injuries. The location of injury therefore influences the degree of benefit derived from training, aerobic capacity, and strength.

Outside of the quads class, persons playing wheelchair tennis compete in the same class regardless of their injury types and levels. This reality requires wheelchair tennis athletes of all disability levels to engage in training to increase their physical strength and game skills, including wheelchair operation, in order to succeed in their sport.

Characteristics of wheelchair tennis wheelchairs

Figure 45.1 shows photographs of wheelchairs for wheelchair tennis, basketball and distance racing. Wheelchairs are tailored to the build and particular disability of their individual users while also being designed according to the characteristics of the event in question.

Wheelchair tennis demands stability and quick response in the game, which in turn demands operability lacking in regular wheelchairs. Competition wheelchairs are lightweight, have wheels with a camber (with the tops inclined toward the seat) to improve pivotability and lack brakes. In contrast to wheelchair distance racing and basketball, no rules govern the specifications of wheelchair tennis wheelchairs. The most widely used type has five tires for greater forward and backward stability. This greater stability comes from the two forward casters on this type of wheelchair, which allows safer, more dynamic movement. A caster (small wheel) in the back prevents backwards falls and provides support during service.

Measuring athletic ability in wheelchair-based sports

Most research on the athletic ability and physical fitness level of wheelchair sports athletes has focused on aerobic capacity. Oxygen uptake is closely correlated to ventilatory threshold during wheelchair tennis play (Bernardi *et al.*, 2010). Increasing aerobic capacity is reported to be important for boosting on-court performance (Roy *et al.*, 2006). These findings suggest that athletes must boost endurance to maintain speedy rallies and quick chairwork through the latter half of a wheelchair tennis match. $\dot{V}O_2$ peak in wheelchair tennis is 30.4 $ml \cdot kg^{-1} \cdot min^{-1}$, which means that exercise intensity is lower than that in wheelchair basketball ($\dot{V}O_2$ peak: 34.1 $ml \cdot kg^{-1} \cdot min^{-1}$) and wheelchair distance racing ($\dot{V}O_2$ peak: 47.6 $ml \cdot kg^{-1} \cdot min^{-1}$) (Bernardi *et al.*, 2010). Roy *et al.* (2006) stated that mean heart rate during a wheelchair tennis game is 121.7 $beats \cdot min^{-1}$ (69.4 per cent of peak heart rate). This figure is not indicative of high exercise intensity. In other words, wheelchair tennis does not demand as high a level of endurance as wheelchair basketball or distance racing.

Investigating wheelchair propulsion techniques for distance racing, Chow *et al.* (2001) found that pushing more and increasing the range over which the hand rim is pushed may allow more efficient propulsion. In addition, while wheelchair hand rim pushing frequency is correlated to pushing efficiency, the optimal frequency depends on the speed and individual movement characteristics (Goosey *et al.*, 2000). The hand rims of competition wheelchairs for distance racing have smaller diameters, differing substantially from competition wheelchairs for basketball and tennis (Figure 45.1).

Wheelchair tennis seldom features the continuous, long-term propulsion at a constant speed associated with wheelchair distance racing, but athletes are required to accelerate their wheelchair through instantaneous movements. Research on the propulsive techniques that wheelchair tennis requires is insufficient.

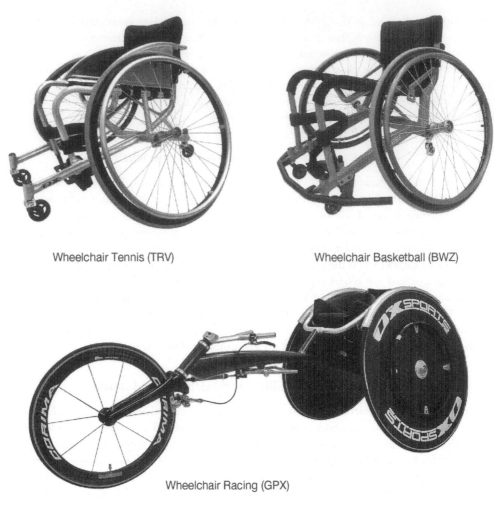

Wheelchair Tennis (TRV)

Wheelchair Basketball (BWZ)

Wheelchair Racing (GPX)

Figure 45.1 Structural difference of wheelchairs among sports-specific (photo by OX Engineering Co., Ltd.).

Physical abilities necessary for wheelchair tennis

Better performance demands both improved skill and physical ability. Athletes in even skill-intensive sports can expect a synergistic boost in their skills by improving their physical ability. Physical ability is closely linked to the performance in the sport.

One major difference between wheelchair tennis and other wheelchair-based sports is the difference in strength needed between the racket hand and the free hand, as athletes must move their wheelchairs while holding their racket in one hand. Wheelchair tennis requires quick movement and chair acceleration not only for forward movements, but also for lunges and turns. Moving the wheelchair well with the racket held in one hand is very difficult, requiring a long time to master. Moreover, athletes are strapped and belted into their wheelchairs, meaning that the chair can be moved through movement of the arms and shifting of body weight. Just as able-bodied athletes increase hit power by twisting their trunks, wheelchair tennis athletes hit the ball or turn with the rotational energy gained from twisting with one of the wheels held stationary. Athletes, with the use of their abdominals and legs, can produce rotational energy by moving their hips or shifting their body weight. It is therefore important to configure competition wheelchairs to be easily manoeuvrable for the level of the user's disability.

Wheelchair tennis coaches in Japan train their athletes with particular emphasis on the movements characterizing the sport. Efficacy is measured with a particular fitness test, and the results are used to raise the level of fitness nationwide. This wheelchair tennis fitness test is a wheelchair tennis-specific field test developed by Dr Horst Guentzel, the fitness director of the Tennis Training Centre (TTC) in Kashiwa, Japan. The test is used to prescribe a fitness training programme based on the current level of fitness of the athlete. The main test components are agility, mobility, speed, power and endurance (Guentzel, 2002).

Wheelchair tennis fitness test

The wheelchair tennis fitness test measures the following eight components:

1   Baseline-net dash (dash).
    Move the distance from the baseline to the net (11.885 m) with the racket held as usual, and the time is measured.
2   Tennis ball throw (ball throw).
    Throw a tennis ball as far as possible, and the distance is measured.
3   T-turns.
    Make a start line 15 cm behind the baseline. Mark two points that are squares of 15 cm and 110 cm right and left of the centre mark (Figure 45.2). Holding the racket as usual, wait at the start line. Touch point A with the front wheels and immediately return to the start line. Then touch point B with the front wheels and again return to the start line. Repeat these actions, finishing when point B has been touched three times, and the time is measured.
4   Grip strength.
    Measure grip strength with an apparatus. In our study, racket hand grip (Grip-R) and freehand grip (Grip-F) were measured.
5   Medicine ball throw (MB throw).
    Lie back down on a mat and extend the arms. Bring the hands, with the medicine ball held, toward the baseline. Without lifting the head from the mat, throw the ball as far as possible toward the leg side as in a soccer throw-in. Males should use a 2 kg medicine ball. Females and quads should use a 1 kg medicine ball. The distance is measured.
6   Resistance dash (r–d).
    Measure the time required for the subject to dash from the baseline to the service line (5.485 m) while pulling a weight. Tie a basket with a weight in it to the back of the wheelchair with a 2 m length of rope. Use three weights. For men, perform the first attempt at 10 kg (r–d 1), the second at 15 kg (r–d 2) and the third at 20 kg (r–d 3). For women and quads, perform the first at 5 kg (r–d 1), the second at 7.5 kg (r–d 2) and the third at 10 kg (r–d 3). Perform without the racket held.
7   Five-point run (5-point).
    Place six cones on the court. Place the cones on the centre mark, where the singles sidelines meet the baseline and service line, and where the service line meets the centreline. Begin from the centre mark. With the racket held as usual, move from the start position (behind

561

the centre mark), move around the cones in order, beginning at cone 1 and going to cone 5 in Figure 45.2. The time is measured.

8   Distance run (1 km time trial: 1 km).

Measure the time required. If using a tennis facility, the 1 km distance may be measured off around two courts. Perform without a racket held.

Perform all components other than the medicine ball throw in a competition wheelchair. As the court surface may affect some measurements, the components are normally performed on a hard court.

Correlation of fitness test results to competitiveness

We analysed fitness test data to determine how the individual test components are correlated with competitiveness (tournament ranking).

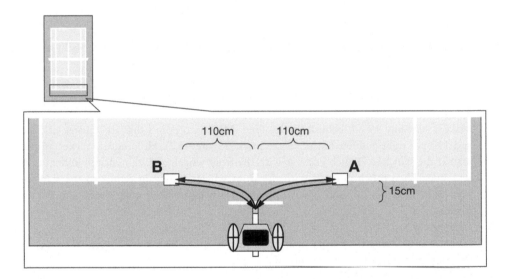

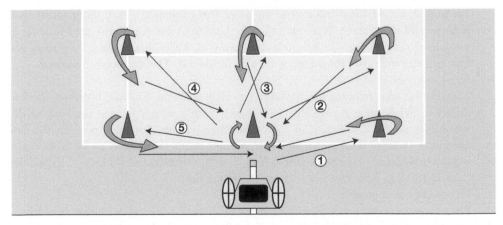

Figure 45.2 Movement for T-turns (top) and five-point (bottom) of Wheelchair Tennis Fitness Test (Guentzel, 2002).

Statistical analysis was performed with a 16-athlete sample of men's wheelchair tennis players. All athletes were non-quad athletes in the men's class. Fifteen were right handed and one was left handed. Two held top-10 JWTA rankings, two were ranked from 11 to 50, three were ranked from 51 to 100, three were ranked from 101 to 150, two were ranked from 151 to 200, two were ranked from 201 to 250 and two, beginners with fewer than one year's experience, were unranked. With the unranked athletes given an arbitrary ranking of 300, the correlation of the test components to the rankings was investigated (Table 45.1).

Five of the eight measured components (and five of the eleven individual items) were correlated to the rankings. Tennis ball throw ($r = -0.810$), baseline-net dash ($r = 0.801$), racket hand grip ($r = -0.736$) and five point run ($r = 0.743$) were closely correlated to the rankings ($p < 0.01$), and T-turns were also correlated ($r = 0.520$, $p < 0.05$). Medicine ball throw, resistance dash and 1 km time were not correlated to the rankings.

Close inter-component correlations were seen for five-point run (9 items), resistance dash attempts one and two (8 items), and resistance dash attempt three and racket hand grip (7 items). The five-point run was correlated with all components and most closely correlated with the ball throw ($r = -0.890$, $p < 0.01$). Thus, the five-point run is closely correlated with both competitiveness ranking and with other measurements.

Wheelchair movements needed for competitiveness

The nature of wheelchair tennis strongly demands that successful athletes have the ability to instantaneously advance and rotate their wheelchair. Analysis of the fitness test data showed the five-point fan run and baseline-net dash to be closely correlated to rankings. Below are data-based descriptions of the movements in these two components characteristic of top athletes.

Movement 1: baseline-net dash

Movement of baseline-net dash in sagittal plane was filmed with a video camera (60 Hz) and analysed. Speed changes and mean power achieved after or during three pushes in the baseline-net dash are shown in Figure 45.3. Athlete A holds the top JWTA ranking, Athlete B is number two, and Athlete C is number three. The 11.88 m dash time of Athlete A was 3.24 seconds. That of Athlete B was 3.25 seconds and that of Athlete C was 3.48 seconds. The athletes travelled a distance of 4.70, 3.88 and 3.41 m, respectively, with three pushes.

As Figure 45.3 shows, top ranked Athlete A had higher peak speeds after pushes 1 to 3 (2.97, 3.85 and 4.31 m.s^{-1}) than the other two athletes. Athletes B and C, in this order, had the next fastest peak speeds. Mean power per push as a function of the combined weight of the athlete and his wheelchair also followed the order of the rankings. The power of Athletes A and B increased stepwise through three pushes, but the power Athlete C achieved with push 3 declined.

The 11.88 m dash times of Athletes A and B differed by 0.01 seconds, but the difference of the three-push distance of the two was 0.82 m, or almost the length of a tennis racket. Although Athlete B appears to have accelerated toward the end of the measurement, athletes seldom quickly travel 11.88 m in a competitive situation. Distances up to 5 m are more frequently travelled, so the first two to three pushes determine whether the athlete reaches the ball. This means that the first three pushes are critical for achieving effective acceleration. In actual competition, the ability to accelerate instantaneously through three pushes may be related to the rankings.

Table 45.1 Correlation coefficient among Wheelchair Tennis Fitness Test result and JWTA ranking

	Mean (SD)	Correlation											
		Ranking	Dash	Ball throw	T-turns	Grip-R	Grip-F	MB throw	r-d 1	r-d 2	r-d 3	5-point	1 km
Ranking	–		##	##	#	##							##	*
Dash (s)	4.50 (0.44)	0.801		**	*				*	*	*	*	**	*
Ball throw (m)	18.48 (4.65)	-0.810	-0.769		*	*			*	**	**	**	**	*
T-turns (s)	19.67 (3.85)	0.520	0.577	-0.631		**	**		*	**	**	**	**	
Grip-R (kg)	48.36 (8.86)	-0.736	-0.491	0.612	-0.817		**	**	**	**	**	**	**	
Grip-F (kg)	44.94 (9.09)	-0.311	-0.183	0.344	-0.703	0.882		*	**	**	**	**	*	
MB-throw (m)	7.42 (1.34)	-0.308	-0.329	0.607	-0.539	0.659	0.560		**	**	**	**	**	**
r-d 1 (s)	2.86 (0.43)	0.485	0.485	-0.594	0.808	-0.807	-0.679	-0.641		**	**	**	**	**
r-d 2 (s)	3.03 (0.57)	0.478	0.468	-0.587	0.821	-0.854	-0.732	-0.632	0.967		**	**	**	*
r-d 3 (s)	3.34 (0.77)	0.399	0.422	-0.578	0.790	-0.838	-0.718	-0.675	0.940	0.942		**	**	
5-point (s)	32.48 (4.99)	0.743	0.745	-0.890	0.889	-0.779	-0.577	-0.663	0.780	0.792	0.781		**
1 km (min.s)	5'39"(1'17")	0.595	0.823	-0.802	0.374	-0.226	0.396	-0.415	0.868	0.760	0.322	0.862	

or **, p < 0.01; # or *, p < 0.05.

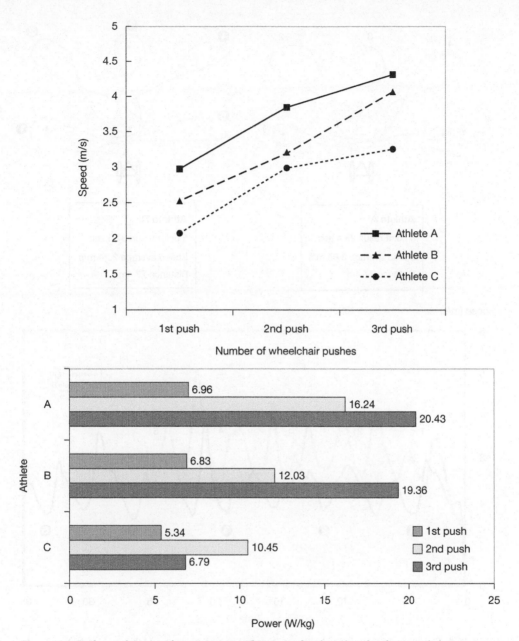

Figure 45.3 Peak speed (top) and average power (bottom) of each push in baseline-net dash test.

Movement 2: five-point run

Movement of five-point run was videotaped with two synchronized video cameras (60 Hz) and was analysed three-dimensionally using DLT (direct linear transformation) procedures. Figure 45.4 shows the speed changes and paths travelled in the five-point run component. Athlete A is the top-ranked athlete in Japan, while Athlete D has a ranking of around 100. The times of Athletes A and D – 25.4 and 34.5 seconds – differed by 9 seconds. Mean speeds

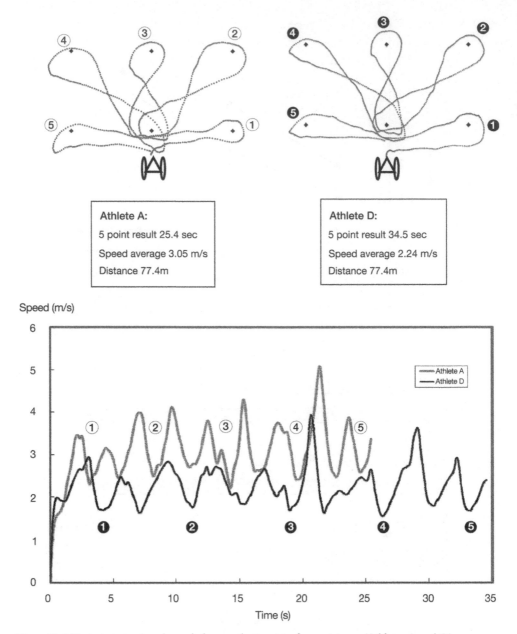

Figure 45.4 Trajectory (top) and speed changes (bottom) in five-point run (Athletes A and D).

were 3.05 m.s^{-1} for Athlete A and 2.24 m.s^{-1} for Athlete D, but both travelled the same distance of 77.4 m.

The wheelchair speed of Athlete A was higher compared to that of Athlete D in general. Moreover, the amplitude of Athlete A's speed changes is clearly substantial. Athlete A slows around turns but soon reaccelerates. Athlete D has smaller speed change amplitudes. He needs time to decelerate when turning and is unable to sufficiently reaccelerate thereafter. Athlete A

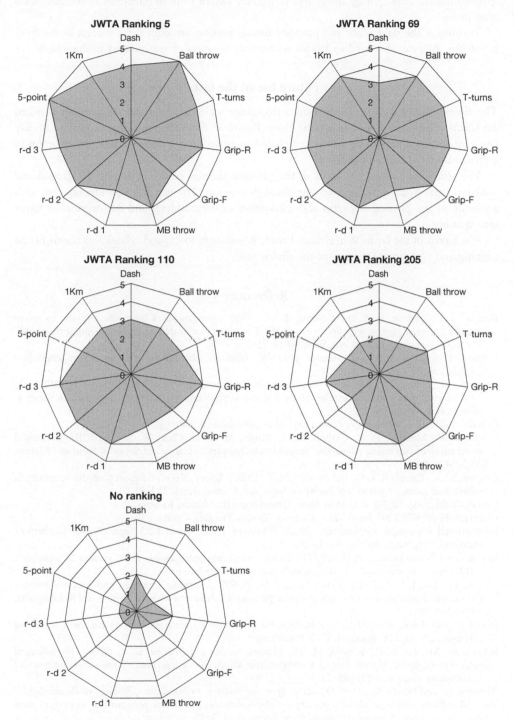

Figure 45.5 Radar chart of Wheelchair Tennis Fitness Test result.

spends minimal time turning and is able to quickly switch from deceleration to reacceleration after turns.

Turning at the right point and properly timing braking are critical for success in the five-point run. Athletes also need to have a wheelchair and tires properly fitted to their body.

Future use of the test

The fitness test data were classified on a five-grade scale based on the average and standard deviation values, and plotted in a radar chart (Figure 45.5). Although differences were already apparent for the components whose correlation increased as the rankings rose, presentation in a chart improved understandability.

The fitness test allows the level of the physical abilities of the athlete to be gauged and indicates areas in need of improvement through training. The test also provides coaches with a picture of the physical strengths and weaknesses of their athletes and information to factor into training.

It is a goal of the Japan Wheelchair Tennis Association to expand wheelchair tennis fitness training and to promote the use of the fitness test.

References

Barfield, J. P., Malone, L. A. and Colema, T. A. (2009) 'Comparison of heart rate response to tennis activity between persons with and without spinal cord injuries: implications for a training threshold', *Research Quarterly for Exercise and Sport*, 80(1): 71–7

Bernard, P. L., Codine, P. and Minaier, J. (2004) 'Isokinetic shoulder rotator muscles in wheelchair athletes', *Spinal Cord*, 42(4): 222–9.

Bernardi, M., Guerra, E., Giacinto, B. D., Cesare, A. D., Castellad, V. and Bhambhani, Y. (2010) 'Field evaluation of paralympic athletes in selected sports: implications for training', *Medicine and Science in Sports and Exercise*, 42(6): 1200–8.

Brittain, I. (2010) *The Paralympic Games Explained*, Abingbon: Routledge.

Chow, J. W., Millikan, T. A., Carlton, L. G., Mores, M. I. and Chae, W. S. (2001) 'Biomechanical comparison of two racing wheelchair propulsion techniques', *Medicine and Science in Sports and Exercise*, 33(3): 476–84.

Goosey, V. L., Campbell, I. G. and Fowler, N. E. (2000) 'Effect of push frequency on the economy of wheelchair racers', *Medicine and Science in Sports and Exercise*, 32(1): 174–81.

Goosey-Tolfrey, V. (2010) *Wheelchair Sport*, Champaign, IL: Human Kinetics.

Guentzel, H. (2002) *TTC Fitness Test*, Kashiwa: Tennis Training Center.

International Paralympic Committee. (2012) *Paralympic games*, viewed 23 September 2012, http://paralympic.org/paralympic-games/london-2012.

International Tennis Federation. (2012) *ITF wheelchair tennis rules and regulations 2012*, viewed 23 September 2012, http://itftennis.com/wheelchair/ambassadors/brad-parks.aspx.

Lin, K. H., Lai, J. S., Kao, M. J, and Lien, I. N. (1993) 'Anaerobic threshold and maximal oxygen consumption during arm cranking exercise in paraplegia', *Archives of Physical Medicine and Rehabilitation*, 74(5): 515–20.

Pluim, B. and Safran, M. (2004) *From breakpoint to advantage: a practical guide to optimal tennis health and performance*, Vista, CA: Racquet Tech Publishing.

Roy, J. L., Menear, K. S., Schmid, M. M., Hunter, G. R. and Malone, L. A. (2006) 'Physiological responses of skilled players during a competitive wheelchair tennis match', *Journal of Strength and Conditioning Research*, 20(3):665–71.

Thomas, N. and Smith, A. (2009) *Disability, Sport and Society: An Introduction*, Abingbon: Routledge.

Yabe, K. (2003) 'Effects of physical activity on physical fitness and motor performance in persons with disabilities', *Japanese Journal of Adapted Sport Science*, 1(1): 2–15.

46

KINEMATICS OF SHOT-PUT, DISCUS AND JAVELIN THROWING IN PARALYMPIC ATHLETES

Justin Keogh[1,2,3] and Brendan Burkett[3]

[1]BOND UNIVERSITY, ROBINA
[2]AUT UNIVERSITY, AUCKLAND
[3]UNIVERSITY OF THE SUNSHINE COAST, SIPPY DOWNS

Introduction

The kinematics of throwing is measured following biomechanical principles, or the study of the human body in motion. Essentially, there are four areas within the biomechanics discipline; developmental biomechanics, biomechanics of exercise and sport, rehabilitative biomechanics and occupational biomechanics. Each of these disciplines relate directly to athletes, either their activities of daily living (when they are not competing) and ultimately their competition. In order to study the human body in motion the kinematic measures rely heavily on technology to quantify this activity.

The discipline of sports biomechanics specifically focuses on the intra-body segment relationships, or posture, in order to minimize risk from injury and to enhance sporting performance. Too often, the exercise science profession concentrates on enhancing sport performance through a combination of generalized and specific training, at the expense of reducing the risk of injury. This may not be optimal as ultimately the 'net gain' from training is the sum of the negative consequence of injury added to the positive outcomes from performance enhancement.

Elite performance enhancement for an athlete with a disability is showcased in the highest level of competition, the Paralympic Games. Paralympic sports evolved from rehabilitation programmes in the 1950s, and as such were built on medical science knowledge with an application to exercise. These programmes initially focused on spinal cord injured athletes who used a wheelchair for their activities of daily living, with the competitive sports programme an extension of their rehabilitation. The objective of a rehabilitation programme is to regain a level of function for the client. In the endeavour to function 'higher, faster and longer', athletes have found that standard wheelchair or prosthetic devices can inhibit their sporting performance. To satisfy the demands of these elite athletes, significant new technological developments in wheelchair design and prostheses have occurred (Burkett *et al.*, 2003), and radical equipment designs such as the J-Leg, seated throwing chairs (Frossard *et al.*, 2007) and racing wheelchairs (Vanlandewijck *et al.*, 2001) have revolutionized sports medicine thinking and Paralympic sports performance. The development of this new 'equipment' was based on the biomechanical analysis when the athlete was performing the throwing event.

Background to athletes with a disability and the Paralympic sports

Paralympic athletes compete in 18 summer sports, 14 of which are the same as Olympic sports. The four sports unique to the Paralympics are goalball, boccia, wheelchair rugby, and powerlifting (International Paralympic Commitee, 2009). Equipment such as prostheses and wheelchairs are fundamental in allowing some people with disabilities to carry out the tasks of daily living (Haisma *et al.*, 2006; Pasquina *et al.*, 2006) and to train for and compete in the Paralympic Games. Advances in technology underpin such assistive devices; for example, the development of the energy-storing prosthetic foot, can make a lower limb amputee's gait more efficient and ambulation faster (Brodtkorb *et al.*, 2008; Nolan and Lees, 2000). When this revolutionary prosthetic technology was specifically applied to sprinters, studies showed that running velocity was significantly increased (Brown *et al.*, 2009; Hsu *et al.*, 2006). However, the application of this technology has been controversial, as clearly demonstrated by the much-publicized Oscar Pistorius or 'Blade Runner' debate before the 2008 Beijing Olympic and Paralympic Games (Burkett, 2008, Burkett *et al.*, 2011; Edwards, 2008; Jones and Wilson, 2009; Lippi and Mattiuzzi, 2008; van Hilvoorde and Landeweerd, 2008). The skill of the athlete, coupled with this new prosthetic technology, enabled Oscar to qualify and compete successfully in the men's 400 m sprint in both the 2012 Olympic and Paralympic Game finals.

Paralympic throwing events are contested by athletes with impairments of strength, range of movement and coordination of varying severity. The events contested comprise javelin, discus and shot-put thrown from a seated or standing position, as well as the club throw. The club is unique to Paralympic sport, and is thrown from a seated position using one of three techniques: over-arm (similar to javelin); round-arm with a straight elbow (similar to the discus action); and a backwards overhead technique.

As there are specific and unique biological requirements (or constraints) associated with particular physical disabilities that directly influences how an athlete can throw the shot put, discus or javelin implements, an overview of the Paralympic classification system will lend clarity to the subsequent discussion. Further, the use of the constraints-led approach of dynamical systems theory may also provide a theoretical construct through which researchers and practitioners can better understand the factors influencing Paralympic sporting performance and injury risk.

The original Paralympic classification system was based on a medical model and athletes competed within five classes of disability (Tweedy, 2003). These class involved athletes with an amputation, defined as having at least one major joint in a limb missing (International Paralympic Committee, 2007); athletes with cerebral palsy, defined as having the cerebellar area of the brain affected (Steenbergen and Gordon, 2006); athletes with a spinal cord injury; athletes with a visual impairment (perception to a visual acuity between 2/60–6/60 and/or a visual field of > 5° and < 20°); and athletes with *les autres*, a French phrase meaning the 'others'. Athletes in the *les autres* group comprises athletes who do not fit within one of the other disability groups, but nevertheless have a permanent physical disability (e.g. one femur shorter than the other, resulting in a significant difference in leg length). Athletes competing in the athletics throwing events therefore may come from four of the five classes; the natural omission is the athlete with a visual impairment.

A contemporary motor control theory that may provide a framework for improving our understanding of the factors influencing performance and injury risk in Paralympic athletes is the constraints-led approach of dynamical system theory. The constraints-led approach states that task performance is affected by the control (coordination) strategy employed by the individual and that the coordination strategy utilized reflects the interaction of the three levels of constraints (environmental, task and organism) and how this alters the perception-action cycle under which movement is performed (see Figure 46.1). The potential environmental and task constraints experienced by Paralympic and able-bodied Olympic athletes within the same sport such as swimming or athletics may be largely the same, as they compete in the same venue under the same rule structure. However, as a wide variety of anatomical and functional differences exist between Paralympic and Olympic athletes, and even between and within Paralympic classification classes, there can be considerable differences in the organism-level constraints under which these movements occur. The nature of the perception-action coupling may also differ as amputations or spinal cord injury may reduce or eliminate various forms of sensory information and the manner in which the task is performed. A further possible application of dynamical systems theory relevant to Paralympic sports is that many athletes (including throwers) require devices such as prosthetic limbs or throwing frames to perform the activity successfully. This means that the organism-level constraints under which they perform and the potential perception-action coupling they receive would reflect the interaction between the athlete and their device(s).

There would appear to be two major implications of the constraint-led approach for improving our understanding of the factors influencing performance and injury risk in Paralympic athletes. The first is that the variety of constraints influencing each athlete during training and competition means that there may exist some subtle-moderate differences in the optimal coordinative strategy for different athletes, even if the environmental and task constraints remain the same. Second, any acute or chronic alterations or changes in the device(s) used during training and/or competition have the potential to alter the organism-level constraints and hence the optimal coordinative strategy to maximize performance and/or reduce injury risk. In order to accommodate this spectrum of possible constraints influencing performance both within and between different competitions, Paralympic athletes may need to be able to alter their coordinative strategies via a process referred to as functional movement variability. Functional movement variability can be considered the ability to utilize a flexible (variant) movement control strategy that allows the athlete to maximize performance even when the interaction of the three levels of constraint under which performance occurs are altered (Bradshaw *et al.*, 2007). Currently, there have been no published constraints-led studies involving Paralympic athletes although two studies (Button *et al.*, 2010; Donker and Beek, 2002) have assessed this question in the relation to the gait patterns of individuals with an

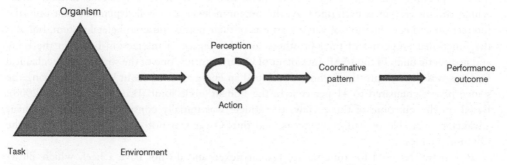

Figure 46.1 A schematic of the constraints-led approach of dynamical systems.

amputation. It is therefore recommended that additional studies in this area be conducted using Paralympic athletes so to gain more insight into what components of performance are critical and require relative invariance of technique and what other technical aspects may benefit from the use of functional variability.

Methods

This book chapter was restricted to a discussion of throwing in the Paralympic summer games for athletes with a locomotor impairment and require the use of a wheelchair or prosthesis. Standard literature searches were performed (in English) using the key words: Paralympic or disabled or disability; wheelchair or spinal cord injured or amputee; shot-put or javelin or discus. Databases searched included EBSCO (CINAHL, Health Source: Nursing/Academic and Sports Discus), as well as PubMed and Google Scholar. The retrieved articles were screened and assessed for relevance to the kinematic and biomechanical aspects. Personal observations of technological developments for athletes competing at the 2004 Athens and 2008 Beijing Paralympic Games were also made by the authors. In addition, specific reviews of the proceedings from key scientific congresses were also conducted. Reference lists of all selected articles were also perused in order to identify any additional relevant articles that were not initially identified.

Prosthesis for throwing

Lower limb amputees rely on the technical attributes of their prosthetic limbs to ambulate, and the specifications of these components have varied considerably in recent years (Camporesi, 2008). For the unique requirements within the three field events of shot put, javelin and discus, athletes may have three sport-specific prostheses built in addition to their day-prosthesis. For example, the need for support during the rotation phase of the shot put or discus requires different properties in a prosthetic device when compared to the need for stability and linear velocity during the run-in when throwing a javelin. The specific rotation requirements for performing the shot put and discus events have resulted in the custom development of the J-Leg technology. This prosthesis essentially has a fixed knee unit to provide stability throughout the rotation, and an energy-storing foot has been mounted at 180° to the standard orientation (i.e. toe facing posteriorly). This alignment facilitates extra stability in rotation and the energy-releasing characteristics of the foot also provide the desired ground push-off before the throw release.

To effectively throw the shot-put, javelin or discus requires the typical projectile motion factors of speed, angle and height of release. The speed of release of the athlete with a lower limb amputation will be affected by the interaction of the three levels of constraint under which the movement is performed. At the organism level, this will depend on not only the interaction and coordination of varying aspects of their neuro-musculoskeletal system, but also the functional properties of their prosthesis and the degree of interaction between the body and prosthetic limb. In the IAAF assessment of Oscar Pistorius, one of the striking biomechanical findings was that the prosthetic limbs developed an energy loss of about 9 per cent during the stance phase, compared to 41 per cent in the human ankle joint (Bruggemann *et al.*, 2008). Based on the outcome of this review, the athlete was initially considered to have an unfair advantage over able-bodied competitors, and thus Oscar was not eligible to compete in the Olympic Games.

Prosthetic feet used for running are plantar-flexed and do not have a heel, which allows the sprinters to stay on their toes. The distal posterior pylon is severely bowed, lengthening the foot plate to increase the moment arm for maximal deflection, propelling the athlete's limb into the acceleration phase of swing as the material energy is returned. To take full advantage of this foot, the athlete lands on the prosthetic toe, extending the hip throughout the support phase and achieving maximal deflection of the foot. The range of individual prosthetic knee and feet, along with the specific alignment and connection of these components, all combine to influence the performance of the athlete, a typical example of this is shown in Figure 46.2 below.

A factor not considered in a laboratory test of mechanical efficiency is the influence of the stump-socket interface on the prosthesis and how this organism-level constraint influences performance and injury risk. This connection is critical to the operation of the prosthesis as any movement of the amputated stump will subsequently swing the prosthetic limb perhaps in directions and rates that are not optimal. Furthermore, once the prosthesis makes contact with the ground, it is the stump-socket interface that transmits the load-bearing ground reaction force back to the amputee. The magnitude, direction and point of application of these ground reaction forces on the stump, as well as the effectiveness of this interface in transferring muscular forces to the ground and in providing proprioception to the amputee, is therefore fundamental for their overall performance and injury risk. These factors must be considered when conducting a kinematic analysis that contains a running component, such as throwing events like the javelin.

Without an effective interface to control the prosthetic device, the potential mechanical efficiency of the technology may not be translated into reality. As a biological structure and an example of organism-level constraint, the anatomical stump can be influenced by a variety of environmental constraints including altitude and humidity. Variation in these factors is likely when travelling overseas to high-level competitions, which will lead to alterations in the volume

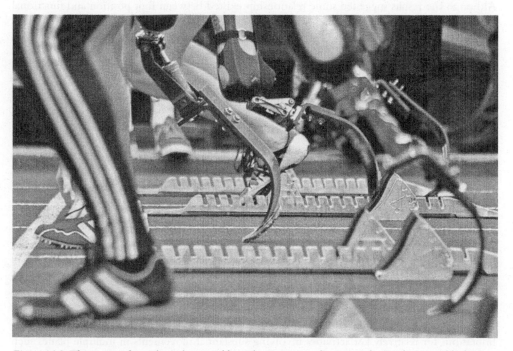

Figure 46.2 The range of prosthetic knee, ankle and connection alignments for Paralympic athletes.

of the stump. As the stump is contained in a volume-specific socket any changes will naturally alter the stump-socket contact points and lead to reduced throwing performance and increased risk of blisters and pressure sores or even injury.

Wheelchairs and frames for throwing

Although some Paralympic throw athletes with an amputation utilize a run-up, many others must throw using specially designed wheelchairs and throwing frames (see Figure 46.3). Traditional wheelchair (day-chair) design consists of two larger wheels at the rear of the chair to allow forward propulsion via the push-rims, and two smaller wheels at the front of the chair to provide stability. The steering of the day-chair is controlled by manipulating the rear wheels, either braking or propelling more on one side to change direction. The unique requirements of sporting use, however, have modified this conventional design dramatically. For more details on the rationale for variations in wheelchair design between, and even within, Paralympic sports, the interested reader is referred to the following papers (Churton and Keogh, 2013; Keogh, 2011).

Consistent with the constraints-led approach, specially designed throwing wheelchairs and throwing frames would appear an important component of the performance of these athletes (Chung *et al.*, 2010), as they comprise part of the organism-level constraint and may provide the athletes with stability and sufficient freedom to rotate the trunk and upper limbs during the throws. While there are several opinion piece articles on the importance of these frames (Curran and Frossard, 2012; O'Riordan and Frossard, 2006), there is very little empirical evidence on what constitutes optimal frame design.

An initial study presented at a national conference by O'Riordan *et al.* (2004) assessed potential relationships between foot position and elite seated wheelchair throwing performance in 12 male discus throwers in the F33/F34 classes at the 2002 IPC World Championships. Although the results suggested some relationship existed between foot position and functional level of the athlete, there was no clear relationship between foot position and distance thrown (O'Riordan *et al.*, 2004). A more recent study by Frossard *et al.* (2010) extended that of O'Riordan *et al.* (2004) and sought to describe the characteristics of throwing frames used by 55 male seated shot putters who competed at the 2006 IPC World Championships. This process involved defining and grouping 26 characteristics of the throwing frames into three main categories (whole body, foot and upper limb) and seven additional sub-categories. Although, the profiling of the athletes and the characteristics of the throwing frames provided information that may be applied to the construction of a throwing frame, as well as coaching, classification and competitive rules for throwing frames, the relationship between frame characteristics and performance were again inconclusive (Frossard *et al.*, 2010).

Kinematic analyses of Paralympic throwers

Several studies have been conducted to examine aspects of the kinematics of throws in track and field events performed by Paralympic athletes (Chow *et al.*, 2000, 2003; Chow and Mindock, 1999; Frossard *et al.*, 2007). As can be seen in Table 46.1, all of these studies were conducted in the field, either during training camps or World Championships. This is a strength of these studies as the constraints underlying performance in laboratory testing can differ markedly from that of the real competitive situation (Churton and Keogh, 2013; Keogh, 2011). Unfortunately, the use of low speed (25–60 Hz) video analysis in all of these studies has many limitations for relatively fast activities involving substantial movements in multiple planes such as the Paralympic throws.

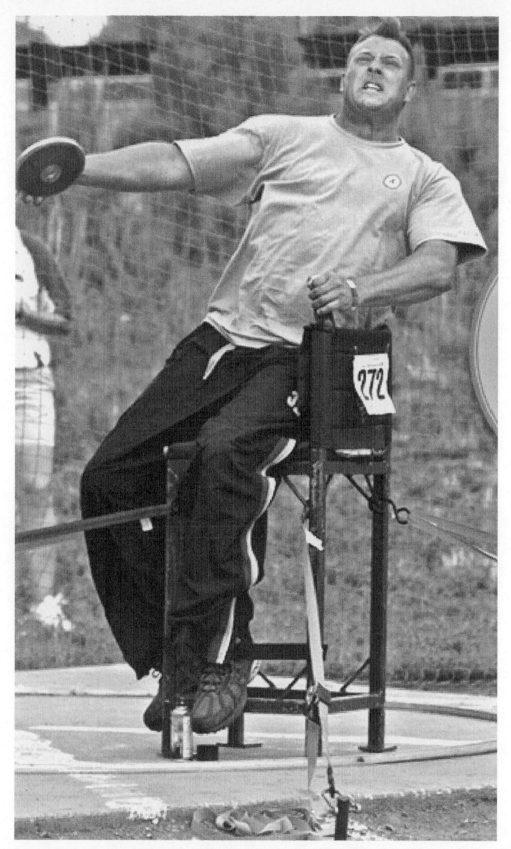

Figure 46.3 A Paralympic athlete using a throwing frame during competition.

Table 46.1 Summary of the peer-reviewed studies examining the kinematics of the discus, javelin and shot-put by Paralympic athletes

Study	Subjects	Event	Type and location of analysis	Primary outcomes assessed
Chow and Mindock (1999)	15 emerging to elite wheelchair males (F2–F8 class)	Discus	3D video field analysis from two cameras operating at 60 Hz during a training camp.	Distance thrown, discus and upper body segments at the instant of release, range of motion and average angular speed of different segments.
Chow et al. (2000)	17 emerging to elite wheelchair males (F2–F8 class)	Shot-put	3D video field analysis from two cameras operating at 60 Hz during a training camp.	Distance thrown, shot and upper body segments at the instant of release, range of motion and average angular speed of different segments.
Chow et al. (2003)	15 emerging to elite wheelchair males (F2–F8 class)	Javelin	3D video field analysis from two cameras operating at 60 Hz during a training camp.	Distance thrown, javelin and upper body segments at the instant of release, range of motion and average angular speed of different segments.
Frossard et al. (2007)	4 elite males and 3 elite wheelchair females (F52–F55) who won their classification	Shot-put	2D video field analysis using one camera at 25 Hz during the 2000 Paralympics and the 2002 IPC World Championships.	Distance thrown, shot, finger and wrist segments speed.

The first study conducted was that of Chow and Mindock (1999), who assessed 14 male discus throwers of different classes over 10 trials with the two longest throws used for analysis. Their three-dimensional analysis indicated that discus' speed of release, which ranged from 9.9–17.2 m.s^{-1}, were substantially less than that of elite male able-bodied throwers. Alternately, the discus' angles of release, which ranged from 25–41° were comparable to what is representative of able-bodied throwers. Inspection of the upper body segment kinematics revealed that the speed and angle of the upper arm at release, the ranges of motion of the shoulder girdle, upper arm, and forearm during the forward swing and the average angular speed of the upper arm and/or shoulder girdle during the forward swing were all significantly correlated to both the classification ($r = 0.55$–0.77) and measured distance ($r = 0.47$–0.84). Between-group comparisons also revealed a tendency for the athletes in the lower classifications (i.e. those with a higher spinal cord lesion) to increase the degree of elbow flexion during the throw, perhaps as a result of their reduced shoulder function. While this difference in technique appears consistent with tenets of the constraints-led approach in that these athletes have to overcome an organism-level constraint, it may explain their reduced performance as the linear velocity of the discus at release reflects the product of arm segment length at release and the summation of angular velocities.

Chow *et al.* (2000) examined the 3D kinematics of 17 wheelchair shot-putters to gain some insight into the primary factors affecting performance and how this might differ between athletes of varying classifications. When compared to normative data for Olympic athletes, the average speed (5.3–7.8 m.s^{-1}) and angles of release (21–34°) for the Paralympic shot-putters were substantially smaller with this especially apparent in the lower classification groups. Significant correlations were also observed between the height of release, angular speed of the upper arm at release, shoulder girdle range of motion during delivery and average angular speeds of the trunk, shoulder girdle and upper arm during delivery to the classification ($r = 0.53$–0.64) and distance thrown ($r = 0.52$–0.79).

When examining the performance of 15 sub-elite/elite wheelchair javelin throwers, Chow *et al.* (2003) found that they produced substantially lower speeds (9.1–14.7 m.s^{-1}) and angles of release (30–36°) than seen in able-bodied athletes, with these differences again greater for the lower classifications. Release height, angular speed of the shoulder girdle, forearm and/or hand at release, range of motion of the shoulder girdle during the forward swing and the average angular speed of the shoulder girdle and hand during the forward swing were significantly correlated to the classification ($r = 0.55$–0.67) and distance thrown ($r = 0.52$–0.67).

Somewhat different to the other studies, Frossard *et al.* (2007) examined the projectile motion characteristics of seven champions at the 2000 Paralympic and 2002 World Championships shot-put events. As expected, the winners of the higher classifications threw the shot greater distances than the lower classifications and the projectile motion release parameters were less than that observed in able-bodied athletes of a similar relative performance level. It was also observed that the greater performances and classification groups had greater shot-put release velocities and angles of release, although differences in the height of release were less consistent.

The kinematic analysis of the discus by Chow and Mindock (1999), shot-put by Chow *et al.* (2000) and Frossard *et al.* (2007) and javelin by Chow *et al.* (2003) therefore appear relatively consistent in their findings and conclusions. These studies all indicate that key release parameters (i.e. speed and angle of release), as well as a number of the upper body segmental angular velocities (if measured), correlated to distance thrown and were able to distinguish higher and lower classification Paralympic throwers as well as Paralympic athletes compared to their able-bodied peers. As these release parameters and segmental velocities appear critical for success in all

Paralympic throws events, one question may be how these variables could be improved through training and what effects on performance these alterations would produce.

One possible way to improve the release parameters of Paralympic throwers could be via improvements in inter-segment coordination patterns, particularly the ability to effectively use the kinetic chain principle. Unfortunately, there appears to be no published research on the inter-segment coordination patterns of Paralympic throwers, so it is unclear how these patterns may differ between different classifications and compare to their able-bodied peers. If improvements in coordination are required, one potential way to achieve this could be via changes in the technical coaching emphasis, particularly if such changes were informed by high-speed, 3D motion analysis. Based on the impulse-momentum or work-energy approaches to understanding human movement, an increase in segmental velocities and overall speed of release might also be obtained by increasing the strength, power and/or range of motion of the primary agonist muscles of the trunk, shoulder girdle and joint and elbow joints. While such a statement would appear sound based on the wider strength and conditioning literature for recreationally active persons with a disability (Hicks *et al.*, 2011) and on the correlational findings of the literature (Chow *et al.*, 2000, 2003; Chow and Mindock, 1999; Frossard *et al.*, 2007), very little research has actually been conducted on the benefits of strength and conditioning in Paralympic athletes. For a review of some the Paralympic strength and conditioning literature, please refer to Churton and Keogh (2013).

Regardless of which approaches are selected, the coaches and support staff should also take into account the wheelchair and/or throwing frames that these athletes use. This would appear important as it is quite possible that increases in muscular strength, power and/or range of motion as well as any changes in inter-segment coordination patterns and projectile release characteristics may alter the requirements of the wheelchair and/or throwing frame. Additional research following on from O'Riordan *et al.* (2004) and Frossard *et al.* (2010) will hopefully assist in this area and contribute to continued performance improvements in Paralympic throwing athletes by better designs and matching of athletes with specific constraints to certain wheelchairs and/or throwing frames.

Recommendation and future directions

The kinematic analysis and primary determinants of performance of the Paralympic throwing event follows similar processes as for analysing able-bodied activities. The subtle, but fundamental difference for the athlete with a disability would appear to reflect the interaction of different levels of constraint under which movement is performed, in particular their disability and their dependence on some form of equipment, such as a wheelchair for the spinal cord injured or lower limb affected athlete, or a prosthesis for the athlete with an amputation. Such an understanding suggests that additional research needs to be conducted to determine whether these Paralympic athletes are indeed compromising their performance by utilizing these lower release angles or if such 'optimal' angles are actually impossible to achieve due to the interaction of constraints that these athletes encounter in competition. As the magnitude of these differences in angle of release appear greater for the lower classifications it further suggests that the optimal angle may be influenced by a variety of organism-level constraints such as the level of trunk control, as well as overall levels of muscular strength, power and range of motion. It is also possible that certain aspects of their wheelchair and/or throwing frame design may also alter their preferred movement patterns and ranges of motion to the extent that lower angles of release may actually become more optimal. Computer simulation, cross-sectional and experimental studies may all play a role in helping to answer this question.

Although many other industries there have shown tremendous technological developments, what is currently lacking is the 'application' of this technology to the Paralympian. It is not a case of needing to reinvent the wheel, but rather to look around at what has been already developed and then determining how this can be applied to improving sporting performance and reducing injury risk in these athletes. It is when this lateral thinking approach is applied to the current issues for people with disabilities the future will really be a better place.

An understandable temptation for researchers is to only research 'hot topics' that are more likely to be funded through research grants. As the majority of people with disabilities are aged, the development of assistive devices has naturally focused on this market. Paralympic athletes have created a new, albeit smaller niche market. Not only are they significantly younger than the traditional aged person with a disability, they are also highly physically active and as such place far greater loads on the assistive devices and musculoskeletal systems. This new market demand, in the long term, will result in a better understanding of the relationship between the three levels of constraint (i.e. the human-machine interface and how this interacts with the environmental and task constraints) to achieve optimal performance while minimizing the risk of injury. However, as can be seen in this chapter, considerable work still needs to be done in this area.

References

Bradshaw, E. J., Maulder, P. S. and Keogh, J. W. L. (2007) 'Biological movement variability during the sprint start: performance enhancement or hindrance?', *Sports Biomechanics*, 6(3): 246–60.

Brodtkorb, T., Henriksson, M., Johannesen-Munk, K. and Thidell, F. (2008) 'Cost-effectiveness of C-leg compared with non-microprocessor-controlled knees: a modeling approach', *Archives of Physical Medicine and Rehabilitation*, 89(1): 24–30.

Brown, M. B., Millard-Stafford, M. L. and Allison, A. R. (2009) 'Running-specific prostheses permit energy cost similar to nonamputees', *Medicine and Science in Sports and Exercise*, 41(5): 1080–7.

Bruggemann, G., Arampatzis, A., Emrich, F. and Potthast, W. (2008) 'Biomechanics of double transtibial amputee sprinting using dedicated sprinting prostheses', *Sports Technology*, 1(4–5): 220–7.

Burkett, B. (2008) 'Technology in sport', *Proceedings of International Convention on Science, Education and Medicine in Sport*, Guangzhou: International Convention on Science, Education and Medicine in Sport.

Burkett, B., Smeathers, J. and Barker, T. (2003) 'Walking and running inter-limb asymmetry for Paralympic trans-femoral amputees, a biomechanical analysis', *Prosthetics and Orthotics International*, 27(1): 36–47.

Burkett, B., Pothast, W. and Mcnamme, M. (2011) 'Shifting boundaries in sports technology and disability: equal rights or unfair advantage in the case of Oscar Pistoruis?', *Disability and Society*, 26(5): 643–53.

Button, C., Moyle, S. and Davids, K. (2010) 'Comparison of below-knee amputee gait performed overground and on a motorized treadmill', *Adapted Physical Activity Quarterly*, 27(2): 96–112.

Camporesi, S. (2008) 'Oscar Pistorius, enhancement and post-humans', *British Medical Journal*, 34(9): 639.

Chow, J. W., Chae, W. S. and Crawford, M. J. (2000) 'Kinematic analysis of shot-putting performed by wheelchair athletes of different medical classes', *Journal of Sport Sciences*, 18(5): 321–30.

Chow, J. W., Kuenster, A. F. and Lim, Y.-T. (2003) 'Kinematic analysis of javelin throw performed by wheelchair athletes of different functional classes', *Journal of Sports Science and Medicine*, 2(2): 36–46.

Chow, J. W. and Mindock, L. A. (1999) 'Discus throwing performances and medical classification of wheelchair athletes', *Medicine and Science in Sports and Exercise*, 31(9): 1272–9.

Chung, C.-S., Lin, J. T., Toro, M. L., Beyene, N. M. and Garcia, Y. (2010) 'Uniform throwing chair for seated throwing sporting events', *Proceedings of Rehabilitation Engineering and Assistive Technology Society of North America Annual Conference*. Las Vegas, NV: Rehabilitation Engineering and Assistive Technology Society of North America, pp. 1–6.

Churton, E. and Keogh, J. W. L. (2013). Constraints influencing sports wheelchair propulsion performance and injury risk. *BMC Sports Science, Medicine, and Rehabilitation*, 5(3). doi: 10.1186/2052-1847-5-3.

Curran, S. A. and Frossard, L. (2012) 'Biomechanical analyses of the performance of Paralympians: from foundation to elite level', *Prosthetics and Orthotics International*, 36(3): 380–95.

Donker, S. F. and Beek, P. J. (2002) 'Interlimb coordination in prosthetic walking: effects of asymmetry and walking velocity', *Acta Psychologica*, 110(2–3): 265–88.

Edwards, S. D. (2008) 'Should Oscar Pistorius be excluded from the 2008 olympic games?', *Sport, Ethics and Philosophy*, 2(2): 112–25.

Frossard, L. A., O'Riordan, A. and Goodman, S. (2010) 'Throwing frame and performance of elite male seated shot-putters', *Sports Technology*, 3(2): 88–101.

Frossard, L. A., Smeathers, J., O'Riordan, A. and Goodman, S. (2007) 'Shot trajectory parameters in gold medal stationary shot-putters during world-class competition', *Adapted Physical Activity Quarterly*, 24(4): 317–31.

Haisma, J., Van Der Woude, L., Stam, H., Bergen, M., Sluis, T. and Bussmann, J. (2006) 'Physical capacity in wheelchair-dependent persons with a spinal cord injury: a critical review of the literature', *Spinal Cord*, 44(11): 642–52.

Hicks, A. L., Martin Ginis, K. A., Pelletier, C. A., Ditor, D. S., Foulon, B. and Wolfe, D. L. (2011) 'The effects of exercise training on physical capacity, strength, body composition and functional performance among adults with spinal cord injury: a systematic review', *Spinal Cord*, 49(11): 1103–27.

Hsu, M. J., Nielsen, D. H., Lin-Chan, S. J. and Shurr, D. (2006) 'The effects of prosthetic foot design on physiologic measurements, self-selected walking velocity, and physical activity in people with transtibial amputation' *Archives of Physical Medicine and Rehabilitation*, 87(1): 123–9.

International Paralympic Committee. (2009) *IPC Sports*, viewed 12 February 2009, http://oldwebsite. paralympic.org/Sport/IPC_Sports/.

International Paralympic Committee. (2007) *Classification*, viewed 26 October 2007, http://paralympic. org/sites/default/files/document/120716152047682_ClassificationGuide_2.pdf.

Jones, C. and Wilson, C. (2009) 'Defining advantage and athletic performance: The case of Oscar Pistorius', *European Journal of Sport Science*, 9(2): 125–31.

Keogh, J. W. L. (2011) 'Paralympic sport: an emerging area for research and consultancy in sports biomechanics', *Sports Biomechanics*, 10(3): 234–53.

Lippi, G. and Mattiuzzi, C. (2008) 'Pistorius ineligible for the Olympic Games: the right decision', *British Journal of Sports Medicine*, 42(3): 160–1.

Nolan, L. and Lees, A. (2000) 'The functional demands on the intact limb during walking for active trans-femoral and trans-tibial amputees', *Prosthetics and Orthotics International*, 24(2): 117–25.

O'Riordan, A. and Frossard, L. (2006) 'Seated shot put – what is it all about?', *Modern Athlete and Coach*, 44(2): 3–8.

O'Riordan, A., Goodman, S. and Frossard, L. (2004) 'Relationship between the parameters describing the feet position and the performance of elite seated discus throwers in Class F33/34 participating in the 2002 IPC World Championships', *Proceedings of AAESS Exercise and Sports Science Conference*, Brisbane: Australian Association for Exercise and Sports Science.

Pasquina, P. F., Bryant, P. R., Huang, M. E., Roberts, T. L., Nelson, V. S. and Flood, K. M. (2006) 'Advances in amputee care', *Archives of Physical Medicine and Rehabilitation*, 87 (3 Suppl 1):S34–43

Steenbergen, B. and Gordon, A. M. (2006) 'Activity limitation in hemiplegic cerebral palsy: evidence for disorders in motor planning', *Developmental Medicine and Child Neurology*, 48(9): 780–3.

Tweedy, S. M. (2003) 'Biomechanical consequences of impairment: a taxonomically valid basis for classification in a unified disability athletics system', *Research Quarterly for Exercise and Sport*, 74(1): 9–16.

van Hilvoorde, I. and Landeweerd, L. (2008) 'Disability or extraordinary talent – Francesco Lentini (three legs) versus Oscar pistorius (no legs)', *Sport, Ethics and Philosophy*, 2(2): 97–111.

Vanlandewijck, Y., Theisen, D. and Daly, D. (2001) 'Wheelchair propulsion biomechanics: implications for wheelchair sports', *Sports Medicine*, 31(5): 339–67.

INDEX

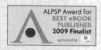 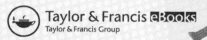